The Science of Mental Health

Volume 1

Bipolar Disorder

Series Content

Volume 1
BIPOLAR DISORDER

Volume 2
AUTISM

Volume 3
SCHIZOPHRENIA

Volume 4
ATTENTION-DEFICIT HYPERACTIVITY DISORDERS

Volume 5
ADDICTION

Volume 6
DEPRESSION

Volume 7
PERSONALITY AND PERSONALITY DISORDER

Volume 8
COMPULSIVE DISORDER AND TOURETTE'S SYNDROME

Volume 9
STRESS AND THE BRAIN

Volume 10
FEAR AND ANXIETY

The Science of Mental Health

Volume 1

Bipolar Disorder

Edited with introductions by

Steven Hyman

National Institute of Mental Health

Published in 2001 by Routledge
2 Park Square, Milton Park, Abingdon, Oxon OX14 4RN
52 Vanderbilt Avenue, New York, NY 10017, USA

Routledge is an imprint of Taylor & Francis Group, an informa business

Library of Congress Cataloging-in-Publication Data

The science of mental health / edited with introductions by Steven Hyman.
p. cm.
Includes bibliographical references.
ISBN 0-8153-3743-4 (set)
1. Mental health. I. Hyman, Steven E.
RA790 .S435 2002
616.89--dc21

2001048491

POD ISBN:	9780415532525
Set ISBN:	9780815337430
Vol 1:	9780815337447
Vol 2:	9780815337454
Vol 3:	9780815337461
Vol 4:	9780815337478
Vol 5:	9780815337485
Vol 6:	9780815337492
Vol 7:	9780815337508
Vol 8:	9780815337515
Vol 9:	9780815337522
Vol 10:	9780815337539

Contents

Introduction

Bipolar disorder, also called manic-depressive illness, is the most severe of the mood disorders. It is distinguished from major (unipolar) depression by the occurrence of manic episodes in addition to depression. Bipolar disorder affects approximately 1 person in 100 worldwide (Kessler et al., 1997). It is a leading cause of disability in both developed and developing countries, and it also leads to excess mortality (Osby et al., 2001) by suicide and other causes. This volume introduces the reader to articles that provide a broad background for understanding bipolar disorder. The introduction includes a description of the illness, which is complemented by a case discussion in the readings (Sachs, 2001). A powerful personal description of bipolar disorder[1] and extensive additional data[2] can be found in other sources. The articles in this collection demonstrate that much has been learned about bipolar disorder, but there is a long way to travel before we fully understand the risk factors, the neural circuitry underlying mood regulation, and the pathogenesis of the disorder and before we have more fully satisfactory treatments for this illness. As is standard in this series, articles have been included that introduce the reader to the epidemiology, genetics, natural history (longitudinal course) of the illness, evolutionary hypotheses (Wilson, 1998), relevant neurobiology, and treatment. The historical basis of this diagnosis can be found in the work of the German psychiatrist Emil Kraepelin.[3]

The lifetime risk of bipolar disorder is 1 percent (Kessler et al., 1997). Unlike major depression, which occurs twice as frequently in females, bipolar disorder occurs equally in females and males in essentially all societies studied. A diagnosis of bipolar disorder requires that the person have had at least one manic episode. If the attack is mild, it is described as hypomania. The dichotomy between unipolar depression and bipolar disorder is supported not only by the phenomenology of the illnesses but also by family studies. The current *Diagnostic and Statistical Manual of Mental Disorders*, 4th edition (DSM-IV),[4] describes patients with full manias and depressions as having bipolar I disorder. Patients with hypomanias (mild manias) and depressions are described as having bipolar II disorder. Individuals who have only hypomanias and milder depressive episodes are said to have cyclothymia rather than bipolar disorder. The depressive episodes of individuals with bipolar disorder are indistinguishable from those of patients with unipolar major depression (see the volume on Depression in this series). The symptoms of mania generally include an elevated mood that may seem cheerful, high, and unselectively enthusiastic. However, the euphoria may be quite brittle, and the person may suddenly become irritable, angry, or sad with little provocation. Indeed, it is characteristic of mania that affect can be markedly labile; thus even if the predominant mood is euphoric, the individual with mania may have brief periods of tearfulness or anger. Some individuals with bipolar disorder do not exhibit euphoria and are predominantly irritable. Mania is also characterized by increased energy and decreased need for sleep. During a manic episode individuals may have marked alterations in behavior and may become intrusive, hypersexual, and impulsive. Inflated self-esteem is common and may become delusional (for example, that the person is the messiah). Cognitively, people with mania tend to be distractible. Their speech is often loud, rapid, and difficult to interrupt (pressured). Often they cannot stick to a topic and may jump rapidly from idea to idea (flight of ideas), making comprehension of their speech difficult.

Psychotic symptoms commonly occur during manic episodes. These symptoms are usually congruent with the elevated mood. For example, patients may have delusions of special powers or hear voices telling them that they are an important religious figure. However, some individuals, especially adolescents, may have florid psychotic symptoms while manic, including bizarre delusions. Bipolar disorder often begins in young adulthood, although onset in childhood is increasingly being recognized. The diagnosis of bipolar disorder in childhood remains difficult, but it connotes a very severe disorder with serious impairments (Geller and Luby, 1998; National Institute of Mental Health Roundtable, 2001; Sanchez et al., 1999). Late onset is less common, but first manic episodes can occur even in the elderly.

The majority of patients with bipolar disorder suffer multiple recurrences that are interspersed with periods of relative health. For a minority, symptoms are unremitting, with continuous cycling or chronic psychotic symptoms (Angst and Sellaro, 2000; Coryell et al., 1998). Individuals who have chronic psychotic symptoms superimposed on unipolar or bipolar disorder are often described as schizoaffective. Manic episodes may in some cases be precipitated by antidepressant therapy and sleep deprivation. The controversial role of life events in the natural history of bipolar disorder is addressed in the article by Ellicott et al. (1990).

The rate of cycling between mania and depression varies widely among individuals. A common pattern of illness is for episodes to become more frequent with age. A minority of patients with bipolar disorder have more than three episodes a year. These patients, termed rapid cyclers, tend to respond poorly to lithium (Kilzieh and Akiskal, 1999; Altshuler et al., 1995). Rapid cycling occurs more commonly in women. A high percentage of patients have onset of rapid cycling while being treated with antidepressants. Individuals with vastly different rates of cycling are frequently found in the same family, which suggests that rapid cycling does not have a genetic basis. Tragically, suicide is a frequent outcome in bipolar disorder, affecting as many as 15 percent of those suffering from the illness (Jamison, 2000).

Genes exert a more powerful effect on the risk of bipolar disorder than they do for major depression. It has long been recognized that bipolar disorder runs in families. Multiple family, twin, and adoption studies have been performed that have established beyond doubt that this family resemblance for bipolar illness is because of shared genes (reviewed in Craddock and Jones, 1999). Some important controversies remain, however. While family studies support the unipolar-bipolar distinction, there is an excess of individuals (over expected population rates) with unipolar depression in families with bipolar disorder. As described, some bipolar individuals, but not others, experience psychotic symptoms during the course of their illness. The relationship between bipolarity and psychosis is explored by Potash et al. (2001). Perhaps most controversial is the significance of finding individuals with well-diagnosed schizophrenia and individuals with bipolar disorder in the same family. The DSM-IV clearly delineates these two disorders, and based on current ideas about classification and etiology, the two disorders should segregate separately in families. Berrettini (2000) raises the question of whether this received wisdom is correct.

While a role for genes in the risk of bipolar disorder is beyond dispute, the way in which genes act remains unclear. As with all mental illnesses, evidence from family studies and from current attempts at gene discovery (for example, by linkage analysis) indicates that the risk of bipolar disorder is a result of complex gene-gene, gene-environment interactions (Craddock and Jones). As with depression, there may be no one gene or no one type of environmental risk factor that is necessary or sufficient to cause bipolar disorder. Because of the potent aggregate effect of genes in the risk of bipolar disorder, the search for risk genes is currently a matter of intense effort.

Neurobiological approaches to bipolar disorder are in their early stages. This volume contains a representative imaging study (Blumberg et al., 2000) and molecular hypotheses based largely on what is known of drug treatment (Ikonomov and Manji, 1999; Manji and Lennox, 2000). One reason for the interest in finding risk genes is the need for clues to the pathophysiologic processes that might lead to bipolar disorder. The relationship between sleep and cycling is one area in which mechanisms are not well understood but in which there are many compelling observations (Leibenluft et al., 1996). The profound effect of sleep deprivation on mood (for example, it can initiate manic episodes) has led to a concern about how to manage sleep patterns when treating bipolar disorder (Frank et al., 2000).

The mainstay of treatment for bipolar disorder is the use of mood-stabilizing agents. Historically, lithium was the first drug to be used (Schou, 1997), and more recently several drugs initially developed as anticonvulsants have proved efficacious; the best studied of these is valproate (Bowden et al., 2000). Despite the routine use of maintenance treatment for bipolar disorder, in naturalistic samples up to 90 percent of patients will experience one or more relapses within five years of diagnosis. Indeed, the management of bipolar disorder is quite complex because breakthrough episodes of mania and depression are all too frequent. Such episodes may require the use of antidepressants (which risk "overshooting" into mania) and antipsychotic drugs to manage acute manic episodes. The atypical antipsychotic drug clozapine has proved useful in the treatment of otherwise refractory bipolar disorder.

Many investigators have addressed the possible mechanisms by which lithium, element number 3 in the periodic table, might treat bipolar disorder. In its charged form (as a monovalent cation), lithium can specifically inhibit a number of enzymes involved in intracellular signaling. The two leading but unproved hypotheses are presented here by seminal articles (Berridge et al., 1989; Klein and Melton, 1996).

References

1. Kay Redfield Jamison. *An Unquiet Mind.* New York: Random House, 1997.
2. Frederick K. Goodwin and Kay Redfield Jamison. *Manic-Depressive Illness.* New York: Oxford University Press, 1990.
3. Emil Kraepelin. *Manic Depressive Insanity and Paranoia.* Edinburgh: Livingston, 1921.
4. American Psychiatric Association. *Diagnostic and Statistical Manual of Mental Disorders,* 4th ed. Washington, D.C.: American Psychiatric Press, 1994.

The Science of Mental Health

Volume 1

Bipolar Disorder

A 25-Year-Old Woman With Bipolar Disorder

Gary S. Sachs, MD, Discussant

Dr Parker: Ms G is a 25-year-old woman who is slowly coming to terms with her diagnosis of bipolar disorder. She lives with her boyfriend and currently attends school. She experienced 2 manic episodes resulting in inpatient psychiatry hospitalizations. Ms G has lost her medical insurance, which is complicating her access to medical and psychiatric care.

In the summer of 1998, Ms G worked in a restaurant, and described the atmosphere as "very tense, pressured, nonsupportive, and demanding." Although she cannot recall all the details, her family brought her to a local emergency department for evaluation of her agitated mental state. She was transferred by ambulance to an inpatient psychiatry unit.

At admission, Ms G described symptoms of hopelessness, difficulty sleeping, emotional lability, decreased appetite, and decreased energy. She denied any suicidal feelings or hallucinations. She complained that "electrical waves" were bothering her. The admitting physician noted her pressured speech and tangential thought processes. Her memory was intact, her affect labile, and her insight and judgment were rated as "fair to poor."

Ms G decided against treatment with lithium carbonate because she feared it would cause weight gain. She was treated with divalproex sodium, 250 mg 4 times daily, and risperidone, 2 mg at bedtime. She started individual psychotherapy. Over time, she discontinued the medications and again became agitated, resulting in a second inpatient stay. During that hospitalization, she was treated with divalproex, 750 mg twice daily, and olanzapine, 5 mg at bedtime.

There is no history of mental illness in first-degree relatives. When Ms G was aged 15 years, her mother died of cancer. She drinks alcohol occasionally and does not use illegal drugs. She smokes cigarettes. Her physical health is good. Her current medications are divalproex, 750 mg twice daily, and bupropion hydrochloride, 150 mg twice daily.

Ms G wonders what her future will bring and whether any other treatment modalities might benefit her, as she does not like the idea of taking medications long-term.

MS G: HER VIEWS

My first experience being treated by a psychiatrist was when I was 15, and I experienced the loss of my mother. My next experience was after I moved to Boston initially, my first year here.

My first episode is difficult to explain because I completely lost a certain amount of mental control. It was a very intense feeling of anxiety and almost paranoia during which I felt completely tense. I had such a heightened anxiety that I felt like I couldn't function in society at all, and people around me became very concerned.

I had a good experience on Depakote (divalproex) after my first hospitalization, but I was not convinced that Depakote was necessarily what had fixed whatever had gone wrong. So, I was very adamant with my psychiatrist that I wanted to be weaned off the medication. Unfortunately, I started having problems again. I had very severe disorientation to the point where I felt that I couldn't remember anything.

I would describe myself as having mood swings several times throughout the day—very irritable would be an understatement—then surges of unbridled anxiety for no apparent reason. It's very hard to describe because that was coupled with disorientation. I was having an incredible amount of difficulty sleeping to the point where I would fall asleep for 15 minutes, then wake up and feel completely awake. It would be some odd hour in the morning, when it was dark outside and no one else was up, and it was very confusing for me. I definitely had feelings of sort of an elevated nature, where I felt like I had a lot more energy than I should be having. I had periods of significant depression, but I was also functioning in the sense of working and going to school.

I think that manic depression in ways has made me stronger in life. But not in the slightest way, shape, or form would I be tempted to go off the medications again until the first

This conference took place at the Combined Longwood Psychiatry Grand Rounds of the Massachusetts Mental Health Center, the Beth Israel Deaconess Medical Center, and the Brigham and Women's Hospital, Boston, Mass, and was held at Beth Israel Deaconess Medical Center on April 25, 2000.

Author Affiliation: Dr Sachs is assistant professor in psychiatry, Harvard Medical School; Director, Harvard Bipolar Research Program, Massachusetts General Hospital, Boston.

Financial Disclosure: Dr Sachs has received research funding from Abbott Laboratories, Glaxo Wellcome, Janssen Pharmaceutica, Eli Lilly, and Scios; has been on the advisory boards of Abbott Laboratories, Glaxo Wellcome, Janssen Pharmaceutica, Eli Lilly, Scios, Solvay Pharmaceuticals, Sanofi-Synthelabo, Novartis, BMS, and UCB; and has been on the speakers' bureau of Abbott Laboratories, Glaxo Wellcome, Janssen Pharmaceutia, Eli Lilly, Scios, Solvay Pharmaceuticals, and BMS.

Reprints: Erin E. Hartman, MS, Division of General Medicine and Primary Care, Beth Israel Deaconess Medical Center, 330 Brookline Ave, LY318, Boston, MA 02215.

Clinical Crossroads at Beth Israel Deaconess Medical Center is produced and edited by Tom Delbanco, MD, Richard A. Parker, MD, and Anne-Marie Audet, MD; Erin E. Hartman, MS, is managing editor.

Clinical Crossroads Section Editor: Margaret A. Winker, MD, Deputy Editor.

complete year of being episode free. I don't ever want to go through another episode again, if it's at all preventable.

DR Z: HER VIEWS

Ms G was hospitalized twice for bipolar disorder. After her second hospitalization, I saw her regularly. During that time, she developed a major depressive episode and had to start taking bupropion for treatment of depression, in addition to the divalproex for mood stabilization. She did well, but she was frightened. She felt that the manic episode and second hospitalization had definitely altered the course of her life, threatened her relationship, and she was afraid to make a job change.

She was receiving insurance through her father's benefits, and it was limited coverage. Once it was denied, she dropped out of treatment, because she could not afford to come in regularly. Part of the problem in working with so many managed care patients is that when they drop out of treatment, it's hard for the physician to reach out to reengage the patient. The personal connection with the patient is weakened as a result of the insurance companies.

The question I have concerning Ms G's treatment is whether or not she should continue receiving divalproex, given that she cannot come in for treatment and that she would have to pay for blood level tests. Does switching to a newer generation of mood stabilizers make sense? Also, is there an antidepressant that doesn't cause a patient to go into a manic episode?

AT THE CROSSROADS: QUESTIONS FOR DR SACHS

What is the epidemiology of bipolar disorder? What is the significance of the age at onset, sex differences, and family history? What is its natural history and effect on patient and family? What other psychiatric illnesses act as comorbidities? How does this complicate diagnosis and treatment? What are the risks and benefits of various treatments? What is on the horizon for treatment of bipolar disorder? What do you recommend for Ms G?

DR SACHS: Ms G is in many ways typical of patients with bipolar disorder. Her history over the past 3 years includes 2 hospitalizations for manic episodes and an episode of major depression. Both her manic episodes began in summer. The recurrences convinced her that she indeed has bipolar illness and needs treatment. Ms G confronts problems far more daunting than those that challenge most other bright women in their 20s. Untreated, she faces a 15% risk of death by suicide.[1] Because of periods of acute illness, the average patient with bipolar disorder will suffer a cumulative 8-year loss of effective function or about 20% of her early and middle adult life.[2] Her attempts to reach adult developmental milestones related to education, occupation, social life, intimacy, and reproduction are all potentially affected by her illness and her treatments.

Ms G lacks the solid supports needed to manage her illness confidently. Finances limit her contact with care providers, and in the little time she has with her treating psychiatrist, she finds communication difficult. Her mother is deceased, her aunt died by suicide, and her father has metastatic cancer. Her boyfriend may be understandably short of full commitment but is her most reliable support. Her care plan provides for minimal contact in the intervals between acute episodes and relies on her to contact her care provider when she experiences the necessity. This means she must cope with the additional terror of knowing she has a potentially deadly illness that has distorted and, at any time, may again distort her judgment and the self-perception she relies on.

She currently is well, but her history indicates a risk of recurrence close to 100%. Ms G apparently responds well to acute treatment but has not yet found a reliable prophylactic regimen. She faces some difficult decisions and will likely ask questions of all the professionals involved in her care: Is there a better treatment regimen to control the illness? Are psychotherapy or closer follow-up worth the price? Must the cost of effective treatment include substantial weight gain or renunciation of the possibility of motherhood?

To help Ms G achieve the best possible outcome, it is useful for her to know as much as possible about her illness and recommended treatments. She also needs help to overcome the additional problem of limited access to care.

What Is Bipolar Disorder?

Bipolar disorder, also known as manic depression, is a common psychiatric disorder that includes periods of abnormal mood elevation. There are no diagnostic laboratory tests for bipolar disorder. Operational criteria for diagnosis are derived from clinical assessment of signs and symptoms. Experienced clinicians and researchers debate whether bipolar disorder is underdiagnosed or overdiagnosed, but there is no debating that it is often poorly diagnosed.[2,3]

The *Diagnostic and Statistical Manual of Mental Disorders, Fourth Edition* (*DSM-IV*)[4] provides criteria for depression, hypomania, mania, and mixed episodes (for a modified summary, see TABLE 1). The *DSM-IV* divides bipolar disorder into 4 subtypes. *Bipolar I* is defined based on the occurrence of a full manic episode. About 90% of bipolar I patients also have episodes of major depression, but these are not required for the diagnosis. The designation *bipolar II* is given to patients who have never experienced a full manic episode but have experienced at least 1 hypomanic episode and at least 1 episode of major depression. *Cyclothymia* refers to forms of bipolar illness that include an index period of chronic mood instability (1 year for children or adolescents, 2 years for adults). During the majority of the index period days, patients experience abnormal mood states including frequent hypomanic symptoms, but never reach full criteria for either mania or major depression. The *DSM-IV* designates patients with period of abnormal mood elevation failing to meet criteria for any of these 3 defined subtypes (eg, hypomanias only) as *bipolar, not otherwise specified*. Ms G's symptoms meet criteria to classify her as a bipolar I–type patient.

Epidemiology and Course of Illness

Epidemiological studies show that the prevalence of bipolar I disorder is about 1%, with a sex ratio close to 1:1.[5] With the inclusion of patients with periods of mood elevation milder than full manic episodes, the reported lifetime prevalence for all subtypes of bipolar illness ranges from 3% to 6%.[6,7]

Typically, the first episode of bipolar disorder has its onset during the second or third decade of life and is followed by a remission of approximately 4.5 years (median).[8] On average, the periods of remission shrink progressively over the course of the first 3 to 5 episodes and then tend to stabilize with an average of about 1 episode per year.[8-11] During the first 10 years, the average patient with bipolar disorder will have about 4 major mood episodes. However, some individuals may have more manic episodes or more depressed episodes, while others may have an equal number of depressive and manic episodes. Coryell et al[12] reported the percentage of weeks during 5-year follow-up that patients with bipolar disorder type 1 experienced depression, hypomania, and mania as 14.3%, 5.6%, and 2.7% respectively. As these data suggest, even among patients who have frequent severe episodes, there may be long periods with normal mood state. Some physicians, patients, and family members may be tempted to interpret prolonged periods of wellness as evidence that the diagnosis of bipolar disorder was incorrect. Unfortunately, this is seldom the case. The natural course of bipolar disorder often includes periods of remission, but without treatment, those who meet criteria for bipolar disorder will usually experience relapse.

Bipolar illness is associated not only with decreased quality of life for patients and their families, but also with high utilization of psychiatric and general medical services[13] and increased mortality rates due to suicide and other medical conditions.[14,15] In a sample of patients with bipolar disorder type I, Kessler[5] found 48% have made at least 1 suicide attempt. Adjusted mortality rates are higher for untreated patients, but are higher still by an order of magnitude for untreated bipolar patients with comorbid alcohol or substance abuse.[15]

Psychiatric Comorbidities

Kessler[5] found 100% of patients with bipolar disorder type I meet criteria for at least 1 other axis I disorder. The most frequent are anxiety disorders, substance abuse, bulimia, and attention-deficit hyperactivity disorder. Successful treatment of bipolar disorder usually improves these other conditions. Likewise, successful treatment of these conditions usually improves the symptoms of bipolar disorder. Unfortunately for some patients, the treatments for other disor-

Table 1. Modified Summary of *DSM-IV* Criteria for Episodes*

Episode Type	Predominant Mood State	Symptom Threshold	Associated Features
		Acute Episodes With Elevated Mood†	
Mania	High, euphoric, expansive, irritable	Present to a significant degree through at least 1 week (any duration if hospitalized) and causes significant social or occupational impairment	1. Increased self-esteem/grandiosity 2. Decreased need for sleep 3. More talkative 4. Racing thought/flight of ideas 5. Distractible 6. Increased goal-directed activities/psychomotor agitation 7. Risk taking
Hypomania	High, euphoric, expansive, irritable	Present to a significant degree through at least 4 days and causes no significant social or occupational impairment	1. Increased self-esteem/grandiosity 2. Decreased need for sleep 3. More talkative 4. Racing thoughts/flight of ideas 5. Distractible 6. Increased goal-directed activities/psychomotor agitation 7. Risk taking
Mixed	Both elevated and depressed	At least 1 week during which symptoms satisfying criteria for depression are present most of the day, nearly every day, and symptoms meeting criteria for mania are present to a significant degree	
		Acute Episodes With Depressed Mood‡	
Depression	Low, dysphoric, sad, disinterested	Present most of the day, nearly every day, through at least 2 weeks	1. Depressed mood 2. Sleep disturbance 3. Diminished interest/anhedonia 4. Inappropriate guilt/low self-esteem 5. Decreased energy/fatigue 6. Inability to concentrate/make simple decisions 7. Appetite disturbance 8. Psychomotor retardation/agitation 9. Suicidal ideation/morbid preoccupation
Mixed	Both elevated and depressed	At least 1 week during which symptoms satisfying criteria for depression are present most of the day, nearly every day, and symptoms meeting criteria for mania are present to a significant degree	

*DSM-IV indicates *Diagnostic and Statistical Manual of Mental Disorders, Fourth Edition*. Adapted with permission from the *Diagnostic and Statistical Manual of Mental Disorders, Fourth Edition*.[4] Copyright 1994 American Psychiatric Association.
†Requires ≥3 associated features in presence of euphoric or expansive mood. If only irritable, ≥4 associated features are required.
‡Requires ≥5 associated features including either depressed mood or diminished interest/anhedonia.

ders can worsen symptoms of bipolar disorder. For example, some medicines used to treat obsessive-compulsive disorder (eg, antidepressants) and attention-deficit hyperactivity disorder (eg, stimulants) may worsen symptoms of bipolar disorder and even cause a manic episode.

How Is Bipolar Disorder Treated?

Although still far from ideal, the armamentarium of available medications (antimanic, antidepressant, and antipsychotic drugs) and psychotherapies with demonstrable benefits has grown impressively during the past 30 years. The irregular course, variety of acute episodes, spectrum of severity, and multiple treatment options bring enormous complexity to the management of bipolar illness.

Despite this complexity, concepts developed by Frank and colleagues[16] for treatment of unipolar depression can simplify the discussion of treatment for bipolar illness. The multiphase treatment strategy directed at the acute, continuation, and discontinuation and maintenance phases facilitates the clinical approach to treatment as well as research. The phases of treatment are summarized in the FIGURE.

Figure. Multiphase Treatment Strategy

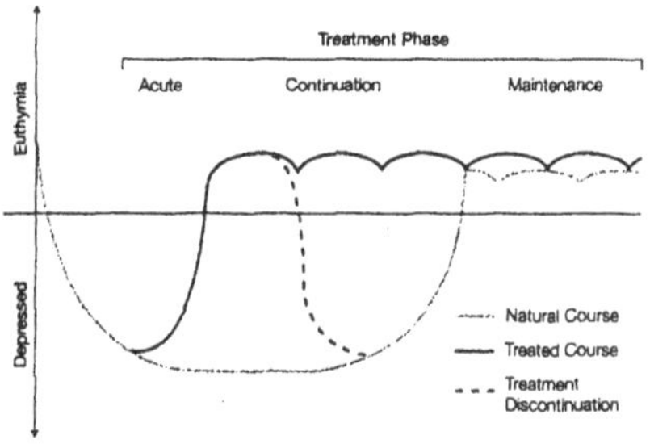

Effective acute phase treatment ameliorates symptoms of the depressive episode, but discontinuation prior to the natural end point (dashed line) is associated with high rates of relapse. Extending treatment beyond the point of initial remission (dark line) is associated with a low relapse rate. The period between initial remission and the estimated natural end point is designated "continuation phase."

Acute Phase

The acute phase begins when the patient meets criteria for an episode (depression, mania, hypomania, or mixed) and treatment is initiated.[16] Each individual acute treatment trial is carried out to 1 of 3 end points: (1) discontinuation because the patient is unable to tolerate adverse effects of treatment; (2) discontinuation because the patient has failed to respond to a maximal trial of the treatment (including, if warranted, augmentation strategies); and (3) the patient improved during treatment.

Problems during the acute phase include treatment intolerance, inadequate dosage, partial response, and nonresponse. Treatments are adjusted or replaced as necessary to manage these problems until the acute symptoms remit, thus ending the acute phase. When Ms G's acute symptoms remitted in response to treatment, the acute phase of her treatment ended.

Continuation Phase

Remission of acute symptoms defines the beginning of the continuation phase, but relapse with full or partial return of symptoms is the most frequently encountered problem during the continuation phase. Successful acute therapies are therefore continued at full dosage for a period (usually 2-6 months) to prevent relapse.[16] With the remission of symptoms, the continuation phase is also a time when denial of illness may foster discordance between the physician's treatment plan and that actually carried out by the patient. Ms G's discontinuation of medication exemplifies this problem.

The length of the continuation phase is based on the clinician's estimate of the period necessary to exceed the natural duration of the episode in the absence of treatment. Expert consensus supports estimating the duration of the continuation phase based on the duration of an individual patient's prior episodes.[17] In the many cases where no reliable history is available, a more general estimate of the likely duration of depressive or manic episodes typically results in a continuation phase of 2 to 12 months.[17] Regardless of how duration is estimated, the purpose of the continuation phase is to avoid relapse.

This is most often accomplished by maintaining treatment at the level required to achieve remission. Much of the art of clinical management relates to dose titration during the continuation and early maintenance phases. Some treatment-responsive patients may benefit from dose reduction during the continuation phase if adverse effects of medications substantially negate the gains due to remission of mood symptoms. A larger group of patients will intermittently experience significant symptoms during the continuation phase that, while not always fulfilling criteria for an acute depressive episode, indicate a full recovery has not occurred. Such a pattern of intermittent symptoms often warrants an increase in antidepressant (or antimanic) treatment but may also respond to more conservative management.[17]

The continuation phase ends and the discontinuation phase and maintenance phases begin when the patient is declared to have recovered from the acute episode.[16]

Discontinuation Phase and Maintenance Phase

The discontinuation phase follows a decision to discontinue a treatment and involves monitoring for recurrence while gradually tapering medication. A decision to redirect the therapeutic focus away from treatment of the acute episode toward maintaining recovery or preventing the recurrence of future acute episodes launches the maintenance phase. Many patients experience intermittent subsyndro-

Table 2. Protective and Risk Factors in Bipolar Disorder*

Protective Factors	
Use of mood-stabilizing medications	Harm-reduction planning
Abstinence from alcohol	Support system
Abstinence from recreational drugs	Professionals
Structured schedule	Family
Regular awakening	Friends
and sleep times	Self-help groups
Schedule of recurring	Learning early warning signs
social activity	Empower executive
Cues to avoid missing	function surrogate
medication	Redundant contingency
Psychotherapy	plans
Risk Factors	
Alcohol	Sleep disruption
Recreational drugs	Intentional
Abrupt discontinuation of medications	Unintentional
Mood stabilizers	Sleep apnea
Antidepressants	Pregnancy
Anxiolytics	Role transition
Antidepressant medication	Negative expressed emotion
Loss of supports	East-west travel
Cognitive distortions	Stress
Interpersonal conflict	

*Table adapted, with permission, from Otto et al.[39]

mal symptoms (roughening) during the discontinuation-to-maintenance phase. The significance of roughening depends on whether it is the harbinger of an impending acute episode or is merely a brief period of mild symptoms with little clear relation to the patient's mood disorder. Studies of such interepisode symptoms done by Keller et al[18] and Fava[19] suggest that roughening with features of depression often resolves without intervention. Symptoms of hypomania carry a higher risk of evolving into a full affective episode. The occurrence of symptoms meeting criteria for an acute episode would be considered a recurrence (new episode) requiring reintroduction of acute treatments.

Who Should Have Maintenance Treatment?

Many experts recommend offering maintenance treatment to all patients who have experienced even a single acute manic episode, while others feel it is appropriate to reserve long-term maintenance treatment for patients who have experienced 3 or more manic episodes.[17] Experts of the former opinion point out the 95% lifetime risk of recurrence after a single manic episode. These experts also point to data showing loss of acute and prophylactic benefit (at least of lithium) among patients with as few as 3 episodes.[20] Experts of the latter opinion point out that the median duration of remission following the first acute episode is more than 4 years[8-11] and the paucity of evidence justifying long-term treatment for bipolar patients beyond 32 weeks.[21]

Another aspect of selecting patients for maintenance treatment relates to the likelihood that patients will discontinue treatment regardless of the psychiatrist's recommendations. Patients who discontinue lithium treatment, particularly when discontinuation is abrupt, appear to be at increased risk for recurrence.[22] Based on the rate of excess relapse associated with abrupt discontinuation, Goodwin[23] calculated the point at which the risks of relapse associated with abrupt discontinuation might outweigh the potential benefits of lithium maintenance. This theoretical calculation suggests it may be counterproductive to offer maintenance treatment to patients unlikely or unwilling to adhere to treatment for at least 2 years.

It is unclear when in the course of treatment the liability to such discontinuation phenomena develops or if similar phenomena apply to other maintenance treatments. In a large prospective study, Bowden et al[24] found no evidence of discontinuation phenomena following discontinuation of acute treatment with lithium or divalproex.

Current literature does not resolve the issue of who should have treatment, but from a practical point of view, the areas of agreement extend so broadly as to largely render the question itself a matter of little clinical significance. First, by the time most patients receive a bipolar diagnosis they have already experienced multiple episodes. Second, since many clinical experts recommend continuation of effective acute phase treatments for 1 year beyond the onset of clinical remission, a substantial proportion of bipolar patients will experience relapse within this period of prudent continuation treatment.[24] Third, a surprisingly large proportion of patients simply never achieve the period of sustained euthymia considered a sufficient prerequisite for consideration of treatment discontinuation.[25] Thus, 2 distinct subgroups exist among the population of patients receiving long-term care: those who have achieved a stable remission and those who have not.

How Well Does Treatment Work?

Like many other chronic medical conditions, bipolar illness is treatable rather than curable. Acute manic episodes generally respond well to treatment with antimanic agents such as lithium, divalproex, carbamazepine, and antipsychotic medications. Double-blind studies reveal that response rates for monotherapy with any of these agents are roughly 50% at 3 weeks compared with about 25% in placebo-treated patients.[26,27] Recent double-blind studies report superior acute response rates when lithium or divalproex is used in combination with antipsychotic medications compared with antipsychotic agents alone (67% vs 40%[28]), or when compared with monotherapy with lithium or divalproex (30% vs 54%,[29] 44.7% vs 67.7%[30]). However, Tohen et al[31] also reported a sharp contrast in the rates of syndromic recovery (eg, no longer meeting criteria for an episode of mania) vs functional recovery (resumption of premorbid level of social and occupational function) at 6 and 24 months. At 6 months, 82% of patients, and at 24 months, 97%, no longer met syndromic criteria for bipolar illness. Functional recovery rates were much less impressive: 30% and 38%, respectively. Ms G's interepisode recovery appears to be excellent, but there is no guarantee that her recovery from further acute episodes will be as full. TABLE 2 lists protective attributes and risk factors in bipolar disorder.

Risks and Benefits of Medication and Psychotherapy

Specialized versions of psychosocial interventions such as family focused therapy,[33] interpersonal social rhythms therapy,[34] Life Goals,[35] and cognitive behavioral therapy[36] have shown promise as adjunctive interventions in the maintenance phase of treatment. The collaborative care model developed at the Massachusetts General Hospital recommends patients use these elements to develop an individualized written management plan that does not rely entirely on the patient for executive function. Samples and directions for constructing treatment contracts can be accessed by Internet (http://www.manicdepressive.org).[37]

Because bipolar illness tends to be understood in biological terms, it is interesting that the data supporting use of psychotherapy for bipolar patients appear to be stronger than for many other psychiatric conditions. While no psychosocial therapies claim acute antimanic benefits, most forms of psychotherapy seem to augment the prophylactic benefit of lithium.[38-43] While the active elements of psychotherapy remain unclear, the prophylactic efficacy of verbal therapies, as with lithium treatment, appears to require continued treatment.[44] The benefit Ms G perceived from therapy often reflects the continuity of care that can only be obtained by maintaining a relationship with a single provider over the course of the illness.

Simple harm-reduction strategies can buffer the social and economic consequences of the illness as well as preserve life. During periods of remission, patients can be encouraged to write a plan that anticipates problems likely to occur during acute episodes and that lays out strategies for management. Most often, this means empowering others to limit the patient's exposure to social scrutiny during periods of illness as well as restricting access to credit cards, firearms, and motor vehicles. Key to the success of any such plan is to avoid sole reliance on the patient to determine when to activate the harm-reduction strategies.[32]

Special Populations

Patients With Psychosis. Roughly 50% to 75% of manic episodes include psychotic features (hallucination, delusions, and formal thought disorder).[45] In most cases, treatment of psychotic mania will consist of mood stabilizing medication in combination with an antipsychotic agent. Most episodes of bipolar depression with psychotic features also require an antipsychotic agent (eg, risperidone, olanzapine, and quetiapine fumarate) in addition to a mood stabilizer such as lithium, divalproex, or carbamazepine and an antidepressant medication.[17] In cases where the immediate need to control psychotic symptoms takes clear precedence over specific treatment for depression or mania, initiation of antipsychotic therapy or electroconvulsive therapy (ECT) precedes other interventions.[17]

Patients responding to acute treatment with ECT can be divided into subgroups based on whether ECT was used as a matter of choice (eg, symptom acuity warranted aggressive treatment) or because the acute episode proved refractory to other interventions.[47] In all cases, mood-stabilizing medications can be offered for prophylaxis, and in the latter case, consideration should be given to use of ECT as a maintenance treatment.[17] In either case, early relapse is common following abrupt discontinuation of ECT.[46,47] Maintenance ECT presents logistical challenges that can make it impractical when treatment is required more frequently than once per month.[46,47]

Women Seeking to Conceive. Bipolar illness is not an absolute contraindication to childbearing. When women with bipolar disorder and their spouses seek counseling prior to conception, the teratogenic potential of the medications should be reviewed as well as the risk of relapse during pregnancy and the postpartum period. Generally, most experts recommend delaying attempts to conceive until patients have experienced a stable remission of at least 6 to 12 months.[48] The management strategy for women with bipolar disorder with stable remission should take into account the severity and frequency of prior episodes, age of the patient, and the quality of available supports. Older women or those with more severe episodes may choose to conceive while maintaining treatment and use fetal ultrasound or amniocentesis to screen for potential teratogenic effects. Younger women and those with milder illness may more reasonably plan to taper some or all medication prior to conception while relying on nonpharmacological strategies at least through the first trimester.[49]

Women Who Have Become Pregnant During the Course of Maintenance Treatment. Management depends largely on when in the course of gestation pregnancy is recognized and which medications are in use. Patient preference is the key determinant in selecting treatment strategies. From the perspective of teratogenicity, once the pregnancy progresses beyond the first 10 weeks, the risk of teratogenicity diminishes and the risk of rapid discontinuation may outweigh the teratogenic risk associated with a slow taper. Tapering medications during a 1- to 2-week period may reduce the risk of early relapse without substantially altering the risk of teratogenicity,[50] but plans should be made in advance for intervention in the event of relapse and close follow-up offered.

Teratogenicity is an issue for all medications. However, recent data indicate the risk of teratogenicity due to fetal exposure to lithium is substantially less than previously feared.[50] Experience with olanzapine is too limited to confidently assess its relative risk for teratogenicity. Conventional antipsychotics appear to be relatively low risk.[51]

New Treatments on the Horizon

Drugs approved for labeling for treatment of epilepsy by the US Food and Drug Administration are often used to treat bipolar disorder. However, evidence of effectiveness of these agents ranges from high-quality double-blind trials to anecdotal, and, in some cases, the only data available are negative. Lamotrigine, gabapentin, topiramate, and oxcarbazepine have been studied in double-blind trials.[52-57] These trials support the use of lamotrigine for the treatment of bipolar depression[52] and rapid cycling,[53] but not acute mania. Gabapentin appears effective for treatment of anxiety disorders, pain syndromes, and insomnia, but for bipolar II disorder double-blind studies indicate no superiority over placebo.[54,55] Reports describing antimanic effects and weight loss have generated interest in topiramate, but the available data for topiramate require careful interpretation.[56] A preliminary analysis (n=36) indicated topiramate was superior to placebo for treatment of acute mania and mixed episodes as measured by the Young Mania Rating Scale (YMRS) as well as secondary measures such as the global assessment of function (GAF) scale. When the full study (n=97) was completed, the advantage over placebo remained according to the GAF scale, but results of the YMRS were no longer statistically significant. A post hoc analysis carried out excluding 36 subjects who discontinued antidepressant medication at the time of study entry again found statistical superiority of topiramate on the YMRS and GAF scale. Successful outcomes have been reported in small samples of patients with bipolar disorder who have been treated in double-blind conditions with oxcarbazepine.[57] Although these preliminary results are encouraging, more data are needed to determine the appropriate role of oxcarbazepine. Other anticonvulsants such as levetriacetam and zonisamide are already in use but have not been studied in a double-blind fashion.

Ziprasidone hydrochloride, a newly approved atypical antipsychotic drug, is reported to be superior to placebo for treatment of acute manic and mixed episodes.[58] Ziprasidone may induce less weight gain and perhaps has greater antidepressant benefits than other atypical antipsychotics, but experience with this drug is limited to controlled clinical trials, and such claims are not yet supported by data.

Recommendations for Ms G

The priority for Ms G is to develop a treatment plan that minimizes the risk of recurrence and makes provisions to reduce the harm to her and her family caused by any future episodes. Ms G's current treatment regimen of divalproex and bupropion should be reviewed to determine whether bupropion will be part of the maintenance regimen as she approaches the summer months. If she relapses while continuing this treatment plan, additional medications should be considered for prophylaxis and the role of bupropion should be reviewed. In developing a prophylactic regimen for Ms G, it is necessary to explore her reservations about using lithium, the only medication with established prophylactic benefit. Ms G, like many patients, rejects treatment with lithium based on her perception of it as a powerful mind-altering drug with high propensity to cause weight gain. These concerns, while entirely understandable, should not preclude use of agents with proven efficacy. Offering patients several treatment options while comparing relative adverse effects and efficacy may help establish the best treatment plan for the individual patient. Expert consensus guidelines suggest carbamazepine as an alternative to lithium and valproate.[17] Ms G will need to manage the weight gain that often complicates long-term use of these medications. Ironically, she has accepted treatment with divalproex and olanzapine, agents that are associated with significantly greater weight gain than lithium.[25,59] At present, evidence of prophylactic benefit is not well established for divalproex or olanzapine, but both drugs appear to have mood-stabilizing properties.

Of course, no treatment plan will work if not properly supervised, and Ms G's options are limited by her insurance status. Continuity of care is highly desirable for management of bipolar illness. Unfortunately, the transfer of her care to a public sector venue such as a community clinic does not ensure continuity in her care. I recommend that Ms G make an agreement to meet with her psychiatrist a minimum of 12 times per year. For some patients, reaching this goal may entail switching insurance providers, applying for disability, or using federal programs designed to help cover the considerable costs of mental health care. Ms G should also consider participation in support groups (eg, National Depressive and Manic-Depressive Association [http://www.ndmda.org]) that provide resources for assistance between visits with her physician.

QUESTIONS AND DISCUSSION

A PHYSICIAN: What is the timing of starting an antidepressant if a patient is not on mood stabilization and comes in with depression?

DR SACHS: When patients have a history of bipolar I disorder, we educate them that mood stabilizers have antidepressant effects equivalent to standard antidepressant drugs. The data are consistent with that.[60-62] I prefer that patients who have had no treatment try a mood stabilizer alone for 3 weeks. Then I add an antidepressant if they don't do well. If they do not want to take a mood stabilizer alone, I will offer the 2 types of drugs together. For very depressed patients, I would certainly break the rule of requiring them to be on a mood stabilizer. Depression, by itself, is life threatening. I treat those patients and try to get them on a mood stabilizer second, if I couldn't do it first.

A PHYSICIAN: With a 100% recurrence rate, my usual policy is to keep patients on the dose of lithium that has cured them. Are you suggesting that it is good to reduce the level of lithium?

DR SACHS: We are deluding ourselves if we think that patients will be on this medicine for a lifetime. Forever is a long time, and patients experience many adverse effects. I would like to give patients optimal treatment. If they have no substantial adverse effects and receive good benefit, then reducing the dose is within reason. I'm not convinced that you need to maintain patients at higher than 0.8 mmol/L of lithium. Many people do fine with a level of 0.4 mmol/L, and I prefer to treat patients as individuals. I want every patient I treat to know that I am completely open to finding a dose that will be consistent with the highest quality of life for them.

Funding/Support: Clinical Crossroads is made possible by a grant from The Robert Wood Johnson Foundation.
Acknowledgment: We thank the patient and her doctor for sharing their stories in person and in print.

REFERENCES

1. Jamison KR. Suicide and bipolar disorders. *Ann N Y Acad Sci*. 1986;487:301-315.
2. Lish JD, Dime-Meenan S, Whybrow PC, Price RA, Hirschfeld RM. The National Depressive and Manic-Depressive Association (DMDA) survey of bipolar members. *J Affect Disord*. 1994;31:281-294.
3. Ghaemi SN, Sachs GS, Chiou AM, Pandurangi AK, Goodwin FK. Is bipolar disorder still underdiagnosed? are antidepressants overutilized? *J Affect Disord*. 1999;52:135-144.
4. American Psychiatric Association. *Diagnostic and Statistical Manual of Mental Disorders, Fourth Edition*. Washington, DC: American Psychiatric Association; 1994.
5. Kessler RC. The National Comorbidity Survey of the United States. *Int Rev Psychiatry*. 1994;6:8-19.
6. Kessler RC, Rubinow DR, Holmes C, Abelson JM, Zhao S. The epidemiology of *DSM-III-R* bipolar I disorder in a general population survey. *Psychol Med*. 1997;27:1079-1089.
7. Hantouche EG, Akiskal HS, Lancrenon S, et al. Systematic clinical methodology for validating bipolar-II disorder: data in mid-stream from a French national multi-site study (EPIDEP). *J Affect Disord*. 1998;50:163-173.
8. Kraepelin E. *Manic-Depressive Insanity and Paranoia*. Edinburgh, Scotland: E & S Livingstone; 1921.
9. Angst J, Lader M, Ralaelson O, Sacher E. The course of affective disorders. In: Van Praag HM, Sachar EJ, eds. *Handbook of Biological Psychiatry*. New York, NY: Marcel Dekker Inc; 1981:225-242.
10. Zis AP, Grof P, Webster M, Goodwin FK. Prediction of relapse in recurrent affective disorder. *Psychopharmacol Bull*. 1980;16:47-49.
11. Roy-Byrne PR, Post RM, Uhde T, Porcu T, Davis D. The longitudinal course of recurrent affective illness: life chart data from research patients at the NIMH. *Acta Psychiatr Scand*. 1985;71:1-34.
12. Coryell W, Keller MB, Endicott J, et al. Bipolar II illness: course and outcome over a 5-year period. *Psychol Med*. 1989;19:129-141.
13. Simon GE, Unuetzer J. Health care utilization and costs among patients treated for bipolar disorder in an insured population. *Psychiatr Serv*. 1999;50:1303-1308.
14. Simpson SG, Jamison KR. The risk of suicide in patients with bipolar disorders. *J Clin Psychiatry*. 1999;60(suppl 2):53-56.
15. Nilsson A. Lithium therapy and suicide risk. *J Clin Psychiatry*. 1999;60 (suppl 2):85-88.
16. Frank E, Prien R, Jarrett R, et al. Conceptualization and rationale for consensus definitions in major depressive disorder: remission, recovery, relapse, and recurrence. *Arch Gen Psychiatry*. 1991;48:851-855.
17. Sachs G, Printz D, Kahn D, Carpenter D, Docherty JP. The expert consensus guideline series: medication treatment of bipolar disorder. *Postgrad Med*. April 2000:1-104.
18. Keller MB, Lavori PW, Kane JM, et al. Subsyndromal symptoms in bipolar disorder: a comparison of standard and low serum levels of lithium. *Arch Gen Psychiatry*. 1992;49:371-376.
19. Fava G. Measurement of prodromal and subclinical symptoms in mood and anxiety disorders. In: Fava M, Rosenbaum J, eds. *Research Designs and Methods in Psychiatry*. New York, NY: Elsevier; 1992:223-230.
20. Gelenberg AJ, Kane JM, Keller MB et al. Comparison of standard and low serum levels of lithium for maintenance treatment of bipolar disorder. *N Engl J Med*. 1989;321:1489-1493.
21. Coryell W, Winokur G, Solomon D, Shea T, Leon A, Keller M. Lithium and recurrence in a long-term follow-up of bipolar affective disorder. *Psychol Med*. 1997;27:281-289.
22. Suppes T, Baldessarini RJ, Faedda GL, Tohen M. Risk of reoccurrence following discontinuation of lithium treatment in bipolar disorder. *Arch Gen Psychiatry*. 1991;48:1082-1088.
23. Goodwin G. Recurrence of mania after lithium withdrawal: implications for the use of lithium in the treatment of bipolar affective disorder. *Br J Psychiatry*. 1994;164:149-152.
24. Bowden CL, Calabrese JR, McElroy SL, et al. Randomized placebo-controlled trial of divalproex versus placebo and lithium in maintenance therapy of bipolar disorder. *Arch Gen Psychiatry*. 2000;57:481-489.
25. Sachs G, Thase M. Bipolar disorder therapies: maintenance treatment. *Biol Psychiatry*. 2000;48:573-581.
26. Bowden C, Brugger A, Swann A, et al. Efficacy of divalproex vs lithium and placebo in the treatment of mania. *JAMA*. 1994;271:918-924.
27. Tohen M, Sanger TM, McElroy SL, et al. Olanzapine versus placebo in the treatment of acute mania. *Am J Psychiatry*. 1999;156:702-709.
28. Muller-Oerlinghausen B, Henn FA, Giedke H, Walden J. Valproate as an adjunct to neuroleptic medication for the treatment of acute episodes of mania: a prospective, randomized, double-blind, placebo-controlled, multicenter study. *J Clin Psychopharmacol*. 2000;20:195-203.
29. Sachs G. Safety and efficacy of resperidone vs placebo vs haloperidol as add-on therapy to mood stabilizers in the treatment of manic phase of bipolar disorder. Paper presented at: 38th Annual Meeting of the American College of Psychopharmacology; May 17, 1999; Acapulco, Mexico.
30. Tohen M, Chengappa KN, Suppes TR, et al. Efficacy of olanzapine added to valproate or lithium in the acute treatment of mania. Paper presented at: 152nd Annual Meeting of the American Psychiatry Association; May 17, 2000; Chicago, Ill.
31. Tohen M, Hennen T, Zarate CM, et al. Two-year syndromal and functional recovery in 219 cases of first-episode major affective disorder with psychotic features. *Am J Psychiatry*. 2000;157:2208-2228.
32. Otto M, Reilly-Harrington N, Sachs G. *Collaborative Care Workbook: A Workbook for Individuals and Families. Partners Bipolar Treatment Center*. Boston: Massachusetts General Hospital; 1999.
33. Miklowitz D. Psychotherapy in combination with drug treatment for bipolar disorder. *J Clin Psychopharmacol*. 1996;16(suppl 1):S56-S66.
34. Frank E, Kupfer, D Ehlers CL, et al. Interpersonal and social rhythm therapy for bipolar disorder: integrating interpersonal and behavioral approaches. *Behav Ther*. 1994;17:143-149.
35. Bauer M, McBride L. *Structured Group Psychotherapy for Bipolar Disorder: The Life Goals Program*. New York, NY: Springer Publishing Co; 1996.
36. Hirshfeld DR, Reilly-Harrington N, Morabito C, Fredman S, Guille C, Sachs G. Short-term adjunctive cognitive-behavioral group therapy for bipolar disorder: preliminary results from a controlled trial. Paper presented at: 106th Annual Meeting of the American Psychological Association; 1998; San Francisco, Calif.
37. Harvard Bipolar Research Program. Available at: http:// www.manicdepressive .org. Accessibility verified December 21, 2000.
38. Mayo JA, O'Connell RA, O'Brien JD. Families of manic-depressive patients: effect of treatement. *Am J Psychiatry*. 1979;136:1525-1529.
39. Lesser AL. Hypomania and marital conflict. *Can J Psychiatry*. 1983;28:362-366.
40. Vasile RG, Samson JA, Bemporad J, et al. A biopsychosocial approach to treating patients with affective disorders. *Am J Psychiatry*. 1987;144:341-344.
41. Miklowitz D, Goldstein M, Nuechterlein K, Snyder K, Mintz J. Family factors and the course of bipolar affective disorder. *Arch Gen Psychiatry*. 1988;45:225-231.
42. Van Gent EM, Vida SL, Zwart FM. Group therapy in addition to lithium therapy in patients with bipolar disorders. *Acta Psychiat Belg*. 1988;88:405-418.
43. Kanas N. Group psychotherapy with bipolar patients : a review and synthesis. *Int J Group Psychother*. 1993;43:321-333.
44. Frank E, Swartz H, Kupfer D. Interpersonal and social rhythms therapy: managing the chaos of bipolar disorder. *Biol Psychiatry*. 2000;48:593-604.
45. Goodwin FK, Jamison KR. *Manic Depressive Illness*. New York, NY: Oxford University Press; 1990.
46. Sackheim HA, Prudic J, Devanand DP, Decina P, Kerr B, Malitz S. The impact of medication resistance and continuation pharmacotherapy on relapse following ECT in major depression. *J Clin Psychopharmacol*. 1990;10:96-104.
47. Gagne G, Furman M, Carpenter L, Price L. Efficacy of continuation ECT and antidepressant drugs compared to long-term antidepressants alone in depressed patients. *Am J Psychiatry*. 2000;157:1960-1965.
48. Sachs G, Cohen L. Update on pharmacologic treatment of mood disorders: bipolar disorder and management through pregnancy and postpartum. *Psychiatr Clin North Am: Ann Drug Ther*. 1995;2:21-75.
49. Cohen LS, Heller VL, Rosenbaum JF. Treatment guidelines for psychotropic drug use in pregnancy. *Psychosomatics*. 1989;30:25-33.
50. Cohen LS, Friedman JM, Jefferson JW, Johnson EM, Weiner ML. A reevaluation of risk of in utero exposure to lithium. *JAMA*. 1994;271:146-150.
51. Altshuler LL, Hendrick V, Cohen LS. Course of mood and anxiety disorders during pregnancy and the postpartum period. *J Clin Psychiatry*. 1998;59(suppl 2):29-33.
52. Calabrese JR, Bowden CL, Sachs GS, Ascher JA, Monaghan E, Rudd GD. A double-blind placebo-controlled study of lamotrigine monotherapy in outpatients with bipolar I depression. *J Clin Psychiatry*. 1999;60:79-88.
53. Calabrese J, Suppes T, Bowden C, et al. A double blind, placebo-controlled, prophylaxis study of lamotrigine in rapid-cycling bipolar disorder. *J Clin Psychopharmacol*. 2000;61:841-850.
54. Pande A, Crockatt J, Janney C, Werth J, Tsaroucha G, for the Group GBDS.

Gabapentin in bipolar disorder: a placebo-controlled trial of adjunctive therapy. *Bipolar Disord.* 2000;2:249-255.
55. Frye M, Ketter T, Kimbrell T, et al. A placebo-controlled study of lamotrigine and gabapentin monotherapy in refractory mood disorders. *J Clin Psychopharmacol.* 2000;20:607-614.
56. Calabrese J. Third generation antiepileptic drugs in bipolar disorder. Paper presented at: 12th Annual Meeting of the European College of Neuropsychopharmacology; 1999; London, England.
57. Wildgrube C. Case studies on prophylactic long-term effects of oxcarbazepine in recurrent affective disorders. *Int Clin Psychopharmacol.* 1990;5(suppl 1):89-94.
58. Keck P, Ice K. A 3-week, double-blind, randomized trial of ziprasidone in the acute treatment of mania. Paper presented at: 40th Annual NCDEU Meeting; May 31, 2000; Boca Raton, Fla.
59. Zajecka J, Weisler R, Swann A, et al. Divalproex sodium vs olanzapine for the treatment of mania in bipolar disorder. Paper presented at: 39th Annual Meeting of the American College of Neuropsychopharmacology; December 10, 2000; San Juan, Puerto Rico.
60. Young L, Joffe R, Robb J, et al. Double-blind comparison of addition of a second mood stabilizer versus an antidepressant to an initial mood stabilizer for treatment of patients with bipolar depression. *Am J Psychiatry.* 2000;157:124-126.
61. Nemeroff C, Evans D, Gyulai L, et al. A double-blind, placebo-controlled comparison of imipramine and paroxetine in the treatment of bipolar depression. *Am J Psychiatry.* In press.
62. Sachs G. Is divalproex appropriate treatment for bipolar depression. *Psychiatr Ann.* 1996;2(suppl):454-459.

Psychological Medicine, 1997, **27**, 1079–1089. Printed in the United Kingdom

The epidemiology of DSM-III-R bipolar I disorder in a general population survey

R. C. KESSLER,[1] D. R. RUBINOW, C. HOLMES, J. M. ABELSON AND S. ZHAO

From the Department of Health Care Policy, Harvard Medical School, Boston, MA; US National Institute of Mental Health, Bethesda, MD; Institute for Social Research, University of Michigan, Ann Arbor, Michigan; and Department of Sociology, Temple University, Philadelphia, PA, USA

ABSTRACT

Background. Data are presented on the general population epidemiology of DSM-III-R bipolar I disorder in the United States.

Methods. Data come from the US National Comorbidity Survey (NCS), a general population survey of DSM-III-R disorders. A modified version of the Composite International Diagnostic Interview was used to make diagnoses.

Results. A small ($N = 59$) clinical reappraisal study showed that the only manic symptom profile that could validly be assessed with the CIDI is characterized by euphoria, grandiosity and the ability to maintain energy without sleep, which described approximately half of all clinically validated bipolar I cases in the NCS. Further analysis focused on this symptom profile, which involved $N =$ 29 cases in the total sample. Lifetime prevalence was estimated to be 0·4% and 12-month prevalence only slightly lower. Caseness was negatively related to income, education and age, positively related to urbanicity, and elevated among the previously married, never married and non-whites. All cases reported at least one other NCS/DSM-III-R disorder and 59·3% reported that their episode of bipolar disorder (either mania or depression) occurred at a later age than at least one other NCS/DSM-III-R disorder. Although 93·2% of lifetime cases reported some lifetime treatment, only 44·7% of recent cases were in treatment.

Conclusions. The type of bipolar disorder examined here is highly chronic, co-morbid and impairing. Increased efforts are required to attract current cases into appropriate treatment. Methodological research is needed to develop more accurate measures of other bipolar symptom profiles for use in general population epidemiological studies.

INTRODUCTION

This report presents data on the descriptive epidemiology of DSM-III-R bipolar I disorder from the National Comorbidity Survey (NCS) (Kessler *et al.* 1994), a nationally representative survey of the United States. Previous general population surveys of bipolar disorder have largely been based on DSM-III criteria (Canino *et al.* 1987; Bland *et al.* 1988*a*; Hwu *et al.* 1989; Wells *et al.* 1989; Lee *et al.* 1990*a*; Wittchen *et al.* 1992; Chen *et al.* 1993). The topics considered include prevalence, age of onset, course, the ratio of manic to depressive episodes, socio-demographic correlates, co-morbidity, impairment and help-seeking.

METHOD

Sample

The NCS is based on a stratified, multi-stage area probability sample of the non-institutionalized civilian population in the 48 coterminous United States with a supplemental sample of students living in campus group

[1] Address for correspondence: Professor Ronald C. Kessler, Department of Health Care Policy, Harvard Medical School, 25 Shattuck Street, Parcel B- 1st Floor, Boston, MA 02115, USA.

housing. Face-to-face in-home interviews with 8098 respondents were administered between 14 September 1990 and 6 February 1992. The response rate was 82·4%. More details about the NCS sample design have been reported previously (Kessler *et al.* 1994, 1995*a*).

Diagnostic assessment

Diagnostic assessment in the NCS was based on a modified version of the Composite International Diagnostic Interview (CIDI) (World Health Organization, 1990*a*; Wittchen, 1994), a fully structured interview developed to generate diagnoses according to the definitions and criteria of both DSM-III-R (American Psychiatric Association, 1987) and ICD-10 (World Health Organization, 1990*b*) from assessments carried out by trained interviewers who are not clinicians. The modifications elaborated the CIDI in a number of ways, while maintaining the CIDI symptom questions that are required to make diagnoses.

There were two main modifications in the assessment of bipolar disorder. First, the diagnostic stem questions were administered early in the interview as part of a special lifetime review section rather than at the beginning of the diagnostic section. This was done in an effort to increase recall among respondents whose most recent episode occurred long before the interview (Kessler *et al.* 1997). Secondly, the organic exclusion questions were administered for symptoms at the episode level rather than before episode clustering. The CIDI approach is to ask separately about the lifetime occurrence of each symptom that might be part of a manic syndrome (e.g. 'Have you ever had a period when thoughts raced through your head so fast that you could not keep track of them?') and probe positive responses to see if they are always due to organic causes. Once this symptom-level probing is finished, respondents are asked if the symptoms judged not to have always been due to organic causes (even if they were sometimes or even usually due to organic causes) ever occurred together in an episode characterized by either euphoria or irritability and, if so, whether the number of symptoms in this episode was sufficient to meet DSM-III-R criteria (which require euphoria plus at least three additional symptoms or irritability plus at least four additional symptoms). No probes are administered at the episode level to determine whether any of the symptoms in these episodes could have been due to organic factors. The NCS corrected this problem by probing each symptom at the episode level. The same questions as in the CIDI were used for this probing.

WHO Field Trials of the CIDI found very good short-term (1–3 day) test–retest reliability (kappa = 0·78) and validity (kappa = 0·83) in comparison with clinical reinterviews for the diagnosis of DSM-III-R bipolar I disorder (Wittchen, 1994). However, virtually all Field Trial cases were from treatment samples. A clinical reappraisal study was carried out of a representative subsample of 59 NCS community respondents consisting of 31 CIDI cases and 28 noncases who endorsed at least one of the two mania stem questions in the NCS to determine whether the Field Trial results can be generalized to the general population. The non-case subsample was confined to those who endorsed a stem question based on the fact that the probability of finding even a single false negative for a disorder as rare as bipolar disorder would be very small in an unrestricted CIDI non-case subsample. While improving our ability to assess the prevalence of false negatives with a fixed sample size, this procedure makes it impossible to compute total-sample validity statistics such as kappa. However, it is possible to compute an unbiased estimate of the CIDI false positive rate with this design.

The reinterviews were administered by trained clinical interviewers who were blind to the NCS diagnoses and used the SCID (Spitzer *et al.* 1990) to arrive at an independent clinical judgement regarding the presence or absence of bipolar disorder. These interviews, which focused on lifetime disorder, were carried out a minimum of 6 months after the NCS in order to avoid respondent fatigue and minimize the possibility of respondents consciously attempting to be consistent with their earlier reports. Clinical diagnoses were based on consensus of the interviewer, a clinical reviewer, the clinical supervisor (J.M.A.) and a senior clinician experienced in the evaluation of mania (D.R.R.).

The correspondence between the NCS diagnoses of bipolar I and the clinical reinterview diagnoses was poor due to the CIDI classifying more people as cases ($N = 31$) than the clinicians ($N = 10$). The false negative rate was quite low, with only one of the 28 CIDI non-cases being classified as a case in the clinical interviews. However, the weighted CIDI false positive rate was very high, 70·8% (with a standard error of 8·5%), which means that 70·8% of the respondents classified as bipolar I by the CIDI were not confirmed by clinical reinterviews. Comparison of symptom-level discrepancies among CIDI cases showed that the major reason for the CIDI false positives was that the CIDI made diagnoses when respondents denied ever having euphoria but reported periods of irritability associated with arousal and role impairments that were not classified as indicative of mania by the clinicians. It was possible to develop a revised CIDI diagnostic algorithm based on *post hoc* comparisons that required euphoria (either a period of abnormally elevated mood or a period of being unusually active to a degree that friends and family members were concerned) and associated symptoms of inflated self-esteem or grandiosity and a decreased need for sleep. About one-fourth of the people originally classified as CIDI cases in the clinical reappraisal study (7 of 31) had this symptom profile, the vast majority of whom (six of seven) were classified as cases in the clinical reinterviews.

This symptom profile is typical of euphoric manics seen clinically. It does not characterize all cases, though, as demonstrated by the fact that only six of the ten respondents diagnosed with bipolar I disorder by the clinicians in the reappraisal study were classified as CIDI cases based on this revised algorithm. This result suggests that only about half of true cases in the household population have this symptom profile even though the vast majority of people with this symptom profile are true cases. We were unable to devise an algorithm for other CIDI cases that had acceptable concordance with the clinical diagnoses. Neither were we able to document any validity for an assessment of bipolar II disorder. As a result, we elected to focus on this single symptom profile of bipolar I disorder in subsequent analyses. As noted below, 29 NCS respondents reported a CIDI symptom profile of this sort. These respondents were defined as cases of bipolar I disorder without diagnostic hierarchy rules for the exclusion of cases superimposed on schizophrenia or other psychotic disorders. This exclusion, if it had been imposed, would have affected only two cases of the 29 in the sample.

Analysis procedures

Most of the analyses reported below were carried out with simple computations of means (prevalences), distributions, and cross-tabulations. Odds-ratios were computed by exponentiating the coefficients obtained from logistic regression models using the SAS logistic regression procedure (SAS Institute, 1989). Cumulative age of onset curves were generated using the SAS lifetest procedure. The effects of earlier disorders in predicting the subsequent onset of mania were estimated in discrete-time survival models (Efron, 1988) based on a person-year data array (Kessler *et al.* 1995*b*). The exponentiated coefficients in these survival models can be interpreted as odds ratios (Allison, 1982).

Because of the weighting and clustering of observations in the NCS, special estimation procedures were used to adjust significance tests. This was accomplished by estimating standard errors for prevalences using the Taylor series linearization method (Woodruff & Causey, 1976; Rust, 1985) implemented in the SUDAAN (Shah *et al.* 1991) software package and confidence intervals for odds-ratios using the method of jackknife repeated replications (Kish & Frankel, 1974) implemented in a SAS macro incorporating the logistic regression procedure (SAS Institute, 1989). There are some cases, noted in the text, where the accuracy of the standard errors or confidence intervals can be questioned because of the small number of cases in the denominator of the calculations.

RESULTS

Prevalence

Prevalences are presented in Table 1. Lifetime (LT) prevalence is estimated to be 0·45% ($N = 29$; 0·42% among men and 0·47% among women, $z = 0{\cdot}2$, $P = 0{\cdot}835$) and 12-month prevalence to be 0·37% ($N = 19$; 0·40% among men and 0·35% among women, $z = 0{\cdot}2$, $P = 0{\cdot}878$). The substantial drop in number of cases with a 12-month disorder compared to a LT disorder without an associated drop in the prevalence estimate is due to the fact that the prevalence estimates are based on weighted data and a handful of cases with large weights can be quite influential in a situation of this sort. As noted above, however, the effect of weighting is taken into consideration in the computation of the standard errors. Median age of onset in the sample is 21 years. The age of onset distribution does not differ significantly by sex ($\chi^2_1 = 0{\cdot}8$, $P = 0{\cdot}383$).

Table 1. *Prevalence of NCS/DSM-III-R Euphoric–Grandiose* bipolar I disorder*

	Male			Female			Total		
	%	(S.E.)	N†	%	(S.E.)	N†	%	(S.E.)	N†
Lifetime	0·42	(0·17)	17	0·47	(0·22)	12	0·45	(0·14)	29
12-Month	0·40	(0·17)	13	0·35	(0·20)	6	0·37	(0·14)	19

* Euphoric-Grandiose bipolar I disorder = a bipolar I symptom profile characterized by euphoria, grandiosity, and decreased need for sleep.

† These are the unweighted number of respondents in the numerators of the prevalence estimates (the prevalence estimates, in comparison, are based on weighted data).

Manic and depressive episodes

One-fifth (20·3%) of LT cases reported never having a depressive episode, a proportion only weakly related to number of years since onset of mania (point-biserial correlation = 0·04, $P =$ 0.832). The average number of manic episodes (mean, 43·4; median, 14) far exceeds the average number of depressive episodes (mean, 23·9; median, 6). Within-person comparisons, however, show that 40·6% of respondents reported having more depressive than manic episodes and that the median proportions of manic and

Table 2. *Co-morbidities between LT Euphoric–Grandiose* bipolar I disorder and other LT NCS/DSM-III-R disorders assessed with cross-sectional odds ratios and with time-lagged discrete-time survival models for prior disorders predicting the subsequent onset of bipolar I disorder*

	LT prevalences of other disorders among respondents with LT bipolar I disorder			Cross-sectional ORs between LT bipolar I disorder other LT disorders	
Other disorders	%	(S.E.)	N†	OR‡	(95% CI)
I Affective disorders					
Major depressive episode	79·7	(7·4)	21	18·4	(3·4–98·7)
Dysthymia	49·6	(9·3)	10	13·6	(8·8–21·1)
Any	90·1	(5·6)	23	36·7	(12·3 – 109·5)
II Anxiety disorders					
Generalized anxiety disorder	42·6	(9·2)	9	13·3	(3·4–52·0)
Agoraphobia	62·4	(8·9)	14	22·7	(10·4–49·4)
Simple phobia	66·6	(8·8)	12	15·3	(4·7–49·2)
Social phobia	47·2	(9·3)	13	5·6	(1·4–22·9)
Panic disorder	33·1	(8·8)	8	13·2	(1·5–114·4)
Post-traumatic stress disorder	38·8	(9·1)	9	7·6	(1·4–42·2)
Any	92·9	(4·7)	25	31·2	(5·0–196·8)
III Substance use disorders					
Alcohol dependence	61·1	(9·0)	15	9·2	(4·9–17·2)
Drug dependence	40·7	(9·1)	11	8·0	(2·2–29·1)
Alcohol abuse	64·2	(8·9)	17	5·8	(2·6–12·8)
Drug abuse	46·1	(9·3)	14	6·6	(1·5–27·9)
Any	71·0	(8·4)	20	6·4	(1·8–22·7)
IV Other disorders					
Conduct disorder	59·4	(9·1)	12	9·6	(1·2–79·3)
Adult anti-social behaviour	29·0	(8·4)	10	7·3	(1·2–44·3)
Any	81·7	(7·1)	18	24·2	(7·2–81·1)
V Aggregate number of disorders					
One +	100·0	(—)	29	(—)	(—)
Three +	95·5	(3·8)	26	69·7	(22·8 – 213·2)

* Euphoric–Grandiose bipolar I disorder = a bipolar I symptom profile characterized by euphoria, grandiosity and decreased need for sleep.

† These are unweighted numbers of respondents classified as manic who also met lifetime criteria for the NCS/DSM-III-R disorder listed in the row heading. The percentage estimates and odds ratios, in comparison, are based on weighted data.

‡ 95% CI does not include 1·0.

OR, odds ratio; CI, confidence interval.

Table 3. *Lifetime prevalences of suicidal thoughts and suicide attempts among NCS respondents with Euphoric–Grandiose* bipolar I disorder (BPI), unipolar major depression (MD), and other NCS respondents by sex*

	BPI			MD			Other NCS respondents		
	%	(S.E.)†	N‡	%	(S.E.)†	N‡	%	(S.E.)†	N‡
I. Suicidal thoughts									
Male	71·8	(13·3)	8	38·6	(3·1)	187	6·1	(0·6)	201
Female	64·7	(23·7)	9	39·6	(2·0)	360	10·1	(1·7)	243
Total	68·0	(9·2)	17	39·2	(1·7)	547	8·1	(0·9)	444
II. Suicide attempts									
Male	48·7	(19·8)	7	14·1	(2·1)	58	1·5	(0·3)	49
Female	48·1	(21·3)	5	16·2	(2·0)	158	3·6	(0·8)	89
Total	48·4	(13·6)	12	15·4	(1·6)	216	2·6	(0·4)	138

* Euphoric-Grandiose bipolar I disorder = a bipolar I symptom profile characterized by euphoria, grandiosity and decreased need for sleep.

† The estimated standard errors are imprecise because of the small numbers of cases on which the percentage estimates are based.

‡ These are the unweighted number of respondents in the numerators of the prevalence estimates (the prevalence estimates, in comparison, are based on weighted data).

depressive episodes as a fraction of all bipolar episodes are virtually identical (50·2% and 49·8%, respectively).

Although male cases were significantly more likely than female cases to report never having a depressive episode (38·9% *v.* 4·0%), the proportion of cases who reported having a larger number of manic than depressive episodes does not differ greatly by sex (60·4% of men and 45·8% of women). Neither is there either a substantial sex difference in mean number of total episodes of mania and depression combined (75·4 among men and 60·4 among women) or a large sex difference in median number of total episodes (38 among men and 30 among women).

Sociodemographic correlates

Bivariate associations between sociodemographic variables and LT prevalence showed significant associations of age and income. The age effect is most plausibly interpreted as a cohort effect due to a significant difference in the age-of-onset distribution of respondents in the age range 15–34 compared to those 35–54 ($\chi^2_1 = 7{\cdot}7$, $P = 0{\cdot}006$), with higher prevalences throughout the comparable age range among the younger respondents. The income effect shows that cases were significantly more likely than non-cases to have incomes less than $20000 (OR = 15·2, 95% CI = 4·7–49·0). There were also non-significant trends suggesting that cases might be more likely than non-cases to be non-white, unmarried, poorly educated, and to live in urbanized rather than rural areas. (Detailed results of these and other analyses reported in the text are available in an appendix that can be obtained either from the senior author or from the NCS WWW home page. See the acknowledgements section for instructions on how to access the home page.)

Co-morbidity

All of the cases considered here reported one or more other lifetime NCS/DSM-III-R disorders, with the majority (59·3%) reporting that at least one of the other disorders occurred at an earlier age than both their mania and depression. These patterns do not differ by sex. The results in the first column of Table 2 show more detailed LT prevalence estimates of individual NCS/DSM-III-R disorders among cases. Virtually all cases (92·9%) reported at least one LT anxiety disorder, while 71·0% reported at least one LT substance use disorder, 81·7% reported a history of either conduct disorder (CD) or adult antisocial behaviour (AAB) and 95·5% reported having three or more of the above disorders in their lifetime. The odds-ratios in the third column of Table 2, ranging between 5·6 for social phobia and 22·7 for agoraphobia, compare the 29 bipolar cases with all other NCS respondents and show that these prevalences are all significantly higher among the former than the latter. The odds-ratio for any LT anxiety disorder (31·2) is especially high.

The results in the last two columns of Table 2

show odds ratios and their confidence intervals obtained from a series of bivariate discrete-time survival models in each of which prior history of one other NCS/DSM-III-R disorder was used as a time-varying predictor of the subsequent onset of bipolar I disorder. The ORs are consistently greater than 1·0 and four are significant at the 0·05 level, indicating that they predict an increased probability of first onset of bipolar disorder. Three of the four significant coefficients are associated with anxiety disorders (GAD, PTSD, any anxiety), while the fourth is associated with prior history of either conduct disorder or adult antisocial behaviour. It is noteworthy that the ORs are all smaller than the comparable values in the second column of the table and that this difference is especially pronounced for the anxiety disorders, indicating that only part of these co-morbidities are due to other disorders predicting the onset of temporally secondary bipolar disorder.

Although the aggregate measures of substance use disorders in Table 2 are not significant predictors of subsequent bipolar disorder, more detailed disaggregated analyses (available from the NCS WWW home page) showed that there are effects of specific substances. Cocaine was the only drug for which prior use had a meaningfully elevated odds ratio (4·2; 95% CI: 0·3–57·2) in predicting subsequent onset of bipolar disorder, a result consistent with a prospective epidemiological investigation by Anthony & Petronis (1991) based on the ECA data. Stimulant abuse (OR = 3·1, 95% CI: 1·0–9·9) and dependence (OR = 5·7, 95% CI: 1·8–18·4) were the only illicit drug use disorders with estimable odds ratios that meaningfully predicted subsequent bipolar disorder.

Suicidality

The results in Table 3 present data on lifetime prevalences of suicidal thoughts and attempts, separately among the 29 NCS respondents with LT bipolar I disorder, those with LT unipolar major depression, and other NCS respondents. More than two-thirds of NCS respondents with LT bipolar I disorder (68·1%) reported having suicidal thoughts ('seriously thinking about committing suicide') at some time in their life, while 48·4% made a suicide attempt. These prevalences are significantly higher than those found among either respondents with unipolar major depression ($z = 1·8$, $P = 0·069$ for thoughts; $z = 3·1$, $P = 0·002$ for attempts) or other NCS respondents ($z = 6·8$, $P < 0·001$ for thoughts; $z = 7·2$, $P < 0·001$ for attempts). There is no meaningful male–female difference in the prevalences of either suicidal thoughts (71·8% *v*. 64·7%) or attempts (48·7% *v* 48·1%) among respondents with LT bipolar I disorder, although the bases on which these differences are computed are too small to assume that the estimates are reliable.

Help-seeking

Virtually all (93·2%) respondents with LT bipolar I disorder reported being in treatment at some time in their life and 44·7% of those with a 12-month disorder reported being in treatment during the year prior to the interview. Approximately half (47·2%) of those in past year treatment were treated in the health care sector (all of them seen by a mental health specialist) compared to 87·0% whose treatment was in the human services sector and/or the self help sector.

DISCUSSION

Limitations

The above results are based on only 29 cases who are believed to represent only about half of bipolar I cases in the population. The small number of cases leads to imprecision in parameter estimates. The incomplete coverage makes it impossible to compare results rigorously with those from other studies. The first of these two limitations is due to the rarity of bipolar I disorder in the population. The only hope of addressing this problem in community samples is to build up a picture across a number of major epidemiological surveys. The present report should be seen as an attempt to begin this process of cumulation for the subset of CIDI cases who can reasonably be considered to be true bipolars. A number of other large CIDI surveys are currently underway in other countries around the world, so the goal of cumulation across studies is a realistic one that could well be realized over a short period of time. The fact that the cumulation will require us to focus on only the subset of bipolars who have a symptom profile characterized by euphoria, grandiosity and the ability to maintain energy without sleep is unfortunate because it limits external validity.

However, this restriction is necessary because this is the only manic symptom profile that is accurately assessed in the current version of the CIDI. Any analysis that studies the broader CIDI definition of bipolar I disorder is, in effect, doing nothing more than studying this subsample of bipolars along with a group of false positives. Improvement in the accuracy of assessment of other bipolars in the CIDI is required to correct this situation. Given the fact that a number of research groups are currently working with this version of the CIDI, we believe that the best option is the one we have taken here; to focus on the validly assessed subsample of bipolars and explicitly acknowledge that we have no way to study other bipolars with this instrument. It is likely that cases with the valid symptom profile differ clinically from others with bipolar disorder due to the very high co-morbidity of this profile with anxiety and the fact that comorbid anxiety is known to be related to a severe illness course of bipolar disorder. Recent research in clinical samples has also shown that there are important differences in the clinical correlates of euphoric versus dysphoric symptom profiles of bipolar disorder (Post *et al.* 1989).

Prevalence

The lifetime prevalence estimate of bipolar I disorder in the NCS using the original CIDI definition is 1·6% (Kessler *et al.* 1994), which is at the upper end of the range of prevalences found in previous epidemiological surveys, which have ranged between 0·5 and 1·6% (Canino et al., 1987; Bland *et al.* 1988*b*; Hwu *et al.* 1989; Wells *et al.* 1989; Lee *et al.* 1990*a*; Wittchen *et al.* 1992; Chen *et al.* 1993). The lifetime prevalence estimate of the narrow definition of bipolar I disorder used in the current report is 0·45%. As this profile characterizes only about half of the respondents in the clinical reappraisal subsample diagnosed by the SCID as having bipolar I, the true LT prevalence of this disorder in the household population is likely to be approximately 0·9%.

Age of onset

Our finding of an average age of onset of 21 is consistent with the median onset ages in the late teens to early twenties found in treatment samples of patients with bipolar I disorder (Goodwin & Jamison, 1990). Our failure to find a sex difference in the age of onset distribution is consistent with the results of previous studies in both treatment samples (Taylor & Abrams, 1981; Coryell & Winokur, 1992) and community samples (Burke *et al.* 1990).

Course

The finding that the vast majority of cases had episodes in the year prior to interview is consistent with evidence from treatment studies that bipolar disorder is a very chronic disease (Coryell & Winokur, 1992). The median numbers of manic (14) and depressive (6) episodes found here are also similar to those in treatment samples (Clayton, 1981). The finding that 20% of cases never had a depressive episode is within the range of 5 to 28% reported in clinical studies (Abrams *et al.* 1979; Andreasen *et al.* 1988; Wolf *et al.* 1988; Fogarty *et al.* 1994). However, the finding that this proportion is much greater for men (38·9%) than women (4·1%) is a new result requiring replication. Our failure to find a strong relationship between number of years since first onset of mania and probability of ever having a depressive episode suggests that few unipolar manics with the symptom profile considered here will subsequently have depressive episodes. Unlike the results of treatment studies (Dunner & Hall, 1980; Taylor & Abrams, 1981; Roy-Byrne *et al.* 1985), we failed to find that women reported either a larger overall number of lifetime episodes of mania and depression combined or a higher proportion of depressive than manic episodes, failures that could be due to our exclusive focus on a single symptom profile.

Sociodemographic correlates

The finding that the symptom profile considered here is negatively related to income and education, while consistent with other epidemiologic surveys (Smith & Weissman, 1992), is inconsistent with the clinical observation of a positive association between bipolar disorder and socioeconomic status (Winokur *et al.* 1969; Woodruff *et al.* 1971; Weissman & Myers, 1978; Krauthammer & Klerman, 1979; Welner *et al.* 1979). This discrepancy could be due to more socially advantaged cases having a higher probability than others of obtaining speciality treatment or to a relationship between socio-economic status and accuracy of diagnosis of bipolar disorder.

The elevated prevalence among respondents in the age range 15–34 compared to older respondents is also consistent with previous research (Canino *et al.* 1987; Bland *et al.* 1988*a*; Wells *et al.* 1989; Wittchen *et al.* 1992). This could be due to bipolar disorder becoming more prevalent in recent cohorts. Or it could be due to selection processes. The latter could include the fact that bipolars have a much higher risk of early death than others in the population due to high rates of suicide (Tsuang *et al.* 1980), accidental death (Weeke & Vaeth, 1986) and cardiovascular and respiratory disorders (Sharma & Markar, 1994). Selection biases associated with differential rates of residence in the household population and differential co-operation could also be involved.

The trend finding that prevalence is elevated among non-whites is consistent with the broader evidence in the NCS that this type of mania is more prevalent among people from disadvantaged sectors of society. The trend finding of elevated prevalences among non-married people is consistent with previous research (Goodwin & Jamison, 1990; Weissman *et al.* 1991) and presumably is due to selection processes. The trend finding of a higher prevalence in urban than rural areas is consistent with the ECA Study (Weissman *et al.* 1991), but inconsistent with epidemiological surveys conducted outside the United States which have consistently failed to find an urban–rural difference in mania (Canino *et al.* 1987; Hwu *et al.* 1989; Lee *et al.* 1990*b*). This discrepancy raises an intriguing question concerning a possible cross-national difference in the relationship between bipolar disorder and urbanicity. Finally, our failure to find a male–female prevalence difference is consistent with previous research (Egeland & Hostetter, 1983; Hwu *et al.* 1989; Wells *et al.* 1989; Burke *et al.* 1990; Lee *et al.* 1990*a*; Weissman *et al.* 1991; Chen *et al.* 1993).

Co-morbidity

The finding that the symptom profile considered here is highly co-morbid with other NCS/DSM-III-R disorders is consistent with evidence of high co-morbidity in bipolar disorder from both treatment samples (Andreasen *et al.* 1988; Black *et al.* 1988; Kutcher *et al.* 1989; Côté & Hodgins, 1990; Brady & Lydiard, 1992) and general population samples (Regier et al., 1990; Robins *et al.* 1991). While alcohol and drug disorders are usually found to be the most prevalent co-morbid disorders in treatment samples, co-morbid anxiety disorders were found to be much more common in our analysis. This difference could reflect an impact of co-morbid substance use disorders on increased probability of help-seeking or an especially high co-morbidity with anxiety among bipolars having the symptom profile that was the focus of our analysis. The evaluation of this second possibility in treatment samples would be of particular interest in light of evidence that high co-morbidity with anxiety disorders is associated with poor treatment response and worse outcome in patients having both unipolar and bipolar disorders (Murphy, 1980; Roth, 1981; Van Valkenburg *et al.* 1984).

The high co-morbidities documented above could be due to an number of causal processes, including the possibility of an impact of earlier disorders on subsequent bipolar disorder, possibly by precipitating mood disorder in genetically predisposed individuals, an effect of bipolar disorder on the subsequent onset of other disorders, an effect of some underlying vulnerability shared by bipolar disorder and other conditions, or some combination of these processes. In the case of co-morbidities involving substance use, it is also possible that substance-related problems could represent attempts to modulate the mood lability associated with bipolar disorder or that they could be symptoms of mood disturbance. Although the NCS design does not allow us to sort out these various possibilities, we were able to examine temporal priority between bipolar disorder and co-morbid disorders. The results showed that first onset of both manic and depressive episodes usually occurred after the prior onset of some other co-morbid disorder. Consistent with this finding, our survival analysis showed that prior anxiety disorders, cocaine use, stimulant abuse or dependence, conduct disorder, and adult anti-social behaviour are associated with an increased risk of the subsequent onset of bipolar disorder.

It is unclear why anxiety disorders should predispose to this type of bipolar disorder, but both genetic and environmental mechanisms are possibilities worthy of future consideration. The finding that cocaine use and stimulant use disorders predict subsequent bipolar disorder is consistent with the suggestion of several authors that drugs can precipitate bipolar illness (El-Guebaly, 1975; Weller *et al.* 1988) as well as with the finding of Post *et al.* (1986) that cocaine is a powerful inducer of kindling, a sensitization-like process that may be a model for the development of bipolar illness. The findings that conduct disorder (CD) and adult antisocial behaviour (AAB) are associated with a significantly increased risk of subsequent mania are, at least superficially, consistent with the findings regarding the effects of drug use disorders. However, it is also important to recognize that the antisocial behaviours giving rise to diagnoses of CD and AAB could be early expressions of bipolar disorder. This sort of symptom overlap is one of a number of diagnostic complexities that makes it difficult to distinguish temporal order of early-onset disorders with subsequent mania in the absence of detailed longitudinal investigation (Bukstein *et al.* 1989).

Impairment and suicidality

Pathogenic speculations notwithstanding, the consequences of high co-morbidity are likely to be untoward. The finding that the cases considered here are 15 times as likely as others to be in the lowest income category at the time of study is consistent with this inference. Another striking indicator of adverse life consequences is the finding that the majority of the cases considered here had serious suicidal thoughts and that close to half made suicide attempts at some time in their life. The 48% rate of suicide attempts is within the range of 20% to 60% reported in 13 clinical studies summarized by Goodwin & Jamison (1990). Our failure to find a sex difference in suicidality is also consistent with the results of clinical studies (Barner-Rasmussen, 1986; Dilsaver *et al.* 1993; Isometsä *et al.* 1994).

Help-seeking

The vast majority of cases reported treatment at some time in their life. However, our results are less encouraging than the ECA Study regarding bipolars in recent treatment. Whereas 60·9% of the people defined as bipolar in the ECA Study reported being in treatment at some time during the year prior to interview and 88·8% of those in treatment were being treated in the health care sector, only 44·7% of the more narrowly defined bipolars in the NCS were in treatment over the past year and only 47·2% of the latter were treated in the health care sector. It is conceivable that this difference in results is due to the fact that the ECA definition of bipolar disorder was broader than the NCS definition, although this would seem to be unlikely in light of the fact that this broader definition presumably includes less impaired people. A more likely possibility, we believe, is that the largely urban sample of the ECA Study produced help-seeking patterns that are atypical of the entire country. Whatever the case may be in this regard, the results of the NCS data are quite clear in showing that only one-fifth of recent cases with a euphoric-grandiose symptom profile in the US household population are in treatment for this disorder with a health care professional in a year. Given the considerable impairment associated with bipolar disorder and the availability of effective pharmacotherapy for those who seek health care treatment, this low rate of service contact suggests that increased efforts are needed to attract and to maintain these patients in appropriate treatment.

The National Comorbidity Survey (NCS) is a collaborative epidemiological investigation of the prevalences, causes, and consequences of psychiatric morbidity and co-morbidity in the United States supported by the National Institute of Mental Health (R01 MH46376, R01 MH49098, and RO1 MH52861) with supplemental support from the National Institute of Drug Abuse (through a supplement to MH46376) and the W. T. Grant Foundation (90135190), R. C. Kessler, Principal Investigator. Preparation for this report was also supported by a Research Scientist Award to R. C. Kessler (K05 MH00507). Collaborating NCS sites and investigators are: The Addiction Research Foundation (Robin Room), Duke University Medical Center (Dan Blazer, Marvin Swartz), Harvard Medical School (Richard Frank, Ronald Kessler), Johns Hopkins University (James Anthony, William Eaton, Philip Leaf), the Max Planck Institute of Psychiatry Clinical Institute (Hans-Ulrich Wittchen), the Medical College of Virginia (Kenneth Kendler), the University of Miami (R. Jay Turner), the University of Michigan (Lloyd Johnston, Roderick Little), New York University (Patrick Shrout), SUNY Stony Brook (Evelyn Bromet), and Washington University School of Medicine (Linda

Cottler, Andrew Heath). A complete list of all NCS publications along with abstracts, study documentation, interview schedules, and the raw NCS public use data files can be obtained directly from the NCS homepage by using the URL: http://www.umich.edu/~ncsum/.

REFERENCES

Abrams, R., Taylor, M. A., Hayman, M. A. & Krishna, N. R. (1979). Unipolar mania revisited. *Journal of Affective Disorders* **1**, 59–68.

Allison, P. D. (1982). Discrete-time methods for the analysis of event histories. In *Sociological Methodology* (ed. S. Leinhardt), pp. 61–98. Jossey-Bass: San Francisco, CA.

American Psychiatric Association. (1987). *Diagnostic and Statistical Manual of Mental Disorders 3rd edn – Revised*). American Psychiatric Association: Washington, DC.

Andreasen, N. C., Grove, W. M., Coryell, W. H., Endicott, J. & Clayton, P. J. (1988). Bipolar versus unipolar and primary versus secondary affective disorder: Which diagnosis takes precedence? *Journal of Affective Disorders* **15**, 69–80.

Antony, J. C. & Petronis, K. R. (1991). Epidemiologic evidence on suspected associations between cocaine use and psychiatric disturbances. *NIDA Research Monograph* **110**, 71–94.

Barner-Rasmussen, P. (1986). Suicide in psychiatric patients in Denmark, 1971–1981: II. Hospital utilization and risk groups. *Acta Psychiatrica Scandinavica* **73**, 449–455.

Black, D. W., Winokur, G., Bell, S., Nasrallah, A. & Hulbert, J. (1988). Complicated mania: Comorbidity and immediate outcome in the treatment of mania. *Archives of General Psychiatry* **45**, 232–236.

Bland, R. C., Orn, H. & Newman, S. C. (1988*a*). Lifetime prevalence of psychiatric disorders in Edmonton. *Acta Psychiatrica Scandinavica, Supplementum* **338**, 24–32.

Bland, R. C., Newman, S. C. & Orn, H. (1988*b*). Period prevalence of psychiatric disorders in Edmonton. *Acta Psychiatrica Scandinavica, Supplementum*, 338, 33–42.

Brady, K. & Lydiard, R. B. (1992). Bipolar affective disorder and substance abuse. *Journal of Clinical Psychopharmacology* **12**, 17S–22S.

Bukstein, O. G., Brent, D. A. & Kaminer, Y. (1989). Comorbidity of substance abuse and other psychiatric disorders in adolescents. *American Journal of Psychiatry* **146**, 1131–1141.

Burke, K. C., Burke, J. D., Regier, D. A. & Rae, D. S. (1990). Age at onset of selected mental disorders in five community populations. *Archives of General Psychiatry* **47**, 511–518.

Canino, G. J., Bird, H. R., Shrout, P. E., Rubio-Stipec, M., Bravo, M., Martinez, R., Sesman, M. & Guevara, L. M. (1987). The prevalence of specific psychiatric disorders in Puerto Rico. *Archives of General Psychiatry* **44**, 727–735.

Chen, C.-N., Wong, J., Lee, N., Chan-Ho, M.-W., Lau, J. T.-F. & Fung, M. (1993). The Shatin Community Mental Health Survey in Hong Kong: II. Major findings. *Archives of General Psychiatry* **50**, 125–133.

Clayton, P. J. (1981). The epidemiology of bipolar affective disorder. *Comprehensive Psychiatry* **22**, 31–43.

Coryell, W. & Winokur, G. (1992). Course and outcome. In *Handbook of Affective Disorders*, 2nd edn. (ed. E. S. Paykel), pp. 89–108. The Guilford Press: New York.

Côté, G. & Hodgins, S. (1990). Co-occurring mental disorders among criminal offenders. *Bulletin of the American Academy of Psychiatry and the Law* **18**, 271–281.

Dilsaver, S. C., Chen, Y.-W., Swann, A. C. & Shoaib, A. M. (1993). Suicidality in patients with pure and depressive mania: 32nd Annual Meeting of the American College of Neuropsychopharmacology (1993, Honolulu, Hawaii). *American Journal of Psychiatry* **151**, 1312–1315.

Dunner, D. L. & Hall, K. S. (1980). Social adjustment and psychological precipitants in mania. In *Mania: An Evolving Concept* (ed. R. H. Belmaker and H. M. van Praag), pp. 337–347. Spectrum Publications: Jamaica, NY.

Efron, B. (1988). Logistic regression, survival analysis, and the Kaplan–Meier Curve. *Journal of the American Statistical Association* **83**, 414–425.

Egeland, J. A. & Hostetter, A. M. (1983). Amish Study, I: Affective disorders among the Amish, 1976–1980. *American Journal of Psychiatry* **140**, 56–61.

El-Guebaly, N. (1975). Manic-depressive psychosis and drug abuse. *Canadian Psychiatric Association Journal* 20, 595–598.

Fogarty, F., Russell, J. M., Newman, S. C. & Bland, R. C. (1994). Mania. *Acta Psychiatrica Scandinavica* **376**, 16–23.

Goodwin, F. K. & Jamison, K. J. (1990). *Manic-Depressive Illness.* Oxford University Press: New York.

Hwu, H.-G., Yeh, E.-K. & Chang, L.-Y. (1989). Prevalence of psychiatric disorders in Taiwan defined by the Chinese Diagnostic Interview Schedule. *Acta Psychiatrica Scandinavica* **79**, 136–147.

Isometsä, E. T., Henriksson, M. M., Aro, H. M. & Lönnqvist, J. K. (1994). Suicide in bipolar disorder in Finland. *American Journal of Psychiatry* **151**, 1020–1024.

Kessler, R. C., McGonagle, K. A., Zhao, S., Nelson, C. B., Hughes, M., Eshleman, S., Wittchen, H.-U. & Kendler, K. S. (1994). Lifetime and 12-month prevalence of DSM-III-R psychiatric disorders in the United States: results from the National Comorbidity Survey. *Archives of General Psychiatry* **51**, 8–19.

Kessler, R. C., Little, R. J. A. & Groves, R. M. (1995*a*). Advances in strategies for minimizing and adjusting for survey nonresponse. *Epidemiologic Reviews* **17**, 192–204.

Kessler, R. C., Sonnega, A., Bromet, E., Hughes, M. & Nelson, C. B. (1995*b*). Posttraumatic stress disorder in the National Comorbidity Survey. *Archives of General Psychiatry* **52**, 1048–1060.

Kessler, R. C., Mroczek, D. K. & Belli R. F. (1997). Retrospective adult assessment of childhood psychopathology. In *Assessment in Child and Adolescent Psychopathology* (ed. D. Shaffer and J. Richters) Guilford Press: New York, NY. (In the press.)

Kish L. & Frankel M. R. (1974). Inferences from complex samples. *Journal of the Royal Statistical Society, Series B*, **36**, 1–37.

Krauthammer, C. & Klerman, G. L. (1979). The epidemiology of mania. *In Manic Illness* (ed. B. Shopsin), pp. 11–28. Raven Press: New York.

Kutcher, S. P., Marton, P. & Korenblum, M. (1989). Relationship between psychiatric illness and conduct disorder in adolescents. *Canadian Journal of Psychiatry* **34**, 526–529.

Lee, C. K., Kwak, Y. S., Yamamoto, J., Rhee, H., Kim, Y. S., Han, J. H., Choi, J. O. & Lee, Y. H. (1990*a*). Psychiatric epidemiology in Korea; Part I: Gender and age differences in Seoul. *Journal of Nervous and Mental Disease* **178**, 242–246.

Lee, C. K., Kwak, Y. S., Yamamoto, J., Rhee, H., Kim, Y. S., Han, J. H., Choi, J. O. & Lee, Y. H. (1990*b*). Psychiatric epidemiology in Korea; Part II: Urban and rural differences. *Journal of Nervous and Mental Disease* **178**, 247–252.

Murphy, J. M. (1980). Continuities in community-based psychiatric epidemiology. *Archives of General Psychiatry* **37**, 1215–1223.

Post, R. M., Rubinow, D. R., Uhre, T. W., Roy-Byrne, P. P., Linnoila, M., Rosoff, A. & Cowdry, R. (1989). Dysphoric mania: clinical and biological correlates. *Archives of General Psychiatry* **46**, 353–358.

Post, R. M., Rubinow, D. R. & Ballenger, J. C. (1986). Conditioning and sensitization in the longitudinal course of affective illness. *British Journal of Psychiatry* **149**, 191–201.

Regier, D. A., Farmer, M. E., Rae, D. S., Locke, B. Z., Kieth, S. J., Judd, L. L. & Goodwin, F. K. (1990). Comorbidity of mental disorders with alcohol and other drug abuse: results from the Epidemiologic Catchment Area (ECA) study. *Journal of the American Medical Association* **265**, 2511–2518.

Robins, L. N., Locke, B. Z. & Regier, D. A. (1991). An overview of psychiatric disorders in America. In *Psychiatric Disorders in America: the Epidemiologic Catchment Area Study* (ed. L. N. Robins and D. A. Regier), pp. 328–366. Free Press: New York.

Roth, M. (1981). Problems in the classification of affective disorders. *Acta Psychiatrica Scandinavica* **290**, 42–57.

Roy-Byrne, P., Post, R. M., Uhde, T. W., Porcu, T. & Davis, D. (1985). The longitudinal course of recurrent affective illness: life chart data from research patients at the NIMH. *Acta Psychiatrica Scandinavica* **71**, 5–34.

Rust, K. (1985). Variance estimation for complex estimators in sample surveys. *Journal of Official Statistics* **1**, 382–397.

SAS Institute. (1989). *SAS/STAT User's Guide, Version 6, Fourth Edition, Volume 2.* SAS Institute: Cary, NC.

Shah, B. V., Barnwell, B. G., Hunt, P. N. & LaVange, L. M. (1991). *SUDAAN User's Manual, Release 5.50.* Research Triangle Institute: Research Triangle Park, NC.

Sharma, R. & Markar, H. R. (1994). Mortality in affective disorder. *Journal of Affective Disorders* **31**, 91–96.

Smith, A. L. & Weissman, M. M. (1992). Epidemiology. In *Handbook of Affective Disorders, 2nd Edition* (ed. E. S. Paykel), pp. 111–129. Guilford Press: New York.

Spitzer, R. L., Williams, J. B. W., Gibbons, M. & First, M. B. (1990). The Structured Clinical Interview for DSM-III-R, I. History, rationale and description. *Archives of General Psychiatry* **49**, 624–629.

Taylor, M. A. & Abrams, R. (1981). Gender differences in bipolar affective disorder. *Journal of Affective Disorders* **3**, 261–277.

Tsuang, M. T., Woolson, R. F. & Fleming, J. A. (1980). Premature deaths in schizophrenia and affective disorders: an analysis of survival curves and variables affecting a shortened survival. *Archives of General Psychiatry* **37**, 979–983.

Van Valkenburg, C. H., Akiskal, H. S., Puzantian, V. & Rosenthal, T. (1984). Anxious depression – clinical family history and naturalistic outcome – comparisons with panic and major depressive disorders. *Journal of Affective Disorders* **6**, 67–82.

Weeke, A. & Vaeth, M. (1986). Excess mortality of bipolar and unipolar manic-depressive patients. *Journal of Affective Disorders* **11**, 227–234.

Weissman, M. M. & Myers, J. K. (1978). Affective disorders in a US urban community. *Archives of General Psychiatry* **35**, 1304–1311.

Weissman, M. M., Livingston, B. M., Leaf, P. J., Florio, L. P. & Holzer, C. III. (1991). Affective disorders. In *Psychiatric Disorders in America: The Epidemiologic Catchment Area Study* (ed. L. N. Robins and D. A. Regier), pp. 53–80. The Free Press: New York.

Weller, M. P. I., Ang, P. C., Latimer-Sayer, D. T. & Zachary, A. (1988). Drug abuse and mental illness. *Lancet* i, 997.

Wells, J. E., Bushnell, J. A., Hornblow, A. R., Joyce, P. R., & Oakley-Brown, M. A. (1989). Christchurch Psychiatric Epidemiology Study, Part I: Methodology and lifetime prevalence for specific psychiatric disorders. *Australian and New Zealand Journal of Psychiatry* **23**, 315–326.

Welner, A., Marten, S., Wochnick, E., Davis, M. A., Fishman, R. & Clayton, P. J. (1979). Psychiatric disorders among professional women. *Archives of General Psychiatry* **36**, 169–173.

Winokur, G., Clayton, C. J. & Reich, T. (1969). *Manic Depressive Illness.* C. V. Mosby Company: St. Louis.

Wittchen, H.-U. (1994). Reliability and validity studies of the WHO-Composite International Diagnostic Interview (CIDI): a critical review. *Journal of Psychiatric Research* **28**, 57–84.

Wittchen, H.-U., Essau, C. A., von Zerrsen, D., Krieg, J.-C. & Zaudig, M. (1992). Lifetime and six-month prevalence of mental disorders in the Munich follow-up study. *European Archives of Psychiatry and Clinical Neuroscience* **241**, 247–258.

Wolf, A. W., Schubert, D. S. P., Patterson, M. B., Grande, T. P., Brocco, K. J. & Pendleton, L. (1988). Associations among major psychiatric diagnoses. *Journal of Consulting and Clinical Psychology* **56**, 292–294.

Woodruff, R. A. Jr., Guze, S. B. & Clayton, P. J. (1971). Unipolar and bipolar primary affective disorder. *British Journal of Psychiatry* **119**, 33–38.

Woodruff, R. S. & Causey, B. D. (1976). Computerized method for approximating the variance of a complicated estimate. *Journal of the American Statistical Association* **71**, 315–321.

World Health Organization. (1990*a*). *Composite International Diagnostic Interview. (CIDI, Version 1.0).* World Health Organization: Geneva, Switzerland.

World Health Organization. (1990*b*). *International Classification of Diseases – Classification of Mental and Behavioural Disorders: Diagnostic Criteria for Research.* World Health Organization: Geneva, Switzerland.

Excess Mortality in Bipolar and Unipolar Disorder in Sweden

Urban Ösby, MD, PhD; Lena Brandt, BSc; Nestor Correia, PhD; Anders Ekbom, MD, PhD; Pär Sparén, PhD

Background: Selected groups of patients with bipolar and unipolar disorder have an increased mortality rate from suicide and natural causes of death. However, there has been no population-based study of mortality of patients followed up from the onset of the illness.

Methods: All patients with a hospital diagnosis of bipolar (n=15386) or unipolar (n=39182) disorder in Sweden from 1973 to 1995 were identified from the inpatient register and linked with the national cause-of-death register to determine the date and cause of death. Overall and cause-specific standardized mortality ratios (SMRs) and numbers of excess deaths were calculated by 5-year age classes and 5-year calendar periods.

Results: The SMRs for suicide were 15.0 for males and 22.4 for females with bipolar disorder, and 20.9 and 27.0, respectively, for unipolar disorder. For all natural causes of death, SMRs were 1.9 for males and 2.1 for females with bipolar disorder, and 1.5 and 1.6, respectively, for unipolar disorder. For bipolar disorder, most excess deaths were from natural causes, whereas for unipolar disorder, most excess deaths were from unnatural causes. The SMR for suicide was especially high for younger patients during the first years after the first diagnosis. Increasing SMR for suicide during the period of study was found for female patients with unipolar disorder.

Conclusions: This population-based study of patients treated in the hospital documented increased SMRs for suicide in patients with bipolar and unipolar disorder. The SMR for all natural causes of death was also increased, causing about half the excess deaths.

Arch Gen Psychiatry. 2001;58:844-850

INCREASED mortality is one of the major adverse effects in individuals with mood disorders. In bipolar disorder, many studies found a mortality rate approximately 2 times[1-8] and a suicide mortality rate approximately 10 times that of the general population, with suicide being the leading single cause of excess mortality. In major depression, several studies found an increased total mortality,[8-16] with a suicide mortality about 20 times that of the general population.

To obtain accurate risk estimates of the increased mortality among patients with bipolar and unipolar disorder, large cohorts are needed to identify small differences in mortality ratios for natural causes of death, which nevertheless may represent large numbers of excess deaths. Patients need to be followed up from their first diagnosis, since suicide mortality is especially likely to be higher in the first phases of the illness and also among younger patients. Cohorts should be population based to enable inferences to be made from the findings to large patient groups.

The aim of the present study was to assess mortality, compared with the general population, in 2 large cohorts comprising all patients in Sweden with an inpatient diagnosis of bipolar or unipolar disorder. Patients were identified from the national patient register during 1973 through 1995, and followed up from the first psychiatric hospital diagnosis. Suicide and other unnatural causes of death were analyzed as well as cardiovascular death and other specific natural causes. Standardized mortality ratios (SMRs) and the numbers of excess deaths were calculated, and the effects of sex, age at first diagnosis, and duration of follow-up were assessed.

RESULTS

A total of 6578 males and 8808 females in Sweden with a bipolar disorder diagnosis during 1973 to 1995 were included in the study (**Table 1**). For unipolar disorder,

From the Departments of Clinical Neuroscience (Dr Ösby and Ms Brandt) and Medical Epidemiology (Drs Ösby, Correia, Ekbom, and Sparén, and Ms Brandt), Karolinska Institutet, Stockholm, Sweden.

SUBJECTS AND METHODS

SUBJECTS

The Swedish psychiatric inpatient register starts in 1971 and covers all inpatient treatments since 1973. For each hospitalization, the unique national registration number, date of admission and discharge, and diagnosis are registered. No private inpatient facilities exist in Sweden, so the psychiatric inpatient register is therefore population based. The diagnoses were recorded according to the *International Classification of Diseases, Eighth Revision (ICD-8)*, from 1971 to 1986, and according to the *International Classification of Diseases, Ninth Revision (ICD-9)*, from 1987 to 1995. All diagnoses in the register are made by a consultant in psychiatry at the time of the patient's discharge from the hospital. Several diagnoses can be recorded at each admission, but only the first (main) diagnosis was used in this study. To exclude readmitted cases, admissions in the inpatient register were observed until the end of 1972, and all individuals with a relevant diagnosis before 1973 were excluded. An upper age limit at the first diagnosis was set at 70 years. All patients with a first diagnosis of bipolar disorder or unipolar disorder from January 1, 1973, to December 31, 1995, were identified in the psychiatric inpatient register. Bipolar disorder was assessed from *ICD-8* as manic-depressive psychosis manic type (296.10), manic-depressive psychosis circular type (296.30), and reactive excitative psychosis (298.10), and from *ICD-9* as unipolar affective psychosis manic form (296 A), bipolar affective psychosis manic phase (296 C), bipolar affective psychosis mixed form (296 E), and reactive excitative psychosis (298 B). Unipolar disorder was defined from *ICD-8* as melancholic involution psychosis (296.00), manic-depressive psychosis depressive type (296.20), manic-depressive psychosis alia definita (296.88), manic-depressive psychosis not otherwise specified (296.99), and reactive depressive psychosis (298.00), and from *ICD-9* as unipolar affective psychosis melancholic form (296 B), bipolar affective psychosis melancholic phase (296 D), unspecified affective psychosis (296 X), and reactive depressive psychosis (298 A).

DEATH REGISTRY

All patients were linked to the national cause-of-death register to determine the date and cause of death, using the national registration number. The cause-of-death register is based on the death certificates. Deaths are classified according to the *ICD* codes, and on each certificate there is one underlying cause of death and a possibility to add contributing causes. For patients who die in the hospital, the death certificate is made by the consultant in charge, and for deaths out of the hospital, the physician in charge of the patient certifies the cause of death. When the cause of death is unclear, an autopsy is performed. In undetermined deaths, there is always a forensic autopsy. If an autopsy is performed, the death certificate is considered preliminary until the information from the autopsy is also included. During 1973-1995, the autopsy frequency for natural causes of death was 86% in persons aged 15 to 49 years, 68% in persons aged 50 to 69 years, and 45% in persons 70 years and older. For unnatural causes of death, the autopsy frequency was 90% in persons aged 15 to 49 years, 88% in persons aged 50 to 69 years, and 53% in persons aged 70 years and older. The cause-of-death register covers more than 99% of all deaths occurring in Sweden (Statistics Sweden [federal agency for national statistics], 1998).

DATA ANALYSES

We calculated person-years of follow-up by sex, 5-year age class, and 5-year calendar period, from the date of admission for a first hospitalization with an eventual bipolar or unipolar disorder diagnosis, occurring from January 1, 1973, until December 31, 1995, or a possible death before this date. Thus, inpatient periods from the first and later admissions were included in the person-years count, and deaths could occur both in and out of the hospital. A bipolar diagnosis was considered more severe than a unipolar diagnosis. Patients with an initial unipolar diagnosis who were discharged later with a bipolar diagnosis were, from the date of admission for a hospitalization with a bipolar diagnosis, excluded from the unipolar group and included among the bipolar patients. Mortality rates for the Swedish population from 1973 through 1995 retrieved from the cause-of-death register (Statistics Sweden, 1998) were used to estimate the expected number of deaths by 5-year age class and 5-year calendar periods. The SMRs were calculated as the observed number of deaths divided by the expected number of deaths, with 95% confidence intervals.[17] We calculated the SMRs for each *ICD* class causes of death and for natural (*ICD* classes I-XVI) and unnatural (*ICD* class XVII; suicide, accidents, homicide, undetermined) causes, in males and females separately. The number of excess deaths for natural and unnatural causes was calculated by subtracting the expected number of deaths from the observed number of deaths.

The SMRs by age at admission and time of follow-up were calculated using Poisson regression models,[18] controlling for calendar time of the first admission. Age at admission and calendar time were divided into 5-year intervals, except for the first calendar interval, which was 3 years. The SMR for suicide was calculated according to age at admission in the following age groups: younger than 30 years, 30 to 44 years, 45 to 64 years, and 65 years and older; time of follow-up was divided into less than 1 year, 1 to 3 years, more than 3 years to 5 years, and more than 5 years. The relative risks for different methods of suicide among patients with bipolar and unipolar disorder compared with methods of suicide in the general population in 1973 to 1995 were calculated. Time trends in suicide mortality for the first 3 years of follow-up were calculated according to 5-year calendar intervals from 1976 to 1995, for bipolar and unipolar disorder groups.

a total of 15829 males and 23353 females were included. The number of deaths for patients with a bipolar disorder was 1716 for males and 1747 for females, while there were 4119 male and 4902 female deaths among patients with unipolar disorder. There was an overlap between the 2 diagnostic groups; 3109 individuals (20% of the patients with bipolar disorder) were initially discharged with a unipolar diagnosis. The mean follow-up was about 10 years, irrespective of sex or psychiatric diagnosis (Table 1).

The most frequent cause of death was cardiovascular disease, followed by suicide and cancer in both bipo-

Table 1. Number of Cases, Person-years, Age at First Admission, Follow-up, and Number of Deaths for Patients With Bipolar or Unipolar Disorder Diagnosis in Sweden, 1973-1995

	Bipolar Disorder		Unipolar Disorder	
	Males	Females	Males	Females
No. of cases	6578	8808	15 829	23 353
No. of person-years	69 222	101 393	148 372	249 366
Age at first admission, mean (SD), y	42.5 (14.4)	43.5 (14.3)	46.2 (14.2)	47.6 (14.4)
Time of follow-up, mean (SD), y	10.52 (6.69)	11.51 (6.73)	9.37 (6.58)	10.68 (6.65)
No. of deaths	1716	1747	4119	4902

Table 2. Standardized Mortality Ratios for Patients With Bipolar or Unipolar Disorder Diagnosis in Sweden, 1973-1995*

		Males			Females		
Cause of Death	*ICD* Class	Obs	Exp	SMR (95% CI)	Obs	Exp	SMR (95% CI)
Bipolar Disorder							
Infectious	I	14	4.08	3.4 (1.9-5.8)	12	5.06	2.4 (1.2-4.1)
Cancer	II	193	176.90	1.1 (0.9-1.3)	282	233.84	1.2 (1.1-1.4)
Endocrine	III	41	12.66	3.2 (2.3-4.4)	40	14.09	2.8 (2.0-3.9)
Mental†	V	50	13.37	3.7 (2.8-4.9)	51	10.66	4.8 (3.6-6.3)
Nervous system	VI	15	9.23	1.6 (0.9-2.7)	26	11.16	2.3 (1.5-3.4)
Cardiovascular	VII	550	283.98	1.9 (1.8-2.1)	523	197.51	2.6 (2.4-2.9)
Cerebrovascular	VII	92	47.92	1.9 (1.5-2.4)	127	63.08	2.0 (1.7-2.4)
Respiratory	VIII	111	35.75	3.1 (2.6-3.7)	113	34.99	3.2 (2.7-3.9)
Gastrointestinal	IX	50	25.12	2.0 (1.5-2.6)	40	21.55	1.9 (1.3-2.5)
Urogenital	X	23	6.26	3.7 (2.3-5.5)	29	6.70	4.3 (2.9-6.2)
Accidents	XVII	93	28.56	3.3 (2.6-4.0)	63	15.88	4.0 (3.0-5.1)
Traffic accidents	XVII	30	6.81	4.4 (3.0-6.3)	14	4.40	3.2 (1.7-5.3)
Suicide	XVII	345	22.93	15.0 (13.5-16.7)	327	14.62	22.4 (20.0-24.9)
Homicide	XVII	6	1.21	5.0 (1.8-10.8)	2	0.87	2.3 (0.3-8.3)
Undetermined‡	XVII	87	8.46	10.3 (8.2-12.7)	75	5.28	14.2 (11.2-17.8)
Natural causes	I-XVI	1185	624.05	1.9 (1.8-2.0)	1280	611.53	2.1 (2.0-2.2)
Unnatural causes§	XVII	531	61.42	8.6 (7.9-9.4)	467	36.76	12.7 (11.6-13.9)
All Causes		**1716**	685.47	2.5 (2.4-2.6)	**1747**	648.28	2.7 (2.6-2.8)
Unipolar Disorder							
Infectious	I	30	12.13	2.5 (1.7-3.5)	38	18.89	2.0 (1.4-2.8)
Cancer	II	547	520.19	1.1 (1.0-1.1)	830	781.97	1.1 (1.0-1.1)
Endocrine	III	61	35.6	1.7 (1.3-2.2)	81	52.3	1.5 (1.2-1.9)
Mental†	V	83	35.19	2.4 (1.9-2.9)	134	44.11	3.0 (2.5-3.6)
Nervous system	VI	49	25.24	1.9 (1.4-2.6)	65	37.05	1.8 (1.4-2.2)
Cardiovascular	VII	1319	871.32	1.5 (1.4-1.6)	1428	819.98	1.7 (1.7-1.8)
Cerebrovascular	VII	230	152.1	1.5 (1.3-1.7)	424	261.45	1.6 (1.5-1.8)
Respiratory	VIII	243	115.3	2.1 (1.9-2.4)	342	141.1	2.4 (2.2-2.7)
Gastrointestinal	IX	96	69.36	1.4 (1.1-1.7)	148	77.85	1.9 (1.6-2.2)
Urogenital	X	39	20.77	1.9 (1.3-2.6)	45	26.99	1.7 (1.2-2.2)
Accidents	XVII	164	68.45	2.4 (2.0-2.8)	135	52.34	2.6 (2.2-3.1)
Traffic accidents	XVII	46	20.07	2.3 (1.7-3.1)	28	15.78	1.8 (1.2-2.6)
Suicide	XVII	1052	50.27	20.9 (19.7-22.2)	993	36.81	27.0 (25.3-28.7)
Homicide	XVII	7	2.90	2.4 (1.0-5.0)	3	2.17	1.4 (0.3-4.0)
Undetermined‡	XVII	149	18	8.3 (7.0-9.7)	156	13.13	11.9 (10.1-13.9)
Natural causes	I-XVI	2747	1881.97	1.5 (1.4-1.5)	3615	2310.01	1.6 (1.5-1.6)
Unnatural causes§	XVII	1372	139.67	9.8 (9.3-10.4)	1287	104.46	12.3 (11.7-13.0)
All Causes		**4119**	2021.64	2.0 (2.0-2.1)	**4902**	2414.47	2.0 (2.0-2.1)

*Standardized mortality ratio (SMR) is calculated by dividing the observed number of deaths (Obs) by the expected number of deaths (Exp). *ICD* indicates *International Classification of Diseases*; CI, confidence interval.

†Mental causes of death for bipolar disorder are dementia (n = 14), psychosis (n = 37), depression (n = 3), alcohol addiction/abuse (n = 40), drug addiction (n = 5), and developmental disorder (n = 2). Mental causes of death for unipolar disorder are dementia (n = 91), psychosis (n = 39), depression (n = 14), alcohol addiction/abuse (n = 61), drug addiction/abuse (n = 9), anorexia nervosa (n = 2), and developmental disorder (n = 1). When the main cause of death is psychosis or depression, there is also an additional somatic cause.

‡Undetermined deaths are unnatural (violent) deaths not classified by a specific cause.

§Unnatural causes of death are accidents, suicide, homicide, and undetermined.

lar and unipolar disorder groups (**Table 2**). For bipolar disorder, the SMRs for all deaths were 2.5 in males and 2.7 in females. All natural causes of death (*ICD* I-XVI) were increased, except cancer and diseases of the nervous system for males. For unipolar disorder, SMRs for all deaths were 2.0 for both sexes. All natural causes

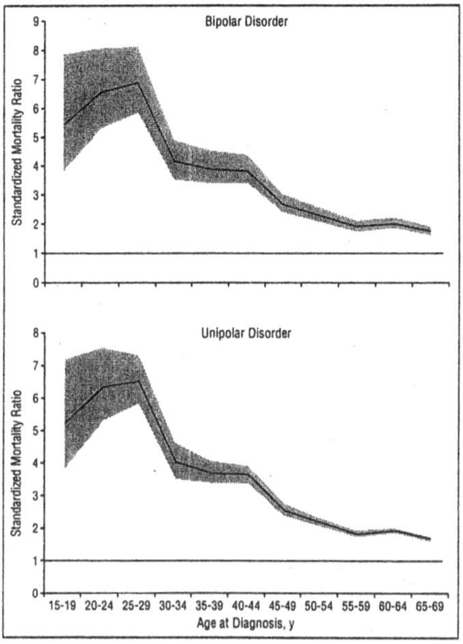

Figure 1. Standardized mortality ratios by age at first admission for patients with bipolar or unipolar disorder in Sweden during 1973 through 1995, controlling for sex, age at admission, and calendar period. Shaded area represents 95% confidence interval.

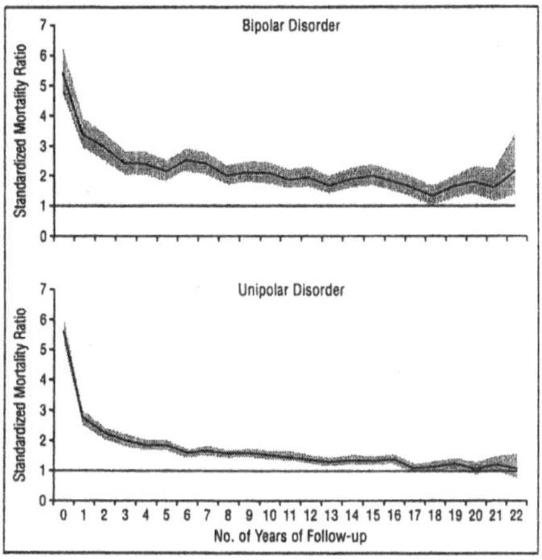

Figure 2. Standardized mortality ratios by time of follow-up for patients with bipolar or unipolar disorder in Sweden during 1973 through 1995, controlling for sex, age at admission, and calendar period. Shaded area represents 95% confidence interval.

of death except cancer were significantly increased. In patients with bipolar disorder, SMRs for death from unnatural causes were highest for suicide (15.0 in males and 22.4 in females) and undetermined violent death (10.3 in males and 14.2 in females). The SMRs for suicide were higher in the unipolar group compared with the bipolar group, while they tended to be lower for deaths due to undetermined violence. There were 2130 excess deaths in patients with bipolar disorder and 4585 in those with unipolar disorder. In the bipolar disorder group, there were more excess deaths from natural than from unnatural causes, both for males (ratio: 561/470 = 1.19) and for females (ratio: 668/430 = 1.55), while in the unipolar disorder group, the number of excess deaths was higher from natural causes for females only (ratio: 1305/1183 = 1.10), but not for males (ratio: 865/1232 = 0.70) (data not shown).

For both bipolar and unipolar disorder, the SMR for all deaths was highest in patients with their first admission at younger ages (**Figure 1**). The SMR decreased with increasing age but was still significantly increased for patients with a first diagnosis at 65 to 69 years of age. An increased SMR was also most pronounced during the first years of follow-up after the first diagnosis, with a significant increase still observed after 15 years of follow-up (**Figure 2**). There were no sex differences in risk ratios by age at first admission or time of follow-up.

The SMRs for suicide were elevated for both bipolar and unipolar disorder in all age classes and follow-up intervals (**Table 3**). In the bipolar disorder group, SMRs for the younger-than-30-year age class in the first year of follow-up were 81.6 for males and 71.7 for females, and SMRs were still 4.7 for males and 13.4 for females in the 65- years-and-older age class with more than 5 years of follow-up. In all age groups, SMR decreased with increasing time of follow-up. An interaction between age and duration of follow-up was observed; the younger the age and shorter the follow-up, the higher the SMR. However, formal tests for multiplicative interaction effects did not render significant results.

Compared with the general population, jumping as a method of suicide was more common in patients with bipolar disorder, whereas shooting was less common for male patients and poisoning less common for female patients (**Table 4**). Hanging and drowning were more common as methods of suicide for male patients with unipolar disorder than in the general population, while shooting was less common. Poisoning was less common in both male and female patients with unipolar disorder.

An increasing time trend in suicide mortality during the first 3 years of follow-up was found for females with unipolar disorder ($P<.001$), but not for males or for those with bipolar disorder (**Table 5**).

COMMENT

The main finding of this study was an increased suicide mortality rate in patients with bipolar and unipolar disorder, which was most pronounced at younger ages and in the first years after the initial diagnosis. In patients with unipolar disorder, suicide mortality for female patients even increased during the study period. The number of excess deaths from natural causes was very high, indi-

Table 3. Standardized Mortality Ratios (SMRs) for Suicide by Age at First Admission and Duration of Follow-up for Patients With Bipolar or Unipolar Disorder Diagnosis in Sweden, 1973-1995

Follow-up, y	No. of Deaths	SMR (95% Confidence Interval)			
		<30 y	30-44 y	45-64 y	≥65 y
Bipolar Males (Interaction $P = .39$)					
<1	96	59.4 (38.7-91.0)	43.5 (30.2-62.6)	44.7 (32.9-60.7)	31.9 (13.3-76.7)
1-3	72	18.3 (10.6-31.6)	21.6 (14.8-31.5)	16.7 (11.5-24.4)	18.3 (7.6-44.0)
>3-5	43	13.2 (6.9-25.4)	15.5 (9.8-24.6)	10.2 (6.1-17.3)	9.0 (2.2-35.9)
>5	134	15.4 (11.7-20.4)	10.7 (8.1-14.0)	6.2 (4.4-8.9)	3.2 (0.8-12.9)
Bipolar Females (Interaction $P = .46$)					
<1	71	43.4 (20.7-91.1)	62.5 (41.5-94.0)	56.7 (40.5-79.4)	65.5 (31.2-137.4)
1-3	75	39.3 (22.8-67.7)	29.5 (19.2-45.2)	31.6 (22.6-44.3)	37.2 (17.7-78.1)
>3-5	37	27.4 (14.3-52.7)	16.3 (9.0-29.4)	16.8 (10.3-27.5)	6.2 (0.9-43.8)
>5	144	25.6 (19.1-34.3)	15.7 (11.9-20.7)	12.1 (9.0-16.4)	12.5 (5.6-27.8)
Unipolar Males (Interaction $P = .76$)					
<1	425	84.1 (63.7-110.9)	84.1 (70.1-101.0)	81.8 (71.4-93.8)	92.6 (71-121.0)
1-3	240	26.7 (18.8-38)	23.3 (18.0-30.1)	28.8 (24.1-34.3)	26.6 (18.2-38.8)
>3-5	117	20.4 (13.4-30.9)	13.4 (9.3-19.1)	13.8 (10.5-18.3)	17.7 (10.7-29.4)
>5	270	11.1 (8.4-14.6)	9.9 (8.0-12.2)	8.9 (7.4-10.7)	8.5 (5.5-13.0)
Unipolar Females (Interaction $P<.09$)					
<1	368	177.3 (134.8-233.3)	131.2 (108.8-158.4)	102.5 (88.5-118.8)	57.9 (40.5-82.9)
1-3	210	52.5 (36.7-75.2)	30.1 (22.6-40.0)	35.0 (29.0-42.2)	27.2 (18.4-40.3)
>3-5	115	19.8 (11.0-35.8)	27.6 (20.2-37.6)	20.8 (16.1-27.0)	8.9 (4.2-18.7)
>5	300	18.2 (13.7-24.2)	13.7 (11.1-17.0)	13.1 (11.1-15.5)	12.0 (8.4-17.1)

Table 4. Relative Risks for Different Methods of Suicide for Patients With Bipolar or Unipolar Disorder Diagnosis in Sweden, 1973-1995*

Method of Suicide	Males			Females		
	Obs	SMR	RR (95% CI)	Obs	SMR	RR (95% CI)
Bipolar Disorder						
Poisoning	95	13.4	0.9 (0.7-1.1)	105	15.8	0.7 (0.6-0.8)
Hanging	124	15.4	1.0 (0.9-1.2)	84	24.6	1.1 (0.9-1.4)
Drowning	20	17.1	1.1 (0.7-1.8)	54	23.6	1.0 (0.8-1.4)
Shooting	31	7.8	0.5 (0.4-0.7)	4	28.6	1.3 (0.5-3.4)
Cutting	13	18.8	1.2 (0.7-2.2)	5	19.2	0.8 (0.4-2.0)
Jumping	39	44.3	2.9 (2.2-4.0)	53	58.2	2.6 (2.0-3.4)
Other	23	21.3	1.4 (0.9-2.1)	22	23.7	1.0 (0.7-1.6)
Late effects	0	...	...	0	...	...
Total	**345**	15.0	1.0 (Reference)	**327**	22.4	1.0 (Reference)
Unipolar Disorder						
Poisoning	234	16.0	0.8 (0.7-0.9)	348	21.7	0.8 (0.7-0.9)
Hanging	484	26.7	1.3 (1.2-1.4)	267	31.0	1.2 (1.0-1.3)
Drowning	92	32.9	1.6 (1.3-1.9)	189	28.9	1.1 (0.9-1.2)
Shooting	90	10.0	0.5 (0.4-0.6)	16	53.3	2.0 (1.2-3.2)
Cutting	41	26.6	1.3 (0.9-1.7)	18	27.3	1.0 (0.6-1.6)
Jumping	49	25.1	1.2 (0.9-1.6)	65	27.3	1.0 (0.8-1.3)
Other	62	27.7	1.3 (1.0-1.7)	88	40.6	1.5 (1.2-1.8)
Late effects	0	...	...	2	40.0	1.6 (0.4-6.2)
Total	**1052**	20.9	1.0 (Reference)	**993**	27.0	1.0 (Reference)

*Obs indicates observed number of deaths; SMR, standardized mortality ratio; RR, relative risk; CI, confidence interval; and ellipses, not applicable.

cating the somatic health of the patients as an important area for improved treatment besides suicide prevention.

Validation of the clinical diagnosis is a problem with register-based studies. The diagnostic system changed in Sweden from *ICD-8* to *ICD-9* in 1987, with accompanying changes in the diagnostic criteria for bipolar and unipolar disorders. It is likely that the patients with bipolar disorder in this study had a history of manic states, since those diagnostic subclassifications were used to define the bipolar group. The psychotic depressive subclassifications used to define the unipolar group may also include some patients with bipolar disorder only diagnosed in a depressive state. Thus, the bipolar group is more strictly defined than the unipolar group.[8] Of the bipolar patients in our study, 20% had a previous diagnosis of unipolar disorder. This may lead to an underesti-

Table 5. Time Trends for Suicide During the First 3 Years of Follow-up for Patients With Bipolar or Unipolar Disorder Diagnosis in Sweden, 1976-1995*

Years	Males			Females		
	Obs	Exp	Relative SMR (95% CI)	Obs	Exp	Relative SMR (95% CI)
			Bipolar Disorder			
1976-1980	115	7.59	1 (Reference)	108	4.86	1 (Reference)
1981-1985	71	4.60	0.92 (0.69-1.24)	68	2.76	1.02 (0.75-1.38)
1986-1990	53	2.63	0.99 (0.71-1.38)	58	1.57	1.28 (0.92-1.78)
1991-1995	24	0.75	1.03 (0.65-1.63)	15	0.41	0.86 (0.49-1.51)
Test for trend		$P = .99$			$P = .57$	
			Unipolar Disorder			
1976-1980	274	15.57	1 (Reference)	281	12.12	1 (Reference)
1981-1985	263	11.72	1.12 (0.94-1.33)	221	8.13	1.04 (0.87-1.24)
1986-1990	209	6.74	1.22 (1.01-1.47)	196	4.27	1.38 (1.14-1.67)
1991-1995	103	2.06	1.14 (0.90-1.45)	93	1.17	1.42 (1.11-1.81)
Test for trend		$P = .07$			$P < .001$	

*Obs indicates observed number of deaths; Exp, expected number of deaths; SMR, standardized mortality ratio; and CI, confidence interval.

mation of suicide mortality for bipolar disorder, since some patients with bipolar disorder who were initially classified as having unipolar disorder will die before they get the correct diagnosis. No validation has been made in Sweden of the clinical affective psychosis diagnoses, but a validation based on medical records of clinical schizophrenia diagnosis in Stockholm County, comprising approximately 20% of the Swedish population, estimated that 80% to 85% of patients with clinical schizophrenia diagnosis met *DSM-III* criteria for schizophrenia.[19] Another problem with this study is that only patients with a hospital admission are included, which leads to a selection of severely ill patients, especially in unipolar disorder, where patients with the less severe forms are expected to have been in outpatient treatment only. Thus, the mortality ratios found in this study for unipolar disorder may be exaggerated by a selection of more severely ill patients, who may have higher mortality rates than patients with unipolar disorder in general.

In the patients with bipolar disorder, suicide mortality was lower and mortality from natural causes was higher than in the patients with unipolar disorder, which is in line with earlier findings.[5,8] When suicide mortality in our bipolar group was compared with the aggregate mortality ratios of a meta-analysis of mortality studies in psychiatric disorders,[20] our rates were several times higher (male-female: 15.05/22.37 vs 5.71/5.88). Only one previous study of mortality in mood disorder has used national population-based patient data, followed up from the first diagnosis,[8] and the reported suicide mortality from that study was in accordance with our findings. Since mortality in suicide is particularly increased in the first years after the first admission and will tend to decline with time of follow-up, first-episode cohort studies provide better estimates of the excess suicide mortality than studies based on cases identified later during the course of the illness. Suicide mortality in our patients with unipolar disorder, however, was not different from that reported in the meta-analysis (male-female: 20.93/26.98 vs 15.73/27.81). The increased mortality rate in undetermined death in both bipolar and unipolar disorder groups is to a large extent likely to be due to suicides.[21,22] In our study, an increase in SMR in suicide during the period of study was apparent among female patients with unipolar disorder. There are other previous findings of increasing time trends in suicide mortality in mood disorders[8] and also in schizophrenia.[23,24] In the Swedish population, suicide as a cause of death has decreased during the past decades, hypothesized to be an effect of increased use of antidepressant drugs.[25] The finding of increasing SMR for suicide indicates that the outcome among patients with unipolar disorder has not improved, although a selection of more severely ill patients with higher suicide risks as inpatients over time cannot be excluded. The proportion of violent methods of suicide such as jumping (bipolar disorder) and hanging and drowning (unipolar disorder) were higher, while the use of poisoning was lower in patients with unipolar disorder. Shooting as a method of suicide was lower for male patients with bipolar and unipolar disorder, which may reflect a reduced access to guns, possibly indicating that the efforts of society and the psychiatric services to reduce access to guns have been successful. A similar result was found for patients with schizophrenia.[26]

There are several studies suggesting that patients with bipolar disorder selected for and compliant with long-term treatment at specialized lithium clinics have lower-than-expected mortality from suicide.[27-32] Unfortunately, there is no information about treatment in the patient registry. However, before such programs are initiated for all patients, one should keep in mind that patients in special lithium programs constitute a selected group, who are probably more compliant compared with other patients with such disorders. Thus, more studies are needed in population-based samples to assess the impact of such measures on the risk of suicide.

Considering natural causes of death, the increased mortality for cardiovascular and respiratory disease found in both bipolar and unipolar disorder patients is in accordance with the findings of other studies.[7,20,33] One possible explanation is higher smoking rates among this population, which also may be the explanation for the increased mortality due to cerebrovascular disease. However, there are also studies that did not find an increased mortality rate from cardiovascular disease,[12] notably studies of patients receiving long-term lithium treatment. Whether this difference is an effect of the specific treatment or the selection of patients is not yet clear. In unipolar disorder, there are findings of an increased risk for coronary heart disease in both men and women.[34-36] Depression must be considered as a risk factor for coronary heart disease, although the mechanism is not known. It may be a direct effect on heart rate or increasing platelet aggregation, or an indirect effect by poor self-care or social isolation.

The number of excess deaths, rather than increased relative mortality, should be the target for preventive programs, since prevention should focus on the number of saved lives. In bipolar disorder, the total number of excess deaths was slightly higher for natural than for unnatural causes of death, while in unipolar disorder the total number of excess deaths was larger for unnatural causes. Suicide was the specific cause of death that caused most excess deaths in both bipolar and unipolar disorder groups, but due to the higher prevalence of unipolar disorder there were approximately 3 times as many excess deaths from suicide in patients with unipolar disorder. Studies of suicide risks have found that the strongest risk factor is mental illness necessitating hospital admission.[37-39] Suicide prevention programs should target patients in the first years after the first diagnosis, but there is also a need for adequate somatic care and general health measures to be improved, especially in bipolar disorder.

In conclusion, this study found a markedly increased mortality rate for patients with bipolar and unipolar disorder. Future studies should focus on the effects of specific interventions such as lithium therapy and other specific treatments. Our results also underscore the need to continuously monitor mortality in those patient groups to improve treatment.

Accepted for publication April 19, 2001.

This study was supported by grant 1998 7289 from the Stockholm County Council.

The study was conducted within the Swedish Schizophrenia Sibling Pair study. We are also indebted to Lars Terenius, MD, PhD, Department of Clinical Neuroscience, Karolinska Institutet, Stockholm, for useful opinions and critical revisions of the manuscript.

Corresponding author and reprints: Urban Ösby, MD, PhD, Karolinska sjukhuset S4, S-171 76 Stockholm, Sweden (e-mail: Urban.Osby@nvso.sll.se).

REFERENCES

1. Astrup C, Fossum A, Holmboe R. A follow-up study of 270 patients with acute affective psychoses. *Acta Psychiatr Neurol Scand.* 1959;34:1-65.
2. Bratfos O, Haug JO. The course of manic-depressive psychosis: a follow up investigation of 215 patients. *Acta Psychiatr Scand.* 1968;44:89-112.
3. Petterson U. Manic-depressive illness: a clinical, social and genetic study. *Acta Psychiatr Scand Suppl.* 1977;269:1-93.
4. Tsuang MT, Woolson RF, Fleming JA. Premature deaths in schizophrenia and affective disorders: an analysis of survival curves and variables affecting the shortened survival. *Arch Gen Psychiatry.* 1980;37:979-983.
5. Weeke A, Vaeth M. Excess mortality of bipolar and unipolar manic-depressive patients. *J Affect Disord.* 1986;11:227-234.
6. Vestergaard P, Aagaard J. Five-year mortality in lithium-treated manic-depressive patients. *J Affect Disord.* 1991;21:33-38.
7. Sharma R, Markar HR. Mortality in affective disorder. *J Affect Disord.* 1994;31:91-96.
8. Høyer EH, Mortensen PB, Olesen AV. Mortality and causes of death in a total national sample of patients with affective disorders admitted for the first time between 1973 and 1993. *Br J Psychiatry.* 2000;176:76-82.
9. Tsuang MT, Woolson RF, Fleming JA. Causes of death in schizophrenia and manic-depression. *Br J Psychiatry.* 1980;136:239-242.
10. Coryell W. Diagnosis-specific mortality: primary unipolar depression and Briquet's syndrome (somatization disorder). *Arch Gen Psychiatry.* 1981;38:939-942.
11. Evans NJ, Whitlock FA. Mortality and late-onset affective disorder. *J Affect Disord.* 1983;5:297-304.
12. Berglund M, Nilsson K. Mortality in severe depression: a prospective study including 103 suicides. *Acta Psychiatr Scand.* 1987;76:372-380.
13. Lee AS, Murray RM. The long-term outcome of Maudsley depressives. *Br J Psychiatry.* 1988;153:741-751.
14. Buchholtz-Hansen PE, Wang AG, Kragh-Sorensen P, for the Danish University Antidepressant Group. Mortality in major affective disorder: relationship to subtype of depression. *Acta Psychiatr Scand.* 1993;87:329-335.
15. Surtees PG, Barkley C. Future imperfect: the long-term outcome of depression. *Br J Psychiatry.* 1994;164:327-341.
16. O'Leary DA, Lee AS. Seven year prognosis in depression: mortality and readmission risk in the Nottingham ECT cohort. *Br J Psychiatry.* 1996;169:423-429.
17. Estève J, Benhamou E, Raymond L. *Descriptive Epidemiology.* Lyon, France; IARC Scientific Publications; 1994.
18. Breslow NE, Day NE. *The Design and Analysis of Cohort Studies.* Lyon, France; IARC Scientific Publications; 1987.
19. Kristjansson E, Allebeck P, Wistedt B. Validity of the diagnoses of schizophrenia in the Stockholm County inpatient register. *Nord J Psychiatry.* 1987;41:229-234.
20. Harris EC, Barraclough B. Excess mortality of mental disorder. *Br J Psychiatry.* 1998;173:11-53.
21. Allebeck P, Varla A, Wistedt B. Suicide and violent death among patients with schizophrenia. *Acta Psychiatr Scand.* 1986;74:43-49.
22. Öhberg A, Lönnqvist J. Suicides hidden among undetermined deaths. *Acta Psychiatr Scand.* 1998;98:214-218.
23. Mortensen PB, Juel K. Mortality and causes of death in first admitted schizophrenic patients. *Br J Psychiatry.* 1993;163:183-189.
24. Ösby U, Correia N, Brandt L, Ekbom A, Sparén P. Time trends in schizophrenia mortality in Sweden: cohort study. *BMJ.* 2000;321:483-484.
25. Isacsson G. Suicide prevention—a medical breakthrough? *Acta Psychiatr Scand.* 2000;102:113-117.
26. Ösby U, Correia N, Brandt L, Ekbom A, Sparén P. Mortality and causes of death in schizophrenia in Stockholm County, Sweden. *Schizophr Res.* 2000;45:21-28.
27. Muller-Oerlinghausen B, Wolf T, Ahrens B, Schou M, Grof E, Grof P, Lenz G, Simhandl C, Thau K, Wolf R. Mortality during initial and during later lithium treatment: a collaborative study by the International Group for the Study of Lithium-Treated Patients. *Acta Psychiatr Scand.* 1994;90:295-297.
28. Nilsson A. Mortality in recurrent mood disorders during periods on and off lithium: a complete population study in 362 patients. *Pharmacopsychiatry.* 1995;28:8-13.
29. Ahrens B, Grof P, Moller HJ, Muller-Oerlinghausen B, Wolf T. Extended survival of patients on long-term lithium treatment. *Can J Psychiatry.* 1995;40:241-246.
30. Wolf T, Muller-Oerlinghausen B, Ahrens B, Grof P, Schou M, Felber W, Grof E, Lenz G, Nilsson A, Simhandl C, Thau K, Vestergaard P, Wolf R. How to interpret findings on mortality of long-term lithium treated manic-depressive patients: critique of different methodological approaches. *J Affect Disord.* 1996;39:127-132.
31. Schou M. The effect of prophylactic lithium treatment on mortality and suicidal behavior: a review for clinicians. *J Affect Disord.* 1998;50:253-259.
32. Nilsson A. Lithium therapy and suicide risk. *J Clin Psychiatry.* 1999;60(suppl 2):85-88. Discussion 111.
33. Weeke A, Juel K, Vaeth M. Cardiovascular death and manic-depressive psychosis. *J Affect Disord.* 1987;13:287-292.
34. Schulz R, Beach SR, Ives DG, Martire LM, Ariyo AA, Kop WJ. Association between depression and mortality in older adults: the Cardiovascular Health Study. *Arch Intern Med.* 2000;160:1761-1768.
35. Ferketich AK, Schwartzbaum JA, Frid DJ, Moeschberger ML. Depression as an antecedent to heart disease among women and men in the NHANES I study: National Health and Nutrition Examination Survey. *Arch Intern Med.* 2000;160:1261-1268.
36. Musselman DL, Evans DL, Nemeroff CB. The relationship of depression to cardiovascular disease: epidemiology, biology, and treatment. *Arch Gen Psychiatry.* 1998;55:580-592.
37. Barner-Rasmussen P, Dupont A, Bille H. Suicide in psychiatric patients in Denmark, 1971-81, I: demographic and diagnostic description. *Acta Psychiatr Scand.* 1986;73:441-448.
38. Goldacre M, Seagroatt V, Hawton K. Suicide after discharge from psychiatric inpatient care. *Lancet.* 1993;342:283-286.
39. Mortensen PB, Agerbo E, Erikson T, Qin P, Westergaard-Nielsen N. Psychiatric illness and risk factors for suicide in Denmark. *Lancet.* 2000;355:9-12.

Genetics of bipolar disorder

Nick Craddock, Ian Jones

Abstract
Bipolar disorder (also known as manic depressive illness) is a complex genetic disorder in which the core feature is pathological disturbance in mood (affect) ranging from extreme elation, or mania, to severe depression usually accompanied by disturbances in thinking and behaviour. The lifetime prevalence of 1% is similar in males and females and family, twin, and adoption studies provide robust evidence for a major genetic contribution to risk. There are methodological impediments to precise quantification, but the approximate lifetime risk of bipolar disorder in relatives of a bipolar proband are: monozygotic co-twin 40-70%; first degree relative 5-10%; unrelated person 0.5-1.5%. Occasional families may exist in which a single gene plays the major role in determining susceptibility, but the majority of bipolar disorder involves the interaction of multiple genes (epistasis) or more complex genetic mechanisms (such as dynamic mutation or imprinting). Molecular genetic positional and candidate gene approaches are being used for the genetic dissection of bipolar disorder. No gene has yet been identified but promising findings are emerging. Regions of interest identified in linkage studies include 4p16, 12q23-q24, 16p13, 21q22, and Xq24-q26. Chromosome 18 is also of interest but the findings are confusing with up to three possible regions implicated. To date most candidate gene studies have focused on neurotransmitter systems influenced by medication used in clinical management of the disorder but no robust positive findings have yet emerged. It is, however, almost certain that over the next few years bipolar susceptibility genes will be identified. This will have a major impact on our understanding of disease pathophysiology and will provide important opportunities to investigate the interaction between genetic and environmental factors involved in pathogenesis. This is likely to lead to major improvements in treatment and patient care but will also raise important ethical issues that will need to be addressed.
(*J Med Genet* 1999;**36**:585–594)

Keywords: bipolar disorder; manic depressive illness

Division of Neuroscience, University of Birmingham, Queen Elizabeth Psychiatric Hospital, Mindelsohn Way, Birmingham B15 2QZ, UK
N Craddock
I Jones

Correspondence to: Professor Craddock.

Bipolar disorder (also known as manic depressive illness) is a complex genetic disorder in which the core feature is pathological disturbance in mood (affect) ranging from extreme elation or mania to severe depression usually accompanied by disturbances in thinking and behaviour, which may include psychotic symptoms, such as delusions and hallucinations. Typically it is an episodic illness, usually with full recovery between episodes. In all modern classifications, such as ICD10[1] or DSMIV[2], the diagnosis of bipolar disorder requires that a person has suffered one or more episodes of mania with or without episodes of depression at other times during the life history. This requirement for the occurrence of an episode of mania at some time during the course of illness distinguishes bipolar disorder from the more common form of mood disorder in the population, namely unipolar disorder (also commonly known as unipolar major depression or simply unipolar depression) in which subjects suffer one or more episodes of depression without ever experiencing episodes of pathologically raised mood. Although bipolar and unipolar disorders are not completely distinct nosological entities, their separation for the purposes of diagnosis and research is supported in evidence from outcome, treatment, and genetic studies.[3,4] In DSMIV, bipolar disorder is subclassified into bipolar I disorder, in which episodes of clear cut mania occur, and bipolar II disorder, in which only milder forms of mania (so-called "hypomania") occur. However, this subclassification awaits robust validation.

Studies using modern operational diagnostic criteria suggest that lifetime prevalence of narrowly defined bipolar disorder is in the region of 0.5-1.5% with similar rates in males and females and a mean age of onset around the age of 21 years.[5] Currently there is no evidence that rates of bipolar disorder vary widely among different populations. Bipolar disorder is associated with high levels of service use and morbidity and it has been estimated that approximately 15% of patients eventually die by suicide.[6] Reasonably effective treatments are available for both manic and depressive phases of illness and lithium, and more recently a variety of anticonvulsants, have been used prophylactically as mood stabilisers to reduce recurrence of acute episodes of depression and mania.[7] However, current treatments have undesirable side effects, are not effective in all patients, and the pathogenesis of bipolar disorder remains poorly understood.

Clinicians have always known that bipolar disorder tends to run in families but recent advances in molecular genetics now provide the tools needed to identify genes influencing susceptibility. Although psychiatric and behavioural traits represent, perhaps, the greatest challenge to molecular investigation of complex genetic disorders, they also offer arguably the greatest potential reward. Identifying susceptibility genes for bipolar disorder will pinpoint biochemical pathways involved in pathogenesis, facilitate development of more effective, better targeted treatments, and offer opportunities for improving the validity of psychiatric diagnosis and classification. In this review article, we start by briefly considering methodological issues involved in genetic studies of bipolar disorder. We will then review the formal evidence that genes are involved in influencing susceptibility to bipolar disorder. We will consider the likely mode of inheritance before discussing current molecular genetic positional and candidate studies. Finally, we will discuss the implications of genetic investigation of bipolar disorder.

Methodological issues

Before reviewing available genetic data, it is important to be aware of several methodological issues that act as impediments to genetic research in bipolar disorder. It should be recognised that some of these apply equally to all complex genetic diseases.

LIFETIME DIAGNOSIS

Although psychiatric diagnoses tend to remain stable, occasionally a change in diagnosis from one episode to another is observed. In genetic studies "lifetime diagnosis" is required in an attempt to classify subjects on the basis of a presumed diathesis for bipolar disorder. This requires that the sum of a person's abnormal behaviour and experience over his/her lifetime be reduced to a small number of diagnostic categories, usually just one. Although this task is non-trivial, a relatively robust methodology of lifetime diagnosis has been developed which allows integration of information from different sources in an unbiased manner in order to produce acceptably reliable diagnoses.[8 9]

VARIABLE AGE AT ONSET

In common with many other diseases, subjects can develop the first episode of bipolar disorder at any time during his or her life. For this reason, unaffected subjects are much less useful in genetic studies than are affected subjects because they provide less information about genetic risk.

SECULAR CHANGES (FOR EXAMPLE, BIRTH COHORT EFFECT)

A change in the measured rate of mood disorder in successive birth cohorts has been described in some studies.[10 11] However, this effect may be an artefact of research methodology[12] and the effect has been less clearly shown in bipolar disorder than in unipolar disorder. This effect complicates prevalence dependent analysis of data that include differing birth cohorts, further reducing the usefulness of unaffected subjects

UNKNOWN DIAGNOSTIC VALIDITY

Clinical, outcome, and genetic studies suggest that bipolar disorder is a relatively distinct nosological entity. However, in the absence of a clear understanding of the biology of psychiatric illnesses the most appropriate boundaries between bipolar disorder and other mood and psychotic disorders remain unclear. The bipolar-unipolar boundary has already been mentioned. At the psychotic end of the spectrum, there are a large number of patients who have illnesses with features both of schizophrenia and bipolar disorder (usually called "schizoaffective disorder"). Current diagnostic boundaries are based on best available evidence,[3 4] but the extent to which they reflect genetic vulnerability will only become clear as susceptibility genes are identified.

Despite these challenges, methodological refinements in both psychiatric diagnosis and complex disease genetics have provided methods and approaches that in large part address most of the methodological issues. Currently the major problem is the unknown biological validity of current psychiatric classifications and it is worth bearing in mind that advances in molecular genetics are likely to be instrumental in providing the first robust validation of our diagnostic schemata.

Family studies

Many of the early studies of mood disorders failed to distinguish between unipolar and bipolar types of illness or failed to provide any description of the clinical features associated with the diagnostic categories used. A review of these early studies (almost all of which showed familial aggregation of mood disorder) can be found in Tsuang and Faraone.[13] Over the last 30 years many studies using the modern concept of bipolar disorder have been conducted and fig 1 provides a graphical summary of the findings. It includes all published studies (1) which use the modern concept of bipolar disorder, (2) measure lifetime risk of bipolar disorder in first degree relatives of a bipolar proband, and (3) in which at least some of the relatives were interviewed directly. There were 21 studies that met these criteria,[14-34] of which eight included a sample of controls.[17 24-26 30-32 34] Fig 1 shows the relative risk of narrowly defined bipolar disorder (equivalent to DSMIV bipolar I disorder) in first degree relatives of bipolar probands as a function of the number of subjects included in the study. Relative risk is defined as the ratio of risk of bipolar disorder in first degree relatives of bipolar probands to the risk in first degree relatives of controls or, for studies that did not include controls, to an assumed general population baseline risk of 1%. As can be seen, all of these studies showed an increased risk of bipolar disorder in the relatives of bipolar probands. Using the eight

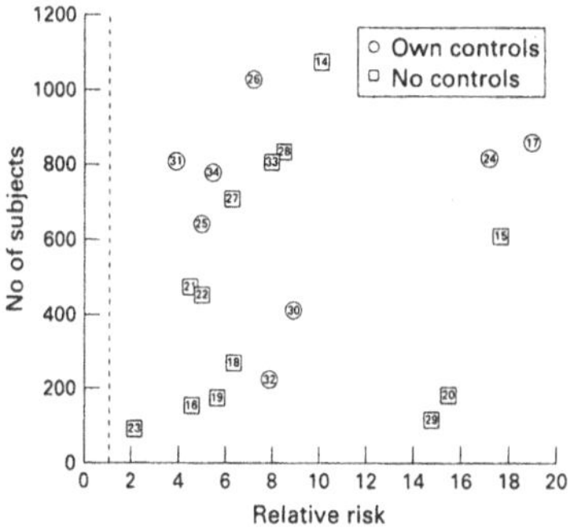

Figure 1 Family studies of bipolar disorder. The relative risk of narrowly defined bipolar disorder (equivalent to DSMIV bipolar I disorder) in first degree relatives of bipolar probands is shown as a function of the number of subjects included in the study. Relative risk is defined as the ratio of risk of bipolar disorder in first degree relatives of bipolar probands to the risk in first degree relatives of controls or, for studies that did not include controls, to an assumed general population baseline risk of 1% (see text for further details). Numbers refer to papers in reference list. All studies can be seen to give a relative risk of greater than one (dashed line) and therefore provide evidence of familial aggregation of bipolar disorder.

studies[17 24-26 30-32 34] that included their own control groups, a meta-analysis[35] showed no evidence of heterogeneity between studies and provided an overall estimate of risk (as measured by odds ratios, OR, and 95% confidence intervals, CI) in first degree relatives of bipolar I probands of OR=7 (CI 5-10).

Family studies are also consistent in showing that first degree relatives of bipolar probands are at increased risk of unipolar major depression when compared with first degree relatives of controls. Indeed, the absolute risk of unipolar depression is higher than the absolute risk of bipolar disorder in the first degree relatives of a bipolar proband. However, because the background population lifetime prevalence of unipolar depression is substantially greater than that of bipolar disorder (of the order of 10% versus 1%), the relative increase in risk is much lower for unipolar disorder (of the order of a doubling of risk).[36] It has been estimated that approximately 2/3-3/4 of cases of unipolar depression in the family of a bipolar proband are genetically bipolar, that is, share a common genetic susceptibility.[37] Bipolar II disorder has been shown to occur with increased frequency in relatives of bipolar I probands compared with the general population[24 27 32] and some workers believe it is the most common manifestation of the bipolar phenotype.[38] However, others have suggested it is a separate disorder.[39] Family studies have not shown an increase in the risk of schizophrenia in the relatives of bipolar probands, but have consistently shown familial aggregation of bipolar disorder and schizoaffective disorder in which manic features occur.[24 27 31 34]

It is an unresolved question as to whether the lifetime rates of illness in first degree relatives of bipolar probands vary according to type of relative (parent, offspring, or sib). Gershon *et al*[17] found the risk in sibs to be greater than that in parents and offspring but in a later study Gershon *et al*[24] found the difference to be reversed. Perhaps because of small sample sizes or because there appears to be no consistent difference between risks in parents, offspring, and sibs, several studies have reported only the pooled estimate of risk for all types of first degree relatives. The lifetime risk of affective disorder in relatives of a bipolar proband does not appear to vary with sex of relative or of the proband.[27 30 32] Lifetime risk of affective disorder in relatives with bipolar probands increases with early age of onset[40] and with number of ill relatives.[24] There are no adequate data to provide meaningful estimates of the rates of affective disorder in second degree relatives of bipolar probands but available evidence suggests that the rates lie between those for first degree relatives and those for the general population.

Twin studies

Early twin studies, which did not distinguish between bipolar and unipolar illness, supported the involvement of genes in broadly defined mood disorders and are reviewed by Tsuang and Faraone.[13] Six twin studies have used a modern concept of bipolar disorder and

Table 1 Lifetime rates of affective disorder in co-twins of bipolar twin probands

Ref No	*Sample*	*Lifetime rates of affective illness in co-twin of bipolar twin probands (probandwise concordance rate)*		*Comment*
41	Norway twin and psychosis register. 6 MZ pairs with BP proband	BP-BP:	MZ: 67%	Small sample and no operationalised diagnostic criteria
42	USA Veteran twin register. 5 MZ, 15 DZ pairs (out of 15 909 twin pairs on register)	BP-BP:	MZ: 20% DZ: 0%	Inferior methodology. Note the very low rate of BP disorder detected in the twin sample (0.07%)
43	Denmark twin and psychiatry registers. 34 MZ, 37 DZ pairs	BP-BP:	MZ: 62% DZ: 8%	Despite lack of operationalised diagnostic criteria this is a detailed study and is the best available
		BP-BP/UP:	MZ: 79% DZ: 19%	
44	Norway twin register. 4 MZ, 6 DZ pairs	BP-BP:	MZ: 75% DZ: 0%	Small sample which may overlap partly with that of ref 41
		BP-BP/UP:	MZ: 100% DZ: 0%	
45	Sweden twin and psychiatric registers. 13 MZ, 22 DZ pairs	BP-BP:	MZ: 39% DZ: 5%	This has the strength of being a large epidemiological twin sample but the weakness of using questionnaire assessments. Likely to underestimate concordance
		BP-BP/UP:	MZ: 62% DZ: 14%	
46	UK psychiatric hospital twin register. 22 MZ, 27 DZ pairs	BP-BP:	MZ: 36% DZ: 7%	Diagnoses based on hospital notes. Likely to underestimate concordance

MZ: monozygotic; DZ: dizygotic. Sample size refers to number of twin pairs in which at least one twin suffered with bipolar disorder. BP-BP refers to twin pairs in which both have narrowly defined bipolar disorder. BP-BP/UP refers to twin pairs in which one has bipolar disorder and the other has broadly defined bipolar phe- [illegible]

Table 2 Approximate lifetime rates of mood disorder in various classes of relative of bipolar probands

Degree of relationship to bipolar proband	*Risk of bipolar disorder (%)*	*(Additional) risk of unipolar depression (%)*
Monozygotic co-twin	40–70	15–25
First degree relative	5–10	10–20
General population (ie, unrelated)	0.5–1.5	5–10

The lifetime risk of major mood disorder in a relative is obtained by adding the risk of bipolar disorder and the risk of unipolar depression. General population lifetime risk of unipolar depression is notoriously difficult to quantify but the figures in the table are based on a definition of clinically significant depression comparable to that used in the genetic studies.

all show an increased probandwise concordance rate in monozygotic (MZ) twins when compared with dizygotic (DZ) twins[41–46] (table 1). Pooling the data from these studies provides an estimate of probandwise MZ concordance for narrowly defined bipolar disorder of 50% (95% confidence intervals 40%-60%). However, three of the studies almost certainly underestimate the concordance so the true MZ concordance is likely to be >50%, probably close to the 60% found in the study of Bertelsen *et al.*[43] Longitudinal study of the offspring of the unaffected members of discordant MZ twin pairs ascertained through a bipolar proband has shown an increase in risk of bipolar illness indistinguishable from that in the offspring of subjects affected by bipolar disorder.[47]

Studies of genetically identical subjects illustrate the phenotypic spectrum that may be associated with bipolar susceptibility genes. In addition to bipolar disorder, unipolar disorder, or absence of illness, MZ co-twins or co-triplets of a bipolar proband have been described who have a diagnosis of schizoaffective disorder[43] or (very rarely) schizophrenia.[48] It should also be recognised that the incomplete phenotypic concordance in MZ twins has provided the most robust evidence that non-genetic factors play an important role in determining susceptibility to bipolar disorder.

Adoption studies

Only two adoption studies have used a modern concept of bipolar disorder. Mendlewicz and Rainer[49] investigated the biological and adoptive parents of 29 bipolar and 22 normal adoptees and the biological parents of 31 bipolar non-adoptees and found significantly ($p<0.05$) greater risk of affective disorder (bipolar, schizoaffective, and unipolar) in the biological parents of bipolar adoptees (18% risk) compared with the adoptive parents (7% risk). This risk in biological relatives of bipolar adoptees was similar to that in the biological relatives of bipolar non-adoptees. The study of Wender *et al*[50] included only 10 bipolar probands but showed a similar (but non-significant) trend for biological relatives of probands to be at increased risk compared with adoptive relatives.

Summary of epidemiological, family, twin, and adoption studies

Family, twin, and adoption studies provide an impressive and consistent body of evidence supporting the existence of genes determining predisposition to bipolar disorder and show a gradation in risk of mood disorder in relatives of bipolar probands in the order (highest to lowest risk) of: monozygotic co-twin, first degree relative, unrelated member of the general population. Although there are many methodological impediments to producing a consistent quantification of risk, the figures given in table 2 may be taken as an "order of magnitude" guide to risk in different classes of relative[51] and, provided appropriate caveats are made, are suitable for providing information to patients and their relatives.

Chromosome studies

Bipolar disorder is not consistently associated with chromosome abnormalities although a number of such published reports have appeared.[52] Perhaps the most interesting observation is that subjects with trisomy 21 appear to be less susceptible to mania than are members of the general population.[53] This is consistent with the existence of a bipolar susceptibility gene on chromosome 21, a possibility that finds support from recent molecular genetic studies (see table 3).

Mode of inheritance

Early linkage studies were predicated on the assumption of single gene inheritance and attempts were made to recruit large unilineal apparently autosomal dominant pedigrees.

Table 3 Some regions of interest from molecular genetic linkage studies of bipolar disorder

Chromosomal location	*Study reference*	*Comment*
4p16	117	Single large UK pedigree with max lod = 4.8
	118	Single moderate size UK pedigree (schizoaffective disorder) with max lod =1.9
12q23-q24	119	Single UK pedigree in which Darier's disease[120 121] and bipolar disorder cosegregate. Max lod = 2.1
	122	29 small-moderate UK pedigrees. Max lod = 2.0. No evidence in 16 German families
	123	Single very large pedigree from an isolated French Canadian community. Max lod = 4.9
	124	2 moderate size Danish pedigrees. Max lod = 3.4
18 centromeric	125	22 moderate size US pedigrees. Max non-parametric evidence p<0.0001
	126	28 moderate size US pedigrees (particularly those showing paternal transmission). Max non-parametric evidence p<0.001
18q22	126	28 moderate size US pedigrees (particularly those showing paternal transmission). Max sib pair evidence p<0.001
18q22-q23	127	2 large Costa Rican pedigrees. Max lod for combined linkage association = 4.06
21q22	128	Single large US pedigree. Max lod = 3.4
	129	22 moderate size US pedigrees (particularly those showing maternal transmission). Max sib pair evidence p<0.001
	130	97 moderate size US pedigrees. Max sib pair evidence p<0.001
	131	23 UK & Icelandic pedigrees. Max lod = 2.2

This table illustrates some current regions of interest. Readers seeking a systematic overview of findings including both negative and positive reports should consult Chromosome Workshop reports (see text).

Table 4 Complex genetic mechanisms that have been suggested in bipolar disorder

Genetic mechanism	*Authors*
Locus heterogeneity	Hodgkinson *et al*[132]
Allelic heterogeneity	Sandkuyl and Ott[133]
Epistasis	Craddock *et al*[60]
Dynamic mutation	McInnis *et al*[134]
Imprinting	McMahon *et al*[135]
Mitochondrial inheritance	McMahon *et al*[135]

Genetic mechanisms causing complex patterns of inheritance and authors who have invoked the mechanisms to explain the inheritance of bipolar disorder.

Although rare, a number of such pedigrees have been identified and it seems likely that in at least some of these a single gene may play a major role in determining disease susceptibility. Some segregation analyses on systematically ascertained pedigree sets have produced results consistent with single gene models,[27 30 54 55] while others have been unable to show major locus transmission.[56-58] However, caution is required in interpreting these results because of the limited power of the studies to distinguish between single gene and oligogenic models and because of the failure to take account of an important parameter, the recurrence risk in MZ cotwins of a bipolar proband.[59] The observed very rapid decrease in recurrence risk from identical co-twins to first degree relatives and back to the general population (as shown in table 2) is not consistent with single gene modes of inheritance.[60] The recurrence risk data are consistent with epistatic interaction of multiple genes or with more complex genetic mechanisms. Several genetic mechanisms that are known to produce complex patterns of inheritance and which have been suggested as possible explanations for bipolar disorder are shown in table 4.

X LINKAGE

The idea that X linkage may explain some forms of affective disorder goes back over half a century[61] and has been debated vigorously over the last 25 years because of several reports of families showing cosegregation between X linked markers (such as colour blindness or glucose-6-phosphate dehydrogenase deficiency) and bipolar disorder, suggesting the possibility of an X linked dominant susceptibility gene.[62-64] However, these reports have been criticised on methodological grounds,[65] particular problems being ascertainment bias and non-blinding to marker status. If X linkage does occur, analyses suggest that it can account for only a minority of cases.[56 66]

In summary, as clinical psychiatrists are well aware, although bipolar disorder tends to aggregate in families, the pattern of inheritance in most pedigrees is not simple. Although it seems likely that occasional families exist in which a single gene plays a major role in determining susceptibility to illness, the evidence indicates that single gene transmission does not occur in most cases. This observation is consistent with the failure to identify genes of major effect in linkage studies predicated on single gene models.

Molecular genetic studies

Linkage and association studies using DNA markers are, of course, the cutting edge of modern approaches to complex genetic diseases. Conceptually, molecular genetic studies can be divided into positional and candidate gene approaches. In positional approaches, chromosomal locations of susceptibility genes are determined, usually by linkage studies. This requires no knowledge of disease pathophysiology and can be considered a purely genetic approach. In contrast, the candidate gene approach presupposes that the researcher has sufficient understanding of disease biology to be able to recognise genes that may be involved in bipolar disorder. These are then examined in linkage or, more usually, association studies. In practice both positional and candidate approaches are often combined.[67] The principles behind, and applications of, these approaches are discussed in detail elsewhere.[68]

LINKAGE STUDIES

Early linkage studies of bipolar disorder used very large families and were based on the implausible assumption that all illness was caused by a single major gene. In the late 1980s there were two high profile claims of linkage published in the journal *Nature*: Baron *et al*[64] reported linkage to X chromosome markers in several Israeli pedigrees and Egeland *et al*[69] reported linkage to markers on chromosome 11p in a large pedigree of the Old Order Amish community in Pennsylvania. Other workers were unable to replicate these findings and eventually in both cases the original groups published updated and extended analyses of their own data in which the significant evidence of linkage all but vanished.[70 71] The reasons for these dramatic reversals in findings included: (1) family members originally diagnosed as unaffected became ill for the first time during follow up; (2) new family members were examined who did not show evidence for linkage; and (3) additional DNA markers were examined which reduced the evidence for linkage. After initial pessimism following these disappointments, the field has moved forward with the development and use of research methodologies more appropriate for the investigation of complex genetic traits. There has been a trend towards use of smaller families (particularly affected sib pairs) and of analytic methods that are less sensitive to diagnostic changes or errors (reviewed by Craddock and Owen[68]).

Several groups around the world are undertaking large scale molecular genetic linkage studies of bipolar disorder and promising findings are beginning to emerge. A variety of different types of sample set are being used ranging from single large densely affected pedigrees in genetic isolates[69] to large numbers of affected sib pairs[72] and systematic genome screens are being undertaken in many of these samples. The pattern of results emerging from these linkage studies supports the view that no single major gene exists that explains the majority of cases of bipolar disorder. Several features are emerging that are to be expected in the search for genes involved in a complex genetic disorder.[73,75] (1) No finding replicates in all data sets. (2) Levels of statistical significance and estimated effect sizes are usually modest. (3) Chromosomal regions of interest are typically broad (often >20-30 cM). (4) The same region may be implicated as (a) containing a susceptibility gene in large samples comprised of small families, and (b) harbouring a potential major locus within one or more large multiply affected pedigrees. (5) Some chromosome regions have been implicated in linkage studies of different psychiatric phenotypes. For example, 15q11-q13 is implicated in studies of both bipolar disorder and schizophrenia.[76]

Table 3 provides information about four regions that are attracting a great deal of interest in linkage studies of bipolar disorder. Of these 12q23-q24 and 21q22 are, perhaps, the most promising (as already mentioned, the reduced incidence of mania in trisomy 21 is consistent with a chromosome 21 locus[53]). Chromosome 18 is the most confusing with positive reports scattered throughout the chromosome in a pattern that is not consistent with a single susceptibility gene.[77] Other regions of interest include 16p13,[78] Xq24-q26,[79] and 15q11-q13.[76] Detailed reviews of linkage data for each chromosome can be found in the chromosome workshop reports of the World Congress of Psychiatric Genetics, held annually. Reports from the Fifth World Congress held in Santa Fe, New Mexico, in 1997 were published in *Psychiatric Genetics* 1998;**8**(2). The report from the Sixth World Congress held in Bonn, Germany, in 1998 will be reported in *American Journal of Medical Genetics (Neuropsychiatric Genetics)* 1999;**88**(3).

As is the case for most complex genetic disorders, methodological differences between linkage studies make conventional meta-analysis all but impossible. However, new methods of meta-analysis are being developed in which the comparison of genome scan results is based on ranking of chromosomal regions according to linkage evidence rather than absolute values of linkage statistics. The application of such approaches to bipolar disorder will provide a more systematic and unified overview of the evidence.

This is a rapidly moving field and new data are becoming available regularly. The reader who is interested in a specific chromosomal region is recommended to consult the most recent chromosome workshop reports and bibliographic databases.

ASSOCIATION STUDIES

For complex genetic disorders such as bipolar disorder, association studies represent an important experimental approach both to follow up regions of interest detected in linkage studies (using both systematic linkage disequilibrium mapping and positional candidate studies) as well as for pure functional candidate gene studies. Important advantages of the association paradigm are relative robustness to genetic heterogeneity and the ability to detect much smaller effect sizes than are detectable using feasible sample sizes in linkage studies.[80] Several research groups are assembling large samples of unrelated probands and appropriate comparison subjects for use in linkage disequilibrium and candidate gene studies but robust positive findings have yet to emerge.

The candidate gene association approach is potentially very powerful, particularly when used within the context of a VAPSE (*V*ariation *A*ffecting *P*rotein *S*equence or *E*xpression) paradigm.[81] This approach involves systematic mutation/polymorphism detection in coding and control regions of candidate genes followed by association studies in disease comparison samples. Conventional association studies are susceptible to spurious associations resulting from inadequate matching of cases and controls, especially when there is population stratification. However, the recent development of family based association methods helps overcome this problem by allowing an artificial well matched notional control sample to be constructed from marker data from the family of each proband.[82] Although several statistical approaches can be used in this design,[83] the transmission disequilibrium test (TDT) has gained popularity.[84] This advance has increased the attractiveness of association studies for genetic dissection of complex diseases and such samples are being developed for investigation of bipolar disorder.

The main problem with candidate gene approaches is that efficiency in the choice of candidates is inevitably a function of the level of previous understanding of disease pathophysiology. To date, most candidate gene studies in bipolar disorder (and in other psychiatric phenotypes) have focused on the major neurotransmitter systems that are influenced by medication used in clinical management of the disorder. Thus, studies of known polymorphisms have been conducted for several genes encoding receptors or proteins and enzymes involved in metabolism or re-uptake of dopamine, serotonin (5HT), and noradrenalin. No convincing positive findings have yet emerged although several studies have provided tantalising, albeit modest, evidence implicating the serotonin transporter gene (*hSERT*).[85-89] This gene is undoubtedly an excellent functional candidate because it is the site of action of selective serotonin re-uptake inhibitors, a major class of antidepressants of which fluoxetine (Prozac™) is a well known member, which are effective in treatment of bipolar depression and can also induce mania in bipolar subjects. The picture is still far from clear[90-94] and *hSERT* is certainly not a gene of major effect, but results are consistent with a modest influence on disease susceptibility. Confirmation of such an effect will require replication in large independent samples from different populations and will ultimately require demonstration of the pathogenic relevance of polymorphisms within tissue and animal systems.

A deeper understanding of the pathogenesis of bipolar disorder will almost certainly include systems involved in signal transduction and modulation of gene expression and, as genes involved in these systems are cloned, candidate gene association studies will offer the opportunity to explore their role in the pathogenesis of bipolar disorder.

TRINUCLEOTIDE REPEAT EXPANSION (DYNAMIC MUTATION)

For several neurological/neuropsychiatric diseases, such as Huntington's disease, myotonic dystrophy, and fragile X syndrome, the clinical phenomenon of anticipation (progressively more severe disease/earlier age at onset as the disease is transmitted through successive generations) occurs and is caused by DNA sequences of trinucleotide repeats that expand as they are passed from parent to offspring.[95] Anticipation has been reported in some recent studies of bipolar disorder and it has been hypothesised that trinucleotide repeat expansion may play a role in the pathogenesis of bipolar disorder (reviewed by O'Donovan and Owen[95]). In agreement with this hypothesis, four independent association studies using the repeat expansion detection (RED) method[96] have shown trinucleotide repeat sequences to be significantly larger in bipolar patients compared with controls.[97-100] However, some studies have failed to find this association.[101] One of the groups with the positive RED finding has reported that most of the large RED products may be explained by two specific loci, CTG18.1 and ERDA7,[102] and that CTG18.1 shows a modest association with bipolar disorder. However, this finding awaits confirmation. Furthermore, if one or more trinucleotide repeat containing loci are confirmed as playing a role in bipolar disorder, it appears likely (1) that the genotype-phenotype correlation in bipolar disorder will prove to be more complicated than is the case for trinucleotide repeat diseases previously described (for example, Huntington's disease), and (2) that trinucleotide repeat containing genes involved in bipolar disorder may operate as susceptibility genes rather than as a single gene of major effect.[103]

Subtypes of bipolar disorder

One of the principles that can be used to increase the power to detect genes involved in complex diseases is to focus investigation on specific phenotypic subtypes known or thought to represent more genetically homogeneous forms of the disorder.[74] A number of such potentially useful subtypes are known in bipolar disorder and researchers are beginning to take an interest in these.

RAPID CYCLING

Rapid cycling, defined as the occurrence of four or more discrete episodes of mood disorder within a 12 month period, occurs in a substantial proportion of bipolar patients, is more common in females, and may be induced by some medications, including antidepressants. Although family studies have produced inconclusive results regarding the familiality of rapid cycling,[104-106] recent candidate gene association studies suggest that the low activity allele at a common polymorphism within the catechol-o-methyl transferase (COMT) gene may be associated with increased susceptibility to rapid cycling within bipolar patients.[107 108] This observation has biological consistency with the observed tendency for antidepressants to induce rapid cycling in that both increase availability of catecholamines at neuronal synapses. However, this genetic finding requires confirmation in large independent samples and, even if confirmed, makes only a modest contribution to rapid cycling.

SEASONAL AFFECTIVE DISORDER

Seasonal affective disorder (SAD) describes mood disorder with a characteristic seasonal variation. Many subjects with SAD are bipolar. Genes have been shown to influence seasonal variation in mood[110] and SAD has been shown to aggregate in families.[111] Biological systems that have been implicated in the pathogenesis of SAD include systems involved in serotonergic neurotransmission and circadian and circannual clocks.[112]

PUERPERAL PSYCHOSIS

Puerperal psychosis refers to severe (usually psychotic) psychiatric disorder occurring within a few weeks of parturition.[113] The vast majority of subjects who suffer episodes of puerperal psychosis have a bipolar disorder diathesis together with a susceptibility to puerperal triggering of episodes (frequently manic). There is strong evidence that the puerperal trigger is familial (Jones and Craddock, unpublished data) and plausible biological systems include steroid hormone pathways.[114]

The future

Several groups around the world are assembling the large clinical samples needed for the genetic dissection of bipolar disorder using currently available methodologies and collaboration will undoubtedly be necessary to identify genes of relatively modest effect. The trend for genotyping methods to become increasingly automated with dramatic increases in efficiency will undoubtedly continue and novel molecular methods may become available that will eventually supersede current linkage and association studies. Such technological advances, in the context of completion of the Human Genome Project in the first years of the next millennium, should facilitate the identification of bipolar susceptibility genes of even small effect. Current biological research in bipolar disorder is constrained by the lack of an animal model. Once susceptibility genes are discovered, it should prove feasible to breed transgenic mice (or other species) that include the abnormal form of the gene, thereby providing a model in which the disease process can be studied in vivo.

Identification of genetic mechanisms conferring susceptibility to bipolar disorder will, of course, be a major achievement. However, this will not be an end in itself but rather the beginning of a path that will lead towards an understanding of the biological underpinnings of bipolar and related mood disorders. It is quite likely that along this path we will learn much about the biological basis of normal affective responses. In this regard it is interesting to note that a recent twin study showed that normal happiness is in large part under genetic influence.[115]

Major benefits will accrue from the research that will follow identification of genes involved in the pathogenesis of bipolar disorder. Knowledge of a gene that confers susceptibility to illness will allow identification of its gene product which will in turn lead to an understanding of the role of the individual protein in disease causation, including its interaction with other substances and the effect of environmental changes on protein level and function. This level of understanding will allow the development of therapeutic agents that are much more specifically targeted at the biochemical lesions involved in disease. It will be possible to develop a rational, aetiology based classification of bipolar and related disorders which will almost certainly provide a much better guide to treatment and prognosis than do current classifications. A new generation of psychiatrists will learn not only to recognise clinical syndromes, as at present, but will be able to perform laboratory tests that will help determine the pathogenesis of the psychopathology which will in turn guide the clinician towards the most appropriate therapy. Importantly, identification of bipolar susceptibility genes will facilitate identification of environmental factors that confer risk or are protective, both in people who are not genetically susceptible and in those who have a high level of genetic risk. Once these environmental factors are characterised, it may prove possible to provide helpful occupational, social, and psychological advice to those at genetic risk of bipolar disorder.

It must not be forgotten that major advances raise major ethical issues. Although many of the issues in psychiatric genetics are no different from those for other common familial disorders, this combination of genetics and mental illness justifiably excites and receives particularly close scrutiny of ethical and psychosocial issues.[116] Areas that will need to be addressed include the availability of services, the right to information, and the possibility of testing of subjects below the age of consent. The challenge to psychiatrists in the 21st century is to ensure that a revolution in understanding of the biology of bipolar disorder is translated into a revolution in clinical care. Our patients deserve nothing less.

Ian Jones is a Wellcome Trust Research Fellow in Mental Health. Nick Craddock is a Wellcome Trust Senior Research Fellow in Clinical Sciences.

1 World Health Organization. *The ICD10 classification of mental and behavioural disorders*. Geneva: WHO, 1993.
2 APA. *Diagnostic and statistical manual for mental disorders*. 4th ed. Washington, DC: American Psychiatric Association, 1994.
3 Kendell RE. Diagnosis and classification of functional psychosis. *Br Med Bull* 1987;43:499-513.
4 Farmer A, McGuffin P. The classification of the depressions contemporary confusion revisited. *Br J Psychiatry* 1989; 155:437-43.
5 Smith AL, Weissman MM. Epidemiology. In: Paykel ES, ed. *Handbook of affective disorders*. Edinburgh: Churchill Livingstone, 1992:111-29.
6 Guze SB, Robins E. Suicide and primary affective disorders. *Br J Psychiatry* 1970;**117**:437-8.
7 Daly I. Mania. Lancet 1997;**349**:1157-60.
8 Leckman JF, Sholomskas D, Thompson D, Belanger A, Weissman MM. Best estimate of lifetime psychiatric diagnosis. *Arch Gen Psychiatry* 1982;**39**:879-3.
9 Farmer AE, Williams J, Jones I. Phenotypic definitions of psychotic illness for molecular genetic research. *Am J Med Genet (Neuropsychiatr Genet)* 1994;**54**:365-71.
10 Klerman GL. The current age of youthful melancholia: evidence for increase in depression among adolescents and young adults. *Br J Psychiatry* 1988;**152**:4-14.
11 Gershon ES, Hamovit JH, Guroff JJ, Nurnberger JI. Birth-cohort changes in manic and depressive disorders in relatives of bipolar and schizoaffective patients. *Arch Gen Psychiatry* 1987;**44**:314-19.
12 Giuffra LA, Risch N. Diminished recall and the cohort effect of major depression: a simulation study. *Psychol Med* 1994;**24**:375-83.
13 Tsuang MT, Faraone SV. *The genetics of mood disorders*. Baltimore: The Johns Hopkins University Press, 1990.
14 Perris C. A study of bipolar (manic-depressive) and unipolar recurrent depressive psychoses. *Acta Psychiatr Scand* 1966;**suppl 42**:15-44.
15 Mendlewicz J, Rainer JD. Morbidity risk and genetic transmission in manic-depressive Illness. *Am J Hum Genet* 1974;**26**:692-701.
16 Helzer JE, Winokur G. Family interview study of male manic depressives. *Arch Gen Psychiatry* 1974;**31**:73-7.
17 Gershon ES, Mark A, Cohen N, Belizon N, Baron M, Knobe KE. Transmitted factors in the morbid risk of affective disorders: a controlled study. *J Psychiatr Res* 1975;**12**: 283-99.
18 James N, Chapman CJ. A genetic study of bipolar affective disorder. *Br J Psychiatry* 1975;**126**:449-56.
19 Smeraldi E, Negri F, Melica AM. A genetic study of affective disorders. *Acta Psychiatr Scand* 1977;**56**:382-98.
20 Johnson GFS, Leeman MM. Analysis of familial factors in bipolar affective illness.*Arch Gen Psychiatry* 1997;**34**:1074-83.
21 Petterson U. Manic-depressive illness: a clinical, social and genetic study. *Acta Psychiatr Scand* 1977;**suppl 269**:1-93.
22 Taylor MA, Abrams R, Hayman MA. The classification of affective disorders—a reassessment of the bipolar-unipolar dichotomy. A clinical, laboratory, and family study. *J Affect Disord* 1980;**2**:95-109.
23 Scharfetter C, Nusperli M. The group of schizophrenias, schizoaffective psychoses, and affective disorders. *Schizophr Bull* 1980;**6**:586-91.
24 Gershon ES, Hamovit J, Guroff JJ, *et al.* A family study of schizoaffective, bipolar I, bipolar II, unipolar, and normal control probands. *Arch Gen Psychiatry* 1982;**39**:1157-67.
25 Winokur G, Tsuang MT, Crowe RR. The Iowa 500—affective disorder in relatives of manic and depressed patients. *Am J Psychiatry* 1982;**139**:209-12.
26 Weissman MM, Gershon ES, Kidd KK, *et al.* Psychiatric disorders in the relatives of probands with affective disorders. *Arch Gen Psychiatry* 1984;**41**:13-21.
27 Rice J, Reich T, Andreasen NC, *et al.* The familial transmission of bipolar illness. *Arch Gen Psychiatry* 1987;**44**:441-7.
28 Andreasen NC, Rice J, Endicott J, Coryell W, Grove WM, Reich T. Familial rates of affective disorder. *Arch Gen Psychiatry* 1987;**44**:461-9.
29 Strober M, Morrell W, Burroughs J, Lampert C, Danforth H, Freeman R. A family study of bipolar I disorder in adolescence. Early onset of symptoms linked to increased familial loading and lithium resistance. *J Affect Disord* 1988;**15**:255-68.
30 Pauls DL, Morton LA, Egeland JA. Risks of affective illness among first-degree relatives of bipolar I Old-Order Amish probands. *Arch Gen Psychiatry* 1992;**49**:703-8.
31 Maier W, Lichtermann D, Minges J, *et al.* Continuity and discontinuity of affective disorders and schizophrenia. Results of a controlled family. *Arch Gen Psychiatry* 1993;**50**:871-83.
32 Heun R, Maier W. The distinction of bipolar II disorder from bipolar I and recurrent unipolar depression: results of a controlled family study. *Acta Psychiatr Scand* 1993;**87**: 279-84.
33 Winokur G, Coryell W, Keller M, Endicott J, Leon A. A family study of manic-depressive (bipolar I) disease. Is it a distinct illness separable from primary unipolar depression? *Arch Gen Psychiatry* 1995;**52**:367-73.
34 Kendler KS, Karkowski LM, Walsh D. The structure of psychosis. *Arch Gen Psychiatry* 1998;**55**:492-9.
35 Woolf B. On estimating the relationship between blood group and disease. *Ann Hum Genet* 1955;**19**:251-3.
36 McGuffin P, Katz R. The genetics of depression and manic-depressive disorder. *Br J Psychiatry* 1989;**155**:294-304.
37 Blacker D, Tsuang MT. Unipolar relatives in bipolar pedigrees: are they bipolar? *Psychiatr Genet* 1993;**3**:5-16.
38 Simpson SG, Folstein SE, Meyers DA, McMahon FJ, Brusco DM, DePaulo JR. Bipolar II: the most common bipolar phenotype? *Am J Psychiatry* 1993;**150**:901-3.
39 Coryell W, Keller M, Endicott J, Andreasen N, Clayton P, Hirschfeld R. Bipolar II illness: course and outcome over a five year period. *Psychol Med* 1989;**19**:129-41.
40 Strober M. Relevance of early age-of-onset in genetic studies of bipolar affective disorder. *J Am Acad Child Adolesc Psychiatry* 1992;**31**:606-10.
41 Kringlen E. *Heredity and environment in the functional psychoses*. London: Heinemann, 1967.
42 Allen MG, Cohen S, Pollin W, Greenspan SI. Affective illness in veteran twins: a diagnostic review. *Am J Psychiatry* 1974;**131**:1234-9.
43 Bertelsen A, Harvald B, Hauge M . A Danish twin study of manic-depressive illness. *Br J Psychiatry* 1977;**130**:330-51.

44 Torgersen S. Genetic factors in moderately severe and mild affective disorders. *Arch Gen Psychiatry* 1986;**43**:222-6.

45 Kendler KS, Pedersen N, Johnson L, Neale MC, Mathe AA. A pilot Swedish twin study of affective illness, including hospital- and population-ascertained subsamples. *Arch Gen Psychiatry* 1993;**50**:699-706.

46 Cardno AG, Marshall EJ, Coid B, *et al.* Heritability estimates for psychotic disorders. *Arch Gen Psychiatry* 1999;**56**:162-8.

47 Gottesman II, Bertelsen A. Confirming unexpressed genotypes for schizophrenia. *Arch Gen Psychiatry* 1989;**46**:867-72.

48 McGuffin P, Reveley A, Holland A. Identical triplets: non-identical psychosis? *Br J Psychiatry* 1982;**140**:1-6.

49 Mendlewicz J, Rainer JD. Adoption study supporting genetic transmission in manic-depressive illness. *Nature* 1977;**268**:327-9.

50 Wender PH, Kety SS, Rosenthal D, Schlusinger F, Ortmann J, Lunde I. Psychiatric disorders in the biological and adoptive families of adopted individuals with affective disorders. *Arch Gen Psychiatry* 1986;**43**:923-9.

51 Craddock N. *Genetic linkage and association studies of bipolar disorder.* PhD thesis, University of Wales, 1995.

52 Craddock N, Owen M. Chromosomal aberrations and bipolar affective disorder. *Br J Psychiatry* 1994;**164**:507-12.

53 Craddock N, Owen M. Is there an inverse relationship between Down's syndrome and bipolar affective disorder? Literature review and genetic implications. *J Intellect Dis Res* 1994;**38**:613-20.

54 Crowe RR, Smouse PE. The genetic implications of age-dependent penetrance in manic-depressive illness. *J Psychiatr Res* 1977;**13**:273.

55 Spence MA, Flodman PL, Sadovnik AD, Bailey-Wilson JE, Ameli H, Remick RA. Bipolar disorder: evidence for a major locus. *Am J Med Genet (Neuropsychiatr Genet)* 1995; **60**:370-6.

56 Bucher KD, Elston RC, Green R, *et al.* The transmission of manic depressive illness—II. Segregation analysis of three sets of family data. *J Psychiatr Res* 1981;**16**:65-78.

57 Goldin LR, Gershon ES, Targum SD, Sparkes RS, McGinnis M. Segregation and linkage analyses in families of patients with bipolar, unipolar, and schizoaffective mood disorders. *Am J Hum Genet* 1983;**45**:274-87.

58 Sham PC, Morton NE, Rice JP. Segregation analysis of the NIMH Collaborative study. Family data on bipolar disorder. *Psychiatr Genet* 1991;**2**:175-84.

59 Craddock N, Van Eerdewegh P, Reich T. Single major locus models for bipolar disorder are implausible. *Am J Med Genet* 1997;**74**:18.

60 Craddock N, Khodel V, Van Eerdewegh P, Reich T. Mathematical limits of multilocus models: the genetic transmission of bipolar disorder. *Am J Hum Genet* 1995;**57**: 690-702.

61 Rosanoff AJ, Handy LM, Plesset IR. The etiology of manic-depressive syndromes with special reference to their occurrence in twins. *Am J Psychiatry* 1935;**91**:725-62.

62 Reich T, Clayton P, Winokur G. Family history studies. V. The genetics of mania. *Am J Psychiatry* 1969;**125**:1358-68.

63 Mendlewicz J, Fleiss JL, Fieve RR. Evidence for X-linkage in the transmission of manic-depressive illness. *JAMA* 1972;**222**:1624.

64 Baron M, Risch N, Hamburger R, *et al.* Genetic linkage between X-chromosome markers and bipolar affective illness. *Nature* 1987;**326**:289-92.

65 Hebebrand J. A critical appraisal of X-linked bipolar illness. Evidence for the assumed mode of inheritance is lacking. *Br J Psychiatry* 1992;**160**:7-11.

66 Risch N, Baron M, Mendlewicz J. Assessing the role of X-linked inheritance in bipolar-related major affective disorder. *J Psychiatr Res* 1986;**20**:275-88.

67 Collins FS. Positional cloning moves from periditional to traditional. *Nat Genet* 1995;**9**:347-50.

68 Craddock N, Owen MJ. Modern molecular genetic approaches to psychiatric disease. *Br Med Bull* 1996;**52**: 434-52.

69 Egeland JA, Gerhard DS, Pauls DL, *et al.* Bipolar affective disorders linked to DNA markers on chromosome 11. *Nature* 1987;**325**:783-7.

70 Kelsoe JR, Ginns EI, Egeland JA, *et al.* Re-evaluation of the linkage relationship between chromosome 11p loci and the gene for bipolar affective disorder in the Old Order Amish. *Nature* 1989;**342**:238-43.

71 Baron M, Freimer NF, Risch N, *et al.* Diminished support for linkage between manic-depressive illness and X-chromosome markers in three Israeli pedigrees. *Nat Genet* 1993;**3**:49-55.

72 Gill M, Craddock N. The Wellcome Trust UK-Irish bipolar sib pair study: sample and study design. *Am J Med Genet* 1998;**81**:461.

73 Suarez BK, Hample CL, Van Eerdewegh P. *Problems of replicating linkage claims in psychiatry. Genetic approaches to mental disorders.* Washington DC: American Psychiatric Press, 1994:23-46.

74 Lander ES, Schork NJ. Genetic dissection of complex traits. *Science* 1994;**265**:2037-48.

75 Kruglyak L, Lander ES. High-resolution genetic mapping of complex traits. *Am J Hum Genet* 1995;**56**:1212-23.

76 Craddock N, Lendon C. Chromosome Workshop. Chromosomes 11, 14, and 15. *Am J Med Genet (Neuropsychiatr Genet)* 1999;**88**:244-54.

77 Van Broeckhoven D, Verheyen G. Chromosome 18 workshop. *Psychiatr Genet* 1998;**8**:97-108.

78 Ewald H, Mors O, Flint T, Koed K, Eiberg H, Kruse TA. A possible locus for manic depressive illness on chromosome 16p13. *Psychiatr Genet* 1995;**5**:71-81.

79 Pekkarinen PJ, Bredbacka PE, Loonqvist J, Peltonen L. Evidence of a predisposing locus to bipolar disorder on Xq24-q27.1 in an extended Finnish pedigree. *Genome Res* 1995; **5**:105-15.

80 Risch N, Merikangas K. The future of genetic studies of complex human diseases. *Science* 1996;**273**:1516-17.

81 Sobell JL, Heston LL, Sommer SS. Delineation of genetic predisposition to multifactorial disease: a general approach on the threshold of feasibility. *Genomics* 1992;**12**:1-6.

82 Falk CT, Rubinstein P. Haplotype relative risks: an easy and reliable way to construct a proper control sample for risk calculations. *Ann Hum Genet* 1987;**51**:227-33.

83 Schaid DJ, Sommer SS. Comparison of statistics for candidate-gene association studies using cases and parents. *Am J Hum Genet* 1994;**55**:402-9.

84 Spielman RS, McGinnis RE, Ewens WJ. Transmission test for linkage disequilibrium: the insulin gene region and insulin-dependent diabetes mellitus (IDDM). *Am J Hum Genet* 1993;**52**:506-16.

85 Collier DA, Stober G, Li T, *et al.* A novel functional polymorphism within the promoter of the serotonin transporter gene: possible role in susceptibility to affective disorder. *Mol Psychiatry* 1996;**1**:453-60.

86 Rees M, Norton N, Jones I, *et al.* Association studies of bipolar disorder at the human serotonin transporter gene (hSERT; 5HTT). *Mol Psychiatry* 1997;**2**:398-402.

87 Kunugi H, Hattori M, Kato T, *et al.* Serotonin transporter gene polymorphisms; ethnic difference and possible association with bipolar affective disorder. *Mol Psychiatry* 1997;**2**:457-62.

88 Kirov G, Rees M, Jones I, McCandless F, Owen MJ, Craddock N. Bipolar disorder and the serotonin transporter gene: a family-based association study. *Psychol Med* (in press).

89 Vincent JB, Masellis M, Lawrence J, *et al.* Genetic association analysis of serotonin system genes in bipolar affective disorder. *Am J Psychiatry* 1999;**156**:136-8.

90 Battersby S, Ogilvie AD, Smith CAD, *et al.* Structure of a variable number tandem repeat of the serotonin transporter gene and association with affective disorder. *Psychiatr Genet* 1996;**6**:177-81.

91 Stöber G, Heils A, Lesch KP. Serotonin transporter gene polymorphism and affective disorder. *Lancet* 1996;**347**: 1340-1.

92 Bellivier F, Laplanche JL, Leboyer M, *et al.* Serotonin transporter gene and manic depressive illness: an association study. *Biol Psychiatry* 1997;**41**:750-2.

93 Furlong RA, Ho L, Walsh C, *et al.* Analysis and meta-analysis of two serotonin transporter gene polymorphisms in bipolar and unipolar affective disorders. *Am J Med Genet (Neuropschiatr Genet)* 1998;**81**:58-63.

94 Hoehe MR, Wendel B, Grunewald I, *et al.* Serotonin transporter (5-HTT) gene polymorphisms are not associated with susceptibility to mood disorders. *Am J Med Genet (Neuropsychiatr Genet)* 1998;**81**:1-3.

95 O'Donovan MC, Owen MJ. Dynamic mutations and psychiatric genetics. *Psychol Med* 1996;**26**:1-6.

96 Schalling M, Hudson TJ, Buetow KH, Houseman DE. Direct detection of novel expanded trinucleotide repeats in the human genome. *Nat Genet* 1993;**4**:135-9.

97 Lindblad K, Nylander PO, De Bruyn A, *et al.* Detection of expanded CAG repeats in bipolar affective disorder using the repeat expansion detection (RED) method. *Neurobiol Dis* 1995;**2**:55-62.

98 O'Donovan MC, Guy C, Craddock N, *et al.* Expanded CAG repeats in schizophrenia and bipolar disorder. *Nat Genet* 1995:**10**:380-1.

99 O'Donovan MC, Guy C, Craddock N, *et al.* Confirmation of association between expanded CAG/CTG repeats and both schizophrenia and bipolar disorder. *Psychol Med* 1996;**26**:1145-53.

100 Oruc L, Lindblad K, Verheyen GR, *et al.* CAG repeat expansions in bipolar and unipolar disorders. *Am J Hum Genet* 1997;**60**:730-2.

101 Vincent JB, Klempan T, Parikh SS, *et al.* Frequency analysis of large CAG/CTG trinucleotide repeats in schizophrenia and bipolar affective disorder. *Mol Psychiatry* 1996;**1**: 141-8.

102 Lindblad K, Nylander PO, Zander C, *et al.* Two commonly expanded CAG/CTG repeat loci: involvement in affective disorders? *Mol Psychiatry* 1998;**3**:405-10.

103 Craddock N, McKeon P, Moorhead S, *et al.* Expanded CAG/CTG repeats in bipolar disorder: no correlation with phenotypic measures of illness severity. *Biol Psychiatry* 1997;**42**:876-81.

104 Coryell W, Endicott J, Keller M. Rapidly cycling affective disorder. Demographics, diagnosis, family history, and course. *Arch Gen Psychiatry* 1992;**49**:126-31.

105 Nurnberger J, Guroff JJ, Hamovit J, Berrettini W, Gershon E. A family study of rapid-cycling bipolar illness. *J Affect Disord* 1988;**15**:87-91.

106 Wehr TA, Sack DA, Rosenthal NE, Cowdry RW. Rapid cycling affective disorder: contributing factors and treatment responses in 51 cases. *Am J Psychiatry* 1988;**145**:179-84.

107 Lachman HM, Morrow B, Shprintzen R, *et al.* Association of codon 108/158 catechol-O-methyltransferase gene polymorphism with the psychiatric manifestations of velo-cardio-facial syndrome. *Am J Med Genet (Neuropsychiat Genet)* 1996;**67**:468-72.

108 Kirov G, Murphy KC, Arranz MJ, *et al.* Low activity allele of catechol-O-methyltransferase gene associated with rapid cycling bipolar disorder. *Mol Psychiatry* 1998;**3**:342-5.
109 Papolos DF, Veit S, Faedda GL, Saito T, Lachman HM. Ultra-ultra rapid cycling bipolar disorder is associated with the low activity catecholamine-O-methyltransferase allele. *Mol Psychiatry* 1998;**3**:346-9.
110 Madden PAF, Heath AC, Rosenthal NE, Martin NG. Seasonal changes in mood and behavior—the role of genetic factors. *Arch Gen Psychiatry* 1996;**53**:47-55.
111 Allen JM, Lam RW, Remick RA, Sadovnick AD. Depressive symptoms and family history in seasonal and nonseasonal mood disorders. *Am J Psychiatry* 1993;**150**: 443-8.
112 Thompson C, Childs PA, Martin NJ, Rodin I, Smythe PJ. Effects of monitoring phototherapy on circadian markers in seasonal affective disorder. *Br J Psychiatry* 1997;**170**:431-5.
113 Brockington IF. Motherhood and mental health. Oxford: Oxford University Press, 1996.
114 Jones IR, McCandless F, Morey J, Benjamin J, Brockington I, Craddock N. Molecular genetic approaches to puerperal psychosis. *Am J Med Genet* 1998;**81**:544.
115 Lykken D, Tellegen A. Happiness is a stochastic phenomenon. *Psychol Science* 1996;**7**:186-9.
116 Nuffield Council on Bioethics. *Mental disorders and genetics: the ethical context*. London: Nuffield Council on Bioethics, 1998.
117 Blackwood DHR, He L, Morris SW, *et al.* A locus for bipolar affective disorder on chromosome 4p. *Nat Genet* 1996;**12**:427-30.
118 Asherson P, Mant R, Williams N, *et al.* A study of chromosome 4p markers and dopamine D5 receptor gene in schizophrenia and bipolar disorder. *Mol Psychiatry* 1998;**3**: 310-20.
119 Craddock N, Owen M, Burge S, Kurian B,Thomas P, McGuffin P. Familial cosegregation of major affective disorder and Darier's disease (keratosis follicularis). *Br J Psychiatry* 1994;**164**:355-8.
120 Craddock N, Dawson E, Burge S, *et al.* The gene for Darier's disease maps to chromosome 12q23-q24.1. *Hum Mol Genet* 1993;**2**:1941-3.
121 Sakuntabhai A, Ruiz-Perez V, Carter S, *et al.* Mutations in ATP2A2, encoding a Ca2+ pump, cause Darier disease. *Nat Genet* 1999;**21**:271-7.
122 Dawson E, Parfitt E, Roberts Q, *et al.* Linkage studies of bipolar disorder in the region of the Darier's disease gene on chromosome 12q23-24.1. *Am J Med Genet (Neuropsychiatr Genet)* 1995;**60**:94-102.
123 Barden N, Plante M, Rochette D, *et al.* Genome-wide microsatellite marker linkage study of bipolar affective disorders in a very large pedigree derived from a homogeneous population in Quebec points to susceptibility locus on chromosome 12. *Psychiatr Genet* 1996;**6**:145-6.
124 Ewald H, Degn B, Mors O, Kruse TA. Significant linkage between bipolar affective disorder and chromosome 12q24. *Psychiatr Genet* 1998;**8**:131-40.
125 Berrettini WH, Ferraro TN, Goldin LR, *et al.* Chromosome 18 DNA markers and manic-depressive illness: evidence for a susceptibility gene. *Proc Natl Acad Sci USA* 1994;**91**:5918-21.
126 Stine OC, Xu J, Koskela R, *et al.* Evidence for linkage of bipolar disorder to chromosome 18 with a parent-of-origin effect. *Am J Hum Genet* 1995;**57**:1384-94.
127 Freimer NB, Reus VI, Escamilla MA, *et al.* Genetic mapping using haplotype, association and linkage methods suggests a locus for severe bipolar disorder (BPI) at 18q22-123. *Nat Genet* 1996;**12**:436-41.
128 Straub RE, Lehner T, Luo Y, *et al.* A possible vulnerability locus for bipolar affective disorder on chromosome 21q22.3. *Nat Genet* 1994;**8**:291-6.
129 Detera-Wadleigh SD, Badner JA, Goldin LR, *et al.* Affected sib-pair analyses reveal support of a prior evidence for a susceptibility locus for bipolar disorder, on 21q. *Am J Hum Genet* 1996;**58**:1279-85.
130 Detera-Wadleigh SD, Badner JA, Yoshikawa T, *et al.* Initial genome scan of the NIMH genetics initiative bipolar pedigrees: chromosomes 4, 7, 9, 18, 19, 20, and 21q. *Am J Med Genet* 1997;**74**:254-62.
131 Smyth C, Kalsi G, Curtis D, *et al.* Two-locus admixture linkage analysis of bipolar and unipolar affective disorder supports the presence of susceptibility loci on chromosomes 11p15 and 21q22. *Genomics* 1997;**39**:271-8.
132 Hodgkinson S, Sherrington R, Gurling H, *et al.* Molecular genetic evidence for heterogeneity in manic depression. *Nature* 1987;**325**:805-6.
133 Sandkuyl LA, Ott J. Affective disorders: evaluation of a three-allele model accounting for clinical heterogeneity. *Genet Epidemiol* 1989;**6**:265-9.
134 McInnis MG, McMahon FJ, Chase GA, Simpson SG, Ross CA, DePaulo JR Jr. Anticipation in bipolar affective disorder. *Am J Hum Genet* 1993;**53**:385-90.
135 McMahon FJ, Stine OC, Meyers DA, Simpson SG, DePaulo JR. Patterns of maternal transmission in bipolar affective disorder. *Am J Hum Genet* 1995;**56**:1277-86.

Are Schizophrenic and Bipolar Disorders *Related*? A Review of Family and Molecular Studies

Wade H. Berrettini

Schizophrenic and bipolar disorders are similar in several epidemiologic respects, including age at onset, lifetime risk, course of illness, worldwide distribution, risk for suicide, gender influence (men and women at equal risk for both groups of disorders), and genetic susceptibility. Despite these similarities, schizophrenia and bipolar disorders are typically considered to be separate entities, with distinguishing clinical characteristics, non-overlapping etiologies, and distinct treatment regimens. Over the past three decades, multiple family studies are consistent with greater nosologic overlap than previously acknowledged. Molecular linkage studies (conducted during the 1990s) reveal that some susceptibility loci may be common to both nosologic classes. This indicates that our nosology will require substantial revision during the next decade, to reflect this shared genetic susceptibility, as specific genes are identified. Biol Psychiatry 2000;48:531–538 *© 2000 Society of Biological Psychiatry*

Key Words: Genetic linkage, schizophrenia, bipolar disorder, family studies

Introduction

The hypothesis that schizophrenic (SZ) and bipolar (BP) syndromes share some genetic risk factors is the subject of this article. To consider this question, epidemiologic, family, and molecular linkage studies are reviewed. If there is shared genetic risk for these syndromes, then we might reasonably expect some similarities in epidemiology. Epidemiologic characteristics common to both BP and SZ disorders are reviewed. Further, if there is shared genetic risk for these syndromes, then family studies should reveal some overlap in familial aggregation. Schizophrenic and BP family studies reveal partial overlap in risk for illness. Finally, if there is shared genetic risk, some susceptibility loci (identified through linkage studies) should be common to both disorders. A review of BP and SZ molecular linkage studies reveals several genomic regions potentially relevant to both nosological classes. It is concluded that SZ and BP disorders share some genetic risk factors. It is not the thesis of this article that the two nosologic categories represent a single entity or a continuum, but that the two groups of disorders are more closely related than previously considered.

Epidemiologic Similarities

Bipolar and SZ disorders are common, chronic groups of illnesses that share many epidemiologic features (for review see Nurnberger and Berrettini 1998). They each affect ~1% of the world's populations, occurring at approximately the same rate across all continents. Although they are common in young adulthood (onset of illness typically occurs prior to age 25 years), these disorders are unusual in prepubertal children. Thus, BP and SZ diagnostic categories have similar ages at onset. These two nosologic classes describe psychotic disorders that often assume episodic courses of illness (with partial to complete remissions and clear exacerbations), although relatively chronic, unremitting SZ disorders are frequently encountered. With rare exceptions, BP and SZ disorders are lifelong conditions. In general, once DSM-4 criteria for BP or SZ diagnoses are met, the disorder persists through life. Spontaneous and lifelong (permanent) remissions of either BP or SZ disorders are very unusual. Increased risk for suicide is another characteristic that these two groups of disorders share. Both syndromes affect men and women equally. Familial aggregation has been demonstrated repeatedly for SZ and for BP. Twin and adoption studies of BP and SZ disorders are consistent with substantial heritability. From twin studies, estimates of heritability for these disorders are quite similar: ~50% for SZ disorders and ~65% for BP disorders.

There are, however, clear clinical distinctions between these two nosologic categories, such that their classic presentations are not often mistaken for one another. The majority of BP individuals benefit from lithium therapy, whereas few persons with SZ are helped substantially. Bipolar disorder manifests as a disturbance of mood, whereas SZ is a primary disorder of cognition. There are

From the Department of Psychiatry and the Center for Neurobiology and Behavior, University of Pennsylvania, Philadelphia.

Address reprint requests to Wade H. Berrettini, M.D., Ph.D., Director, Center for Neurobiology and Behavior, University of Pennsylvania School of Medicine, Room 111, Clinical Research Building, 415 Curie Blvd, Philadelphia PA 19104.

Received January 12, 2000; revised March 18, 2000; accepted March 20, 2000.

0006-3223/00/$20.00
PII S0006-3223(00)00883-0

several electrophysiologic (Adler et al 1999; Freedman et al 1997; Ford 1999) abnormalities in SZ that do not characterize BP disorder. In the context of these shared epidemiologic characteristics, is there any evidence that these two syndromal classifications share genetic risk factors? If this hypothesis is true, then we would expect to find increased risk for SZ syndromes among the first-degree relatives of BP probands, and, conversely, increased risk for BP syndromes among the first-degree relatives of SZ probands.

Review of Family Studies

A review of BP family studies reveals the following: First-degree relatives of BP probands are at increased risk for several nosologically related disorders: BPI, BPII (hypomanic and recurrent unipolar [RUP] episodes in the same person), schizoaffective (SA) and RUP (Angst et al 1980; Baron et al 1983; Gershon et al 1982; Helzer and Winokur 1974; James and Chapman 1975; Johnson and Leeman 1977; Maier et al 1993; Weissman et al 1984; Winokur et al 1982, 1995). Despite numerous careful investigations, no study of the first-degree relatives of BP probands reveals increased risk for SZ.

Similarly, a review of SZ family studies reveals that the first-degree relatives of SZ probands are at increased risk for SZ, SA, and RUP disorders (Gershon et al 1988; Maier et al 1993). Kendler et al (1993) describe increased risk for psychotic affective illness among relatives of SZ probands. Despite numerous carefully conducted investigations, no family study of SZ reports increased risk for BP disorders among first-degree relatives of SZ probands; however, the first-degree relatives of SZ probands *and* the first-degree relatives of BP probands are at increased risk for SA and RUP disorders. The overlap in elevated risk for SA and RUP diagnoses is evident. Therefore, these family studies are consistent with *partial* overlap in familial susceptibility for BP and SZ disorders; however, these family studies are limited in size and power. A small increase in risk for SZ among the first-degree relatives of BP probands might have been undetected. There is a need for large, systematic family studies of SA probands.

It is argued here that the epidemiologic and family study similarities suggest that these two *groups* of disorders are more closely related than previously considered. Because BP and SZ nosologic classes each represent multiple disease entities (with some clinical similarities), it is hypothesized here that some of these disease entities might produce syndromes that may be assigned to either nosologic group (BP or SZ), depending on the genetic background on which they arise. This hypothesis implies that the partial overlap in epidemiologic and family studies may originate in genetic susceptibility.

Given the evidence for *partial* overlap in familial susceptibility for BP and SZ disorders, one may ask whether the overlap may have genetic origins. If this partial overlap is genetic, then molecular linkage studies of BP and SZ disorders should have detected some loci in common. The next section will review BP and SZ molecular linkage studies.

Review of BP and SZ Molecular Linkage Studies

In genetic linkage analysis of common complex disorders, failure of subsequent studies to confirm previously nominated susceptibility loci has become commonplace. This is as true for diabetes mellitus (Concannon et al 1998; Hanis et al 1996) as it is for SZ and BP disorders. This failure to confirm has multiple origins. The most important origin is power to detect a susceptibility locus of limited effect size in the presence of genetic heterogeneity. Common, complex disorders (e.g., asthma, epilepsy, diabetes mellitus, and SZ disorders) are most probably the manifestations of multiple susceptibility loci, within an affected individual, which interact with each other and the environment to produce these well-known syndromes. For these disorders, no single susceptibility locus has a major effect on risk for illness in a majority of the ill population. Loci that increase risk by factors greater than 2 are unusual for common, complex disorders. Despite Herculean efforts in numerous disorders, only two loci that increase risk by a factor of >2 in a large fraction of ill people have been detected: one is HLA for insulin-dependent diabetes mellitus (increased risk = ~3 [Davies et al 1994]; the other is apolipoprotein E in late onset Alzheimer's disease (Corder et al 1993; Mayeux et al 1993; Tsai et al 1994). Substantial sample sizes are required to detect such loci which increase risk by factors of ≤2. As Hauser et al (1996) have shown, ~400 affected sibling pairs are needed to have >90% power to detect ($p < .0001$ or log of the odds ratio [LOD] > 3) loci that increase risk by a factor of 2. No single linkage study of BP or SZ disorders published in the 1990s has exceeded this sample size, although meta-analyses of multiple independent data sets have larger sample sizes.

A second major reason for lack of confirmation is a failure to appreciate the limited ability of linkage methods to localize susceptibility genes to small (~5 million base pairs of DNA or ~5 cM) genomic regions. Linkage analyses of complex traits are not able to localize disease genes to narrow (<5 cM) genomic regions with currently available (<2000 affected sibling pairs) sample sizes (Kruglyak and Lander 1995). For example, the BRCA1 gene was cloned (Futreal et al 1994) ~15 cM from the peak of the original LOD score (Hall et al 1990). Roberts et al (1999) simulated linkage studies for a complex, genetically heterogeneous disorder. They found that the 95% confidence interval for location estimates (from simulated linkage studies of 200 affected sibling pairs) is ~30 cM.

A third major reason for lack of confirmation in linkage studies of common complex disorders has been delineated by Suarez et al (1994), who conducted simulation studies to evaluate the power to replicate linkage. They simulated linkage data for a complex disease caused in part by six equally frequent independent (unlinked) disease loci. They found that a larger sample size was required to confirm linkage of a previously detected locus, because independent pedigree samples might (through sampling variation) contain an over-representation of different susceptibility loci, rather than the locus initially detected. Given that investigators often draw their pedigrees from different ethnic backgrounds (in which prevalence of a particular susceptibility locus might vary), sampling variation is an important origin of confirmation failure. Thus, expectations of universal agreement (even when sample size is adequate) regarding susceptibility loci for common complex traits are unrealistic.

Although validity (through confirmation) of previously reported linkages is difficult for common, complex disorders, some guidelines for validity have been proposed (Lander and Kruglyak 1995; Lander and Schork 1994). These guidelines include a threshold for an initial report of "significant" linkage (LOD score = ~3.6 or nominal p = ~.00002) and for confirmation (LOD score = 1.2 or p = ~.01). These guidelines should limit false positives to less than 5%. These thresholds for statistical significance assume analysis of one affection status model (phenotypic definition of caseness), for example BPI, SA, and BPII disorders. If several (overlapping) affection status models are used in multiple linkage analyses (dominant, recessive, and nonparametric approaches) then some "Bonferroni" correction for multiple hypothesis testing may be necessary.

The Lander and Kruglyak (1995) guidelines for statistical significance in linkage studies (LOD score = ~3.6 or nominal p = ~.00002 and one confirmation LOD score = 1.2 or p = ~.01) were determined through simulation to represent a false positive rate less than 5% (one in 20 genome scans). It seems logical that three or more independent studies, each with $p \leq .001$, should provide a similar level of statistical confidence, although this has not been tested through simulation.

If analysis is limited to "confirmed" BP and SZ linkage susceptibility loci, then the risk for false positive conclusions should be minimized. Our approach will have two facets. First, confirmed BP susceptibility loci will be examined, asking the question: Is there at least one report, in this same region, of linkage to SZ with a p value $\leq$ .001? Second, we will examine all confirmed SZ susceptibility loci, asking the question: Is there at least one report, in this same region, of linkage to BP disorder with a p value $\leq$ .001?

Evidence for Linkage of BP and SZ Disorders to 18p11

Berrettini et al (1994, 1997) reported evidence for a BP susceptibility locus on 18p11 using affected sibling pair (ASP) and affected pedigree member (APM) methods ($p = 10^{-4} - 10^{-6}$). Independent evidence of confirmation of this finding was reported by Stine et al (1995), Nothen et al (1999), and Turecki et al (1999). Evidence for linkage was found most often among those families with paternally transmitted illness (Gershon et al 1996; Nothen et al 1999; Stine et al 1995). As part of Genetic Analysis Workshop #10, independent BP chromosome 18 linkage data sets, including ~1200 samples, were assembled for meta-analyses (Goldin et al 1997). An affected sibling pair (n = 382 sibling pairs) meta-analysis yielded $p = 2.8 \times 10^{-8}$ at marker D18S37 (Lin and Bale 1997).

Schwab et al (1998) employed ~20 chromosome 18 markers in a linkage study of 59 multiplex German and Israeli SZ pedigrees, in which there were 24 affective disorder cases (two were BP). When these data were analyzed in two-point parametric methods, the maximum LOD score was 3.1 at D18S53. A multipoint nonparametric analysis revealed p = .002, at D18S53.

One may be concerned that Schwab et al (1998) studied kindreds whose probands were misdiagnosed or unusual in some undetected characteristics; however, the SZ kindreds studied for 18p11 linkage by Schwab et al (1998) are not nosologically or genetically distinct from other multiplex SZ kindreds. If the SZ kindreds of Schwab et al (1998, 1995, 1999) were nosologically unique (perhaps misclassified affective disorder kindreds), then one would not expect to find confirmations of other SZ loci in those kindreds. These kindreds show linkage to chromosome 6p (Schwab et al 1995), as reported in other series of multiplex SZ kindreds (Straub et al 1995; Maziade et al 1997; Moises et al 1995). Similarly, Faraone et al (1998) and Straub et al (1998) report SZ linkage to 10p14, as did Schwab et al (1999). Nosological misclassification does not explain the chromosome 18p11.2 linkage to SZ detected by Schwab et al (1998). Thus, one region of potential overlap in susceptibility for BP and SZ syndromes is 18p11.2.

Evidence for Linkage of SZ and BP Disorders to 13q32

Lin et al (1997) observed a LOD score of 2.58 (p = ~0.001) at 13q32 markers (D13S122 and D13S128) in a linkage study of SZ. Blouin et al (1998), studying independent SZ kindreds, report a p value of .00002 (LOD = 3.6) at the 13q32 marker, D13S174, in 54 SZ kindreds. Subsequently, Brzustowicz et al (1999) confirmed these reports in 21 Canadian SZ families, with a maximal LOD score of 3.92 at the 13q marker D13S793. Thus, there are at least three independent reports, with substantial statistical significance, consistent with a 13q32 SZ susceptibility locus.

Detera-Wadleigh et al (1999) described linkage (p = .00003) to 13q32 markers (D13S1271 and D13S779) in 22 BP kindreds of European ancestry. One may be concerned that the kindreds studied by Detera-Wadleigh et al (1999) were misclassified; however, these kindreds reveal evidence for linkage to 21q21 (Detera-Wadleigh et al 1996), a BP susceptibility locus (see below). Kelsoe et al (1998) reported linkage of BP disorder to 13q32 markers, with LOD = 2.4 at D13S154. Thus, the 13q32 region has a confirmed SZ susceptibility locus, and there are statistically impressive reports of linkage at this locus in BP disorder.

Evidence for Linkage of SZ and BP Disorders to 10p14

In a recent series of articles, Faraone et al (1998), Straub et al (1998) and Schwab et al (1998) reported evidence for linkage of SZ to 10p14 markers. Faraone et al (1998) reported p = .0004 for marker D10S1423 and p = .0006 for D10S582, in a study of 43 American SZ kindreds of European ancestry. Straub et al (1998), in a study of Irish SZ kindreds, reported p = .006 for this region in a multipoint analysis. For marker D10S582, Schwab et al (1998) reported p = .0058 for German SZ kindreds. These three groups of investigators studied independent sets of kindreds that were of general European ancestry. Although no single report was consistent with significant linkage (p = .00002), these three reports probably constitute a true positive linkage, nonetheless.

Foroud et al (2000) studied BP kindreds from the National Institute of Mental Health Genetics Initiative. They found LOD = 2.5 (p = .001) for marker D10S1423. Thus, the 10p14 region may represent a third region of the genome at which there is shared susceptibility for BP and SZ disorders.

Evidence for Linkage of SZ and BP Disorders to 22q11-13

Lachman et al (1996), Edenberg et al (1997), Kelsoe et al (1998), and Detera-Wadleigh et al (1997) described evidence for a BP susceptibility locus on chromosome 22q11-13, near the velo- cardiofacial syndrome (VCFS) locus. Kelsoe et al (1999) report an LOD score of 3.8 at D22S278. Detera-Wadleigh et al (1999) report p = .008 for markers in this region. This VCFS has been associated with microdeletions of the 22q region. These individuals have a psychosis in ~30% of cases. The syndromal form of the psychosis has been termed schizophrenia-like (Pulver et al 1994b), whereas others have described it in terms of bipolar disorder (Carlson et al 1997; Papolos et al 1996). This region of 22q has been implicated in risk for schizophrenia (Gill et al 1996; Pulver et al 1994a). This region represents a fourth area of overlap for BP and SZ susceptibility loci.

Confirmed Susceptibility Loci Unique to BP Disorders

Although there are four regions of the genome (18p11.2, 13q32, 22q11-13, and 10p14) where BP and SZ susceptibility loci may overlap, the reader should not be left with the impression that this is true for all confirmed BP susceptibility loci. In fact, there are multiple other confirmed BP susceptibility loci at which no report is consistent with a SZ susceptibility locus. The "uniquely BP" susceptibility loci are summarized as follows.

Morissette et al (1999) reported evidence for a chromosome 12q24 BP susceptibility locus, detected through study of a population isolate (French ancestry) from the Saguenay River region of Quebec province. The LOD score exceeds 8 in a recent abstract (Barden et al 1998), clearly exceeding guidelines for significant linkage. Independent confirmation of this BP susceptibility locus has been observed by Ewald et al (1998a) in a study of Danish BP kindreds, with LOD = 3.3. Detera-Wadleigh et al (1999) observed modest support for this locus in a study of 22 American kindreds of European origin. There have been no reports of SZ linkage to this region. Thus, the 12q24 region represents a confirmed BP susceptibility locus.

Straub et al (1994) initially described linkage of BP disorder to 21q21 markers, in a study of American and Israeli BP kindreds. One BP pedigree with a LOD score of 3.41 was reported from a series of 57 BP kindreds; further, nonparametric analysis provided evidence for linkage ($p < .0003$ for the phosphofructokinase locus). An emendation of this original work has been published by Aita et al (1999). A confirmation has been described in a two-locus analysis of genotypic data from 21q21 and 11p15.5 (Smyth et al 1996). This 21q21 BP susceptibility locus has been confirmed by Detera-Wadleigh et al (1996), who employed multipoint nonparametric analyses ($p < .001$). Kwok et al (1999) described confirmatory evidence for linkage to this region in nonparametric analyses. Kelsoe et al (1999) reports an LOD of >2 in this region. Morisette et al (1999) also report a confirmation for this locus in a population isolate of French ancestry. There are no reports of SZ susceptibility to this region, suggesting that the 21q21 region harbors a locus that increases risk for BP disorder.

An extended Scottish kindred showed linkage (LOD 4.1 at D4S394) to 4p16 DNA markers (Blackwood et al 1996). Confirmation of the 4p locus has been reported in a paper by Nothen et al (1997), in which increased allele sharing was noted at D4S394 (p = .0009). Another confirmation was described by Ewald et al (1998b), who noted a LOD of 2.0 at D4S394. Ginns et al (1998) reported linkage to this region for a *mental health locus,* meaning absence of any psychiatric disorder. This requires additional investigation. Thus, the 4p16 region has a confirmed BP susceptibility locus. No reports of SZ linkage are known.

A fourth region of the genome that harbors a BP susceptibility locus is 18q22. Stine et al (1995) initially reported linkage to this region in 28 American BP kindreds (LOD is 3.51 for D18S41) and the ASP method (0.00002 at D18S41). In an extension of this work, McMahon et al (1997) provided additional evidence for linkage to 18q21-2 in 30 new BP kindreds. This locus may have been detected by Freimer et al (1996) and McInnes et al (1996) who studied Costa Rican BP kindreds. McInnes et al (1996) described evidence for increased allele sharing at some of the same markers identified by McMahon et al (1997). For example, at D18S55, McMahon et al (1997) reported a nonparametric LOD score of 2.2, whereas McInnes et al (1996) at this same marker report a maximum likelihood estimate of the LOD score as 1.67. Although the genetic map position of greatest significance for these two studies are not identical (see Roberts et al 1999), there is sufficient map location overlap to conclude tentatively that the two studies detect the same locus.

In summary, there are four regions of the genome that appear to harbor unique BP susceptibility loci, including 21q21, 18q22, 12q24, and 4p16. For each of these four regions there are several consistent reports of linkage, indicating that these loci are probably true positives.

Confirmed Susceptibility Loci Unique to SZ Disorders

In parallel to the BP disorders linkage literature, there are SZ susceptibility loci that appear to be unique to that nosologic classification, in that there are no reports of BP disorders linkage to these genomic regions. Straub et al (1995) initially identified SZ linkage in Irish multiplex families to 6p22-24. Confirmations were published by Schwab et al (1995), who studied German SZ kindreds, and by Moises et al (1995). Levinson et al (1996), in a collaborative venture, noted support for this locus in a large data set. Maziade et al (1997) also confirmed this locus. Although no single report among these studies provides significant linkage (Lander and Kruglyak 1995), there is sufficient evidence in the original report and the several confirmations, that this is likely to be a true positive SZ locus on 6p22-24. There are no molecular reports of BP disorders linkage to this region.

A second "unique" SZ susceptibility locus is found on 8p. Blouin et al (1998) reported evidence for a SZ locus at 8p22, in 54 multiplex kindreds. The LOD score, assuming heterogeneity, was 4.5. Nonparametric analysis yielded p = .0001. Brzustowicz et al (1999) studied 21 extended Canadian SZ pedigrees with 8p markers. The maximum multipoint LOD score was 2.1 at D8S136, providing an additional confirmation of an 8p22 SZ locus. Levinson et al (1996), in a multicenter collaborative effort, reported independent results (that did not include the pedigrees of Blouin et al 1998), yielding p = .00018 in this same region of 8p22. Gurling et al (1999), in a study of 13 extended European SZ kindreds, reported an LOD of 3.6 for 8p22 markers. Thus, these reports constitute a confirmed SZ linkage, and there is no report of BP disorders linkage to this region.

A third unique SZ susceptibility locus may be found on 6q21 (Cao et al 1997; Martinez et al 1999). There is no statistically robust ($p \geq .001$) report of BP linkage at this locus.

Summary

A review of epidemiology and family studies suggests some similarities between SZ and BP disorders. Family studies, in particular, suggest partial overlap in risk for SA diagnoses and some affective disorders (Gershon et al 1988; Kendler et al 1993; Maier et al 1993). This overlap is consistent with shared genetic risk.

A review of molecular linkage studies reveals evidence for shared genetic loci at 18p11.2, 22q11-13, 13q32, and 10p14. This is consistent with the family studies. There remain independent BP susceptibility loci at 18q22, 21q21, 4p16, and 12q24, where there are no prominent reports of SZ susceptibility. Similarly, there are confirmed SZ susceptibility loci at 6p22, 6q21, and 8p22, where there are no reports of BP susceptibility. Thus, the molecular reports are consistent with the family studies, in suggesting partial shared genetic risk. The confirmed BP *and/or* SZ susceptibility loci, identified through linkage studies, are summarized in Figure 1.

If there were only a single genomic region of overlap, this might occur randomly; however, there are four genomic regions of overlap for BP and SZ susceptibility loci, observations that are consistent with the family study data. It is possible, however, that these regions of overlap are secondary to sources of error that are *common* to the several BP and

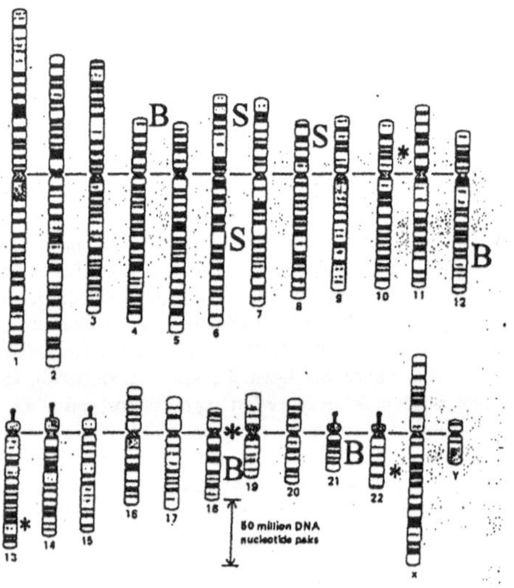

Figure 1. Ideograms of human chromosomes are marked *to the right* with *B* to indicate the location of susceptibility loci unique to bipolar disorder, with *S* to indicate schizophrenic loci, and with * for both bipolar disorder and schizophrenia.

SZ linkage studies. Although this seems improbable, it should be considered carefully in future studies.

It is expected that novel genes, corresponding to these loci, will be identified in the next several years. Direct study of these susceptibility alleles will allow for correlation between genotype and phenotype. Nosology for these disorders must be redefined accordingly, and this will require that we relinquish long-held (mis)conceptions about these disorders. In the bright light of new genetic knowledge concerning the origins of these disorders, we will be able to ask refined questions concerning environmental risk factors. Because environment drives gene expression, knowledge of the environmental risk factors will certainly enhance comprehension at the molecular level. This complex evolution of our understanding of SZ and BP disorder will require several decades at least. As a result of this effort, we can anticipate marked improvements in the outcomes for these disorders, which now shatter the lives of so many.

This article was prepared with the support of NIH Grant MH59553 and a NARSAD Distinguished Investigator Award.

Aspects of this work were presented at the conference, "Bipolar Disorder: From Preclinical to Clinical, Facing the New Millennium," January 19–21, 2000, Scottsdale, Arizona. The conference was sponsored by the Society of Biological Psychiatry through an unrestricted educational grant provided by Eli Lilly and Company.

References

Adler LE, Freedman R, Ross RG, Olincy A, Waldo MC (1999): Elementary phenotypes in the neurobiological and genetic study of schizophrenia. *Biol Psychiatry* 46:8–18.

Aita VM, Liu J, Knowles JA, Terwilliger JD, Baltazar R, Grunn A, et al (1999): A comprehensive linkage analysis of chromosome 21q22 supports prior evidence for a putative bipolar affective disorder locus. *Am J Hum Genet* 64:210–217.

Angst J, Frey R, Lohmeyer R, Zerben-Rubin E (1980): Bipolar manic depressive psychoses: Results of a genetic investigation. *Hum Genet* 55:237–254.

Barden N, Morisette J, Shink E, et al (1998): Confirmation of bipolar affective disorder susceptibility locus on chromosome 12 in the region of the Darier disease gene. *Am J Med Genet* 81:475.

Baron M, Gruen R, Anis L, Kane J (1983): Schizoaffective illness, schizophrenia and affective disorders: Morbidity risk and genetic transmission. *Acta Psychiatr Scand* 65:253–262.

Berrettini W, Ferraro T, Choi H, Goldin L, Detera-Wadleigh SD, Muniec D, et al (1997): Linkage studies of bipolar illness. *Arch Gen Psychiatry* 54:32–39.

Berrettini W, Ferraro T, Goldin L, Weeks D, Detera-Wadleigh SD, Nurnberger JI Jr, Gershon E (1994): Chromosome 18 DNA markers and manic depressive illness: Evidence for a susceptibility gene. *Proc Natl Acad Sci U S A* 91:5918–5921.

Blackwood DHR, He L, Morris SW, McLean A, Whitton C, Thomson M, et al (1996): A locus for bipolar affective disorder on chromosome 4p. *Nat Genet* 12:427–430.

Blouin J-L, Dombroski B, Nath SK, Lasseter VK, Wolyniec PS, Nestadt G, et al: Schizophrenia susceptibility loci on chromosomes 13q32 and 8p21. *Nat Genet* 20:70.

Brzustowicz LM, Honer WG, Chow EWC, Little D, Hogan J, Hodgkinson K, et al (1999): Linkage of famlial schizophrenia to chromosome 13q32. *Am J Hum Genet* 65:1096–1103.

Cao Q, Martinez M, Zhang J, Sanders AR, Badner JA, Cravchik A,et al (1997): Suggestive evidence for a schizophrenia susceptibility locus on chromosome 6q and a confirmation in an independent series of pedigrees. *Genomics* 43:1–8.

Carlson C, Papolos D, Pandita RK, Faedda GL, Veit S, Goldberg R, et al (1997): Molecular analysis of VCFS patients with psychiatric disorders. *Am J Med Genet* 60:851–859.

Concannon P, Gogolin-Ewens KJ, Hinds DA, Wapelhorst B, Morrison VA, Stirling B, et al (1998): A second-generation screen of the human genome for susceptibility to insulin-dependent diabetes mellitus. *Nat Genet* 19:292–296.

Corder EH, Saunders AM, Strittmatter WJ, Schmechel DE, Gaskell PC, Small GW, et al (1993): Gene dose of apolipoprotein E type 4 allele and the risk of Alzheimer's disease in late onset families. *Science* 261:921–923.

Davies JL, Kawaguchi Y, Bennett ST, Copeman JB, Cordell HJ, Pritchard LE, et al (1994): A genome-wide search for human type 1 diabetes susceptibility genes. *Nature* 371:130–136.

Detera-Wadleigh SD, Badner JA, Berrettini WH, Yoshikawa T, Goldin LR, Turner G, et al (1999): Evidence for a bipolar susceptibility locus on 13q32 and other potential loci on 1q32 and 18p11.2. *Proc Natl Acad Sci U S A* 96:5604–5609.

Detera-Wadleigh SD, Badner JA, Goldin LR, Berrettini WH, Sanders AR, Rollins DY, et al (1996): Affected sib-pair analyses reveal support of prior evidence for a susceptibility locus for bipolar disorder on 21q. *Am J Hum Genet* 58:1279–1285.

Detera-Wadleigh SD, Hsieh W-T, Berrettini WH, Goldin LR, Rollins DY, Muniec D, et al (1997): Genetic linkage mapping for a susceptibility locus to bipolar illness: Chromosomes 2, 3, 4, 7, 9, 10p, 11p, 22, and Xpter. *Neuropsychiatr Genet* 74:206–218.

Edenberg H, Foroud T, Conneally M, Sorbel J, Carr K, Crose C, et al (1997): Initial genomic scan of the NIMH genetics initiative bipolar pedigrees: chromosomes 3,5,15,16,17, and 22. *Neuropsychiatr Genet* 74:238–246.

Ewald H, Degn B, Mors B, Kruse TA (1998a): Significant linkage between bipolar affective disorder and chromosome 12q24. *Psychiatr Genet* 8:131–140.

Ewald H, Degn B, Mors B, Kruse TA (1998b): Support for the possible locus on chromosome 4p15 for bipolar affective disorder. *Mol Psychiatry* 3:442–448.

Faraone SV, Matise T, Svrakic D, Pepple J, Malaspina D, Suarez B, et al (1998): Genome scan of European-American schizophrenia kindreds: Results of the NIMH Genetics Initiative and Millenium consortium. *Am J Med Genet* 81:290–295.

Ford J (1999): Schizophrenia: The broken P300 and beyond. *Psychophysiology* 36:667–682.

Foroud T, Castelluccio PF, Keller DL, Edenberg HJ, Mill M, Bowman E, et al (2000): Suggestive evidence of a locus on chromosome 10p using the NIMH Genetics Initiative bipolar affective disorder pedigrees. *Am J Med Genet* 96:18–23.

Freedman R, Coon H, Myles-Worsley M, Orr-Urtreger A, Olincy A, Davis A, et al (1997): Linkage of neurophysiological deficit in schizophrenia to a chromosome 15 locus. *Proc Natl Acad Sci U S A* 94:587–592.

Freimer NB, Reus VI, Escamilla MA, McInnes LA, Spesny M, Leon P, et al (1996): Genetic maping using haplotype, association and linkage methods suggests a locus for severe bipolar disorder (BPI) at 18q22–q23. *Nat Genet* 12:436–441.

Futreal PA, Liu Q, Shattuck-Eidens D, Cochran C, Harshman K, Tavtigian S, et al (1994): BRCA1 mutations in primary breast and ovarian carcinomas. *Science* 266:120–122.

Gershon ES, Badner JA, Ferraro TN, Detera-Wadleigh S, Berrettini WH (1996): Maternal inheritance and chromosome 18 allele sharing in unilineal bipolar illness pedigrees. *Neuropsychiatr Genet* 67:1–8.

Gershon ES, DeLisi LE, Hamovit J, Nurnberger JI Jr, Maxwell ME, Schreiber J, et al (1988): A controlled family study of chronic psychoses. *Arch Gen Psychiatry* 45:328–336.

Gershon ES, Hamovit J, Guroff JJ, Dibble E, Leckman JF, Sceery W, et al (1982): A family study of schizoaffective, bipolar I, bipolar II, unipolar, and normal control probands. *Arch Gen Psychiatry* 39:1157–1167.

Gill M, Vallada H, Collier D, Sham P, Holmans P, Murray R, et al (1996): A combined analysis of D22S278 marker alleles in affected sib-pairs: Support for a susceptibility locus for schizophrenia at chromosome 22q12. *Am J Med Genet* 67:40–45.

Ginns EI, St Jean P, Philibert RA, Galdzicka M, Damschroder-Williams P, Thiel B, et al (1998): A genome search for chromosomal loci linked to mental health wellness in relatives at high risk for bipolar affective disorder among the Old Order Amish. *Proc Natl Acad Sci U S A* 95:15531–15536.

Goldin LR, Gershon ES, Berrettini WH, Stine OC, DePaulo R, McMahon F, et al (1997): Description of the Genetic Analysis Workshop 10 bipolar disorder linkage data sets. *Genet Epidemiol* 14:563–568.

Gurling HMD, Kalsi G, Blaveri E, McQuillin A, Read I, Murphy P, et al (1999): Initial genome wide parametric genetic linkage analysis of schizophrenia and schizophrenia spectrum disorders finds LOD scores above 3.00 on four chromosomes at 1q22–23, 5q22–35, 8p21–23 and 11q14–24. *Mol Psychiatry* 4(suppl):S4.

Hall JM, Lee MK, Newman B, Morrow JE, Anderson LE, Nuey B, et al (1990): Linkage of early-onset familial breast cancer to chromosome 17q21. *Science* 250:1684–1690.

Hanis CL, Boerwinkle E, Chakraborty R, Ellsworth DL, Concannon P, Stirling B, et al (1996): A genome-wide search for human non-insulin-dependent (type 2) diabetes genes reveals a major susceptibility locus on chromosome 2. *Nat Genet* 13:161–166.

Hauser ER, Boehnke M, Guo S-W, Risch N (1996): Affected sib pair interval mapping and exclusion for complex genetic traits. *Genet Epidemiol* 13:117–137.

Helzer JE, Winokur G (1974): A family interview study of male manic-depressives. *Arch Gen Psychiatry* 31:73–77.

James NM, Chapman CJ (1975). A genetic study of bipolar affective disorder. *Br J Psychiatry* 126:449–456.

Johnson GFS, Leeman MM (1977): Analysis of familial factors in bipolar affective illness. *Arch Gen Psychiatry* 34:1074–1083.

Kelsoe JR, Loetscher E, Spence MA, Foguet M, Sadovnick AD, Remick RA, et al (1998): A susceptibility locus for bipolar disorder on chromosome 22: Results of a genome survey. *Am J Hum Genet* 63(suppl):A295.

Kelsoe JR, Spence MA, Loetscher E, Sadovnick AD, Remick RA, Keck PE, et al (1999): A genome survey indicates a susceptibility locus for bipolar disorder on chromosome 22. *Mol Psychiatry* 4(suppl 1):S74.

Kendler KS, McGuire M, Gruenberg AM, O'Hare A, Spellman M, Walsh D (1993): The Roscommon family study. *Arch Gen Psychiatry* 50:527–540.

Kruglyak L, Lander ES (1995): High-resolution genetic mapping of complex traits. *Am J Hum Genet* 57:1212–1223.

Kwok JB, Adams LJ, Salmon JA, Donald JA, Mitchell PB, Schofield PR (1999): Non-parametric simulaton-based statistical analyses for bipolar affective disorder locus on chromosome 21q22.3. *Am J Med Genet* 88:99–102.

Lachman HM, Kelsoe JR, Remick RA, Sadovnick AD, Rapaport MH, Lin M, et al (1996): Linkage studies support a possible locus for bipolar disorder in the velocardiofacial syndrome region on chromosome 22. *Am J Med Genet* 74:121–128.

Lander E, Kruglyak L (1995): Genetic dissection of complex traits: Guidelines for interpreting and reporting linkage results. *Nat Genet* 11:241–247.

Lander E, Schork N (1994): Genetic dissection of complex traits. *Science* 265:2037–2048.

Levinson DF, Schizophrenia Linkage Collaborative Group (1996): Additional support for schizophrenia linkage for chromosomes 6 and 8. *Am J Med Genet* 67:580–594.

Lin JP, Bale SJ (1997): Parental transmission and D18S37 allele sharing in bipolar affective disorder. *Genet Epidemiol* 14:665–668.

Maier W, Lichtermann D, Minges J, Hallmayer J, Heun R, Benkert O, et al (1993): Continuity and discontinuity of affective disorders and schizophrenia. Results of a controlled family study. *Arch Gen Psychiatry* 50:871–883.

Martinez M, Goldin LR, Cao Q, Zhang J, Sanders AR, Nancarrow DJ, et al (1999): Follow-up study on a susceptibility locus for schizophrenia on chromosome 6q. *Am J Med Genet* 88:337–343.

Mayeux R, Stern Y, Ottman R, Tatemichi TK, Tang MX, Maestre G, et al (1993): The apolipoprotein E4 allele in patients with Alzheimer's disease. *Ann Neurol* 34:752–754.

Maziade M, Bissonnette L, Rouillard E, Martinez M, Turgeon M, Charron L, et al (1997): 6p24–22 region and major psychoses in the eastern Quebec population. *Am J Med Genet* 74:311–318.

McInnes LA, Escamilla MA, Service SK, Reus VI, Leon P, Silva S, et al (1996): A complete genome screen for genes predisposing to severe bipolar disorder in two Costa Rican pedigrees. *Proc Natl Acad Sci U S A* 93:13060–13065.

McMahon FJ, Hopkins PJ, Xu J, McInnis MG, Shaw S, Cardon L, et al (1997): Linkage of bipolar affective disorder to chromosome 18 markers in a new pedigree series. *Am J Hum Genet* 61:1397–1404.

Moises HW, Yang L, Kristbjarnarson H, Wiese C, Byerley W, Macciardi F, et al (1995): An international two-stage genome-wide search for schizophrenia susceptibility genes. *Nat Genet* 11:321–324.

Morissette J, Villeneuve A, Bordeleau L, Rochette D, Laberge C, Gagne B, et al (1999): Genome-wide search for linkage of bipolar affective disorders in a very large pedigree derived from a homogeneous population in Quebec points to a locus of major effect on chromosome 12q23–q24. *Am J Med Genet* 88:567–587.

Nothen MM, Cichon S, Franzek E, Albus M, Bormann M, Rietschel R, et al (1997): Systematic search for susceptibility genes in bipolar affective disorder—evidence for disease loci at 18p and 4 p. *Am J Hum Genet* 61S:A288.

Nothen MM, Cichon S, Rohleder H, Hemmer S, Franzek E, Fritze J, et al (1999): Evaluation of linkage of bipolar affective disorder to chromosome 18 in a sample of 57 German families. *Mol Psychiatry* 4:76.

Nurnberger JI Jr, Berrettini WH (1998): *Psychiatric Genetics.* London: Chapman and Hall.

Papolos DF, Faedda GL, Veit S, Goldberg R, Morrow B, Kucherlapati R, et al (1996): Bipolar spectrum disorders in patients diagnoses with VCFS: Does a hemizygous deletion of chromosome 22q11 result in bipolar affective disorder? *Am J Psychiatry* 153:1541–1547.

Pulver AE, Karayiorgou M, Wolyniec PS, Lasseter VK, Kasch L, Nestadt G, et al (1994a): Sequential strategy to identify a susceptibility gene for schizophrenia: report of potential linkage on chromosome 22q12–q13.1: Part 1. *Am J Med Genet* 54:36–43.

Pulver AE, Nestadt G, Goldberg R, Shprintzen RJ, Lamacz M, Wolyniec PS, et al (1994b): Psychotic illness in patients diagnosed with velo-cardio-facial syndrome and their relatives. *J Nerv Ment Dis* 182:476–478.

Roberts SB, MacLean CJ, Neale MC, Eaves LJ, Kendler KS (1999): Replication of linkage studies of complex traits: An examination of variation in location estimates. *Am J Hum Genet* 65:876–884.

Schwab SG, Albus M, Hallmayer J, Honig S, Borrmann, Lichtermann D, et al (1995): Evaluation of a susceptibility gene for schizophrenia on chromosome 6p by multipoint affected sib-pair linkage analysis. *Nat Genet* 11:325–327.

Schwab SG, Hallmayer J, Albus M, Lerer B, Hanses C, Kanyas K, et al (1999): Further evidence for a susceptibility locus on chromosome 10p14–p11 in 72 families with schizophrenia by non-parametric linkage analysis. *Am J Med Genet* 81:302–307.

Schwab SG, Hallmayer J, Lerer B, Albus M, Borrmann M, Honig S, et al (1998): Support for a chromosome 18p locus conferring susceptibility to functional psychoses in families with schizophrenia, by association and linkage analysis. *Am J Hum Genet* 63:1139.

Smyth C, Kalsi G, Brynjolfsson J, O'Neill J, Curtis D, Rifkin L, et al (1996): Further tests for linkage of bipolar affective disorder to the tyrosine hydroxylase gene locus on chromosome 11p15 in a new series of multiplex British affective disorder pedigrees. *Am J Psychiatry* 153:271–274.

Stine OC, Xu J, Koskela R, McMahon FJ, Geschwend M, Friddle C, et al (1995): Evidence for linkage of bipolar disorder to chromosome 18 with a parent-of-origin effect. *Am J Hum Genet* 57:1384–1394.

Straub RE, Lehner T, Luo Y, Loth JE, Shao W, Sharpe L, et al (1994): A possible vulnerability locus for bipolar affective disorder on chromosome 21q22.3. *Nat Genet* 8:291–296.

Straub RE, MacLean CJ, Martin RB, Ma Y, Myakishev MV, Harris-Kerr C, et al (1998): A schizophrenia locus may be located in region 10p15–p11. *Am J Med Genet* 81:296–301.

Straub RE, MacLean CJ, O'Neill FA, Burke J, Murphy B, Duke F, et al (1995): A potential vulnerability locus for schzophrenia on chromosome 6p22–24: Evidence for genetic heterogeneity. *Nat Genet* 11:287–293.

Suarez B, Harpe CL, Van Eerdewegh P (1994): Problems of replicating linkage claims in psychiatry. In: Gershon ES, Cloninger CR, editors. *Genetic Approaches to Mental Disorders. Proceedings of the 82nd Annual Meeting of the American Psychopathological Association.* Washington, DC: American Psychiatric Press, 23–46.

Tsai M-S, Tangalos EG, Petersen RC, Smith GE, Schaid DJ, Kokmen E, et al (1994): Apolipoprotein E: Risk factor for Alzheimer disease. *Am J Hum Genet* 54:643–649.

Turecki G, Grof P, Cavazzoni P, Duffy A, Grof E, Martin R, et al (1999): Lithium responsive bipolar disorder, unilineality and chromosome 18: A linkage study. *Am J Med Genet* 88:411–415.

Weissman MM, Gershon ES, Kidd KK, Prusoff BA, Leckman JF, Dibble E, et al (1984): Psychiatric disorders in the relatives of probands with affective disorder. *Arch Gen Psychiatry* 41:13–21.

Winokur G, Coryell W, Keller M, Endicott J, Leon A (1995): A family study of manic-depressive (bipolar I) disease. Is it a distinct illness separable from primary unipolar depression? *Arch Gen Psychiatry* 52:367–373.

Winokur G, Tsuang MT, Crowe RR (1982): The Iowa 500: Affective disorder in relatives of manic and depressed patients. *Am J Psychiatry* 139:209–212.

Article

The Familial Aggregation of Psychotic Symptoms in Bipolar Disorder Pedigrees

James B. Potash, M.D., M.P.H.

Virginia L. Willour, Ph.D.

Yen-Feng Chiu, Ph.D.

Sylvia G. Simpson, M.D., M.P.H.

Dean F. MacKinnon, M.D.

Godfrey D. Pearlson, M.D.

J. Raymond DePaulo, Jr., M.D.

Melvin G. McInnis, M.D.

Objective: Symptomatic overlap between affective disorders and schizophrenia has long been noted. More recently, family and linkage studies have provided some evidence for overlapping genetic susceptibility between bipolar disorder and schizophrenia. If shared genes are responsible for the psychotic manifestations of both disorders, these genes may result in clustering of psychotic symptoms in some bipolar disorder pedigrees. The authors tested this hypothesis in families ascertained for a genetic study of bipolar disorder.

Method: Rates of psychotic symptoms—defined as hallucinations or delusions—during affective episodes were compared in families of 47 psychotic and 18 nonpsychotic probands with bipolar I disorder. The analysis included 202 first-degree relatives with major affective disorder.

Results: Significantly more families of psychotic probands than families of nonpsychotic probands (64% versus 28%) contained at least one relative who had affective disorder with psychotic symptoms. Significantly more affectively ill relatives of psychotic probands than of nonpsychotic probands (34% versus 11%) had psychotic symptoms. An analysis of clustering of psychotic subjects across all families revealed significant familial aggregation. Clustering of psychosis was also apparent when only bipolar I disorder was considered the affected phenotype.

Conclusions: Psychotic bipolar disorder may delineate a subtype of value for genetic and biological investigations. Families with this subtype should be used to search for linkage in chromosomal regions 10p12–13, 13q32, 18p11.2, and 22q11–13, where susceptibility genes common to bipolar disorder and schizophrenia may reside. Putative schizophrenia-associated biological markers, such as abnormal evoked response, oculomotor, and neuroimaging measures, could similarly be explored in such families.

(Am J Psychiatry 2001; 158:1258–1264)

Symptomatic overlap between affective disorders and schizophrenia has long been noted. Even the psychotic, or "positive," symptoms most closely identified with schizophrenia—Schneider's first-rank symptoms—also occur in patients with affective disorder (1). This overlap and other considerations have led some investigators to challenge the dichotomous Kraepelinian classification of the psychoses (2, 3). Recently, overlap has also been noted in the findings from genetic linkage studies of bipolar disorder and schizophrenia. Four chromosomal regions that could potentially harbor susceptibility genes for both disorders have been identified: 10p12–13, 13q32, 18p11.2, and 22q11–13 (reviewed in reference 4). In spite of the limitation imposed by the generally low resolution of linkage data, this overlap has renewed interest in the hypothesis that there are susceptibility genes that contribute to the psychotic manifestations of both bipolar disorder and schizophrenia.

If psychosis genes exist, they may lead to familial aggregation of psychotic symptoms in subjects with familial bipolar disorder. There are suggestions from prior studies that psychotic symptoms cluster in some families with affective disorder, although the evidence to date has been limited. To our knowledge, only one prior study (5) has specifically addressed the hypothesis that psychotic bipolar disorder aggregates in families; the finding was negative in a small study group. In another study (6), in which bipolar disorder and major depression were grouped together, relatives of probands with psychotic affective disorder had a higher rate of psychotic affective disorder than did relatives of nonpsychotic probands, although the difference was not statistically significant. Two studies (7, 8) have provided evidence of familial aggregation of psychotic symptoms in major depression, although in only one of these (7) did the finding reach significance. A follow-up study (9) failed to replicate this significant finding.

We have previously used clinical features in an effort to define a more genetically homogenous group of bipolar disorder families. Bipolar II disorder (10) and comorbid panic disorder (11) have been investigated within our group and have been found to enhance evidence for linkage to chromosome 18q. Here we assess the familial aggregation of psychotic symptoms within bipolar disorder pedigrees to determine whether this feature may increase homogeneity and inform the discussion of possible overlap in genetic susceptibility to bipolar disorder and schizophrenia.

Method

Subjects

Aspects of family ascertainment have been described in detail previously (12). Probands were selected from inpatients and outpatients screened in Baltimore and Iowa City and from individuals who contacted us to volunteer. The ascertainment criteria required a treated proband with bipolar I disorder who had two first-degree relatives who were affected with bipolar I disorder, bipolar II disorder with at least two major depressive episodes, recurrent unipolar depression, or schizoaffective disorder, manic type. In addition, the families had to be unilineal: only one parent could be affected and the unaffected parent could not have any affected first-degree relatives. Five families included in the analysis had only two affected members each. They were ascertained and studied because they had initially appeared to meet the inclusion criterion of three affected members according to family history. Because many useful clinical and genotype data on these families had already been obtained, we included them in the genome-wide scan analysis under way by our group. The 65 families in the genome-wide scan provide the basis for the analyses in this paper.

All available first- and second-degree relatives 14 years old or older, as well as probands themselves, were interviewed by psychiatrists using the Schedule for Affective Disorders and Schizophrenia—Lifetime Version (SADS-L) (13). After complete description of the study to the subjects, written informed consent was obtained. Collateral information from multiple family informants was obtained, and medical records were added whenever possible. Diagnoses of affective disorders were made independently by two psychiatrists using a best-estimate procedure and the Research Diagnostic Criteria (RDC) (14).

First-degree relatives with diagnoses of major affective disorder—bipolar I disorder, bipolar II disorder with at least two major depressive episodes, schizoaffective disorder, manic type, and recurrent unipolar depression—were analyzed in this study. Schizoaffective disorder, manic type, and recurrent unipolar depression were included in addition to bipolar disorder because of genetic epidemiological evidence suggesting that liability to these disorders may be higher than normal in both familial schizophrenia and familial bipolar disorder (see Discussion). In addition, analyses using only relatives with bipolar I disorder were performed. No subjects in the data set were diagnosed with schizophrenia or schizoaffective disorder, depressed type. The presence of psychotic symptoms—defined as hallucinations or delusions (mood-congruent and/or mood-incongruent)—during mania and during depression were assessed by using the SADS-L interview, which elicits information regarding the most severe manic and most severe depressive episode. A total of 45 probands and 52 first-degree relatives were identified as psychotic on the basis of the SADS-L interview alone. Data from family informants and medical records were reviewed to increase the sensitivity of detection of psychotic symptoms. This resulted in the identification of an additional two probands and three relatives as psychotic.

Statistical Analysis

Pearson's chi-square analysis, Fisher's exact test, and Student's t test were used to test differences between the psychotic and nonpsychotic proband groups on diagnostic, demographic, and clinical variables. Three tests of the hypothesis of familial aggregation of psychotic symptoms were performed. The first was a comparison of the proportion of psychotic probands having at least one psychotic relative with affective disorder to the proportion of nonpsychotic probands with at least one such relative; the chi-square test was employed for this comparison. In the second analysis, the odds of being psychotic for first-degree affectively ill relatives of psychotic probands were compared to the odds for those relatives of nonpsychotic probands. This was implemented by using the generalized estimating equation approach (15), which uses logistic regression but has the added advantage of taking into account potential correlation between observations when multiple members of the same family are considered. In these analyses we controlled for sex, age at interview, and duration of illness. A third analysis of familial clustering of psychotic symptoms was performed by testing the distribution of psychosis among the affectively ill subjects (including probands) across all 65 families. The null hypothesis of no familial aggregation of psychotic symptoms was tested by using Tarone's one-sided score test for binomial distributions (16). A low and nonsignificant score indicates the expected random distribution of a variable, in this case psychosis, whereas a high and significant score suggests that the variable clusters more in some families than in others. We repeated these three analyses using only bipolar I disorder as the affected phenotype.

TABLE 1. Percentage of Families Containing First-Degree Relatives With Any Psychotic Affective Disorder and With Psychotic Bipolar I Disorder for Probands With Psychotic and Nonpsychotic Bipolar I Disorder

Family Characteristic	Families of Psychotic Probands (47 families)		Families of Nonpsychotic Probands (18 families)	
	Mean	*SD*	*Mean*	*SD*
First-degree relatives interviewed per family	5.9	2.1	6.3	2.1
First-degree relatives with affective disorder per family	3.1	1.5	3.1	1.3
First-degree relatives with bipolar I disorder per family	1.1	1.2	0.6	0.9
Age of relatives at interview (years)	42.9	14.7	42.0	13.5
	N	*%*	*N*	*%*
Families with one or more first-degree relatives with any psychotic affective disorder[a]	30	63.8	5	27.8
Families with one or more first-degree relatives with psychotic bipolar I disorder[b]	23	48.9	4	22.2

[a] Significant difference between groups (χ^2=6.81, df=1, p=0.009).
[b] Nonsignificant difference between groups (χ^2=3.83, df=1, p<0.06).

Results

Group Characteristics

The subjects included 65 bipolar I disorder probands and 202 affected first-degree relatives. The diagnoses for the affected relatives were as follows: bipolar I disorder, N=60; schizoaffective disorder, manic type, N=6; bipolar II disorder, N=77; and recurrent unipolar depression, N=59. Among the subjects with bipolar I disorder, 71.2% (89 of 125) had psychosis, whereas the figures were 3.9% (three of 77) for bipolar II disorder and 6.8% (four of 59) for recurrent unipolar depression. By definition, all six subjects with schizoaffective disorder, manic type, had psychosis. There were 47 probands with psychotic symptoms and 18 probands with no psychotic symptoms. The psychotic probands had 146 first-degree relatives with affective disorder, and the nonpsychotic probands had 56 such relatives. The two sets of families did not substantially differ in

TABLE 2. Odds of Psychotic Symptoms in First-Degree Relatives With Any Affective Disorder and With Bipolar I Disorder in Families of Probands With Psychotic or Nonpsychotic Bipolar I Disorder

Variable	Odds of Psychotic Symptoms, With Control for Age, Sex, and Duration of Illness, Analyzed With Generalized Estimating Equation					
	Parameter Estimate	SE	z	p	Odds Ratio	95% CI
Relatives with any affective disorder						
Intercept	–2.38	0.72	–3.32	0.0009		
Psychotic proband	1.44	0.48	3.01	0.003	4.22	1.65–10.78
Age	–0.01	0.02	–0.26	0.80	0.99	0.96–1.04
Sex	–0.36	0.28	–1.28	0.20	0.70	0.40–1.21
Duration of illness	0.04	0.02	1.61	0.11	1.04	0.99–1.08
Relatives with bipolar I disorder						
Intercept	–1.20	1.30	–0.92	0.36		
Psychotic proband	1.27	0.69	1.83	0.07	3.56	0.92–13.86
Age	0.01	0.03	0.24	0.81	1.01	0.94–1.08
Sex	–0.26	0.46	–0.56	0.58	0.77	0.31–1.91
Duration of illness	0.04	0.03	1.37	0.17	1.04	0.98–1.11

number of first-degree relatives interviewed per family, number of affected first-degree relatives per family, or age of relatives at the time of interview (Table 1). The proportion of relatives with affective disorder whose specific diagnosis was bipolar I disorder was higher in the families of psychotic probands than in the families of nonpsychotic probands: 50 (34.2%) of 146 versus 10 (17.9%) of 56 (χ^2= 5.21, df=1, p=0.02). The affectively ill relatives of the psychotic probands included six individuals diagnosed with schizoaffective disorder, manic type, while no one with this diagnosis was found among the relatives of nonpsychotic probands; this difference was not significant (six of 146 versus none of 56; Fisher's exact test, p=0.15). The affected relatives of the psychotic probands had significantly more hospitalizations (mean=2.23, SD=4.86) than did the affected relatives of the nonpsychotic probands (mean=0.81, SD=2.01) (t=2.91, df=201, p=0.004). No statistically significant differences were found between affected members of the families of the psychotic and nonpsychotic probands in the following severity indicators: age at onset of affective disorder, duration of longest mood disorder episode, rate of attempted suicide, and rates of alcoholism and substance abuse.

Analysis by Family

Among the families of the psychotic probands, 63.8% contained at least one first-degree relative with psychotic affective disorder (Table 1). Among the families of the nonpsychotic probands, the proportion with psychotic affective disorder in at least one relative was significantly lower, 27.8%. We also did the analysis by considering only subjects with bipolar I disorder as affected. Of the families with psychotic probands, 48.9% contained at least one first-degree relative with psychotic bipolar I disorder, compared to 22.2% of the families of nonpsychotic probands (Table 1).

Analysis by Individuals

Among all first-degree relatives with major affective disorder, 27.2% (55 of 202) had a lifetime history of psychotic symptoms during an affective episode. In the families of psychotic probands, 33.6% (49 of 146) of the relatives with major affective disorder had psychotic symptoms, compared to only 10.7% (six of 56) of those in nonpsychotic families; the difference was statistically significant (Table 2). Psychosis was a feature of 74.0% (37 of 50) of the relatives with bipolar I disorder in the families of the psychotic probands and of 50.0% (five of 10) of the relatives with bipolar I disorder in the families of the nonpsychotic probands. This difference was not statistically significant.

Analysis by Distribution of Family Clusters

Of all probands and their first-degree affected relatives, 38.2% (102 of 267) were psychotic. Analysis of familial clustering was performed to determine whether the distribution of psychotic individuals was uniform throughout the 65 families (the null hypothesis) or, conversely, whether these individuals clustered in some families but not in others. The results indicated significant clustering (Table 3). A subset of 31 families were found to contain two or more psychotic affected subjects; 30 of these families had a psychotic proband. Ten families with three or more psychotic affected members were identified; all of these included a psychotic proband. When we considered only subjects with bipolar I disorder as affected, the evidence for the clustering of psychotic disorder was stronger than in the analysis of all subjects with major affective disorder (Table 4).

Discussion

We have found evidence for the familial aggregation of psychotic symptoms, defined as hallucinations or delusions, in bipolar disorder pedigrees. Four analyses support this: 1) more families with psychotic probands than with nonpsychotic probands had at least one first-degree relative with psychotic affective disorder; 2) among the first-degree affectively ill relatives of psychotic probands, there was a higher rate of psychosis than among comparable relatives of nonpsychotic probands; 3) psychotic affective disorder clustered disproportionately in a subset of families; and 4) the clustering of psychosis was also apparent

TABLE 3. Observed and Expected Distribution of Psychotic Affective Disorder in Families of Probands With Bipolar I Disorder, by Number of Subjects With Any Affective Disorder in a Family (Cluster Size)[a]

Cluster Size and Type of Value	Number of Families Containing Members With Psychotic Affective Disorder, by Number of Psychotic Subjects in Cluster										Total Number of Families
	0	1	2	3	4	5	6	7	8	9	
2											
Observed	0	3	2								5
Expected	1.9	2.4	0.7								
3											
Observed	5	7	4	1							17
Expected	4.0	7.4	4.6	1.0							
4											
Observed	5	5	11	3	2						26
Expected	3.8	9.4	8.7	3.6	0.5						
5											
Observed	3	4	2	0	0	0					9
Expected	0.8	2.5	3.1	1.9	0.6	0.1					
6											
Observed	0	1	1	0	0	0	0				2
Expected[b]	0.1	0.4	0.6	0.5	0.2	0.1	0.0				
7											
Observed	0	0	1	0	2	1	0	0			4
Expected	0.1	0.6	1.1	1.1	0.7	0.3	0.1	0.0			
8											
Observed	0	1	0	0	0	0	0	0	0		1
Expected[b]	0.0	0.1	0.2	0.3	0.2	0.1	0.0	0.0	0.0		
9											
Observed	0	0	0	0	0	0	1	0	0	0	1
Expected	0.0	0.1	0.2	0.3	0.2	0.1	0.1	0.0	0.0	0.0	
All families	13	21	21	4	4	1	1	0	0	0	65

[a] Tarone's one-sided score test for binomial distributions was used to compare the observed and expected values under the null hypothesis of a random distribution of psychotic subjects in these families. The result showed a significant deviation from the expected distribution (χ^2= 13.17, df=1, p=0.0003).

[b] The sum of the values in this row does not equal the sum of the respective observed values because of rounding.

when only subjects with bipolar I disorder were considered as affected.

A strength of this study is that all of the diagnostic interviews were done by psychiatrists, thus maximizing the chance of eliciting valid reports of psychotic symptoms. In addition, the reliability of the assessment of hallucinations and delusions with the SADS-L has previously been demonstrated to be excellent (13). The test-retest reliability for the diagnosis of psychotic bipolar disorder was also found to be good to excellent in another study using the SADS-L (17). Even so, the SADS-L assesses only the most severe manic and depressive episodes; it does not require the interviewer to ask about each lifetime episode, so that a psychotic affective episode could be missed.

This study used a narrow definition of psychosis. We did not assess formal thought disorder or disorganized behavior even though these features are often considered psychotic. Although formal thought disorder is assessed by the SADS-L, it has been shown to have lower reliability than hallucinations and delusions (13). Prior analyses of the structure of psychosis (18) have suggested that hallucinations and delusions may be independent of thought disorder and disorganization, however, so that our narrow definition of psychosis may be helpful in our pursuit of a genetically more homogeneous subtype of bipolar disorder.

We considered whether hallucinations and delusions were just one aspect of a broader severity that was familial. No statistically significant differences in most severity indicators were found between relatives in the families of psychotic and nonpsychotic probands. However, two significant differences were found: an excess of bipolar I disorder subjects and more hospitalizations in the families of psychotic probands. The higher rate of hospitalization is not surprising given that psychotic symptoms generally lead to impaired judgment and thus to potential dangerousness. The finding that a higher rate of psychosis is associated with a higher rate of bipolar I disorder is not unexpected given that mania is associated with a substantially higher rate of psychosis than is depression (19). Among the relatives with psychotic bipolar I disorder, all but two experienced psychosis during mania (the two exceptions were psychotic only during depression). In order to assess whether the clustering of psychosis in families was independent of the clustering of bipolar I disorder in families, we did separate analyses in which we considered only bipolar I disorder as the affected phenotype. Analysis by family and analysis by individual relative yielded differences in the rate of psychosis between proband groups that were not statistically significant. Application of the third analytic method to the phenotype of bipolar I disorder only, however, resulted in a highly significant clustering of psychosis; this latter method had more power than the first two to detect familial aggregation of psychotic symptoms because, by including probands, it took into ac-

TABLE 4. Observed and Expected Distribution of Psychotic Bipolar I Disorder in Families of Probands With Bipolar I Disorder, by Number of Subjects With Bipolar I Disorder in a Family (Cluster Size)[a]

Cluster Size and Type of Value	Number of Families Containing Members With Psychotic Bipolar I Disorder, by Number of Psychotic Subjects in Cluster							Total Number of Families
	0	1	2	3	4	5	6	
1								
Observed	12	17						29
Expected	8.3	20.7						
2								
Observed	2	7	13					22
Expected	1.8	9.0	11.2					
3								
Observed	0	2	2	4				8
Expected	0.2	1.4	3.5	2.9				
4								
Observed	0	1	1	0	1			3
Expected	0.0	0.2	0.8	1.2	0.8			
5								
Observed	0	0	0	0	1	1		2
Expected[b]	0.0	0.0	0.2	0.6	0.7	0.4		
6								
Observed	0	0	0	0	0	1	0	1
Expected	0.0	0.0	0.1	0.2	0.3	0.3	0.1	
All families	14	27	16	4	2	2	0	65

[a] Tarone's one-sided score test for binomial distributions was used to compare the observed values to those expected under the null hypothesis of a random distribution of psychotic subjects in these families. The result showed a significant deviation from the expected distribution (χ^2=21.36, df=1, p=0.000004).

[b] The sum of the values in this row does not equal the sum of the respective observed values because of rounding.

count more than double the number of subjects with bipolar I disorder.

These results are consistent with some (6–8), but not all (5, 9), previous findings on familial aggregation of psychotic affective disorder. One study, by Winokur et al. (5), specifically had a negative result in a study group restricted to bipolar disorder. One explanation for the difference between that result and ours may lie in the different inclusion criteria used: the Winokur et al. study used only relatives with psychiatric records (N=43), whereas we assessed all available relatives. Our study group therefore included 108 relatives without psychiatric records among 137 total relatives with bipolar disorder (after exclusion of relatives of probands with schizoaffective disorder, manic type, and recurrent unipolar depression, as in the study by Winokur et al.). The relatives with records were significantly more likely to be psychotic than those without records. Among our bipolar disorder relatives with records, 48.3% (14 of 29) were psychotic, whereas among those without records the figure was 28.7% (31 of 108) (χ^2= 3.97, df=1, p=0.05). Because the Winokur et al. analysis omitted those without records, many nonpsychotic relatives may have been excluded, and, in the presence of familial aggregation of psychotic symptoms, those excluded would have been disproportionately relatives of nonpsychotic probands, thus biasing the study group toward a negative finding.

Our findings should be considered in the context of other studies of several types that have yielded evidence to support the utility of subtyping by the presence of psychosis. These can be grouped into clinical studies, family studies, and biological studies.

1. Clinical studies have included those that assessed symptoms, course of illness, and treatment response. Two studies using factor analysis to assess the underlying structure of symptoms in mania have demonstrated an independent psychotic factor based on the presence of hallucinations and delusions (20, 21). One study (22) was an assessment of the factor structure of familial bipolar disorder and produced evidence for the three-factor model of negative, psychotic, and disorganized dimensions. Investigations on the course of illness have shown that, compared to nonpsychotic bipolar subjects, subjects with psychosis have an earlier onset (23), more impaired functioning over time (24–26), and a higher rate of relapse at 4-year follow-up (24). One study, however, did not show differences in functioning (27). The findings of studies assessing treatment response have been more equivocal (28–31).

2. Family studies have suggested shared liability between psychotic affective disorder and schizophrenia, although the evidence for overlapping liability between bipolar disorder (irrespective of psychotic symptoms) and schizophrenia is less strong. Three large data sets have been studied to address the issue of overlap between schizophrenia and psychotic affective disorder (6, 32–35). In all three, higher than expected rates of psychotic affective disorder in relatives of schizophrenic probands, and vice versa, were found. Methodologically rigorous studies (36–38), however, have not shown an excess of schizophrenic relatives in families of probands with bipolar disorder or an excess of relatives with bipolar disorder in families of probands with schizophrenia; excess rates of major depression and of schizoaffective disorder were found in both types of families.

3. Biological studies have focused on brain imaging and on neurophysiology. One study (39) indicated anomalous brain asymmetry in the postcentral gyrus in psychotic, but not nonpsychotic, subjects with bipolar disorder. A functional imaging study (40) demonstrated high dopamine D_2 receptor densities in patients with psychotic, but not nonpsychotic, bipolar disorder; the high levels were similar to those seen in schizophrenia patients. Evidence for shorter REM latency in psychotic than in nonpsychotic subjects with depressive episodes (some of whom had bipolar disorder) has been found (41). In two brain imaging studies (42, 43) subjects with psychotic affective disorder and those with schizophrenia had abnormally low volumes of similar regions: the left hippocampus in one study (42) and the left posterior amygdala-hippocampal complex in the other (43).

If subtyping bipolar disorder by the presence of psychosis is biologically meaningful, at least two scenarios seem plausible: there might be a vulnerability to psychosis and a separate vulnerability to bipolar disorder, or there might be a particular vulnerability to psychotic bipolar disorder. Given that psychosis is familial in our study group, either the separate vulnerabilities or the particular vulnerability may be the result of genetic influences. Either scenario would be consistent with the hypothesis that genes increase susceptibility to both psychotic bipolar disorder and to schizophrenia: the separate psychosis vulnerabilities might reflect shared psychosis genes because delusions and hallucinations occur in both disorders; the particular psychotic bipolar disorder vulnerability might reflect genes that predispose to psychotic symptoms and to affective symptoms because affective symptoms frequently co-occur with psychosis not only in bipolar disorder, but also in schizophrenia—there is a high rate of depressive symptoms in schizophrenia (44), and this co-occurrence may be familial (45, 46). Studying bipolar disorder families enriched for the psychotic bipolar disorder subtype could yield greater power to detect genes leading to either of the vulnerabilities described. In this regard, the chromosomal regions 10p12–13, 13q32, 18p11.2, and 22q11–13, which have been implicated in both bipolar disorder and schizophrenia (4), are of particular interest. Further study of families with psychotic bipolar disorder should also focus on putative schizophrenia-associated biological markers, including abnormalities in evoked response, oculomotor, neuroimaging, and cognitive measures (47).

In summary, our data demonstrate that hallucinations and delusions during affective episodes show familial aggregation in bipolar disorder pedigrees. This finding suggests the value of using the psychotic bipolar disorder subtype in genetic and biological investigations. Such investigations may inform the discussion about possible etiologic overlap between bipolar disorder and schizophrenia.

Presented in part at the VIII World Congress of Psychiatric Genetics, Versailles, France, Aug. 17–21, 2000. Received Aug. 16, 2000; revision received Jan. 12, 2001; accepted Feb. 7, 2001. From the Department of Psychiatry and Behavioral Sciences, The Johns Hopkins School of Medicine; and the Department of Biostatistics, School of Public Health, University of North Carolina, Chapel Hill. Address reprint requests to Dr. Potash, Meyer 3-181, Johns Hopkins Hospital, 600 North Wolfe St., Baltimore, MD 21287-7381; jpotash@jhmi.edu (e-mail).

Supported by grants from the Theodore and Veda Stanley Foundation, the Charles A. Dana Foundation Consortium on the Genetic Basis of Manic Depressive Illness, and the National Alliance for Research on Schizophrenia and Depression; by NIMH grant MH-42243 to Dr. DePaulo; and by the Affective Disorders Fund, the George Browne Laboratory Fund, and the Alexander Wilson Schweizer Fund at Johns Hopkins University.

The authors thank Drs. Francis McMahon, Susan Folstein, Phillip Slavney, and Paul McHugh; Barbara Schweizer, R.N., Jo Thomas, Erin Miller, Krista Vishio, Katie Aman, and Jen Chellis; and members of the study families who volunteered their time.

References

1. Carpenter WT Jr, Strauss JS, Muleh S: Are there pathognomonic symptoms in schizophrenia? an empiric investigation of Schneider's first-rank symptoms. Arch Gen Psychiatry 1973; 28:847–852
2. Crow TJ: The continuum of psychosis and its implication for the structure of the gene. Br J Psychiatry 1986; 149:419–429
3. Kendler KS, Karkowski LM, Walsh D: The structure of psychosis: latent class analysis of probands from the Roscommon Family Study. Arch Gen Psychiatry 1998; 55:492–499
4. Berrettini WH: Are schizophrenic and bipolar disorders related? a review of family and molecular studies. Biol Psychiatry 2000; 48:531–538
5. Winokur G, Scharfetter C, Angst J: A family study of psychotic symptomatology in schizophrenia, schizoaffective disorder, unipolar depression, and bipolar disorder. Eur Arch Psychiatry Neurol Sci 1985; 234:295–298
6. Kendler KS, McGuire M, Gruenberg AM, O'Hare A, Spellman M, Walsh D: The Roscommon Family Study, IV: affective illness, anxiety disorders, and alcoholism in relatives. Arch Gen Psychiatry 1993; 50:952–960
7. Leckman JF, Weissman MM, Prusoff BA, Caruso KA, Merikangas KR, Pauls DL, Kidd KK: Subtypes of depression: family study perspective. Arch Gen Psychiatry 1984; 41:833–838
8. Coryell W: Do psychotic, minor and intermittent depressive disorders exist on a continuum? J Affect Disord 1997; 45:75–83
9. Goldstein RB, Horwath E, Wickramaratne PJ, Wolk SI, Warner V, Weissman MM: Familial aggregation of delusional depression: re-examination in a recent family study. Depress Anxiety 1998; 8:160–165
10. McMahon FJ, Simpson SG, McInnis MG, Badner JA, MacKinnon DF, DePaulo JR: Linkage of bipolar disorder to chromosome 18q and the validity of bipolar II disorder. Arch Gen Psychiatry (in press)
11. MacKinnon DF, Xu J, McMahon FJ, Simpson SG, Stine OC, McInnis MG, DePaulo JR: Bipolar disorder and panic disorder in families: an analysis of chromosome 18 data. Am J Psychiatry 1998; 155:829–831
12. Simpson SG, Folstein SE, Meyers DA, DePaulo JR: Assessment of lineality in bipolar I linkage studies. Am J Psychiatry 1992; 149:1660–1665
13. Endicott J, Spitzer RL: A diagnostic interview: the Schedule for Affective Disorders and Schizophrenia. Arch Gen Psychiatry 1978; 35:837–844
14. Spitzer RL, Endicott J, Robins E: Research Diagnostic Criteria (RDC) for a Selected Group of Functional Disorders, 2nd ed.

New York, New York State Psychiatric Institute, Biometrics Research, 1975

15. Liang KY, Zeger SL: Longitudinal data analysis using generalized linear models. Biometrika 1986; 73:13–22
16. Tarone RE: Testing the goodness-of-fit of the binomial distribution. Biometrika 1979; 66:585–590
17. Leboyer M, Maier W, Teherani M, Lichtermann D, d'Amato T, Franke P, Lepine JP, Minges J, McGuffin P: The reliability of the SADS-LA in a family study setting. Eur Arch Psychiatry Clin Neurosci 1991; 241:165–169
18. Arndt S, Alliger RJ, Andreasen NC: The distinction of positive and negative symptoms: the failure of a two-dimensional model. Br J Psychiatry 1991; 158:317–322
19. Black DW, Nasrallah A: Hallucinations and delusions in 1,715 patients with unipolar and bipolar affective disorders. Psychopathology 1989; 22:28–34
20. Cassidy F, Forest K, Murry E, Carroll BJ: A factor analysis of the signs and symptoms of mania. Arch Gen Psychiatry 1998; 55: 27–32
21. Serretti A, Rietschel M, Lattuada E, Krauss H, Held T, Nothen MM, Smeraldi E: Factor analysis of mania (letter). Arch Gen Psychiatry 1999; 56:671–672
22. Maziade M, Roy MA, Martinez M, Cliche D, Fournier JP, Garneau Y, Nicole L, Montgrain N, Dion C, Ponton AM: Negative, psychoticism, and disorganized dimensions in patients with familial schizophrenia or bipolar disorder: continuity and discontinuity between the major psychoses. Am J Psychiatry 1995; 152:1458–1463
23. Black DW, Winokur G, Nasrallah A, Brewin A: Psychotic symptoms and age of onset in affective disorders. Psychopathology 1992; 25:19–22
24. Tohen M, Waternaux CM, Tsuang MT: Outcome in mania: a 4-year prospective follow-up of 75 patients utilizing survival analysis. Arch Gen Psychiatry 1990; 47:1106–1111
25. Rosen LN, Rosenthal NE, Dunner DL, Fieve RR: Social outcome compared in psychotic and nonpsychotic bipolar I patients. J Nerv Ment Dis 1983; 171:272–275
26. Coryell W, Leon AC, Turvey C, Akiskal H, Mueller T, Endicott J: The significance of psychotic features in manic episodes. J Affect Disord (in press)
27. MacQueen GM, Young LT, Robb JC, Cooke RG, Joffe RT: Levels of functioning and well-being in recovered psychotic versus nonpsychotic mania. J Affect Disord 1997; 46:69–72
28. Rosenthal NE, Rosenthal LN, Stallone F, Fleiss J, Dunner DL, Fieve RR: Psychosis as a predictor of response to lithium maintenance treatment in bipolar affective disorder. J Affect Disord 1979; 1:237–245
29. Maj M, Pirozzi R, Magliano L, Bartoli L: Long-term outcome of lithium prophylaxis in bipolar disorder: a 5-year prospective study of 402 patients at a lithium clinic. Am J Psychiatry 1998; 155:30–35
30. Suppes T, Webb A, Paul B, Carmody T, Kraemer H, Rush AJ: Clinical outcome in a randomized 1-year trial of clozapine versus treatment as usual for patients with treatment-resistant illness and a history of mania. Am J Psychiatry 1999; 156:1164–1169
31. Tohen M, Sanger TM, McElroy SL, Tollefson GD, Chengappa KNR, Daniel DG, Petty F, Centorrino F, Wang R, Grundy SL, Greaney MG, Jacobs TG, David SR, Toma V (Olanzapine HGEH Study Group): Olanzapine versus placebo in the treatment of acute mania. Am J Psychiatry 1999; 156:702–709
32. Kendler KS, Gruenberg AM, Tsuang MT: A DSM-III family study of the nonschizophrenic psychotic disorders. Am J Psychiatry 1986; 143:1098–1105
33. Kendler KS, Gruenberg AM, Tsuang MT: Psychiatric illness in first-degree relatives of schizophrenic and surgical control patients: a family study using DSM-III criteria. Arch Gen Psychiatry 1985; 42:770–779
34. Kendler KS, McGuire M, Gruenberg AM, O'Hare A, Spellman M, Walsh D: The Roscommon Family Study, I: methods, diagnosis of probands, and risk of schizophrenia in relatives. Arch Gen Psychiatry 1993; 50:527–540
35. Erlenmeyer-Kimling L, Adamo UH, Rock D, Roberts SA, Bassett AS, Squires-Wheeler E, Cornblatt BA, Endicott J, Pape S, Gottesman II: The New York High-Risk Project: prevalence and comorbidity of axis I disorders in offspring of schizophrenic parents at 25-year follow-up. Arch Gen Psychiatry 1997; 54:1096–1102
36. Gershon ES, Hamovit J, Guroff JJ, Dibble E, Leckman JF, Sceery W, Targum SD, Nurnberger JI Jr, Goldin LR, Bunney WE Jr: A family study of schizoaffective, bipolar I, bipolar II, unipolar, and normal control probands. Arch Gen Psychiatry 1982; 39: 1157–1167
37. Gershon ES, DeLisi LE, Hamovit J, Nurnberger JI Jr, Maxwell ME, Schreiber J, Dauphinais D, Dingman CW, Guroff JJ: A controlled family study of chronic psychoses: schizophrenia and schizoaffective disorder. Arch Gen Psychiatry 1988; 45:328–336
38. Maier W, Lichtermann D, Minges J, Hallmayer J, Heun R, Benkert O, Levinson DF: Continuity and discontinuity of affective disorders and schizophrenia: results of a controlled family study. Arch Gen Psychiatry 1993; 50:871–883
39. Reite M, Teale P, Rojas DC, Arciniegas D, Sheeder J: Bipolar disorder: anomalous brain asymmetry associated with psychosis. Am J Psychiatry 1999; 156:1159–1163
40. Pearlson GD, Wong DF, Tune LE, Ross CA, Chase GA, Links JM, Dannals RF, Wilson AA, Ravert HT, Wagner HNJ: In vivo D2 dopamine receptor density in psychotic and nonpsychotic patients with bipolar disorder. Arch Gen Psychiatry 1995; 52:471–477
41. Stefos G, Staner L, Kerkhofs M, Hubain P, Mendlewicz J, Linkowski P: Shortened REM latency as a psychobiological marker for psychotic depression? an age-, gender-, and polarity-controlled study. Biol Psychiatry 1998; 44:1314–1320
42. Velakoulis D, Pantelis C, McGorry PD, Dudgeon P, Brewer W, Cook M, Desmond P, Bridle N, Tierney P, Murrie V, Singh B, Copolov D: Hippocampal volume in first-episode psychoses and chronic schizophrenia: a high-resolution magnetic resonance imaging study. Arch Gen Psychiatry 1999; 56:133–141
43. Hirayasu Y, Shenton ME, Salisbury DF, Dickey CC, Fischer IA, Mazzoni P, Kisler T, Arakaki H, Kwon JS, Anderson JE, Yurgelun-Todd D, Tohen M, McCarley R: Lower left temporal lobe MRI volumes in patients with first-episode schizophrenia compared with psychotic patients with first-episode affective disorder and normal subjects. Am J Psychiatry 1998; 155:1384–1391
44. Koreen AR, Siris SG, Chakos M, Alvir J, Mayerhoff D, Lieberman J: Depression in first-episode schizophrenia. Am J Psychiatry 1993; 150:1643–1648
45. DeLisi LE, Goldin LR, Maxwell ME, Kazuba DM, Gershon ES: Clinical features of illness in siblings with schizophrenia or schizoaffective disorder. Arch Gen Psychiatry 1987; 44:891–896
46. Kendler KS, Karkowski-Shuman L, O'Neill FA, Straub RE, MacLean CJ, Walsh D: Resemblance of psychotic symptoms and syndromes in affected sibling pairs from the Irish Study of High-Density Schizophrenia Families: evidence for possible etiologic heterogeneity. Am J Psychiatry 1997; 154:191–198
47. Pearlson GD: Neurobiology of schizophrenia. Ann Neurol 2000; 48:556–566

Historical Perspectives and Natural History of Bipolar Disorder

Jules Angst and Robert Sellaro

A review of two centuries' literature on the natural history of bipolar disorder, including modern naturalistic studies and new data from a lifelong follow-up study of 220 bipolar patients, reaches the following conclusions: the findings of modern follow-up studies are closely compatible with those of studies conducted before the introduction of modern antidepressant and mood-stabilizing treatments. Bipolar disorder has always been highly recurrent and considered to have a poor prognosis.

Bipolar patients who have been hospitalized spend about 20% of their lifetime from the onset of their disorder in episodes. Fifty percent of bipolar episodes last between 2 and 7 months (median 3 months). The intervals between the first few episodes tend to shorten; later the episodes return at an irregular rhythm of about 0.4 episodes per year with high interindividual variability. Switches from mania into mild depression and from depression into hypomania were frequently reported in the 19th century and the first half of the 20th.

Antidepressant and antimanic drugs have to be given as long as the natural episode lasts. Given the poor outcome of bipolar disorders found in naturalistic follow-up studies and our lifelong investigation, intensive antidepressant, antimanic, and mood-stabilizing treatments are required in most cases. Despite modern treatments the outcome into old age is still poor, full recovery without further episodes rare, recurrence of episodes with incomplete remission the rule, and the development of chronicity and suicide still frequent. Biol Psychiatry 2000;48:445–457 © *2000 Society of Biological Psychiatry*

Key Words: Bipolar disorder, natural history, course, recurrence, outcome

Introduction

This article briefly reviews the natural history of bipolar disorder, giving special weight to historical studies before the era of antidepressants; integrates the results of modern naturalistic follow-up studies; and from our own findings 1) reanalyzes data from an early multicenter study (Angst et al 1968b, 1973) and 2) includes some new data from our lifelong Zurich follow-up study (Angst and Preisig 1995a, 1995b). The article focuses mainly on episodes and recurrence and, to a lesser extent, outcome; it does not deal with rapid cycling and seasonal depression. Recent reviews of the course of bipolar disorder have been published by Lavori et al (1984), Keller (1987), Goodwin and Jamison (1990), Coryell and Winokur (1992), Verdoux and Bourgeois (1995), Kessing et al (1998), Goldberg and Harrow (1999), Marneros (1999), and Bourgeois and Marneros (in press).

The Concept of Bipolar Disorder

We owe the categorization of bipolar disorder as an illness to Falret, who in 1851 and 1854 on the basis of longitudinal observations developed the entity of "folie circulaire" (circular madness), defined by manic and melancholic episodes separated by symptom-free intervals. In 1854 Baillarger used the term *folie à double forme* to describe cyclic (manic–melancholic) episodes (Pichot 1995; Ritti 1879). Kraepelin called such cyclic episodes "double attacks." In both French diagnoses the prognosis was considered to be "desperate, terrible and incurable" (Bourgeois and Marneros, in press). Circular illness was described by most authors as a recurrent condition; it became the prototype of the larger group of periodic psychoses embracing periodic mania, periodic melancholia, and periodic cyclic disorders (Ballet 1903; Mendel 1881; Pilcz 1901; Ziehen 1902, 1907).

The Concept of Mixed States

The history of the concept of mixed states has been extensively studied by Marneros (in press): what we today call "mixed states" were probably already known at the beginning of the 19th century and named "mixtures" (*Mischungen*) by Heinroth in 1818 and "middle forms" (*Mittelformen*) by Griesinger (1845). Guislain (1852) gave clear descriptions of different syndromes of mixed states. The history of bipolar disorder by Haustgen (1995) traces the term *mixed states* to J.P. Falret's son Jules Falret (1861).

Very influential in this field was Weygandt (1899), who worked with Kraepelin and whose monograph distinguished three forms of mixed states: manic stupor, agitated

From the Zurich University Psychiatric Hospital, Zurich, Switzerland.
Address reprint requests to Jules Angst, M.D., Zurich University Psychiatric Hospital, Box 68, Lenggstrect 31, Zurich 8029, Switzerland.
Received January 13, 2000; revised April 13, 2000; accepted April 20, 2000.

0006-3223/00/$20.00
PII S0006-3223(00)00909-4

melancholia (depression with flight of ideas and agitation), and unproductive mania (elated mood, increased motor activity, and inhibition of thinking). Kraepelin's (1899) textbook descriptions of mixed states were founded on Weygandt's monograph. Further progress was made by Rehm's monograph (1919, 113), which classified mixed states systematically on the basis of the permutations of the three elements that had been defined by Kraepelin: thought disorder, mood, and psychomotor activity (identified as a, b, and c for mania and as A, B, and C for depression).

Kraepelin's Manic–Depressive Insanity

At the turn of the 19th century Kraepelin's unifying approach to the classification of mood disorders (1899) resulted in bipolar disorders being subsumed within manic–depressive insanity (MDI), a broad group that included single-episode and recurrent depression. Kraepelin (1913, 1183) was later himself to raise the possibility of the heterogeneity of MDI. Unlike the French concepts, Kraepelin's MDI had a good prognosis and did not develop into severe dementia, although Kraepelin conceded the existence of mild residual states after recovery from the episodes themselves (*Schwächezustände;* Kraepelin 1913, 1349) and of mild fluctuations between episodes. Kraepelin considered periodicity to be unimportant for the diagnosis (Pilcz 1901). As a consequence of Kraepelin's unification of affective disorders, research on their course frequently failed to distinguish between depression, mania, and bipolar disorder (Bratfos and Haug 1968; Fuller 1935; Paskind 1930; Pollock 1931a, 1931b, 1931c; Poort 1945; Rennie 1942; Tomasson 1947).

Notable contemporary authors nevertheless disagreed with Kraepelin's unitarian approach, and their studies of the natural history of affective disorders maintained the distinction between mania, depression, and bipolar disorder (Ballet 1903; Pilcz 1901; Ziehen 1902, 1907). This data on the course of bipolar disorder collected in the 19th century and the first half of the 20th, before the introduction of modern antidepressants and mood stabilizers, is of special value in that it represents the disorder's untreated natural history.

Onset of Bipolar Disorder

The dating of the age of onset is to a certain extent unreliable because it is usually retrospective and dependent on insecure recall. Bipolar disorder begins about 10 years earlier than recurrent depression, as shown by a review of the literature (Angst 1988). Earlier studies indicated a mean age of 28 to 33 years; epidemiologic and newer clinical studies show that bipolar symptoms start frequently in adolescence (Weissman et al 1988) and that manic episodes manifest usually in the early 20s (Fogarty et al 1994).

Periodic Mania and Switches of Polarity

There is considerable interest today in data on the course of single and multiple episodes, which can answer questions about the psychopathology, duration, and frequency of episodes; the syndromal stability over lifetime; and the frequency with which initial major depression develops into bipolar disorder. Today the switch of an episode from depression to hypomania is often assumed to be drug induced, but the phenomenon was already very common as "reactive hyperthymia" before the introduction of antidepressants.

A century ago the concept of periodic mania was well known and the diagnosis much more frequent, quite simply because it was applied to cases that today would be considered bipolar disorders. For instance, an initial depressive syndrome cycling into a manic episode, although frequently observed, was not considered an indication of bipolarity (Mendel 1881; Ziehen 1902). Similarly, "postmelancholic reactive hyperthymia" with clear hypomanic symptoms was compatible with the diagnosis of pure periodic melancholia (Ziehen 1907, 26).

Mania switching into depression was likewise very commonly reported as "reactive depression" (Ziehen 1902, 546, 554; Wernicke 1906, 355). Postmanic depression lasted a few days or a few weeks according to Wernicke (1906, 355). Mild depression was observed preceding or terminating manic attacks in most of the 128 manic patients studied by MacDonald (1918).

Modern naturalistic and treatment studies have also found that mania frequently cycles into depression: the rates of cycling observed in follow-up studies over 8 weeks vary from 17% (Tohen et al 1990) to 30% (Keller et al 1986a). Our earlier retrospective record study of 300 manic patients (admitted between 1920 and 1970) found that 21% of manic episodes cycled into depression, a rate that did not change significantly during the intervening decades (Angst 1987).

In a retrospective record study, depression switching into hypomania was found in 29% of bipolar patients hospitalised between 1920 and 1959 (Angst 1987).

Diagnostic Change from Depression to Bipolar Illness

The syndromal course over lifetime has been little investigated. It was frequently assumed that mania was predominant in earlier years and depression in the second half of life. Kinkelin (1954) followed-up 146 hospital first admis-

Table 1. Length of Episodes (Months) of Patient Samples

	Mean	Median	Q_1	Q_3
Mendel (1881)		5–6	3–4	6–7
Kraepelin (1913)	6–8			
Panse (1924)	7			
Wertham (1929)		4–6	2–4	8–10
Rennie (1942)	3.5[a]–5.8[b]			
Kinkelin (1954)	3.5–8.4			
Angst and Preisig (1995a)	4.3[c]	3[d]	2	5

[a]First episode.
[b]Third episode.
[c]Mean after logarithmic transformation.
[d]Median of Table 2.

Natural Length of Episodes

Valuable data on the natural length of episodes were published before the introduction of effective treatments (Table 1).

Mendel (1881, 155) reported data on the length of manic episodes ($N = 43$), from which a median duration of 5–6 months ($Q_1 = 3$–4 months, $Q_3 = 6$–7 months) can be computed; Mendel found only one episode which lasted 10–12 months and one over 1 year. Kraepelin (1913) stressed the great variability in episode length but estimated that most episodes lasted between 6 and 8 months.

Panse's follow-up study (1924) of 205 hospitalized bipolar patients found an identical mean length of 7 months for manic and depressive episodes.

Wertham (1929) provided the most conclusive data on episode length with his investigation of 1000 male and 1000 female first admissions for mania. From his published histograms we can today estimate the length of episodes as lognormally distributed, with a mode between 2–4 months and a median duration of 4–6 months ($Q_1 = 2$–4 months, $Q_3 = 8$–10 months). There was no follow-up; most of these manic cases may therefore have been bipolars.

Rennie (1942) found that there was a lengthening of repeated manic episodes, with the first episode lasting 3.5 months, the second 5.2 months, the third 5.8 months, and the fourth and fifth even longer. Rennie ascribed this to a prolonging effect of aging, since before the age of 45 episode length remained constant.

Unlike Rennie, Kinkelin (1954), in a longitudinal study, found no systematic change in episode length between the first and seventh episodes. Among 347 bipolar patients the mean length of depressive episodes varied impressively from 3.5 to 8.4 months, and of manic episodes from 4 to 11.6 months. Kinkelin, too, concluded that later episodes tended to be longer.

In the NIMH Collaborative Study on the Psychobiology of Depression Clinical Studies (Keller et al 1986a) survival analysis demonstrated that mixed or cycling episodes were slower to recover than pure depressed or pure manic episodes. Perugi et al (1997) also reported that episodes involving mixed states lasted significantly longer (mean 13.4 months) than manic episodes (8.8 months).

The computation of the length of episodes has to take into account their lognormal distribution (Angst and Weis 1967) and to control for the individual number of episodes (Slater 1938). In patients experiencing multiple cyclic (bipolar) episodes, the episodes tend to be slightly shorter, whereas in general the latest episode tends to be longer because of the development of chronicity in some cases, as found in our multicenter study on the course of mood disorders (Angst et al 1973).

In the Baltimore Epidemiologic Catchment Area Follow-Up Eaton et al (1997) found a median length of episodes of approximately 8 to 12 weeks; this is shorter than that reported in treated populations, but similar to the median episode length of 8 weeks reported in a community study of adolescents in Oregon (Lewinsohn et al 1994).

The most recent data from the Zurich follow-up study (Angst and Preisig 1995a) showed a mean episode length of 4.3 months ($s = 5.44$) calculated on the basis of intraindividual means. The median length of episodes is not obviously dependent on the total number of episodes—see Table 2, where subgroups with two to 10 episodes are computed separately (following Slater's [1938] suggestion). On the whole, the median length of episodes in bipolar illness (on the basis of individual medians) was 3 months ($Q_1 = 2$ months, $Q_3 = 5$ months). There is a difference in length dependent on psychopathology. Pure manic and pure depressive episodes lasted 3 months ($Q_1 = 2$, $Q_3 = 5$), as did mixed episodes ($M = 3$; $Q_1 = 2$, $Q_3 = 7$); in contrast, cyclic episodes lasted almost 50% longer ($M = 4.19$; $Q_1 = 2.5$, $Q_3 = 7.75$). These figures are based on intraindividual medians. We found no gender differences in median episode length.

The shorter episode length reported by modern studies may be a result of their including milder cases or, what is more probable, a consequence of antidepressant therapy: medication has usually to be maintained for a further 6 months after recovery to avoid relapse into the still persistent latent episode, which represents the natural history.

Recurrence of Bipolar Disorder

The total number of episodes experienced by patients is amply reported. Findings regarding the occurrence of single episode cases vary widely, ranging from 0% to 55%

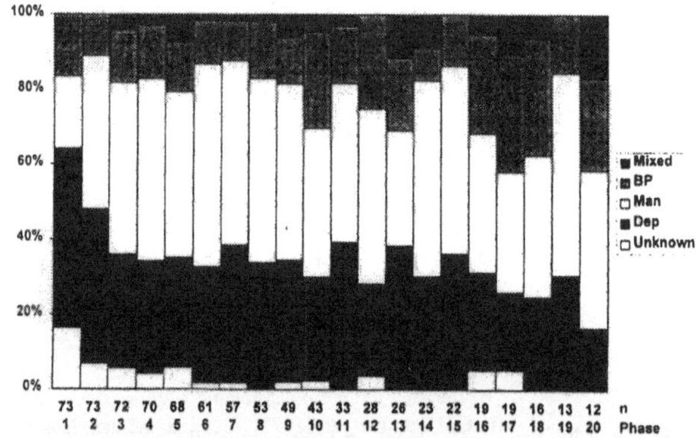

Figure 1. Proportion of syndromes across 20 episodes in male subjects. BP, bipolar; Man, mania; Dep, depression.

sions suffering from MDI (1929–1947) until 1948 in a study covering an average of 21.8 years of the total course of the disorder. Of the 146 cases, 125 began with depression and 21 with mania. During the follow-up period 36 (28.8%) of the 125 depressive patients developed manic episodes, a figure that would correspond to a diagnostic change from depression to bipolar illness of 1.3% per year of observation. Marneros et al (1991b) reported that the initial diagnosis of depression remained stable in 79% of cases over 27 years. In our preponderantly prospective study we found a rate of diagnostic change from depression to hypomania/mania of about 1% per year (Angst and Preisig 1995a). Coryell and colleagues' (1995a) intensive prospective follow-up study of 381 depressive subjects over 10 years found that 10.2% developed into mania (5.2%) and hypomania (5.0%), which also corresponds to a 1% change per year of observation.

In their monograph, Marneros et al (1991a) found that mania frequently developed into schizomania or mixed states.

Syndromal Stability of the Course

New data from our Zurich follow-up study confirmed a major gender difference in the psychopathology of bipolar patients over the first 20 episodes (Angst 1978): female subjects manifested significantly more depressed episodes and male subjects more cyclic episodes (mania and depression), whereas pure manic and mixed episodes were equally frequent in both genders (Figures 1 and 2). The syndromal proportions were found to remain remarkably stable over 20 episodes (Angst and Weis 1967), which also means, for instance, that aging brings no increase in the depressive component of bipolar illness.

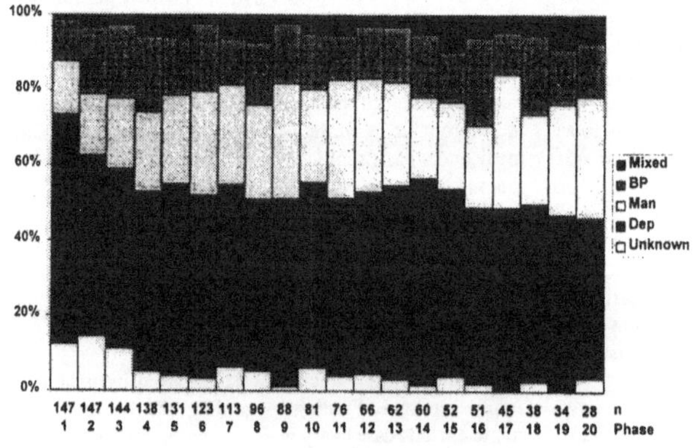

Figure 2. Proportion of syndromes across 20 episodes in female subjects. BP, bipolar; Man, mania; Dep, depression.

Table 2. Total Number of Episodes and Length (Zurich Study)

Episodes	Patients	Median length of episodes (months)									
2	4	1.5	5.8								
3	8	6.0	2.8	9.0							
4	9	3.0	5.0	6.0	9.0						
5	15	5.5	4.5	4.6	4.0	5.8					
6	14	2.5	5.5	5.0	3.8	2.8	2.9				
7	21	3.0	5.0	4.0	4.3	3.5	3.0	4.0			
8	12	2.9	3.0	2.0	3.0	2.4	2.5	4.0	4.0		
9	13	3.5	4.5	4.0	4.0	3.0	2.5	2.5	2.0	1.0	
10	15	4.5	3.5	3.0	3.5	4.5	3.0	3.0	3.0	3.0	6.0
Episodes		1	2	3	4	5	6	7	8	9	10

(Goodwin and Jamison 1990), with five of 11 studies reporting rates between 0% and 8%. It is clear that any loss of information will inflate nonrecurrence rates; furthermore, the length of follow-up and development into chronicity have to be taken into account in assessing findings.

The earlier literature assumed that periodic mania had a better prognosis with fewer episodes and better outcome than periodic melancholia or circular disorder, the latter having the worst outcome (Rehm 1919, 107); however, Rehm also found twice as many manic cases (53%) than circular cases (26%) with short free intervals between episodes (up to 1 year), reflecting a higher periodicity of mania (it is unclear whether the length of observation in these cases was the same).

Certain methodological advances contributed to the investigation of the question of recurrence. One was the introduction of a more precise terminology and clear definitions of remission, recovery, relapse, and recurrence (Frank et al 1991). Another was the introduction of life table analyses into psychiatry, a method first used for length of hospitalization (Kramer 1969) and for follow-up data after recovery from depression (Klerman et al 1974) and soon also applied in longitudinal studies of bipolar disorder (Dunner et al 1976, 1979; Fleiss et al 1976, 1978). Lavori et al (1984) applied life table methods to reanalyze 40 earlier studies on the relapse/recurrence of affective disorders; the results varied considerably between the studies, and the authors formulated the hypothesis of the heterogeneity of patients' courses in terms of low or high hazard with a low or high risk of relapse. More recently, survival analysis was applied to prospective data on recurrence after remission (Fleiss et al 1978; Gitlin et al 1995; Keller et al 1993; Lavori et al 1984).

In a 2-year placebo-controlled lithium study Fleiss et al (1978) found that under placebo 80% of bipolar I patients experienced recurrences within about 70 weeks. (Admittedly a treatment study of this type dealt with a selected sample of patients, who, for instance, had had a mean number of two episodes in the previous 2 years.) The 4-year follow-up of a naturalistic study of mania showed recurrence in 72% of patients, with a mere 28% remaining in remission (Tohen et al 1990). Patients who were symptomatic at the 6-month follow-up had a 45% greater chance of a recurrence within the next 3.5 years.

Course of Subtypes of Bipolar Disorder

Important findings from a naturalistic study, the National Institute of Mental Health (NIMH) Collaborative Program on the Psychobiology of Depression, Clinical Studies (Keller et al 1993), showed a high rate of recurrence for pure mania (48% by 1 year and 81% by 5 years) and even higher rates for the mixed cycling group (57% by 1 year and 91% by 5 years). Over 7 years the rate of recurrence was 81%. The length of sustained recovery was associated with a lower risk for recurrence over the subsequent 4 years, but over a period of 10 years this predictive power decreased considerably (Coryell et al 1995b); the authors showed that even under sustained lithium prophylaxis recurrences were present in more than 70% of cases within 5 years of recovery. This finding is consistent with the outpatient study of Gitlin et al (1995), in which 73% of 82 bipolar patients had relapses/recurrences over an average of 4.3 years despite maintenance pharmacotherapy (two thirds of patients who relapsed experienced multiple relapses). Among the 26 patients who suffered no relapse 46% continued to show significant symptoms of mania or depression.

The NIMH Collaborative Program on the Psychobiology of Depression, Clinical Studies (Coryell et al 1989) provided no evidence that the course of bipolar II disorder differed from that of bipolar I, which confirms our own findings (Angst 1986).

A recent study comparing patients suffering from bipolar II disorder with major depressive subjects under fluoxetine showed similar relapse/recurrence rates of 36% versus 35% after 50 weeks and 44% versus 49% after 62 weeks (Amsterdam et al 1998). This study provides no indication of a deterioration in the course of bipolar II disorder due to antidepressant medication; on the contrary, the disorder had a better course than under placebos.

Marneros et al (1991a) reported that bipolar disorder and schizo-bipolar disorder had very similar course characteristics.

Is Recurrence of Bipolar Illness Progressive?

Describing the intervals between episodes, Kraepelin (1913, 1365) found a progressive shortening of the first three intervals (first interval of male/female subjects 4.6/4.3 years, second interval 2.8/2.0 years, third interval 1.2/1.4 years). His data, like that of some other authors, are not controlled for the total number of episodes: clearly the intervals between episodes in patients having few episodes over a lifetime will be longer than in patients who experience many. We owe this particular methodological breakthrough to Eliot Slater (1938), who, in his paper on the periodicity of manic–depressive insanity, investigated 116 patients of the Forschungsanstalt für Psychiatrie in Munich who had been personally diagnosed by Kraepelin. Studying the length of intervals between episodes, Slater made his major methodological contribution by controlling for the total number of episodes and analyzing separately the subgroups with 1, 2, 3, . . . , *n* intervals. He showed that there was indeed a shortening of the intervals, but only between the first few manifestations of the illness. Investigating the individual periodicity, he concluded that every patient had his or her own rhythm.

In 1968 Bratfos and Haug applied Slater's method to the follow-up data on 215 cases of manic–depressive disorder (including depression) in an analysis of the length of the intervals between episodes. Correcting for the number of episodes, the authors found that the first interval length was 2.1 years, the second was 4.8 years, and the third was 2.2 years; thus no clear tendency emerged from these data.

Again following Slater's method of correcting for the number of episodes, Angst et al (1973) published the results of a multinational retrospective and partially prospective hospital record study on the course of 393 bipolar and 634 unipolar depressive patients. Analyzing cycle lengths, they indirectly confirmed Slater's finding that the intervals shortened as the number of recurrences increased; however, the median cycle lengths gave clear evidence only for continuous shortening of the first three cycles; the pattern of later recurrences seemed to be unpredictable. On the other hand, nonparametric tests between successive cycle lengths showed a significant shortening from cycle one to cycle 11 (Angst et al 1973, 499). Marneros et al (1991a) confirmed the shortening of cycles on the basis of the Cologne naturalistic follow-up study of 30 bipolar and 56 schizo-bipolar patients. Zis et al (1980) and Zis and Goodwin (1979) arrived at similar conclusions. This seemed to confirm earlier findings that had suggested decreasing cycle length (e.g., those of Kraepelin [1913, 1325] or Kinkelin [1954], although not controlled for number of cycles—see Figure 6-3 in Goodwin and Jamison [1990]). All these results, together with the finding that precipitation rates decrease (Angst 1966, 41) with increasing recurrence, led Roy-Byrne et al (1985) to speak of sensitization and Post et al (Post 1992; Post et al 1984, 1986) to develop the theory that vulnerability grows with the number of episodes and the theory of conditioning, sensitization, and kindling (by analogy with electrophysiologic kindling).

National data on hospital admissions and readmissions can also provide a rough estimate of the natural history of severe cases. Kessing et al (1998a, 1998b) recently described the course of Danish hospital admissions on the basis of a nationwide register of ICD-8 diagnoses. Rehospitalizations were taken as a measure of recurrence. The authors found, on the basis of 2903 bipolar cases, a progressive shortening of the interval between discharge from hospital and the next rehospitalization and, therefore, a deteriorating course. Selection bias did not completely explain the shortening intervals between hospital admissions, and control for gender and age did not alter the conclusions. So far, then, it would seem to have been established that the course of bipolar disorder is recurrent and progressive, but this aspect is still surrounded by considerable controversy, which may partially be due to the possibility "that recent studies deal with different, more broadly diagnosed populations than the seminal, earlier studies" (Grof et al 1995).

The Lithium Controversy: Does Recurrence Improve Spontaneously?

One controversy about the natural history of bipolar disorder dates back to 1968 and the criticism by two reputed British authors, Blackwell and Shepherd of lithium trials. They assumed not only the inefficacy of lithium but also that bipolar disorder had a good prognosis, making long-term prophylaxis unnecessary. This view was supported theoretically by Lader (1968) and empirically by Saran (1969), who found no evidence for high recurrence in his follow-up data and who concluded that past recurrence was not predictive for recurrence in the future. Saran's findings were of critical importance because the early work on lithium had been based statistically on the assumption that high recurrence in a patient's previous history should be expected to repeat itself in the future. Saran concluded that his findings on the spontaneous course corresponded to the course as observed under lithium treatment by Baastrup and Schou (1968). Saran's findings have not been confirmed by other studies: a methodological investigation by Isaaksson et al (1969) demonstrated the persistence of recurrence for bipolar and unipolar depression, and the same conclusion was reached by Laurell and Ottosson (1968).

Stability of Recurrence after Initial Deterioration

Another debated question is whether the course of bipolar disorder is really progressive, characterized by unlimited shortening of cycles throughout (Angst et al 1973). This model is disconfirmed by a number of new studies. The recent summary of the literature by Kessing et al (1998b) shows that Fukuda et al (1983), who investigated not the early but the later course of the illness, could find no shortening of cycles (a finding that would still be compatible with the hypothesis that shortening is a feature of the first few cycles only). This aspect of the systematic shortening of cycle length was also very seriously questioned in the reviews by Coryell and Winokur (1992) and Solomon et al (1995), which drew mainly on Winokur and colleagues' findings (1994) from the prospective naturalistic NIMH study covering 10 years (Turvey et al 1999). This study found that the second cycle was clearly shorter than the first, the third a little longer than the second, but the fourth and fifth cycles were again shorter. On the other hand, Winokur et al (1993) stressed that bipolar illness was highly recurrent, with an "inexorable continuation of episodes and hospitalisations," and could find no data suggesting that the illness burned out at a later stage.

On the basis of prospective data Coryell and Winokur (1992) found that rapid cycling, which is observed in 20% to 25% of bipolar patients, is usually a transient manifestation and not therefore a characteristic of the long-term course.

Meta-Analysis of Two Studies on the Course

Samples and Methodology

Here we reanalyze some data from our two studies, the mainly retrospective multicenter study published by Angst et al (1973) and the Zurich follow-up study described by Angst and Preisig (1995a).

1. The multicenter study (Angst et al 1968a, 1973) consisted of consecutive hospital admissions of bipolar and unipolar depressive patients from Basel (103); Berlin (104); Hamilton, Canada (69); Prague (132); Zurich (392); Glostrup, Denmark (100); and Landeck, Germany (140). For the present analysis the Zurich sample was excluded, to avoid any overlap with the Zurich follow-up study. The remaining sample consisted of 329 bipolar patients. The data collection was mainly of the retrospective type based on case histories and verbal information. The documentation of the course was carried out by means of a standardized form of protocol in which all data were entered separately for each episode and subsequent interval (Angst and Weis 1968). In retrospect the onset (date) and length (months, weeks) of previous episodes and aspects of treatment (none, ambulatory, hospital) were assessed. The degree of remission was coded as full, partial, or unknown. Psychopathology was coded with a list of 10 syndromes. The data were reanalyzed for this study.
2. The Zurich follow-up study consisted of 406 consecutive hospital admissions for severe depression or mania from 1959 to 1963. Regular follow-up investigations (by telephone, interviews, and record collection) were conducted in 1963, 1965, 1979, 1975, 1980, and 1985. In 1991 and 1997 mortality data were available from the Swiss federal office of statistics. Seventy-six percent of patients had died by the end of 1997. The sample and the methodology of assessments were described in detail by Angst and Preisig (1995a). The principal data collected were comparable to the multicenter study, but psychopathology and treatment were assessed in more detail. The 220 bipolar patients were reanalyzed for this article.

Results

Table 3 presents the data from the mainly retrospective multicenter study and demonstrates a systematic shortening of the first four cycles. The predominantly prospective data from the Zurich sample (Table 4) shows a significant shortening between cycles 1 and 2 only, with no systematic change thereafter. In both studies the conclusions were confirmed by t tests for dependent measures.

In a survival analysis of the Zurich follow-up data significant differences were found between cycles 1–5 but were difficult to interpret. The first cycle was longer and the second cycle shorter than all the others. Otherwise the survival curves were very similar (Figure 3). The mean cycle length was 28.7 months (s = 30.93) but the median length, which is much more representative, only 18 months (Q_1 = 3, Q_3 = 18); exclusion of the first longer cycle does not change this median.

In conclusion, we found a shortening of cycle length at the beginning of the disorder only; later episodes were persistently recurrent but occurred at irregular intervals without any systematic deterioration or amelioration, thus

Table 3. Total Number of Cycles and Length (Multicenter Study)

Cycles	Patients	Median length of cycles (months)								
1	18	23								
2	35	26	15							
3	38	38	20	15						
4	45	21	27	13	14					
5	39	35	18	19	13	11				
6	31	42	31	19	15	15	9			
7	26	28	18	16	12	13	15	12		
8	27	42	17	14	14	9	11	9	10	
9	17	37	20	18	9	8	12	15	15	12
Cycles		1	2	3	4	5	6	7	8	9

This table does not include Zurich data.

confirming Winokur and colleagues' (1993, 1994) findings.

Episode Frequency per Year

Periodicity can also be expressed by the episode frequency per year. In a follow-up of 140 bipolar I patients over 11.4 years Dunner et al (1979) found 0.54 episodes per year; we found 0.37 (Angst and Preisig 1995a). Marneros' group found 0.41 episodes per year (Marneros 1999; Marneros et al 1991a) for bipolar disorder and about half as many in the case of recurrent depression. These figures included the first cycle, which is considerably longer than later ones. Dunner et al (1979) found no relationship between episode frequency and age of onset (which was not consistent with our early results; Angst and Weis 1967). The question of a gender difference in episode frequency per year remained open. After the onset of their disorder, bipolar patients spent on the average about 19% of their lives in affective episodes over an observation period of 27 years (Angst and Preisig 1995a).

In the present analysis the median cycle length (on the basis of individual medians) was 18 months (Q_1 = 12 months, Q_3 = 33.5 months), a length that corresponds to a recurrence rate of 0.66 episodes per year. On the basis of an episode length of 3 months (median), bipolar patients spent about 2 months/year in episodes. We could not find any gender differences (Mann–Whitney *U* test) in episode frequency measured by cycle length. Recently Gottschalk et al (1995) found some evidence for a nonlinear deterministic structure in long-term daily mood records of six out of seven bipolar patients, something not found in normal control subjects. Further research on a chaotic course is certainly desirable.

Correlates of Recurrence

For the analysis of correlates with long-term recurrence we excluded the first two cycles and entered the median of all intraindividual medians of cycle length as the dependent variable into a multiple regression analysis. Cycle length did not correlate with gender, retrospective versus prospective data collection, or long-term administration of tricyclic antidepressants. This finding does not confirm the assumed deterioration of the course of bipolar illness under tricyclics (Arnold and Kryspin-Exner 1965; Koukopoulos et al 1980; Till and Vuckovik 1970; Tondo et al 1981). Unsurprisingly, long-term lithium and antipsy-

Table 4. Total Number of Cycles and Length (Zurich Study)

Cycles	Patients	Median length of cycles (months)								
1	4	64								
2	8	105	12							
3	9	55	21	34						
4	15	78	25	33	45					
5	14	30	22	37	19	20				
6	21	44	35	36	24	24	17			
7	12	42	23	34	16	17	30	17		
8	13	34	22	23	30	23	12	17	28	
9+	124	26	19	21	15	15	12	12	12	12
Cycles		1	2	3	4	5	6	7	8	9+

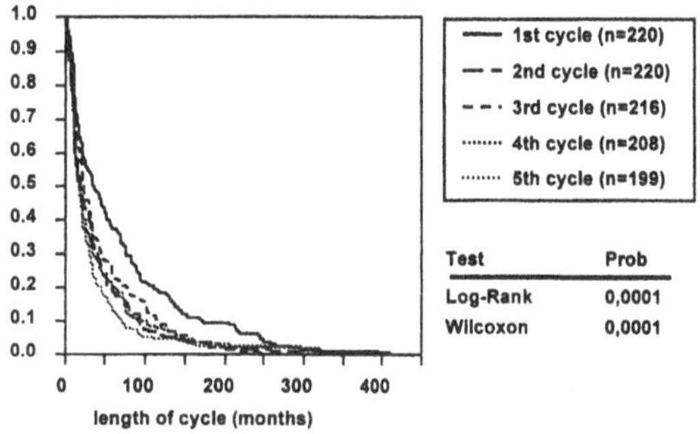

Figure 3. Survival analysis of cycle lengths (first to fifth).

chotic medication correlated with shorter cycles; this result is explicable by the selection of highly recurrent cases for prophylaxis. The syndromal characteristics of episodes had some impact on cycle length: it was significantly shorter in cases with cyclic versus pure (manic or depressive) episodes and in those with more manic than depressive episodes.

Poor Outcome of Bipolar Disorder in Early Follow-Up Studies

In the predrug era most bipolar cases were described as manifesting residual symptoms after recovery from episodes. Their state was described as "unsteady, moody, irritable, indolent, egocentric" (Pilcz 1901, 61–62), a symptom that often preceded the episodes or had even been present since childhood. Kraepelin (1913, 1185), too, although assuming a good prognosis, admitted the existence of mild residual "debility states." Ziehen (1902) estimated complete recovery in periodic mania to occur at most in 20% of cases.

In a follow-up of first admissions from 1920 to 1947 over a mean of 22 years Kinkelin (1954) found chronicity (including severe residual states) in 14.6% of depressive subjects ($N = 89$) and in 41% of circular cases ($N = 51$).

An important follow-up study of 297 bipolar and 945 unipolar patients in the Phipps Clinic (admissions from 1913 to 1940) was published by Stephens and McHugh (1991). Compared with depressive subjects, bipolar patients had an earlier age of onset on admission and were more likely to be psychotic; they also had more serious premorbid characteristics, more sudden onsets (44%), more previous admissions (62% for depression and 67% for mania), and more problems with alcohol, but more bipolar than depressed patients were discharged in a recovered state. In bipolar disorders they found a lifetime average of 3.6 hospitalizations, and in their follow-up they observed 0.19 episodes of depression and 0.29 episodes of mania per year followed up. Only 2% of all patients had manic episodes with no lifetime depressions; this small group had the best outcome. Bipolar patients ($N = 301$) had the poorest outcome: 7% were recovered, 50% improved, and 43% unimproved at the follow-up rating. The rates of recovered, improved, and unimproved patients were 19%, 56%, and 25% for pure mania ($N = 16$) and 25%, 44%, and 32% for pure depression ($N = 700$).

In a follow-up of 86 manic patients over 30 to 40 years, outcome (measured by psychiatric symptoms) was good in 43% of cases, fair in 18%, and poor in 25% (Tsuang et al 1979).

Poor Outcome in Recent Follow-Up Studies

Modern studies (e.g., a 4.5-year follow-up study by Goldberg et al [1995]) showed that only 41% of bipolar patients had a good overall outcome, the remainder being moderately impaired (37%) or showing poor functioning (22%). Gitlin et al (1995) found a poor outcome even under prophylactic medication (mainly lithium); poor outcome was more closely associated with the number of depressive episodes than the number of manic episodes. In their above-mentioned NIMH Collaborative Program on the Psychobiology of Depression with a 15-year intensive follow-up, Coryell et al (1998) found that 56.6% of 113 bipolar I patients had had no symptoms over the past 12 months, 22.1% had had symptoms for fewer than 52 weeks, and 20.4% had had symptoms in all 52 weeks, representing a poor outcome (defined as having had symptoms of major depressive disorder, mania, or schizoaffective disorder in all 52 weeks of year 15).

The short-term outcome, 12 months after discharge from hospital, was similar in patients with manic episodes or mixed episodes (Keck et al 1998), whereas in Keller and colleagues' (1986b) study after 18 months of follow-up mixed episodes also developed more frequently

Table 5. Outcome of 219 Patients in the Zurich Follow-Up Study (Median Age at Follow-Up or Death, 68 Years)

Recovered (GAS score > 60, no episodes over the past 5 years)	16.0%
Remitted (GAS score > 60) but still recurrent (<5 years since last episode)	25.5%
Incomplete remission (GAS score 1–60) over more than 5 years	7.8%
Incomplete remission, course still recurrent	27.0%
Chronic (last episode without remission, minimum length 2 years)	15.9%
Suicide	7.8%

GAS, Global Assessment Scale.

into chronicity (32%) than pure manic episodes (7%). In bipolar I patients poor outcome did not correlate clearly with early onset of the disorder or cycling per se (Coryell et al 1998), but persistence of depressive symptoms in years 1 and 2 was correlated with impairment after 15 years (household duties, recreational activities, overall satisfaction, and global social adjustment). Such early persistence of depressive symptoms predicted a poor prognosis of a bipolar subtype, whereas this was not the case for early persistence of manic symptoms.

The lifetime outcome of bipolar disorder in our Zurich follow-up study is given in Table 5 and demonstrates a poor prognosis despite modern treatments. Up to a median age of 68 years only 16% of patients had recovered; 52% still suffered from recurrent episodes and the remaining patients had become chronically ill or had committed suicide. These data underline the poor outcome into old age and the need for intensive treatment. This table shows the outcome of bipolar disorder before the occurrence of an organic brain syndrome in the elderly, which was found in 14.5% of cases. The previous number of affective episodes was not correlated with the development of an organic brain syndrome (Angst and Preisig 1995b).

Future studies on outcome should clearly distinguish between different outcome measures, since Tohen et al (2000) have shown that functional recovery can be much worse than syndromal recovery.

Conclusions

Several important conclusions regarding episodes, recurrence, and outcome have emerged from this review and data analysis of the natural history of bipolar disorder:

1. Before the introduction of modern drugs, spontaneous mild depression following a manic episode and spontaneous hypomania following a melancholic episode were very common; they were interpreted as "reactive" and had no effect on the principal diagnosis of pure mania or pure melancholia. This historical fact has to be taken into account in today's hypothesis of drug-induced hypomania or drug-induced depression; these have to be proven statistically by placebo-controlled trials.
2. Our decades-long prospective study shows that over lifetime the proportions of mania and depression in bipolar disorder remain stable into old age. Bipolar female subjects manifest more depression than bipolar male subjects.
3. Mixed states have been described since the early 19th century. Modern studies have demonstrated that they have a poorer prognosis than other bipolar conditions, with slower remissions and higher risk for chronicity.
4. The natural length of affective episodes has probably not changed over the past 120 years. Patients responding to antidepressants still require a maintenance treatment throughout the underlying episode. In clinical studies the median length of episodes is 3 to 6 months; in epidemiological studies it is 2 to 3 months.
5. The recurrence of bipolar disorder was always the rule; it now seems to be established that there is some initial shortening of intervals/cycles, followed by an irregular persistent recurrence, with a median cycling of 18 months. In contrast to earlier reports, the new studies show that there is no unlimited shortening of cycle length—not therefore supporting the kindling model. In several studies rapid cycling has been found to be relatively frequent, but usually transient.
6. Lifelong outcome has rarely been studied, and precise data on the natural outcome are scarce. Some new prospective studies demonstrate that most patients continue to suffer from residual depressive or hypomanic symptoms between episodes, and many are functionally impaired.
7. Overall research into the natural history of bipolar illness shows that it has a poor prognosis, as reflected by high recurrence, chronicity of episodes or residual symptoms, and premature death by suicide and somatic disorders; however, unlike schizophrenia, which is characterized by much higher chronicity and the predominance of negative and psychotic symptoms, chronicity in bipolar disorders is rarer (10–20%) and the more frequent residual states are limited to characteristic depressive and hypomanic symptoms.

The authors thank Professor Andreas Marneros (University of Halle) and Dr. Mauricio Tohen (Lilly Company) for their contribution to this article in the form of comments and suggestions.

Aspects of this work were presented at the conference "Bipolar Disorder: From Pre-Clinical to Clinical, Facing the New Millennium," January 19–21, 2000, Scottsdale, Arizona. The conference was sponsored by the Society of Biological Psychiatry through an unrestricted educational grant provided by Eli Lilly and Company.

References

Amsterdam JD, Garcia-Espana F, Fawcett J, Quitkin FM, Reimherr FW, Rosenbaum JF, et al (1998): Efficacy and safety of fluoxetine in treating bipolar II major depressive episode. *J Clin Psychopharmacol* 18:435–440.

Angst J (1966): *Zur Aetiologie und Nosologie Endogener Depressiver Psychosen. Eine Genetische, Soziologische und Klinische Studie.* Berlin: Springer.

Angst J (1978): The course of affective disorders. II. Typology of bipolar manic-depressive illness. *Arch Psychiatr Nervenkr* 226:65–73.

Angst J (1986): The course of major depression, atypical bipolar disorder, and bipolar disorder. In: Hippius H, Klerman GL, Matussek N, editors. *New Results in Depression Research.* Berlin: Springer, 26–35.

Angst J (1987): Switch from depression to mania, or from mania to depression. *J Psychopharmacol* 1:13–19.

Angst J (1988): Clinical course of affective disorders. In: Helgason T, Daly RJ, editors. *Depressive Illness: Prediction of Course and Outcome.* Berlin: Springer, 1–48.

Angst J, Baastrup PC, Grof P, Hippius H, Poeldinger W, Weis P (1973): The course of monopolar depression and bipolar psychoses. *Psychiatr Neurol Neurochir* 76:489–500.

Angst J, Battegay R, Bente D, Berner P, Broeren W, Cornu F, et al (1968a): Das Dokumentationssystem der Arbeitsgemeinschaft für Methodik und Dokumentation in der Psychiatrie (AMP). *Arzneimittelforschung* 18:3–8.

Angst J, Grof P, Hippius H, Poeldinger W, Weis P (1968b): La psychose maniaco-depressive est-elle periodique ou intermittente? Dans: Cycles biologiques et psychiatrie. In: de Ajuriaguerra J, editor. *Symposium Bel-Air III, Geneve 1967.* Geneva: Georg et Cie, 339–351.

Angst J, Preisig M (1995a): Course of a clinical cohort of unipolar, bipolar and schizoaffective patients. Results of a prospective study from 1959 to 1985. *Schweiz Arch Neurol Psychiatr* 146:5–16.

Angst J, Preisig M (1995b): Outcome of a clinical cohort of unipolar, bipolar and schizoaffective patients. Results of a prospective study from 1959 to 1985. *Schweiz Arch Neurol Psychiatr* 146:17–23.

Angst J, Weis P (1967): Periodicity of depressive psychoses. In: Brill H, Cole JO, Deniker P, Hippius H, Bradley PB, editors. *Neuro-Psychopharmacology. Proceedings of the Fifth International Congress of the Collegium Internationale Neuro-Psychopharmacologicum, Washington, D.C. 1966,* International Congress Series No 129. Amsterdam: Excerpta Medica, 703–710.

Angst J, Weis P (1968): Aetiologie und Verlauf endogener Depressionen. In: Rémy M, editor. *Depressionen und ihre Behandlung. Fortbildungskurse der SGP,* Vol 1. Basel, Switzerland: Karger, 8–16.

Arnold OH, Kryspin-Exner K (1965): Zur Frage der Beeinflussung des Verlaufes des manisch-depressiven Krankheitsgeschehens durch Antidepressiva. *Wien Med Wochenschr* 115: 929–934.

Baastrup PC, Schou M (1968): Prophylactic lithium. *Lancet* I:1419–1422.

Baillarger J (1854): De la folie à double forme. *Ann Med Psychol* 6:369–384.

Ballet G (1903): *Traité de Pathologie Mentale.* Paris: Doin.

Blackwell B, Shepherd M (1968): Prophylactic lithium: Another therapeutic myth? An examination of the evidence to date. *Lancet* 1(7549):968–971.

Bourgeois ML, Marneros A (in press): Course and prognosis of bipolar disorders. In: Marneros A, Angst J, editors. *Bipolar Affective Disorders.* Dordrecht, The Netherlands: Kluwer.

Bratfos O, Haug JO (1968): Course of manic-depressive psychosis. A follow-up investigation of 215 patients. *Acta Psychiatr Scand* 44:89–112.

Coryell W, Endicott J, Maser JD, Keller MB, Leon AC, Akiskal HS (1995a): Long-term stability of polarity disinctions in the affective disorders. *Am J Psychiatry* 152:385–390.

Coryell W, Endicott J, Maser JD, Mueller T, Lavori P, Keller M (1995b): The likelihood of recurrence in bipolar affective disorder: The importance of episode recency. *J Affect Disord* 33:201–206.

Coryell W, Keller M, Endicott J, Andreasen N, Clayton P, Hirschfeld R (1989): Bipolar II illness: Course and outcome over a five-year period. *Psychol Med* 19:129–141.

Coryell W, Turvey C, Endicott J, Leon AC, Mueller T, Solomon D, Keller M (1998): Bipolar I affective disorder: Predictors of outcome after 15 years. *J Affect Disord* 50:109–116.

Coryell W, Winokur G (1992): Course and outcome. In: Paykel ES, editor. *Handbook of Affective Disorders,* 2nd ed. London: Churchill Livingstone, 89–108.

Dunner DL, Fleiss JL, Fieve RR (1976): The course of development of mania in patients with recurrent depression. *Am J Psychiatry* 133:905–908.

Dunner DL, Murphy D, Stallone F, Fieve RR (1979): Episode frequency prior to lithium treatment in bipolar manic-depressive patients. *Compr Psychiatry* 20:511–515.

Eaton WW, Anthony JC, Gallo J, Cai G, Tien A, Romanoski A, et al (1997): Natural history of Diagnostic Interview Schedule DSM-IV major depression. The Baltimore Epidemiologic Catchment area follow-up. *Arch Gen Psychiatry* 54:993–999.

Falret J (1861): Principes à suivre dans la classification des maladies mentales. *Ann Med Psychol* 19:145.

Falret JP (1851): Marche de la folie. *Gazette Hopitaux* 24:18–19.

Falret JP (1854): De la folie circulaire ou forme de maladie mentale caractérisée par l'alternative régulière de la manie et de la mélancholie. *Bull Acad Med (Paris)* 19:382.

Fleiss JL, Dunner DL, Stallone F, Fieve RR (1976): The life table: A method for analyzing longitudinal studies. *Arch Gen Psychiatry* 33:107–112.

Fleiss JL, Prien RF, Dunner DL, Fieve RR (1978): Actuarial studies of the course of manic-depressive illness. *Compr Psychiatry* 19:355–362.

Fogarty F, Russell JM, Newman SC, Bland RC (1994): Mania. *Acta Psychiatr Scand Suppl* 376:16–23.

Frank E, Prien RF, Jarrett RB, Keller MB, Kupfer DJ, Lavori PW, et al (1991): Conceptualisation and rationale for consensus definitions of terms in major depressive disorder. Remission, recovery, relapse, and recurrence. *Arch Gen Psychiatr* 48:851–855.

Fukuda K, Etoh T, Iwadate T, Ishii A (1983): The course and prognosis of manic-depressive psychosis: A quantitative analysis of episodes and intervals. *Tohoku J Exp Med* 139:299–307.

Fuller RG (1935): What happens to mental patients after discharge from hospital. *Psychiatr Q* 9:95–104.

Gitlin MJ, Swendsen J, Heller TL, Hammen C (1995): Relapse and impairment in bipolar disorder. *Am J Psychiatry* 152: 1635–1640.

Goldberg JF, Harrow M (1999): Poor-outcome bipolar disorders. In: Goldberg JF, Harrow M, editors. *Bipolar Disorders. Clinical Course and Outcome.* Washington, DC: American Psychiatric Press, 1–20.

Goldberg JF, Harrow M, Grossman LS (1995): Course and outcome in bipolar affective disorder: A longitudinal follow-up study. *Am J Psychiatry* 152:379–384.

Goodwin FK, Jamison KR (1990): *Manic-Depressive Illness.* New York: Oxford University Press.

Gottschalk A, Bauer MS, Whybrow PC (1995): Evidence of chaotic mood variation in bipolar disorder. *Arch Gen Psychiatry* 52:947–959.

Griesinger W (1845): *Pathologie und Therapie der Psychischen Krankheiten für Aerzte und Studierende,* 1st ed. Stuttgart: A. Krabbe.

Grof P, Alda M, Ahrens B (1995): Clinical course of affective disorders: Were Emil Kraepelin and Jules Angst wrong? *Psychopathology* 28(suppl 1):73–80.

Guislain J (1852): *Leçons Orales sur les Phrénopathies, ou Traité Théorique et Pratique des Maladies Mentales.* Ghent, Belgium: Hebbelynck.

Haustgen T (1995): Aspects historiques des troubles bipolaires dans la psychiatrie Française. *Encephale* 21(suppl 6):13–20.

Heinroth JCA (1918): *Lehrbuch der Störungen des Seelenlebens Oder der Seelenstörungen und Ihre Behandlung, vom Rationalen Standpunkt aus Entworfen.* Leipzig, Germany: Vogel.

Isaaksson A, Ottosson J-O, Perris C (1969): Methodologische Aspekte der Forschung über prophylaktische Behandlung bei affektiven Psychosen. In: Hippius H, Selbach H, editors. *Das Depressive Syndrom. Internationales Symposion Berlin am 16. und 17. Februar 1968.* Munich: Urban & Schwarzenberg, 561–574.

Keck PE Jr, McElroy SL, Strakowski SM, West SA, Sax KW, Hawkins JM, et al (1998): 12-Month outcome of patients with bipolar disorder following hospitalization for a manic or mixed episode. *Am J Psychiatry* 155:646–652.

Keller MB (1987): Differential diagnosis, natural course, and epidemiology of bipolar disorders. *Annu Rev* 6:10–31.

Keller MB, Lavori PW, Coryell W, Andreasen NC, Endicott J, Clayton PJ, et al (1986a): Differential outcome of pure manic, mixed/cycling, and pure depressive episodes in patients with bipolar illness. *JAMA* 255:3138–3142.

Keller MB, Lavori PW, Coryell W, Endicott J, Mueller TI (1993): Bipolar I: A five-year prospective follow-up. *J Nerv Ment Dis* 181:238–245.

Keller MB, Lavori PW, Rice J, Coryell W, Hirschfeld RMA (1986b): The persistent risk of chronicity in recurrent episodes of nonbipolar major depressive disorder: A prospective follow-up. *Am J Psychiatry* 143:24–28.

Kessing LV, Andersen PK, Mortensen PB (1998a): Predictors of recurrence in affective disorder. A case register study. *J Affect Disord* 49:101–108.

Kessing LV, Andersen PK, Mortensen PB, Bolwig TG (1998b): Recurrence in affective disorder. I. Case register study. *Br J Psychiatry* 172:23–28.

Kinkelin M (1954): Verlauf und Prognose des Manisch-Depressiven Irreseins. *Schweiz Arch Neurol Neurochir Psychiatr* 73:100–146.

Klerman GL, DiMascio A, Weissman MM, Prusoff B, Paykel ES (1974): Treatment of depression by drugs and psychotherapy. *Am J Psychiatry* 131:186–191.

Koukopoulos A, Reginaldi D, Laddomada P, Floris G, Serra G, Tondo L (1980): Course of manic-depressive cycle and changes caused by treatments. *Pharmacopsychiatry* 13:156–167.

Kraepelin E (1899): *Psychiatrie. Ein Lehrbuch für Studierende und Ärzte,* 6th ed, Vol 2. Leipzig, Germany: Barth.

Kraepelin E (1913): *Psychiatrie. Ein Lehrbuch für Studierende und Aerzte,* 8th ed, Vol III. Leipzig, Germany: Barth.

Kramer M (1969): *Application of Mental Health Statistics.* Geneva: World Health Organization.

Lader MH (1968): Prophylactic lithium? *Lancet* II:103.

Laurell B, Ottosson JO (1968): Prophylactic lithium? *Lancet* 2:1245–1246.

Lavori PW, Keller MB, Klerman GL (1984): Relapse in affective disorders: A reanalysis of the literature using life table methods. *J Psychiatr Res* 18:13–25.

Lewinsohn PM, Clarke GN, Seeley JR, Rohde P (1994): Major depression in community adolescents: Age at onset, episode duration, and time to recurrence. *J Am Acad Child Adolesc Psychiatry* 33:809–818.

MacDonald JB (1918): Prognosis in manic-depressive insanity. *J Nerv Ment Dis* 47:20–30.

Marneros A (1999): *Handbuch der Unipolaren und Bipolaren Erkrankungen.* Stuttgart: Thieme.

Marneros A (in press): Origin and development of the concept of "mixed states". *J Affect Disord.*

Marneros A, Deister A, Rohde A (1991a): *Affektive, Schizoaffektive und Schizophrene Psychosen. Eine Vergleichende Langzeitstudie.* Berlin: Springer.

Marneros A, Deister A, Rohde A (1991b): Stability of diagnoses in affective, schizoaffective and schizophrenic disorders. Cross-sectional versus longitudinal diagnosis. *Eur Arch Psychiatry Clin Neurosci* 241:187–192.

Mendel E (1881): *Die Manie. Eine Monographie.* Vienna: Urban & Schwarzenberg.

Panse F (1924): Untersuchungen über Verlauf und Prognose beim Manisch-Depressiven Irresein. *Monatsschr Psychiatr Neurol* 56:15–82.

Paskind HA (1930): Manic-depressive psychosis as seen in private praxis. Length of the attack and length of the interval. *Arch Neurol* 23:789–794.

Perugi G, Akiskal HS, Micheli C, Musetti L, Paiano A, Quilici C, et al (1997): Clinical subtypes of bipolar mixed states: Validating a broader European definition in 143 cases. *J Affect Disord* 43:169–180.

Pichot P (1995): The birth of the bipolar disorder. *Eur Psychiatry* 10:1–10.

Pilcz A (1901): Die Periodischen Geistesstörungen. Eine Klinische Studie. Jena, Germany: G. Fischer.

Pollock HM (1931a): Prevalence of manic-depressive psychoses in relation to sex, age, environment, nativity and race. In: White WA, Davis TK, Frantz AM, editors. *Manic-Depressive Psychosis.* Baltimore: Williams & Wilkins, 655–667.

Pollock HM (1931b): Recurrence of attacks in manic-depressive psychoses. *Am J Psychiatry* 11:567–574.

Pollock HM (1931c): Recurrence of attacks in manic-depressive psychoses. In: White WA, Davis TK, Frantz AM, editors. *Manic-Depressive Psychosis.* Baltimore: William & Wilkins, 668–675.

Poort R (1945): Catamnestic investigations on manic-depressive psychoses with special reference to the prognosis. *Acta Psychiatr Scand* 20:59–74.

Post RM (1992): Transduction of psychosocial stress into the neurobiology of recurrent affective disorder. *Am J Psychiatry* 149:999–1010.

Post RM, Rubinow DR, Ballenger JC (1984): Conditioning, sensitization, and kindling: Implications for the course of affective illness. In: Post RM, Ballenger JC, editors. *Neurobiology of Mood Disorders. Frontiers of Clinical Neurosciences,* Vol 2. Baltimore: Williams & Wilkins, 432–466.

Post RM, Rubinow DR, Ballenger JC (1986): Conditioning and sensitisation in the longitudinal course of affective illness. *Br J Psychiatry* 149:191–201.

Rehm O (1919): *Das Manisch Melancholische Irresein,* Monographien aus dem Gesamtgebiete der Neurologie und Psychiatrie, Vol 17. Berlin: Springer.

Rennie TAC (1942): Prognosis in manic-depressive psychoses. *Am J Psychiatry* 98:801–814.

Ritti A (1879): Folie avec conscience. In: Dechambre A, editor. *Dictionnaire Encyclopédique des Sciences Médicales.* Paris: P. Asselin, G. Masson, 520–559.

Roy-Byrne P, Post RM, Uhde TW, Porcu T, Davos D (1985): The longitudinal course of recurrent affective illness: Life chart data from research patients at the NIMH. *Acta Psychiatr Scand Suppl* 317:1–34.

Saran BM (1969): Lithium. *Lancet* I:1208–1209.

Slater E (1938): Zur Periodik des manisch-depressiven Irreseins. *Z Ges Neurol Psychiatr* 162:794–801.

Solomon DA, Keitner GI, Miller IW, Shea MT, Keller MB (1995): Course of illness and maintenance treatments for patients with bipolar disorder. *J Clin Psychiatry* 56:5–13.

Stephens JH, McHugh PR (1991): Characteristics and long-term follow-up of patients hospitalized for mood disorders in the Phipps Clinic, 1913–1940. *J Nerv Ment Dis* 179:64–73.

Till E, Vuckovik S (1970): Ueber den Einfluss der thymoleptischen Behandlung auf den Verlauf endogener Depressionen. *Int Pharmacopsychiatry* 4:210–219.

Tohen M, Hennen J, Zarate CM Jr, Baldessarini RJ, Strakowski SM, Stoll AL, et al (2000): Two-year syndromal and functional recovery in 219 cases of first-episode major affective disorder with psychotic features. *Am J Psychiatry* 157:220–228.

Tohen M, Waternaux C, Tsuang MT (1990): Outcome in mania. A 4-year prospective follow-up of 75 patients utilizing survival analysis. *Arch Gen Psychiatry* 47:1106–1111.

Tomasson H (1947): Investigations on manic depressive psychosis. *Acta Psychiatr Scand* 47:472–480.

Tondo L, Laddomada P, Serra G, Minnai G, Kukopoulos A (1981): Rapid cyclers and antidepressants. *Int Pharmacopsychiatry* 16:119–123.

Tsuang MT, Woolson RF, Fleming JA (1979): Long-term outcome of major psychoses. I. Schizophrenia and affective disorders compared with psychiatrically symptom-free surgical conditions. *Arch Gen Psychiatry* 36:1295–1301.

Turvey CL, Coryell WH, Solomon DA, Leon AC, Endicott J, Keller MB, Akiskal H (1999): Long-term prognosis of bipolar I disorder. *Acta Psychiatr Scand* 99:110–119.

Verdoux H, Bourgeois ML (1995): Evolution pronostic des troubles bipolaires. In: Bourgeois ML, Verdoux H, editors. *Les Troubles Bipolaires de l'Humeur.* Paris: Masson, 197–207.

Weissman MM, Leaf PJ, Tischler GL, Blazer DG, Karno M, Bruce ML, Florio LP (1988): Affective disorders in five United States communities. *Psychol Med* 18:141–153.

Wernicke C (1906): *Grundriss der Psychiatrie in Klinischen Vorlesungen.* Leipzig, Germany: Thieme.

Wertham FI (1929): A group of benign chronic psychoses: Prolonged manic excitements. With a statistical study of age, duration and frequency in 2000 manic attacks. *Am J Psychiatry* 9:17–78.

Weygandt W (1899): *Uber die Mischzustände des manisch-depressiven Irreseins. Medizinische Fakultät.* Würzburg, Germany: Königliche Julius-Maximilians-Universität.

Winokur G, Coryell W, Akiskal HS, Endicott J, Keller M, Mueller T (1994): Manic-depressive (bipolar) disorder: The course in light of a prospective ten-year follow-up of 131 patients. *Acta Psychiatr Scand* 89:102–110.

Winokur G, Coryell W, Keller M, Endicott J, Akiskal H (1993): A prospective follow-up of patients with bipolar and primary unipolar affective disorder. *Arch Gen Psychiatry* 50:457–465.

Ziehen T (1902): *Psychiatrie für Ärzte und Studirende.* Leipzig, Germany: S. Hirzel.

Ziehen T (1907): *Die Erkennung und Behandlung der Melancholie in der Praxis.* Halle, Germany: Carl Marhold.

Zis AP, Goodwin FK (1979): Major affective disorders as a recurrent illness. *Arch Gen Psychiatry* 36:835–839.

Zis AP, Grof P, Webster M, Goodwin FK (1980): Prediction of relapse in recurrent affective disorder. *Psychopharmacol Bull* 16:47–49.

ELSEVIER

Journal of Affective Disorders 50 (1998) 109–116

JOURNAL OF AFFECTIVE DISORDERS

Research report

Bipolar I affective disorder: predictors of outcome after 15 years

William Coryell*, Carolyn Turvey, Jean Endicott, Andrew C. Leon, Timothy Mueller, David Solomon, Martin Keller

University of Iowa College of Medicine, Psychiatry Research–MEB, Rm. 2-205, Iowa City, IA 52242-1000, USA

Abstract

Background: Robust predictors of long-term outcome in bipolar affective disorder would have substantial importance to both clinicians and researchers. Such predictors are not available, however, perhaps because of the limitations of previous efforts to find them. *Methods*: In this study, 113 patients with bipolar affective disorder were followed semiannually for 5 years and annually for a subsequent 15 years. Of these, 23 (20.4%) had a poor long-term outcome indicated by the presence of mania or major depressive disorder throughout the 15th year. *Results*: Among the baseline demographic and clinical variables tested, only active alcoholism and low levels of optimum functioning in the preceding 5 years characterized poor outcome patients. The persistence of depressive symptoms in the first 2 years of follow-up predicted depressive symptoms 15 years later but the early persistence of manic symptoms seemed to have no predictive value. A regression analysis eliminated alcoholism as an independent predictor. Thus, only poor optimal functioning in the 5 years before baseline assessment, and the persistence of depressive symptoms in the two subsequent years, were independently associated with poor, long-term prognosis. *Limitations*: Patients were recruited at tertiary care centers and sampling was therefore biased toward greater severity and chronicity. As is true of all naturalistic studies of course, treatment was not controlled. *Conclusion*: These findings suggest the existence of a poor outcome, depression-prone subtype of bipolar affective disorder.

1. Introduction

Psychiatrically ill patients often have an intense, and understandable, interest in what the long-term outcome of their illness is likely to be. The existence of long-term predictors is essential to this estimation. Researchers, too, need robust outcome predictors, though for different reasons. Clear relationships between outcome categories and gender, age at onset, premorbid measures, or diagnostic subtypes would suggest subgroupings with greater homogeneity. This, in turn, would facilitate the search for pathogenesis. Yet, there is scant knowledge with which to make such predictions. Despite a number of efforts to characterize the eventual outcomes of particular disorders, and to identify robust predictors, conclusions are severely limited by methodological weaknesses and by inconsistencies across studies.

Bipolar affective disorder offers an important example. With the exception of the study described below, none of the follow-ups of 10 years or longer began with a structured interview of all patients and potential predictors were therefore not uniformly ascertained (Rennie, 1942; Poort, 1945; Lundquist,

*Corresponding author.

0165-0327/98/$ – see front matter
PII: S0165-0327(98)00043-3

1945; Stenstedt, 1952; Bratfos and Haug, 1968; Shobe and Brion, 1971; Tsuang et al., 1979; Fukuda et al., 1983; McGlashan, 1984). Five of these long-term studies (Bratfos and Haug, 1968; Fukuda et al., 1983; Poort, 1945; Rennie, 1942; Shobe and Brion, 1971) used mailed questionnaires rather than direct interviews for follow-up assessments and only the more recent studies provided operational definitions of bipolar illness.

The NIMH Collaborative Program on the Psychobiology Of Depression-Clinical Studies (CDS) is a multicenter, prospective study of the phenomenology and natural history of the major affective disorders. The baseline evaluations of probands took place over 15 years ago and follow-up continues. Earlier reports from this group have described various aspects of the course in bipolar patients at 2 years (Keller et al., 1986a,b; Coryell et al., 1987), 5 years (Coryell et al., 1989, 1990, 1992, 1993; Winokur et al., 1993a,b; Keller et al., 1993; Winokur et al., 1995; Coryell et al., 1997) and 10 years (Winokur et al., 1994; Coryell et al., 1995a,b). Nearly all of these reports focused on phenomenology and on the timing of episodes. Coryell et al. (1993) emphasized psychosocial outcome but only after 5 years. The following will focus instead on outcomes after 15 years of follow-up. It will include as potential predictors not only the conventional demographic and clinical variables assessed at baseline, but also symptom persistence during the first 2 years of follow-up.

2. Methods

Clinically experienced raters recruited probands within a week of hospital admission, or within 1 month of their initial outpatient contact at any of five academic centers—Massachusetts General Hospital and Harvard University in Boston, Rush Presbyterian–St. Luke's Medical Center in Chicago, University of Iowa College of Medicine in Iowa City, New York State Psychiatric Institute and Columbia University in New York and Washington University School of Medicine in St. Louis. All probands met Research Diagnostic Criteria (RDC) (Spitzer et al., 1978) for major depressive disorder, mania or schizo-affective disorder, were white and were 17 years of age or older. All provided informed consent before participating.

Raters completed the Schedule for Affective Disorders and Schizophrenia (SADS) (Endicott and Spitzer, 1978) on the basis of direct interviews, medical records and, often, interviews with informants. They then reassessed probands at 6-month intervals, first with the Longitudinal Interval Follow-up Evaluation (LIFE) (Keller et al., 1987) and then, in Years 3–5, with the somewhat shorter LIFE II (available upon request). Subsequent follow-ups were annual and used a similar but shorter instrument, the Streamlined Longitudinal Interval Continuation Evaluation or SLICE (available upon request).

All three instruments tracked psychopathology by syndrome and provided a week-by-week quantification of symptom levels. For the major affective syndromes (manic disorder, major depressive disorder and schizo-affective disorder), the six-point scale used ranged from 1, indicating no symptoms of the corresponding syndrome, to 6, indicating the full syndrome at a severe level. Minor depressive disorder, intermittent depressive disorder, hypomania and other, non-affective, RDC disorders were tracked with a three-point scales on which 3 represented the full syndrome and 1 the absence of symptoms.

These instruments included six-point scales to quantify psychosocial adjustment in the specific areas of employment, household duties, friendships, overall satisfaction, marital adjustment and recreational activities. After assessing these particular areas, interviewers rendered a global rating of social adjustment. Psychosocial ratings ranged from 1 or 'very good' to 6 or 'very poor (markedly impaired)' adjustment. Some subjects missed individual follow-up interviews, but were assessed at a later date. In these cases, the weekly ratings of symptom levels for individual syndromes was maintained. However, because psychosocial ratings referred only to the month preceding the interview, these were not rendered for years in which an interview was missed.

Participation in this study did not determine or influence treatment. All somatic treatments directed at mental disorders were carefully quantified on a week-by-week basis, though, and raters recorded individual drugs and their doses (Keller et al., 1986a,b). These data were later condensed to dose equivalencies in major classes (i.e. chlorpromazine, imipramine, phenelzine, diazepam) and then to composite scores intended to reflect the overall intensity of treatment. A UNICAD score quantified the intensity of treatment considered appropriate for acute and prophylactic management of depression. Patients with a 2 on this 4-point scale had been treated with the equivalent of 100–199 mg of imipramine per day. The PURCAM score reflected the intensity of treatment appropriate for mania or mixed states. A 2 on this 4-point scale indicated treatment with an antipsychotic equivalent to 300–800 mg of chlorpromazine and a 3 indicated treatment with lithium, ECT and/or higher levels of antipsychotics.

The following analyses describe probands who completed 15 years of follow-up and who, at intake, described a current or past history of RDC mania or schizo-affective mania, other than the mainly schizophrenic subtype. This combination of RDC disorders closely approximates the DSM-IV definition of mania, inclusive of cases with mood-incongruent psychotic features. For simplicity, the following text will refer to this combination as 'bipolar I'.

Poor outcome was arbitrarily defined by the presence of symptoms of MDD, mania or schizo-affective disorder throughout the 15th year of follow-up at PSR levels of 3, 4, 5 or 6. Because some among the remaining patients were symptomatic for much, though not all, of this year, we labeled all those not in the poor outcome group as 'others' rather than as 'good outcome'. The analyses compared these two groups by the demographic and clinical variables listed in Table 1, and by morbidity indexes based on the first 2 years of follow-up. A two-year interval corresponds to the current convention which defines chronicity as at least 2 years of persistent symptoms (Endicott and Spitzer, 1978). The MDD morbidity index (MI), was the number of weeks in the first 2 years of follow-up with PSR

Table 1
Baseline characteristics of Bipolar I patients by outcome 15 years later

	Poor outcome	Others
n	23	90
No. (%) male	15 (65.2)	54 (60.0)
Age, mean (*S.D.*)	32.4 (10.0)	35.0 (11.4)
Marital status:		
Never married	37 (41.1)	13 (56.5)
Married	8 (34.8)	33 (35.7)
Divorced	2 (8.7)	20 (22.2)
Age at first episode, mean years (*S.D.*)	26.3 (10.1)	28.2 (11.5)
No. of prior episodes, mean (*S.D.*)	2.8 (4.5)	4.3 (10.5)
Healthiest functioning in previous 5 years, (1–6, 6 = poorest functioning), mean (*S.D.*)[a]	3.0 (1.1)	2.2 (1.0)
Adolescent friendship patterns (1–6, 6 = grossly inadequate), mean (*S.D.*)	3.2 (1.1)	2.7 (1.2)
Occupation of subject (1–8, 8 = lowest), mean (*S.D.*)	4.1 (1.5)	3.9 (1.6)
Education of subject (1–7, 7 = lowest), mean (*S.D.*)	3.3 (1.4)	3.2 (1.2)
Annual income of subject (1–8, 8 = highest), mean (*S.D.*)	3.4 (2.5)	3.8 (1.9)
Duration, mean weeks (*S.D.*):		
Of manic syndrome	24.3 (46.3)	16.5 (22.2)
Of affective syndrome	91.1 (152.1)	29.5 (70.3)
No. (%) with cycling during episode	14 (60.9)	42 (46.7)
No. (%) with psychotic features	15 (65.2)	51 (56.7)
No. (%) with schizo-affective diagnosis	4 (17.4)	7 (7.8)
No. (%) with current:		
Alcoholism[b]	5 (21.7)	5 (5.6)
Drug use disorder	0–	3 (3.3)
Phobic disorder	1 (4.3)	2 (2.2)
Panic disorder	0–	2 (2.2)

[a] Wilcoxon rank sum test, $z = 3.25$, $p = 0.0012$.
[b] $x^2 = 6.0$, $df = 1$, $p = 0.015$.

ratings of 3 (obvious evidence of the disorder was present) or greater for major depressive disorder, or schizo-affective disorder, depressive type. The mania MI reflected the number of weeks with manic, or schizo-affective manic, disorder. Both poles were combined in the 'all major affective MI'.

These analyses used *t*-tests or dimensional variables, Wilcoxon rank-sum tests for ordered categorical variables, and chi square tests for 2 × 2 categorical comparisons. Pearson product–moment correlation coefficients tested the strength of linear relationships between two variables and a two-tailed alpha level of 0.05 was used for all tests.

3. Results

Of the 206 patients who began the study with bipolar I disorder, 26 were known to have died during the next 15 years. Of the other 180, 113 (62.8%) are described below. Some of the remaining 67 have refused further follow-up but others have not been located and efforts continue to complete follow-up for these individuals. As a consequence, follow-up rates will be somewhat higher in future reports. After the exclusion of subjects who died, those who completed follow-up did not differ from the remainder by the baseline variables listed in Table 1.

Sixty-five (56.6%) had no symptoms of RDC major depressive disorder, mania or schizo-affective disorder during any week of the final year and 25 (22.1%) had symptoms for fewer than 52 weeks. Twenty-three (20.4%), on the other hand, had a 'poor outcome' as defined above in that they had symptoms of one or more of these disorders in all 52 weeks of year 15. The poor outcome patients did not differ from the remaining 90 patients by baseline demographic or socio-economic measures (Table 1). Results of more detailed analyses of ages at onset did not associate a particularly early age at onset with poor outcome; of 23 with an onset before age 18, 4 (17.4%) proved to have a poor outcome. Only 5 had an onset of illness past age 50 years and 1 (20.0%) of these had a poor outcome.

The two outcome groups had similar levels of treatment in their first 2 years of follow-up. The mean (*S.D.*) number of weeks with UNICAD scores of two or more were 62.4 (39.7) and 74.1 (38.0), respectively, for poor outcome and for other patients. The mean (*S.D.*) numbers of weeks with PURCAM scores of two or more were 73.5 (37.1) and 72.3 (39.2), respectively. In Year 15, the groups again the groups did not differ in this regard. Individuals in the poor prognosis group had a mean of 34.9 weeks (*S.D.* = 22.2) with UNICAD scores of 2 or more and 32.2 weeks (*S.D.* = 22.8) with PURCAM scores of 2 or more. The remaining patients had mean numbers of weeks of 34.8 (*S.D.* = 24.0) and 33.2 (*S.D.* = 24.5), respectively.

Among the baseline historical and clinical measures considered, only two distinguished those who were to have sustained symptoms during the 15th year of follow-up. Poor outcome individuals had been significantly more impaired when functioning at their best in the 5 years preceding intake and were nearly four times more likely to have had active alcoholism when they entered the study. Of the five poor outcome patients with active alcoholism at intake, one met criteria for definite alcoholism at any point in the 15th year of follow-up. None of the five 'other outcome' patients with alcoholism at intake had active alcoholism in the 15th year. Only one of the ten patients with alcoholism at intake had developed alcoholism prior to the first manic episode.

The variables which were statistically significant predictors of outcome status in the univariate analyses were entered as independent variables in an analysis of covariance. For the entire model R^2 = 0.22, $F = 10.05$ and $p = 0.0001$. Both 'healthiest level of functioning in previous 5 years' ($F = 8.35$, $df = 1$, $p = 0.0047$) and the depression morbidity index in Years 1 and 2 ($F = 16.3$, $df = 1$, $p = 0.0001$) were robustly predictive but the presence or absence of current alcoholism at intake was not ($F = 0.36$, $df = 1$, $p = 0.5474$).

Among the 113 who completed 15 years of follow-up, one-sixth to one-third were rated as psychosocially impaired at the end of that year, depending on the specific area considered, and employment was the most heavily impacted area (Table 2). Psychosocial impairment ratings overlapped substantially with symptom-based outcome categories. All of the 14 individuals with moderate or marked impairment in social adjustment were in the poor outcome group. Of those with very good (8)

Table 2
Proportions with moderate to marked impairment in specific areas after 15 years

	Number rated	Percentage impaired
Employment or self-employment	73	34.2
Household duties	84	17.9
Friendships	88	27.3
Recreation	88	17.0
Global social adjustment	90	15.6

or good (34) overall social adjustment, none were in the poor outcome group.

The number of weeks in which symptoms of MDD were present in the first 2 years of follow-up correlated with the persistence of depressive symptoms 15 years later (Table 3). No linear relationship emerged for manic symptoms, however; the number of weeks that manic symptoms were present in Years 1 and 2 was unrelated to the weeks ill with either manic or depressive symptoms in Year 15. The distribution of depression morbidity indexes in the first 2 years did not reveal a clear threshold with which an ultimately poor outcome might be predicted (Fig. 1).

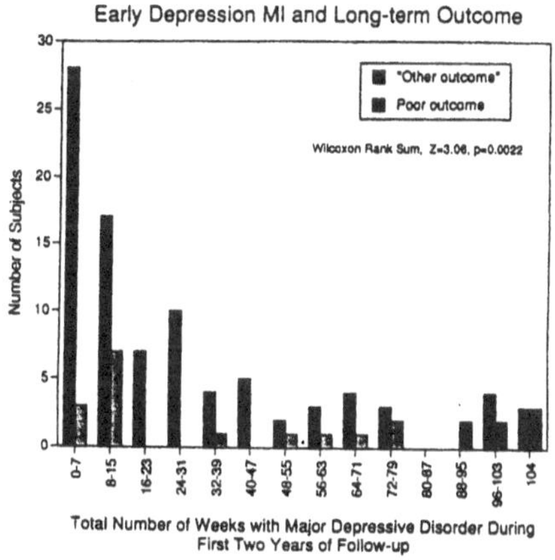

Fig. 1. Early depression MI and long-term outcome.

An alternative calculation of the depression morbidity index included symptom severity. This morbidity index was the product of the number of weeks ill and the symptom levels for each week. Thus, a year in which the PSR was five for 13 weeks, three for another 13 weeks, and two for the remaining 26 weeks would have an MI of 156. The depression morbidity indexes for Years 1 and 2 and Year 15, calculated in this way, were not as strongly correlated ($r = 0.19$, $p = 0.025$) as were the morbidity indexes which reflected simply the number of weeks with MDD.

The persistence of depressive symptoms in Years 1 and 2 (MDD-MI) was also significantly associated with the degree of impairment present 15 years later in the areas of household duties, recreational activities, overall satisfaction and globally rated social adjustment (Table 4). Only one correlation reached significance, this between the number of weeks with manic symptoms in the first 2 years of follow-up and psychosocial ratings at 15 years. The direction was counter-intuitive, however; a greater number of

Table 3
Pearson correlation coefficients between Morbidity Indexes (MI) early and late in follow-up

	Year 15 for:		
	MDD	Mania	All major affective disorders
MI in years 1 and 2 for:			
MDD	0.38*	0.05	0.32*
Mania	0.06	−0.02	0.05
All major affective	0.036	0.04	0.31*

* $p < 0.001$.

Table 4
Morbidity Indexes (MIs) early in follow-up and psychosocial impairment 15 years later (Pearson correlation coefficients)

	Morbidity Index in Years 1 and 2 for:		
	MDD	Mania	All major affective
Employment	0.18	−0.13	0.09
Household duties	0.32**	−0.23*	0.17
Friends	0.16	0.14	0.23*
Recreational activities	0.30**	0.04	0.28**
Overall satisfaction	0.22*	0.01	0.22**
Overall social adjustment	0.33**	0.15	0.38

*$p < 0.05$.
**$p < 0.01$.

weeks with manic symptoms in Years 1 and 2 were associated with lesser impairment in household duties at a modest level of significance.

4. Discussion

The current study's design avoided several of the methodological limitations of earlier efforts. The use of structured interviews insured the uniform assessment of potential predictors, baseline diagnostic groupings were fully operationalized, and the direct interview of subjects determined all outcome measures. On the other hand, the generalizability of these findings is limited by the sampling methods used. All probands were recruited as they sought treatment at tertiary care centers and, within the universe of individuals with bipolar affective disorder, those in the current sample were suffering from a relatively severe and relatively treatment-resistant illness.

One-fifth of patients who entered this study with bipolar I disorder were symptomatic throughout the final year of a 15-year follow-up. Though grouped as 'poor outcome' purely on the basis of symptom persistence throughout this year, none of these individuals were judged to have had good social adjustment at the end of follow-up and nearly all were considered markedly impaired. Thus, though bipolar affective disorder is a remitting illness, and has a prognosis which compares favorably to certain other psychiatric illnesses, a substantial number of those with this disorder face an unfavorable long-term outcome.

Clear predictors of such an outcome are not available though the literature contains many relevant follow-up studies. While methodological differences and deficiencies have undoubtedly undermined consensus on outcome predictors, the fact that simple demographic variables have not proven important suggests that these measures, in fact, lack dependable prognostic significance. Likewise, age of onset has been included in many studies as a potential correlate of outcome and has not proven useful as such.

The other baseline variables assessed in this cohort have not been so consistently described in earlier follow-up studies. Among these, the average duration of the index episode at the time of intake, though three times longer in the poor prognosis group, did not significantly differentiate the outcome groups. The standard deviations were quite large, though, and the duration of a specific episode is often an inaccurate reflection of chronicity. The onset of a current episode may have been preceded by a relatively brief period of remission which, in turn, may have been preceded by a very lengthy episode. In this respect, the level of optimal functioning in the preceding 5 years is probably a more valid measure of chronicity. This item robustly separated the two outcome groups.

Though cycling (Keller et al., 1993) and, in particular, rapid cycling (Maj et al., 1994; Wehr et al., 1988) has been associated with greater morbidity in the short-term, cycling per se did not predict a poor 15-year outcome in these analyses. Earlier analyses of data from this cohort have shown that, though rapid cycling anticipates greater morbidity in the ensuing year, its prognostic significance may not be more sustained than that (Coryell et al., 1992). However, though cycling within a given episode may have only temporary prognostic significance, a recurrent tendency to polyphasic episodes appears to indicate an illness with greater long-term morbidity (Turvey et al., in press).

The persistence of depressive symptoms in the first 2 years of follow-up predicted the persistence of depressive symptoms 15 years later in patients with bipolar I disorder. No such relationship emerged for manic symptoms early and late in follow-up. This suggests the existence of a poor prognosis subtype of bipolar disorder marked by a relative persistence of depressive symptoms. Such a subtype may, in turn, correspond to the 'prevailingly depressed type' of bipolar patient described by Angst (1978), or the 'depression prone' form characterized by Quitkin et al. (1986). The reliable dominance of depressive symptoms in each year of follow-up, and a clear tendency for such a pattern to be over-represented among affected relatives of probands with this pattern, would comprise evidence for the validity of this subtype. This would enable clinicians to advise their patients accordingly, and to be particularly systematic in determining which antidepressant appears most effective over time.

Very few researchers have attempted to classify bipolar patients on this basis and little can be said about the probable validity of this subtype. Unfortunately, the distribution of weeks ill in the first 2 years was not clearly discontinuous and, thus, did not offer a means to identify such patients early in follow-up. A future analysis will seek to determine whether such a subtype can be more efficiently identified.

Acknowledgements

From the National Institute of Mental Health Collaborative Program on the Psychobiology of Depression-Clinical Studies, conduction with the participation of the following investigators: M.B. Keller, M.D. (Chairperson, Providence); W. Coryell, M.D. (Co-Chairperson, Iowa City); J.D. Maser, Ph.D. (Washington, DC); T.I. Mueller, M.D., M.T. Shea Ph.D. (Providence); J. Fawcett, M.D., W.A. Scheftner, M.D. (Chicago); W. Coryell, M.D., James Haley (Iowa City); J. Endicott Ph.D., A.C. Leon, Ph.D., J. Loth, M.S.W. (New York); J. Rice, Ph.D., T. Reich, M.D. (St. Louis). Other contributors include: H.S. Akiskal, M.D., N.C. Andreasen, M.D., Ph.D., P.J. Clayton, M.D., J. Croughan, M.D., R.M.A. Hirschfeld, M.D., L. Ludd, M.D., M.M. Katz, Ph.D., P.W. Lavori, Ph.D., D. Solomon, M.D., R.L. Spitzer, M.D., M.A. Young, Ph.D. Deceased: G.L. Klerman, M.D., E. Robins, M.D., R.W. Shapiro, M.D. and G. Winokur, M.D. This manuscript has been reviewed by the Publication Committee of the Collaborative Depression Study and has its endorsement.

References

Angst, J., 1978. The course of affective disorders II. Typology of bipolar manic depressive illness. Arch. Psychiat. Nervenkr. 226, 65–73.

Bratfos, O., Haug, J.O., 1968. The course of manic depressive psychosis: A follow-up investigation of 215 patients. Acta Psychiatrica Scandinavia 44, 89–112.

Coryell, W., Andreasen, N., Endicott, J., et al., 1987. The significance of past mania or hypomania in the course and outcome of major depression. American Journal of Psychiatry 144, 309–315.

Coryell, W., Keller, M., Endicott, J., et al., 1989. Bipolar II illness: Course and outcome over a five-year period. Psychological Medicine 19, 129–141.

Coryell, W., Keller, M., Lavori, P., et al., 1990. Affective syndromes, psychotic features and prognosis II Mania. Archives of General Psychiatry 47, 658–664.

Coryell, W., Endicott, J., Keller, M., 1992. Rapidly cycling affective disorder: Demographics, diagnosis, family history, and course. Archives of General Psychiatry 49, 126–131.

Coryell, W., Scheftner, W., Keller, M., et al., 1993. The enduring psychosocial consequences of mania and depression. American Journal of Psychiatry 150, 720–727.

Coryell, W., Endicott, J., Maser, J.D. et al., 1995a. The likelihood of recurrence in bipolar affective disorder: The importance of episode recency. Journal of Affective Disorders 33, 201–206.

Coryell, W., Endicott, J., Maser, J.D., et al., 1995. Long-term stability of polarity distinctions in the affective disorders. American Journal of Psychiatry 152, 385–390.

Coryell, W., Winokur, G., Solomon, D., et al., 1997. Lithium and recurrence in a long-term follow-up of bipolar affective disorder. Psychological Medicine 27, 281–290.

Endicott, J., Spitzer, A.L., 1978. A diagnostic interview: The schedule for affective disorders and schizophrenia. Archives of General Psychiatry 35, 837–844.

Fukuda, K., Etoh, T., Iwadate, T., et al., 1983. The course and prognosis of manic depressive psychosis: A quantitative analysis of episodes and intervals. Tohoku Journal of Experimental Medicine 139, 299–307.

Keller, M.B., Lavori, P.W., Coryell, W., et al., 1986. Differential outcome of pure manic, mixed/cycling, and pure depressive episodes in patients with bipolar illness. JAMA 255, 3138–3142.

Keller, M.B., Lavori, P.W., Ikerman, G.L., et al., 1986. Low levels and lack of predictors of somatotherapy and psychotherapy received by depressed patients. Archives of General Psychiatry 43, 458–466.

Keller, M.B., Lavori, P.W., Friedman, B., et al., 1987. The Longitudinal Interval Follow-up Evaluation. Archives of General Psychiatry 44, 540–548.

Keller, M.B., Lavori, P.W., Coryell, W., et al., 1993. Bipolar I: A five-year prospective follow-up. Journal of Nervous and Mental Disease 181, 238–245.

Lundquist, G., 1945. Prognosis and course in manic depressive psychoses: A follow-up study of 319 first admissions. Acta Psychiatrica et Neurologica 35, 1–96.

Maj, M., Magliano, L., Pirozzi, R., et al., 1994. Validity of rapid cycling as a course specifier for bipolar disorder. American Journal of Psychiatry 151, 1015–1029.

McGlashan, T.H., 1984. The Chestnut Lodge follow-up study. II. Long-term outcome of schizophrenia and the affective disorders. Archives of General Psychiatry 41, 586–601.

Poort, R., 1945. Catamnestic investigations on manic-depressive psychoses with special reference to the prognosis. Acta Psychiatrica et Neurologica 20, 59–74.

Quitkin, F.M., Rabkin, J.G., Prien, R.F., 1986. Bipolar disorder: Are there manic-prone and depressive-prone forms?. J. Clin. Psychopharmacol. 6, 167–172.

Rennie, T.A.C., 1942. Prognosis in manic-depressive psychosis. American Journal of Psychiatry 98, 801–814.

Shobe, F.O., Brion, P., 1971. Long-term prognosis in manic depressive illness. Archives of General Psychiatry 24, 334–337.

Spitzer, R.L., Endicott, J., Robins, E., 1978. Research Diagnostic Criteria, 3rd ed., Biometrics Research, New York State Department of Mental Hygiene, New York, New York.

Stenstedt, A., 1952. A study in manic depressive psychosis. Acta Psychiatrica et Neurologica 79, 3–85.

Tsuang, M.T., Woolson, R.F., Fleming, J.A., 1979. Long-term outcome of major psychosis. I. Schizophrenia and affective disorders compared with psychiatrically symptom free surgical controls. Archives of General Psychiatry 36, 1296–1301.

Turvey, C.L., Coryell, W.H., Solomon, D.A., Leon, A.C., Endicott, J., Akiskal, H. Long-term prognosis of bipolar I disorder (in press).

Wehr, T., Sack, D., Rosenthal, N., 1988. Rapid cycling affective disorder: Contributing factors and treatment responses in fifty-one patients. American Journal of Psychiatry 145, 179–184.

Winokur, G., Coryell, W., Endicott, J., et al., 1993. Further distinctions between manic depressive illness (bipolar disorder) and primary depressive disorder (unipolar depression). American Journal of Psychiatry 150, 1176–1181.

Winokur, G., Coryell, W., Keller, M., et al., 1993. A prospective follow-up of patients with bipolar and primary unipolar affective disorder. Archives of General Psychiatry 50, 457–465.

Winokur, G., Coryell, W., Akiskal, H., et al., 1994. Manic depressive (bipolar) disorder: The course in light of a prospective 10-year follow-up of 131 patients. Acta Psychiatrica Scandinavia 89, 103–110.

Winokur, G., Coryell, W., Akiskal, H.S., et al., 1995. Alcoholism in manic depressive (bipolar) illness: Familial illness, course of illness, and the primary-secondary distinction. American Journal of Psychiatry 152, 365–372.

Life Events and the Course of Bipolar Disorder

Aimee Ellicott, Ph.D., Constance Hammen, Ph.D.,
Michael Gitlin, M.D., Gary Brown, and Kay Jamison, Ph.D.

The authors examined the impact of life stress on the course of bipolar disorder over a 2-year period in a group of 61 outpatients. The patients were followed prospectively with ongoing assessments of stressful life events, symptoms, levels of maintenance medication, and compliance with treatment regimens. As predicted, survival analyses indicated a significant association between life events and relapse or recurrence of the disorder. These effects could not be explained by differences in levels of medication or compliance. Further research is recommended to examine which specific subgroups of bipolar patients are most susceptible to stress.

(Am J Psychiatry 1990; 147:1194–1198)

Despite the consistent finding of modest but significant associations between stress and unipolar depressive symptoms (1–5) and recent theoretical and methodological improvements in research on stress and illness, there have been few rigorous investigations of the impact of stress on the course of bipolar illness. Given that bipolar illness is a recurrent disorder (6), with high rates of considerable exacerbation of symptoms over a 1- to 2-year period even when patients apparently comply with lithium carbonate treatment regimens (7), studies examining the factors that predict recurrence and relapse are essential. While genetic and biological components are undoubtedly important in the etiology of bipolar disorder, such factors alone do not entirely explain the variance in the expression of the illness or the timing and frequency of symptoms (8). Psychosocial factors are likely to affect the onset, course, and resolution of this disorder.

Hirschfeld and Cross (9) surveyed the results of controlled and uncontrolled studies of stress and bipolar disorder and concluded that most studies reported that the subjects experienced increased stress before onset or subsequent episodes of the disorder. Results from these studies must be interpreted cautiously, however, given the pervasive methodological flaws and theoretical limitations. First, the use of retrospective designs with lengthy recall periods and questionnaire methods may have contributed to biased or incomplete reporting, errors in memory, inadequate sampling of relevant events, and inaccuracies in dating event onset and duration (5, 10, 11). The only study that used a prospective design to assess stress and symptom levels in 38 patients during a 7-month observation period found few differences in frequency or type of stress between the patients who remained well and those who relapsed (12). However, this investigation may not have used an adequately long observation period and did not control for the effects of medication or compliance with medication regimens, despite the possible effect of these variables on stress-illness relationships.

Received Nov. 7, 1989; revision received March 7, 1990; accepted March 23, 1990. From the Departments of Psychology and Psychiatry, University of California, Los Angeles. Address reprint requests to Dr. Hammen, Department of Psychology, UCLA, 405 Hilgard Ave., Los Angeles, CA 90024.

The present study examined the impact of life stress on the course of bipolar illness over a 2-year period in carefully diagnosed bipolar patients in treatment at an outpatient medication clinic. Prospective methods of assessing symptoms and life stress that have been effective in elucidating the relationships between life stress and unipolar illness were used. In particular, interviews about stressful events and their context, based on methods developed by Brown, Harris, and colleagues (1), were used to obtain careful dating of events and to yield reliable, objective ratings of stressfulness. Symptom levels, diagnoses, and medication and compliance levels were ascertained, independent of the life stress interviews, during the patients' ongoing medication visits to the clinic. The longitudinal design permitted the use of sophisticated techniques such as survival analysis, which incorporates life table and regression analyses, to evaluate the association between probability of relapse and life events. It was hypothesized that patients experiencing increased life stress would have a higher likelihood of relapse as time passed than would patients having lower levels of stress.

METHOD

The participants were outpatients at an affective disorders clinic who were receiving medication for bipolar disorders. Patients were recruited into the ongoing longitudinal study of life stress and course of affective disorder after being followed at the clinic for at least 4 months and after achieving remission status (defined as no episodes of major depression, mania, or hypomania for at least 2 months) or, for a minority of patients, best clinical state (defined as a stable symptom picture for at least the past 6 months).

The subjects were 61 adults (28 men and 33 women) who were followed for at least 1 year. Forty-six were diagnosed as having bipolar I disorder and 15 as having bipolar II disorder. All had experienced prior episodes. Their mean±SD age was 39.6±10.2 years. Eighty-five percent (N=52) of the group was white; 26% (N=16) were currently married or cohabiting, 51% (N=31) were single, and 23% (N=14) were divorced. Forty-one percent (N=25) had at least a college education, and 59% (N=36) had completed high school or less.

Procedures

Initial diagnostic evaluation. Upon admission to the clinic for treatment, each patient received a 3- to 5-hour standard evaluation by a psychiatrist and a psychologist or psychology intern. Detailed information regarding the nature, duration, and dates of current and past symptoms, pharmacologic and psychosocial treatment and treatment response, and family history was obtained from diagnostic interviews (clinical interview, Family History Research Diagnostic Criteria [13]) and self-report questionnaires. Each patient agreed to be contacted in the future for research purposes. Supplementary information for some patients was provided by interviews with family members and review of past medical records. The kappa coefficient of agreement on *DSM-III-R* axis I diagnoses was 0.80 for a random sample of 39 of the patients.

Ongoing symptom assessment. The ongoing symptom status of the patients was assessed when they attended the medication clinic, at intervals (depending on individual need) of 3 days to 3 months. At each visit the patient's psychiatrist evaluated both current symptoms and symptom status throughout the period since the last medication visit, using the *DSM-III-R* criteria for mania, hypomania, major depression, dysthymia, and mixed states. The duration and dates of any diagnosable episodes and subsyndromal disturbances were carefully noted on clinical research forms, and these data were transferred onto individual symptom time lines that indicated the onset and end of all affective episodes during the observation period.

In addition, psychiatrists used a 4-point scale to rate the patient's current diagnosis, current medication regimen, any medication changes or laboratory results, and compliance with the treatment regimen. The research staff monitored the records closely for completeness and accuracy.

Life stress assessment. Life stress that had occurred during the past 6 months was first assessed with a 45- to 90-minute semistructured face-to-face interview when the patient entered the study. Every 3 months thereafter, all subjects were interviewed by telephone or in person about the occurrence of life events since the last contact.

Life stress interviews were based on the methods of Brown, Harris, and colleagues (1) and were conducted to minimize the patients' reporting biases and forgetfulness, while also evaluating the impact of each event in the context in which the event occurred. The 3-month interval minimized the time period over which the subject had to remember, and the accuracy of life event dating was enhanced by the use of cues to aid the subject's memory. Distortions due to selective recall and symptoms were minimized by the prospective design of the study and by conducting the first interview while the subject was in a state of remission.

The life stress interview included standardized probes to obtain detailed information about the date, duration, nature, and circumstances of each event, including the expectedness, the subjective impact, the desirability, and the resources for coping with the event. Definitions of what constituted an event were based on guidelines from Paykel and Mangen's Interview for Recent Life Events (unpublished manuscript, 1981). Each event was described in a written summary prepared by the interviewer, specifically omitting descriptions of the individual's reactions to the event.

Following procedures described by Brown and Harris (1) and Paykel and Mangen (unpublished manuscript, 1981), after the interview a research team eval-

TABLE 1. Maintenance Treatment Scale Used to Rate Treatment Level of 61 Patients With Bipolar Disorder

Maintenance Treatment Level[a]	Lithium (meq/liter)	Carbamazepine (mg/day)	Valproate (mg/day)	Neuroleptics (mg/day)[b]
0	0.00	0	0	0
1	≤0.54	≤499	≤749	≤299
2	0.55–0.69	500–699	750–1249	300–599
3	0.70–0.89	700–999	1250–1999	600–899
4	≥0.90	≥1000	≥2000	≥900

[a]Each level indicates treatment with one kind of drug at the dose shown.
[b]In chlorpromazine equivalents, according to Hollister's conversion table (15).

TABLE 2. Relative Hazard for Relapse at Various Levels of Stress Compared to Baseline Level for 61 Patients With Bipolar Disorder

Stress Level	Coefficient[a]	Standard Error	t (df=25)[b]	Relative Hazard
2	0.07	0.60	0.12	1.08
3	−0.10	0.63	−0.15	0.91
4	1.51	0.44	3.41[c]	4.53

[a]Comparison with baseline level of stress (level 1).
[b]df equals number of relapse points minus 3, where "relapse points" refers to the number of days on which relapse occurred relative to entry into the study.
[c]$p<0.001$.

uated each event and made an "objective" rating of its threat or severity (defined as the way the average person would be likely to experience the impact of the event under similar conditions) on a scale ranging from 1 (no threat) to 5 (severe threat). The research team, which consisted of at least two persons blind to the subject's symptom status who had been extensively trained in the use of contextual-threat interviewing techniques, also rated each event along several dimensions. Reliability calculations based on a total of 45 events from 16 patients yielded an intraclass correlation coefficient of 0.77 ($p\leq0.0001$) for overall objective ratings of threat by two independent teams of raters.

Medication and compliance assessment. Since the adequacy of a maintenance medication regimen and the patient's compliance with this regimen can easily affect relapse rates, medication regimens and compliance were noted at each outpatient visit. Medication regimens were evaluated by using a 5-point scale modeled after Keller's summary scales for treatment of acute affective disorder (14). Table 1 shows the maintenance treatment scale, which ranges from 0 (no maintenance treatment) to 4 (a high level of treatment) with regard to the four most common forms of maintenance treatment in bipolar disorder. Ratings of combination medication regimens were computed by adding the levels of the components.

At each outpatient visit, the psychiatrist rated his or her impression of the patient's degree of adherence to the prescribed regimen since the last visit on a scale ranging from 1 (complete adherence) to 4 (refused recommended treatment). Mean ratings across visits were determined for each patient for the various time periods of interest. The resulting scores yielded a rough compliance rating suitable for assessing the role of differences in compliance as an alternative to the role of stressful events in explaining changes in symptom status.

Analysis

The symptom time lines of the patients were inspected, and the date of relapse or recurrence was noted. Thirty-two of the 61 patients experienced hypomania or mania (N=21) or a major depressive episode (N=11) according to the *DSM-III-R* criteria. If a subject experienced multiple episodes, the first was arbitrarily chosen for examination. These episodes represented recurrences in 22 patients (who had been symptom free for at least 1 month before onset of diagnosable disorder) and relapses in 10 (who went into an episode representing exacerbation of mild previous symptoms). For these 32 patients, the total of objective ratings of stress for events occurring in the 3 months before symptom change was calculated. Of the remaining subjects, 21 experienced no episode, and seven dropped out of the study before completing the first year. Of the no-episode patients, 11 were symptom free over the entire period, and 10 experienced minor, nondiagnosable symptoms. For this group, the final 3 months of the observation period were used to compute totals of objective ratings of life event stress.

We used survival analysis to evaluate the association between stress and symptoms in terms of the probability of symptom change given the stress level, measured by time to episode onset. A variation of Cox's proportional hazards model (16), incorporating stress as a time-dependent covariate, was used. Following the method of Gail (17), we divided the total objective ratings of stress before relapse into quartiles and then calculated coefficients comparing the hazard for the baseline level of stress to the hazard for higher levels.

RESULTS

There was a significant relationship between the highest levels of stress and the likelihood of relapse (see table 2). As table 2 indicates, the patients with low and average levels of stress did not have a greater risk of relapse than those without stress, but those with the highest levels had a risk 4.53 times higher than the patients without stress.

To rule out the confounding effects of differences in the intensity of medication treatment or the level of compliance with regimens, patients who did experience new affective episodes were compared to patients who did not. When the mean medication ratings shown in table 1 for the 3-month comparison periods were used, a t test indicated no significant difference in treatment between those who had an episode and those who did not ($t=1.16$, $df=45$, $p=0.25$, two-tailed test). Similarly, mean compliance ratings for the comparable periods did not differ for the two symptom group ($t<1$, $df=38$, $p=0.40$). Thus, level of medication and compliance with medication regimens did not explain the differential relapse/recurrence rates of the two groups.

DISCUSSION

The longitudinal analysis of symptom changes in bipolar patients indicated a significantly greater likelihood of relapse in the patients with high stress levels than in the patients with lower stress levels and the patients who did not relapse. The subjects who had no stress or low or average levels of stress did not show a greater risk of relapse than those who stayed well. The following representative case example highlights the importance of this finding.

Case 1. Mr. A, a 30-year-old man, had been given a diagnosis of bipolar I disorder at age 21. He had had two manic episodes and multiple minor depressions and hypomanic episodes before treatment at the affective disorders clinic. After entering the study, he remained asymptomatic on a regimen of lithium carbonate and had no severely threatening life events (those rated 4 or 5 on the objective threat scale) during the first 6 months of observation. Then the patient reported a severely threatening event that involved a month-long financial investigation at his workplace. Directly afterward he experienced a mild subsyndromal depression, which spontaneously resolved after 18 days. Several weeks later, however, Mr. A reported three severely threatening events over the course of a month, two of which were employment-related changes that jeopardized his job, and one of which involved a major estrangement from his live-in girlfriend. One week after these events, he had a 2-week manic episode, which was controlled on an outpatient basis with an increased dose of lithium and which subsided into hypomania that persisted for over 3 months.

In this patient's case, each severe event occurred during an asymptomatic period, and several were closely associated with his subsequent manic relapse. He also reported milder stressful events throughout the observation period, which may have added to his risk of relapse.

The results of this study are consistent with those of studies based on retrospective event reporting that have indicated an association in some bipolar patients between stressors and episodes of illness. However, this study is the first to demonstrate this association between symptoms and stress by using a prospective design, systematic interview procedures, and survival analysis. Although the sample size was limited, the results are particularly suggestive because of the longitudinal design of the study. The results have both theoretical and clinical implications.

Theoretically, the results affirm the impact of psychosocial factors on the course of an affective disorder with a presumed biological base. At present there is no complete model for integrating psychological and biological factors in the course of bipolar disorder. One promising approach, however, is that of Goplerud and Depue (18), who argued that some forms of bipolar disorder may involve weak inhibitory modulation in certain CNS systems which control behavioral and biological variables and that stress contributes to dysregulation of such variables. A different model has been proposed by Wehr et al. (19), who suggested that sleep reduction, often a concomitant of stressful life circumstances, may be a final common pathway precipitating mania. Clearly, future efforts to integrate biological and psychosocial factors will improve the prediction of the course of bipolar disorder.

Clinically, an important implication of our findings is the possibility that reducing the impact of stressful life events on patients' lives may help to prevent episodes of affective disorder. Both psychological and medical interventions might need to be increased at times of stress, and it might be important for clinicians to carefully monitor the occurrence of stressors in patients' lives and to be alert to the effects of the events over a period of several months.

It is noteworthy that the results could not be explained by differences in the adequacy of medication regimens or by differences in the level of compliance with these regimens. There were no significant differences between the group that relapsed and the group that did not in maintenance medication levels or in medication compliance ratings, which could account for changes in symptoms and thus provide an alternative explanation to the effects of stress. Nevertheless, in some individuals it is likely that the effects of stressful events may indeed be mediated by changes in compliance with medication regimens. In individual cases, stressors may have a complex interaction with symptoms and compliance behavior, sometimes leading to the exacerbation of symptoms because of the patient's failure to adhere to the medication regimen.

It is also important to note that relapse was more likely only in patients who experienced high levels of stress over the observation period. It appears that there may be a threshold at which a patient becomes more vulnerable to the impact of threatening events. Individuals with lower levels of stress did not differ in risk of relapse from individuals who remained episode free. This finding is consistent with research on associations between life stress and unipolar disorder, suggesting that episodes and symptoms are associated with severely threatening events or chronic strain (1, 5).

Although there was a significant overall effect linking changes in symptoms and high degrees of stress, a larger sample size is necessary to replicate the results of this pilot study. Further, the demonstrated relationship between stress and relapse is not invariable for all bipolar patients. There appeared to be some subjects who experienced major stressors but did not have an increase in symptoms, while some individuals had an increase in symptoms apparently in the absence of major life events. In a previous study (20), we showed that, at least for unipolar patients, the personal meaning of events, rather than simply the occurrence of the events, is associated with depression. In addition to the personal meaning of events, there are a number of factors, such as psychiatric history and family history of affective disorders, that might affect reactions to stress in bipolar patients. Further exploration of these issues is underway and promises to help clarify the impact of stressful life events on the individual course of disorder and to aid in the construction of models that predict the course of bipolar illness from various combinations of psychosocial, genetic, and psychiatric factors.

REFERENCES

1. Brown GW, Harris T: Social Origins of Depression: A Study of Psychiatric Disorder in Women. New York, Free Press, 1978
2. Paykel ES: Life stress and psychiatric disorder: applications of the clinical approach, in Stressful Life Events. Edited by Dohrenwend BS, Dohrenwend BP. New York, John Wiley & Sons, 1974
3. Lloyd C: Life events and depressive disorder reviewed, I: events as predisposing factors. Arch Gen Psychiatry 1980; 37:529–535
4. Lloyd C: Life events and depressive disorder reviewed, II: events as precipitating factors. Arch Gen Psychiatry 1980; 37:541–548
5. Thoits PA: Dimensions of life events that influence psychological distress: an evaluation and synthesis of the literature, in Psychosocial Stress: Trends in Theory and Research. Edited by Kaplan HP. New York, Academic Press, 1983
6. Zis AP, Goodwin FK: Major affective disorder as a recurrent illness: a critical review. Arch Gen Psychiatry 1979; 36:835–839
7. Prien RF, Kupfer DJ, Mansky PA, et al: Drug therapy in the prevention of recurrences in unipolar and bipolar disorders. Arch Gen Psychiatry 1984; 41:1096–1104
8. O'Connell RA: Psychosocial factors in a model of manic-depressive disease. Integrative Psychiatry 1986; 4:150–161
9. Hirschfeld RMA, Cross CK: Epidemiology of affective categories. Arch Gen Psychiatry 1982; 39:35–46
10. Monroe SM: Major and minor life events as predictors of psychological distress: further issues and findings. J Behav Med 1983; 6:189–205
11. Tausig M: Measuring life events. J Health Soc Behav 1983; 23:52–64
12. Hall KS, Dunner DL, Zeller G, et al: A prospective study of life events. Compr Psychiatry 1977; 18:497–502
13. Andreasen NC, Endicott J, Spitzer RL, et al: The family history method using diagnostic criteria: reliability and validity. Arch Gen Psychiatry 1977; 34:1229–1235
14. Keller MB: Undertreatment of major depression. Psychopharmacol Bull 1988; 24:75–80
15. Hollister LE: Antipsychotic medications and the treatment of schizophrenia, in Psychopharmacology: From Theory to Practice. Edited by Barchas JD, Berger PA, Ciaranello RD, et al. New York, Oxford University Press, 1977
16. Cox DR: Regression models and life-tables. J Royal Statistical Society 1972; series B, 34:187–220
17. Gail MH: Evaluating serial cancer marker studies in patients at risk of recurrent disease. Biometrics 1981; 37:66–78
18. Goplerud E, Depue R: Behavioral response to naturally occurring stress in cyclothymia and dysthymia. J Abnorm Psychol 1985; 94:128–139
19. Wehr TA, Sack DA, Rosenthal NE: Sleep reduction as a final common pathway in the genesis of mania. Am J Psychiatry 1987; 144:201–204
20. Hammen CL, Ellicott AG, Gitlin MT, et al: Sociotrophy/autonomy and vulnerability to specific life events in unipolar and bipolar patients. J Abnorm Psychol 1989; 98:154–160

RAPID-CYCLING BIPOLAR DISORDER

An Overview of Research and Clinical Experience

Nael Kilzieh, MD, and Hagop S. Akiskal, MD

> At times the malady begins with a closed series of very short attacks following very quickly one after the other . . . that is especially the case in a small group of youthful patients, preferably, as it seems, women.
>
> KRAEPELIN[62]

Bipolar disorder is a chronic illness characterized by recurrent episodes of depression and mania or hypomania. Cycle length can range from years to only a few days or even hours. *Rapid cycling* (RC) was arbitrarily defined by Dunner and Fieve[36] as having four or more full length affective episodes per year. This work, conducted at Columbia University, showed that RC was overrepresented in patients who had failed lithium. Subsequently, Koukopoulos et al[61] in Rome and Wehr and Goodwin[102] at the National Institute of Mental Health (NIMH) proposed that antidepressant use was involved in RC.

Unipolar RC is extremely rare, and when it occurs, family history is positive for bipolar disorder.[99] Hence the focus in this article is on rapid-cycling bipolar disorder (RCBD). Although there has been more attention paid to this topic in recent years, it was already described by Kraepelin[62] as a temporary phase in the course of manic-depressive illness. This

From the VA Puget Sound Health Care Services, Tacoma, Washington (NK); and the International Mood Center, Department of Psychiatry, The University of California at San Diego, La Jolla, San Diego VA Medical Center, San Diego, California (HSA)

classic viewpoint is endorsed by the *Diagnostic and Statistical Manual of Mental Disorders*, fourth edition (DSM-IV), which included RC as a *specifier* of longitudinal course[8] rather than a specific mood disorder subtype. These criteria stipulate that episodes are demarcated by partial or full remission for at least 2 months or a switch to an episode of the opposite polarity. In practice this definition means that RCBD represents an alternation between major depression on the one hand and manic, hypomanic, or mixed episodes. *Partial remission* is not defined, thus increasing the possibility of including heterogeneous populations.

This article focuses on demographics; putative risk factors, including hypothyroidism and antidepressants; family history; treatment; and outcome. Developments of the greatest clinical relevance are covered. For the early literature on RCBD, the reader is referred to Alarcon's masterful review.[5] (Rapid-cycling can have early- and late-onset.[45] Although it is not uncommonly seen in juvenile patients[46, 55] and sometimes in elderly patients,[26, 30, 75] these topics are covered elsewhere in this issue.)

DEFINITION

DSM-IV accepted the threshold of four episodes or more per year. Attempts to establish a less arbitrary cutoff or to support the current established threshold, revert to examining the distribution of cycle lengths in bipolar patients. If cycle length does separate bipolar patients into two groups (i.e., RC and non-RC), one would expect cycle length to be bimodally distributed. Coryell et al[31] reviewed data from the Collaborative Program on the Psychobiology of Depression, and found a continuous rather than bimodal distribution. Several caveats could be raised here, however. Coryell et al analyzed cycles over a 5-year period, not a 1-year period, which dilutes clustering because RC was a temporary phase in that data set; furthermore, short cycles were probably underestimated because "shifts in polarity did not constitute new episodes and were not recorded as such."[31] All these factors make it less likely to discover bimodality, even if it existed in that cohort. Goodwin and Jamison[49] reported an unpublished study by Zis et al addressing this question: The study revealed a "continuum of cycle lengths," but there were "too few short cycles to determine whether RC exists on a continuum with longer cycles or whether it represents a discontinuity." Meanwhile, in a more recent study, Bauer et al[13] found a trend in female patients only that supports a cutoff point at four episodes per year. This cutoff was based on frequency of episodes on follow-up of the RC subgroup. Bauer et al emphasized that the small cell size dictates a cautious interpretation of the data.

A related problem to address is the nature of the interepisodic period. Studies differ on the duration and level of symptoms. Researchers have used 4 or 8 weeks, some allowing for one or two symptoms[31, 74] and others requiring a period of euthymia "lasting as long as the proximate episodes."[13] Some studies fail to mention their criteria. Therefore, although RCBD is operationally defined, further delineation might prove useful. Ultra-RC (cycling every few days) might be one such category.[63]

DEMOGRAPHIC ASPECTS

RCBD has been reported in both sexes across different age groups. Studies have mostly been done at tertiary centers or clinics where patients sought treatment. Thus, reported data reflect inherent bias seen in such referred populations. No community-based studies have yet been conducted, and the true prevalence of RC in an unselected bipolar patient population remains unknown. This deficiency in our knowledge is in part due to the fact that epidemiologic methodology and current structured interviewing tools do not adequately capture bipolar subtypes.[90]

With the aforementioned caveats in mind, several demographic features of clinical interest emerge from existing studies (Table 1). The prevalence is less than 20% in most studies with some exceptions. For example, Cowdry et al[32] report 56% at a specialized center, such as NIMH. The age of these patients at onset or index episode is not different from patients with non-RC. Koukopoulos et al[61] made the observation that RC appeared in the 40s whether the illness began with a RC course or switched from a previous non-RC course. Others have reported onset before and after age 25, with shorter episodes in the former.[44]

The gender difference is the most replicated finding: A preponderance of females is cited (range, 70% to 92%) except in one study.[57] One possible explanation for the exception in the latter study is that the

Table 1. DEMOGRAPHICS OF RAPID CYCLING (RC) VS NON-RAPID CYCLING (NRC) BIPOLAR DISORDER

	N		Age		% Female		%BP-II		%RC
Study	***RC***	***NRC***	***RC***	***NRC***	***RC***	***NRC***	***RC***	***NRC***	
Dunner et al[38]	33	215	29	30	71	47	40	36	13
Koukopoulos et al[61]	87	347			70	57	82	43	20
Cowdry et al[32]	24	19	45	41	83	53*			56
Joffe et al[57]	17	25			41	80*			40
Nurnberger et al[77]	29	29			86	53*	41	28	15
Wehr et al[103]	51	19	30	27	92	44*	47	47	
Coryell et al[31]	45	198	26	25	71	50*	36	18*	18
Lish et al[72]	45	44	39	44	82	64*			
Maj et al[74]	37	74	43.3	37.7*	64.9	51.4	40.5	24.3	13.6
Bauer et al[13]	120	119	39.3	37.8	70	50.4*	45	37.8	

$^{*}P \leq 0.05$.
RC = Rapid cycling; NRC = nonrapid cycling.

larger sample from which the group of RCBD was drawn had an 80% male bias. In a meta-analysis, Tondo et al[100a] reported RC in 29.6% of women and 16.5% of men. Thus, greater cyclicity appears to be characteristic of being female, and this is particularly marked for ultra-RC.

As for bipolar subtype, Coryell et al[31] found that RCBD was almost exclusively from a bipolar II base. The same finding has emerged from a Chinese study.[95] Although some authors describe unipolar RC,[105] these patients are probably best considered *pseudo-unipolar* or cryptic bipolar whose hypomanic features have been inadequately characterized.[99] Given that bipolar II RC is dominated by depressive episodes, the results of the foregoing investigations overall reflect the well-known female tendency for depressive recurrence, whether in the setting of unipolar or bipolar disorders.[10, 84]

HYPOTHYROIDISM

The relationship between thyroid function and affective illness has long been recognized.[53] Hypothyroidism has been classified into grades I through III according to severity into overt, mild, and subclinical.[48] Hypothyroidism is more common in females in the general population. Clinical hypothyroidism occurs in 2% of women compared with 0.1% of men; subclinical hypothyroidism is reported to occur in approximately 7.5% in women compared to 3% in men.[53] Rates of hypothyroidism in lithium clinics range from 4% to 30%,[67] with women showing more sensitivity to its antithyroid effects.[89] Studies on RC and thyroid function reported in the literature thus far are retrospective, and many are nonblind. Thyroid status was usually assessed after lithium treatment and only a few at baseline. The relationship between hypothyroidism and RC remains controversial. These studies are summarized in Table 2. The studies show mixed significant as well as nonsignificant results. Several points can be raised about these studies. Cho et al[28] included *unipolar* patients and showed 31% of those who became rapid cyclers developed postlithium hypothyroidism versus 2% of those who did not become rapid cyclers. The Cowdry et al[32] study supports this finding in a subgroup (8 RC and 5 non-RC): Rapid cyclers had a significantly larger increase in thyroid-stimulating hormone after lithium. They noted a high prevalence of grade II hypothyroidism (92%). This prevalence could be related to selection bias (patients referred to NIMH) and broad criteria for diagnosing hypothyroidism (thyroid-stimulating hormone > 4). Bauer et al[15] also reported a positive correlation with hypothyroidism, which curiously included overt or grade I hypothyroidism; a limitation of this study is that the authors used a literature-based comparison group.

Joffe et al[57] found mean thyroid-stimulating hormone to be significantly higher in non-RC than in RC patients. This significance disappeared when patients on thyroid medication were not included, most of

Table 2. HYPOTHYROIDISM IN RAPID-CYCLING (RC) VS NON-RAPID CYCLING (NRC) MOOD DISORDER

	N		Grade-I		Grade II	
Study	***RC***	***NRC***	***%RC***	***%NRC***	***%RC***	***%NRC***
Cho et al[23]	1699		31	2*		
Cowdry et al[32]	2419		50	0	92	32*
	8	5	4†	0.5†*		
Joffe et al[57]	1725		2.1†	2.3†	3 ± 1.2‡	7.4 ± 8.5†
Wehr et al[103]	5119		47	39		
Bartalena et al[12]	1111		36	27		
Bauer et al[15]	30508		23	4-15*	27	1–32
Maj et al[74]	3774		5.4	1.3	10.8	9.5

RC = Rapid cycling; NRC = nonrapid cycling.
*$P \leq 0.05$.
†Thyroid-stimulating hormone value.
‡Delta thyroid-stimulating hormone value in thyrotropin-releasing hormone stimulation test.

whom were in the non-RC group. Their sample (significantly more women in non-RC group; M : F = 5 : 20) would be expected to bias the results against finding a relationship to hypothyroidism because hypothyroidism is more common in women, and the preponderance of rapid cyclers in this study was unexpectedly male (M : F = 10 : 7). Even in positive studies, no relationship was found between thyroid status and response to thyroid replacement. There are only sparse data from nonpsychiatric settings. In one study among patients in an endocrinology clinic,[79] those with abnormal thyroid tests (especially those with high antithyroid antibodies), RCBD was significantly overrepresented. This study from a psychiatrically unbiased sample gives legitimacy to the notion that the thyroid gland is somehow involved in RCBD. An authority as prominent as Post,[87] however, remains skeptical of the direction of causability.

ANTIDEPRESSANTS

Antidepressants, including tricyclic antidepressants (TCAs) and monoamine oxidase inhibitors, have been implicated in causing a switch into hypomania or mania and inducing RC in bipolar patients.[20, 101] These issues, which are of the utmost importance for clinicians, are still debated in the literature. That antidepressants are a contributory cause—neither necessary nor sufficient—can be inferred from the fact that many cases of de novo RCBD (i.e. without prior antidepressant use) do exist, as, for example, those beginning after menopause. That antidepressants can aggravate the course of mood disorders and eventually cause RCBD originally came from the work of Wehr and Goodwin[102] and Koukopoulos et al.[61] For obvious reasons, this work and much of subsequent work on the role of antidepressants in RC are based on retrospective methodology.

Review of records spanning over several decades reveals an increase in switch rates[11] and RC[105] that coincides with the introduction of antidepressants. Goodwin and Jamison[49] reviewed this controversy and highlighted the disparity between different studies. Switch rates with antidepressants range from 3% (same as spontaneous switch) to 50%. This wide range has been attributed—to name only a few confounding factors—to different designs, criteria for hypomania (lower rates with more stringent criteria), and latency between initiation of antidepressants and the onset of hypomania.

Kupfer et al[65] reported low switch rates in bipolar II patients. They had 230 patients with recurrent depression (average six episodes) in an imipramine treatment study, of whom 15% were bipolar II. The switch rate was 3% in the bipolar II group and 2.5% in the unipolar group. This difference was not statistically significant. Bipolar II diagnosis was based on RDC criteria, the SADS was the diagnostic instrument used, and the criteria for hypomania were Raskin mania score of 4 or more supported with a note of hypomanic symptoms in the chart. The design of the study, which required patients to be stable on TCAs before follow-up, biased any likelihood of finding TCA-induced course aggravation; also, 67% of the switches occurred when imipramine was discontinued (which might suggest anicholinergic rebound[35]).

Altshuler et al,[6] in a retrospective nonblind design in a refractory bipolar group (every other patient was RC), estimated that 35% of the switching into mania was due to antidepressants. No variable was a predictor of vulnerability to this switch. Meanwhile, Calabrese et al[24] noted a 25% drug-induced hypomania or mania in their sample of RC bipolar patients. Of those who improved but relapsed into depression, reinstating an antidepressant resulted in reintroduction of RC in 25%.

Medication type has also been implicated as a variable. In a 2-year prospective study conducted by Haykal and Akiskal,[52] bupropion was suggested as a preferred agent in bipolar II patients. Rather than inducing RC, bupropion was reported to be effective in the treatment of RC in refractory patients. Altshuler et al[6] found similar rates of switching and cycle acceleration between monoamine oxidase inhibitors and heterocyclic antidepressants. In a related finding, Maj et al[74] noted that there was no difference in switch rates between TCAs and a non-TCA group (fluoxetine, fluvoxamine, mianserin, and maprotiline) in a bipolar RC population. Although a meta-analysis done by Peet[83] suggests that selective serotonin reuptake inhibitors induce a manic switch less often than TCA's, these data do not necessarily indicate that SSRI's are safer from the standpoint of RC induction.

Another area of importance is switch rates in different bipolar subtypes. Cassano et al[27] reported a higher switch rate in bipolar I disorder compared to bipolar II, whereas Altshuler et al[6] did not find this difference; it would appear that it is easier to detect—because of more systematic follow-up—a switch in the former than in the latter. In a Memphis study, Akiskal et al[2] found a switch rate in cyclothymics on antidepressants to be similar to bipolar I patients; it is uncertain what percent of the bipolar I patients were also cyclothymic. Again, although the issue of induction of hypomania or mania reviewed earlier could reasonably be related to the induction of RC, such a correlation has not been conclusively established.

Many studies have shown a relationship between initiating antidepressants and subsequent development of RC.[61, 103] Interestingly, Koukopoulos et al[61] reported electroconvulsive therapy to be rather innocent in this respect. Wehr et al[103] reported that recovery could be attained by discontinuing antidepressants. Bauer et al[13] found that spontaneous and antidepressant-induced RC had similar gender distribution (70.8%). Altshuler et al[6] found 26% of bipolars had cycle acceleration on antidepressants: Younger age of onset predicted such an outcome, and there was a trend toward female gender and bipolar II as predictors. A caveat has been raised by Coryell et al,[31] who pointed out that the relationship between antidepressants and RC could be epiphenomenal, not causal. They argued that because rapid cyclers have more depressive episodes, they are more likely to be treated with antidepressants, leading to a spurious statistical finding; they further argued that although a relationship with antidepressants and depression was found, in a log linear model "the presence of depression and not antidepressants determined subsequent RC."[31] This interpretation was criticized by Wehr,[101] who objected that the Coryell et al study[31] was a naturalistic one, not designed to test this question specifically. Wehr and Goodwin,[102] using a prospective double-blind design, had shown that cycle length significantly decreased with antidepressants using patients as their own controls; because these patients were originally rapid cyclers, this study does not prove that nonrapid cyclers become rapid cyclers with antidepressants; rather it indicates that rapid cyclers can have acceleration in cycling on antidepressants. A relationship between switch and RC has been observed by Koukopoulos et al,[60] in which the first onset of hypomania after depression heralded subsequent RC course.

This area—linking switching and RC to antidepressants—is virtually impossible to study with the requisite methodologic purity: Much of it is after the fact because to attempt prospective induction would not be ethically acceptable. In the authors' experience,[4] the link, although not present in every case of RCBD, is clinically persuasive. RCBD is such a pernicious phenomenon that it makes good clinical sense to refrain from using most existing antidepressants in such patients. Caution must in particular be exercised in the offspring of manic–depressives who, more often than not, begin their illness with depressive episodes.[3] Bupropion might be the only exception, but this must be qualified as largely pertinent to RCBD from a bipolar II baseline.[52]

COURSE OF EPISODES

There have been few observations addressing the type of first episode and course of episodes as they relate to RCBD. Some investigators[92, 103] have noted that rapid cyclers were more likely to have an onset of illness with a depressive episode. Also, in a prospective follow-up study[3] of juvenile offspring of bipolars, the authors found that cycling course—including two rapid cyclers—was greater in those who had an onset with depression: This finding could be related to these patients being more likely to receive antidepressants, compared to those whose onset was with mania (the latter group would be more likely to have received lithium).

The extent to which gender differences could explain this relationship is unclear. In one study, bipolar illness started with mania in about 50% of cases, with a range of 34% to 79% depending on the criteria[49]; because the sex distribution was not reported, it is not known whether women were more likely to start with a depressive episode. Indirect evidence indicates that this might be the case because studies have shown that women have more depressive episodes, whereas men tend to have an equal number of depressions and manias.[49] Therefore, the increased likelihood of onset with a depressive episode could be merely a reflection of the preponderance of women with RCBD.

Some studies have shown a tendency for bipolar patients to have shorter cycles as their illness progresses. This tendency stabilizes after four to six episodes.[49] In a study by Roy-Byrne et al,[92] bipolars were classified into two groups, sensitizers and nonsensitizers, depending on whether they developed shorter cycles as their illness progressed or not; sensitizer status bore no relationship to ultimate RC. These data overall tend to contradict a kindling hypothesis, as do related data by Coryell et al.[31]

As for the phenomenology of RC, episodes appear reproducible lethargic-hypoactive versus activated periods from one cycle to another.[68] RC and mixed states appear to be distinct processes.[54] RC represents depression alternating with hypomania or mania; mixed states represent simultaneous mixtures of depressive and hypomanic or manic symptoms. In ultra-RC patients, however, this distinction may, in part, blur.[1]

PATTERN OF EPISODES

Another interesting yet poorly studied feature of bipolar illness is sequence of episodes. Koukopoulos et al[61] presented data on this topic from their mostly outpatient probands. Patients with a depression–

mania–hypomania-free interval (D-M-I) course were overrepresented in the RC group. Although they constituted 24% of the total sample (106 of 434), they comprised 62% of those whose illness started with a RC course (43% of total RC) and 47% of those who switched later to RC (57% of total RCBD). There was no sex difference in D-M-I or mania-depression-interval (M-D-I). Angst[10] analyzed the number of total episodes in different patterns (95 patients and 1176 episodes) and found no sex differences in sequence of episodes. The results of these two studies are presented in Table 3. Should the finding by Koukopoulos' group be replicated (i.e., those with D-M-I are more vulnerable to RC), it cannot be explained by a gender difference. The relationship of this pattern to RC becomes particularly interesting because Faeda and colleagues[41] have shown a poor response in D-M-I pattern to lithium, a treatment response profile most similar to that of RCBD.

SUBTYPES

The sex ratio for bipolar illness is slightly higher in women (F : M = 1.2 : 1).[104] Angst[10] and Perugi et al[84] have shown a higher rate of bipolar II disorder in women, whereas Koukopoulos et al[61] and Endicott et al[39] failed to find such an increased ratio. Coryell et al[31] found that hypomania and bipolar II predicted RC, whereas mania was *protective.* Similar data were published by Maj et al.[74]

Another interesting observation is the high rate of bipolar II disorder among D-M-I patients (78%), although they represented only 52% of the sample in a report by Koukopoulos et al.[61] The higher rate of RC in bipolar II may be related to the higher incidence of D-M-I pattern in this population. The answer is not likely to be so simple, however. For instance, several investigators[37, 39] have found that bipolar II women, but not men, were more likely to have alcohol abuse compared with their bipolar I counterparts. Therefore, a comorbid condition, such as alcoholism, could be a mediating factor that would indirectly explain the relationship of type and gender to RC.

Table 3. GENDER AND EPISODE PATTERN

	Depression Mania-Interval		Mania-Depression-Interval	
Study	***% Male***	***% Female***	***% Male***	***% Female***
Angst[10]	15.3	16.6	12.6	9.2
Koukopoulos et al[61]	9.4	14.9	12.2	15.2

TEMPERAMENT

Kraepelin[62] described four basic temperaments, which he considered the *fundamental states* from which manic-depressive illness arose. He considered these to lie on the boundary of manic-depressive illness with normality. In research conducted in Memphis,[4] the authors operationalized these concepts by Kraepelin as well as those of other classic German psychiatrists. There is convincing evidence to include cyclothymia into the rubric of bipolar spectrum on the basis of work conducted in Memphis.[2] It would thus be logical to assume that RC represents a natural accentuation of the cyclothymic's tendency toward cycling on a lower plane of severity.

The data available in this area are limited. Koukopoulos et al[61] noted that patients with cyclothymic and hyperthymic temperament were more likely to become rapid cyclers (in younger and older patients). Similar data, from the same clinic, were reported by Tondo et al.[100] Meanwhile, Cassano et al[27] found bipolar I probands more likely to have a depressive temperament, whereas bipolar II probands are more likely to have a hyperthymic one; cyclothymic temperament was not measured in that study, and what was registered as hyperthymic may have represented repeated hypomanic bursts of a cyclic nature. Tentatively, these data are compatible with the hypothesis that cyclic mood changes of the cyclothymic type might predispose to depressive cycling. This impression is further strengthened by the fact that women—who have higher rates of RC—outnumber men 2:1 in rates of cyclothymia in the general population.[85] In brief, cyclothymia could hypothetically represent the mediating factor between gender and RC. The few men who develop RC might come, again hypothetically, from the rank of hyperthymic temperament that is favored by male gender.[3a, 85]

FAMILIAL ASPECTS

Family history constitutes an important tool in validation of psychiatric disorders.[43] There are several published family studies of RCBD (Table 4). Dunner et al[38] found similar family history in rapid cyclers compared to nonrapid cyclers. Among bipolar I patients, 35.3% and 29.4% of rapid cyclers had a positive family history of bipolar and unipolar illness; this was not significantly different from their non-RC counterparts (33.3% and 24.4%). This finding held true for the bipolar II group (RC 45.5% and 36.3% versus non-RC 25% and 33.8%). Wehr et al[103] noted a nonsignificant trend for more RC in first-degree relatives of RC probands (13% versus 0%). Both studies did not interview relatives. Other studies with more systematic assessment of relatives with structured interviews are listed in Table 4. The Nurnberger et al[77] study found no difference when bipolar I and bipolar II were considered separately, and it did not report any familial aggregation of RC. Therefore, all the

Table 4. RISK OF AFFECTIVE DISORDER IN FIRST-DEGREE RELATIVES OF RAPID-CYCLING (RC) VERSUS NONRAPID-CYCLING (NR) BIPOLAR (BP) PATIENTS

		RC Proband			NRC Proband		
Study	**Method**	**N *(rel)***	***%M***	***%D***	**N *(rel)***	***%M***	***%D***
Nurnberger et al[77]*	SADS-L and Records	179	5.6	11.7	189	5.5	18.7
Coryell et al[31]*	FH-RDC SADS-L	268	4.1	20.1	1273	4.2	19.6
Lish et al[72]*	Modified FH-RDC	221	11	27	190	15	25
Maj et al[74]†	FH-RDC	37	13.6	29.7	74	8.1	21.6
Bauer et al[13]†	Nonstructured	81	28.4	39.5	91	23.1	53.8
Wehr et al[103]†	Nonstructured	47	26	40	19	37	26
Dunner et al[38]†	Nonstructured	17 (BP I)	35.3	29.4	123	33.3	24.4
		11 (BP II)	45.5	36.3	68	25	33.8

M = mania; D = depression; Rel = first-degree relative; FH-RDC = Family history–research diagnostic criteria.
*Morbid risk in interviewed relatives.
† = Percent of affected relatives reported by proband.

family studies done to date indicate a similar family history in RC and do not lend support to classifying them separately. A genetic finding from two centers,[59, 81] however, suggests that ultra-RC might be associated with low activity of the catechol-*O*-methyltransferase allele. Even if this finding were further replicated, it would pertain to a relatively small percentage of RC.

TREATMENT

Treatment resistance to lithium was noted in the landmark paper by Dunner and Fieve[36] that initially defined RCBD. In that study, 82% of RC patients did not respond compared with 41% of non-RC patients. Even with such a high failure rate, some patients exhibited greater percent time in remission while on lithium. Since then, many studies have been published, with focus on anticonvulsants. Although these have been open studies, some conclusions can be drawn regarding response to medications and are summarized subsequently. Further details can be obtained from reviews[5, 9, 25, 64, 66, 86, 91, 92a, 96] as well as the Expert Consensus Guidelines[40] for the treatment of bipolar disorder.

Lithium

Resistance of bipolar disorder to lithium has been noted by several investigators over the years.[61, 88] Other investigators, however, such as

Schou,[93] reported fair response to lithium. Most studies have concluded that lithium failure rates are high in RC patients. Koukopoulos et al[61] indicated that those with D-M-I and with continuous circular patterns are particularly likely to be lithium nonresponders. In a follow-up study to test this hypothesis, Faedda et al[41] analyzed five studies, and their conclusion supported poorer response in D-M-I by an odds ratio of 4.4. They also noted that bipolar II patients had a higher response rate compared to bipolar I (49.3% versus 37.6%). Lastly, some investigators contend that lithium may shorten episodes and thus exacerbate an RC course.[61]; this could reflect the fact that tertiary care centers attract treatment failures.

Although most reports indicate poor response to lithium in RCBD, necessitating use of other agents, at least one report[103] contended that, in a substantial minority, the mere removal of antidepressants might permit lithium to act as an effective anticycling agent. This situation does occur in selected patients and represents a viable initial approach to RCBD.

Valproate

An open trial of the efficacy of divalproex versus lithium in the treatment of mania found divalproex to be equally effective in RC and non-RC manic patients.[21] This finding has been replicated.[64] Calabrese et al[22, 24] concluded that valproate has a marked antimanic effect and a poor to moderate antidepressant effect. Predictors of positive outcome for acute and prophylactic mania were bipolar II and mixed states, no prior lithium treatment, and a positive family history of affective disorder. Negative outcome predictors were increase in frequency and severity of mania in the course of the illness and presumably borderline personality. Combination treatment with lithium has been shown to improve response rate,[21, 94] Although Hayes[51] was unable to detect such a finding. On the basis of the available clinical data, valproate appears to be the most effective agent in the treatment of this refractory group; it probably works even in those with borderline personality to the extent that some of the latter might represent complex subaffective ultra-rapid cycling bipolar variants.[1, 2, 33, 70]

Carbamazepine

Previous reviews[25, 64] note that 196 patients were included in a total of 23 studies. Response rate for acute depression was 32% and for acute mania 52%. Prophylactic response rates for depression and mania were 57% and 59%.[25] Controlled or semicontrolled studies, however, included only 10 patients. Okuma[78] refuted the utility of carbamazepine in the treatment of RCBD. Meanwhile, Joffe[56] reported an observation that continuous cyclers benefited from lithium and carbamazepine combination. Others have reported similar data about the necessity of combining carbamazepine with lithium.[34]

Levothyroxine

Controversy about the higher prevalence of hypothyroidism in RC bipolar patients has already been discussed. This controversy extends to the response to thyroid replacement. Several investigators documented a positive response in RC patients to L-thyroxine.[14, 80, 97] Stancer and Persad[97] and Bauer and Wybrow[14] used doses of 0.5 mg of L-thyroxine daily. Typically the dose was increased 0.05 to 0.1 mg every 1 to 2 weeks until response was obtained. Therefore, it is not known whether a slower rate of increase to achieve normal dosing would have resulted in a similar outcome. Meanwhile, Cowdry et al[32] reported *inconsistent results* with thyroid replacement in this population. This view is upheld in a review that found no relationship between hypothyroidism and RCBD.[12, 57] The aforementioned treatment studies were open and retrospective. Bauer and Wybrow[14] added a single-blinded or double-blinded phase in 4 of their 10 patients and had outcomes supportive of their open phase conclusions. Although the data to date are inconclusive, clinical experience supports that bipolar II patients who became rapid cyclers as a result of lithium failure might benefit from thyroid augmentation in selected cases. This approach can be attempted even in patients with normal baseline thyroid function, as positive response in these studies was not related to thyroid status. In the authors clinical experience, thyroid augmentation is more likely to work in women. Nonetheless, the potential for cardiac arrhythmias and osteoporosis tends to limit the more widespread use of thyroid augmentation in RC. At least one recent report[49b] suggests that the risk for osteoporosis may have been overestimated.

Neuroleptics

Because psychotic symptoms are common in bipolar disorder, the use of neuroleptics in this population is prevalent in clinical practice. Concern has been raised about conventional neuroleptics prolonging depressive episodes[61] and increased risk of tardive dyskinesia in affectively ill individuals.[7] In a report of two cases,[23] clozapine reduced the frequency, duration, and amplitude of episodes in refractory RC patients, who had failed to respond to conventional neuroleptics in combination with other treatments. Anectodal use of atypical neuroleptics in RC has been published.[76] In the authors' clinical experience, olanzapine is useful adjunctively in the early stabilization phase of treating refractory RCBD; such use is supported in secondary analyses in the Tohen et al study[100b] of olanzapine in mania.

Calcium-Channel Blockers

Evidence for the utility of these agents in the treatment of bipolar disorder at large is presently inconclusive. The authors have not observed successes in RCBD patients under their care with verapamil or nifedipine. A controlled preliminary trial[82] indicates the utility of nimodipine in RCBD. In this report, the patients who responded best were *ultrarapid* cyclers. They were defined as those with affective episodes lasting *as short as a week*. The authors' limited clinical experience since this report was published has been encouraging. More studies are needed to clarify further the role of these agents in RCBD.

Newer Anticonvulsants

In an open naturalistic study[42] of five women with refractory RCBD, lamotrigine monotherapy or augmentation showed a mood-stabilizing and antidepressant effect. The mean dose used was 185 ± 33.5 mg/d, and treatment was tolerated in four out of five patients. This being a preliminary open study with a small number of patients, one should proceed with caution to this step, after having exhausted other better-studied options. Given the specter of a potentially life-threatening rash, lamotrigine should be started at 25 mg and increased on a weekly basis until 300 mg is achieved; it should not be combined with valproate, which rapidly increases the blood level of lamotrigine. Patients must be alerted about the rash; it is best to interrupt the trial at the first sign of a pruritic rash on the trunk. The authors have seen several RC patients—refractory to all other approaches—respond to lamotrigine. In the authors' clinical experience, lamotrigine is well tolerated by bipolar patients.

Other Agents

Bupropion has been reported[52] as an effective add-on treatment in five of six patients who had severe RC bipolar type II disorder; all previously used antidepressants—mostly TCAs and monoamine oxidase inhibitors—and had failed lithium with thyroid augmentation. Chouinard et al[29] reported benefit from magnesium in an open study of nine RC patients. Choline has been used experimentally.[98]

Electroconvulsive Therapy

Electroconvulsive therapy has been less implicated than antidepressants in the induction of RC; if this happens, it is in cases in which electroconvulsive therapy is combined with antidepressants.[61] Berman and Wolpert[17] reported a case of an adolescent patient who had developed RC after treatment with an antidepressant who responded well to electroconvulsive therapy. No systematic studies are available to delineate the role of electroconvulsive therapy in RCBD.

Light Therapy

NIMH research[44, 69] in open design involving nine RC bipolar patients concluded that midday light was beneficial in improving mood and even reducing hypomania, whereas morning light led to instability and exacerbation in some patients. They speculated that midday light might stabilize diurnal rhythms and make them more resistant to shift by increasing the amplitude of nocturnal melatonin secretion. They recommended that light therapy be avoided in the morning during the depressive phase and withheld during hypomanic phases.

OUTCOME

Although RCBD is more refractory to treatment, this does not necessarily indicate a poor long-term outcome. Kraepelin[62] observed that having rapid cycles is a transient phase of the illness. In their original paper describing lithium refractoriness, Dunner and Fieve[36] reported mean percent time in remission in the second and third year of lithium treatment in 11 rapid cyclers at 47% and 43%. Meanwhile, Wehr et al[103] reported data on 51 RC patients with follow-up of nearly 5 years. The non-RC cohort ($n = 19$) had a follow-up period of 10 years. The remission rates in non-RC versus RC women were 63% versus 34%. There were two suicides (4%) in the RC group and none in the non-RC group, a difference that was not statistically significant; also, RC patients who failed to improve were more likely to have attempted suicide than RC patients who improved (78% versus 37%).

In a prospective study, Coryell et al[31] found only 1 of 39 RC patients who completed 5 years of follow-up to have RC in all of the subsequent 4 years, whereas 64% had no RC after the first year. Although RC patients were less likely to be recovered from the index episode in the second year, this finding did not extend into years 3, 4, and 5. Nevertheless, these patients were less likely to have the entire last year of follow-up free of affective symptoms (25.6% versus 40.5%). There was no difference in suicide attempts or completed suicides (2.6% versus 4.1% in RC and non-RC).

Maj et al[74] found that at 5-year follow-up, 34.8% of RC patients continued to be rapid cyclers, as opposed to only 2.1% of non-RC patients; they noted 18.9% had RC throughout their follow-up period *whatever its duration* (62.2% of RC patients completed 5-year follow-up). Lastly, Bauer et al[13] in a follow-up of *12 months or more* found only 8.6% of RC patients to be episode-free during that time, compared to 25% of non-RC patients; 53.4% of RC subjects converted to non-RC during follow-up. Comparing these patients to those who did not convert, there were no differences in gender, bipolar type, age of evaluation, age of onset of affective symptoms, or age of onset of RC.

In these data sets, several studies suggest that in a 2- to 5-year follow-up period, RC patients are less likely to be symptom free. There is also an indication that RC patients are more likely than non-RC patients to be rapid cyclers at 5-year follow-up, although this is not as strongly supported. Nonetheless, given time, most RC patients tend to convert to non-RC course.

METHODOLOGIC CONSIDERATIONS FOR FUTURE RESEARCH

To explore the multitude of important, unanswered questions, several areas should be addressed in prospectively designed studies. Detailed phenomenologic assessment of bipolar patients, including temperament, subtype, and pattern and distribution of episodes, should be pursued. DSM-IV is insufficiently useful in this regard.[1, 96] Studying the switch process, separating spontaneous versus induced, early versus late onset, and continuous (i.e., no euthymia between episodes) versus noncontinuous RC might enhance understanding of all maniform phenomena. An attempt to separate true mixed states (i.e., coexistence—rather than rapid change—of depressive and manic symptoms) should be made. In all these areas, special attention should be paid to gender differences.

Another extremely important yet underexplored area is the relationship of substance abuse to RC. The rates of substance abuse in this group should be carefully examined. This factor could partly explain refractoriness to treatment. A variety of drugs, both abused (e.g., cocaine) and prescribed (e.g., levodopa), have been reported as possible risk factors. Clinicians who report case series must record all potentially *cyclogenic* drugs.

Because cerebral factors have been implicated,[47, 71, 73] clinicians are also admonished to record any neurologic, electroencephalographic, or neuropsychological conditions among RC patients. RCBD represents a *natural experiment*, providing the opportunity to examine peripheral and central metabolic changes. For instance, depression and mania have been shown to be associated with decreased and increased brain glucose utilization.[16] Finally, high plasma cortisol levels preceded the switch into depression, and higher urinary dopamine preceded the switch into mania.[58] Such data also exist for urinary methoxyhydroxy-phenyl-glycol.[19] These are exciting vistas into the biologic basis of the switch process and one day might inform clinicians better about the pathophysiology of RC, paving the way for more rational treatments.

Proneness to switching might prove to be an essential ingredient in cyclicity, which, when combined with gender-related and other factors, ultimately leads to rapid cycling. It is conceivable that antidepressant-induced switching represents an initial step in a cascade of events, which might include changes in seasonal patterns, rapid cycling, or chronicity of cyclic depressions.[4]

Because prospective experimental manipulation of this process poses the risk of aggravating the course of illness, the authors do not foresee much progress in the near future: Clinicians must use their judgment based on available naturalistic observations. The authors are convinced on clinical grounds that in a selected group of patients within the bipolar spectrum nearly all antidepressants can accentuate the instability that underlies their illness. Therefore, future research should focus on identifying those depressed (cryptic bipolar) patients who are at the highest risk for such an outcome; in this regard, the concept of bipolar spectrum proposed by Akiskal[1] represents an effort to expand the grossly underinclusive bipolar categorization in DSM-IV.[8] Caution should be exercised in using antidepressants in soft bipolar conditions,[4] and the use of anticonvulsant mood stabilizers can be defended as a viable clinical strategy in opposing cycle acceleration and chronicity in these conditions.

SUMMARY

Although many studies of RCBD have been reported over the last 2 decades, knowledge remains limited. Higher incidence in women is the sole clearly replicated finding in most studies. This finding might be mediated by cyclothymia, a temperament that is of higher prevalence in women and that might be considered as a *normal* variant of RC. Many questions remain unanswered.

Review of putative risk factors, such as hypothyroidism and treatment with antidepressants, provides no conclusive answers. There is clinical evidence to implicate both factors. In principle, the thyroid connection can be approached rationally, yet there seems to be no relationship between thyroid status and response to thyroid augmentation. For this reason and given the potential risks of long-term thyroid use, this strategy should not be the first one to be tried in RC. Cumulatively, naturalistic studies over the past 30 years have strongly implicated antidepressants in switching and cycle acceleration, yet the double-blind, controlled, prospective studies that are needed to provide definitive answers are unlikely to be conducted for ethical reasons discussed in this article. Bipolar family history of RC probands appears indistinguishable from non-RC probands, indicating that most likely RCBD *does not breed true*. Although RC seems to be more lithium resistant with less likelihood of being symptom-free after 2 to 5 years of follow-up, many of these patients nonetheless have resolution of the RC course. There is no marked difference in suicide rates.

An association of RC with bipolar type II, D-M-I pattern and those who switch into mania or hypomania on antidepressants is a provocative possibility: Antidepressants might introduce RC by first inducing a switch during a depressive episode, creating a D-M-I pattern, a pattern that is poorly responsive to lithium, which eventually degenerates into RC. Again, this sequence might be mediated by the high prevalence of cyclothymia in bipolar II patients.[50]

Thus, data from phenomenology, family history, and long-term outcome do not support RC as a separate entity. RC appears to be a temporary complicated phase in the illness, not a stable feature. This was noted by Kraepelin:[62]

> I think I am convinced that that kind of classification must of necessity wreck on the irregularity of the disease. The kind and duration of the attacks and the intervals by no means remain the same in the individual case but may frequently change, so that the case must be reckoned always to new forms.

Data by Gottschalk et al[49a] testify to the chaotic mood swings of contemporary bipolar disorder. Moreover RC is seen in other medical diseases, such as epilepsy, in which patients have phases of increase in frequency of episodes (seizures) that become refractory to treatment. Further longitudinal prospective studies are required to understand the complexity of this intriguing phenomenon and to provide better treatments. Algorithms[25, 92a] deriving from tertiary research or university-based clinical experience may not generalize to RC or otherwise treatment-resistant bipolar patients seen in more routine practice. Illness severity in RCBD generally precludes double-blind controlled investigations. Meanwhile, clinicians may rely on discontinuing antidepressants, maintaining patients on combined mood stabilizers—of which valproate is probably the most useful—and making judicious use of atypical neuroleptics. Benzodiazepines and alcohol (which produce withdrawal), caffeine, stimulants, exposure to bright light, and sleep deprivation during excited phases should be avoided. Thyroid and nimodipine augmentation can be considered in those with the most malignant course. These are patients who need the maximal support that their psychiatrist can provide them. Office visits must be arranged as the last appointment of the day.

References

1. Akiskal HS: The prevalent clinical spectrum of bipolar disorders: Beyond DSM-IV. J Clin Psychopharmacology 16(suppl 1):4S–14S, 1996
2. Akiskal HS, Djenderedjian AH, Rosenthal RH, et al: Cyclothymic disorder: Validating criteria for inclusion in the bipolar affective group. Am J Psychiatry 134:1227–1233, 1977
3. Akiskal HS, Downs J, Jordan P, et al: Affective disorders in referred children and

younger siblings of manic-depressives: Mode of onset and prospective course. Arch Gen Psychiatry 42:996–1003, 1985
3a. Akiskal HS: Delineating irritable and hyperthymic variants of the cyclothymic temperament. J Person Disord 6:326–342, 1992
4. Akiskal HS, Mallya G: Criteria for the "soft" bipolar spectrum: Treatment implications. Psychopharmacol Bull 23:68–73, 1987
5. Alarcon RD: Rapid cycling affective disorders: A clinical review. Compr Psychiatry 26:522–540, 1985
6. Altshuler L, Post RM, Leverich GS, et al: Antidepressant-induced mania and cycle acceleration: A controversy revisited. Am J Psychiatry 152:1130–1138, 1995
7. American Psychiatric Association: Tardive Dyskinesia. A Task Force Report of the American Psychiatric Association. Washington, DC, American Psychiatric Association, 1992
8. American Psychiatric Association: Diagnostic and Statistical Manual of Mental Disorders, ed 4. Washington, DC, American Psychiatric Association, 1994
9. Ananth J, Wohl M, Ranganath V, et al: Rapid cycling patients: Conceptual and etiological factors. Neuropsychobiology 27:193–198, 1993
10. Angst J: The course of affective disorders: II. Typology of bipolar manic-depressive illness. Arch Psychiatr Nervenkr 226:65–73, 1978
11. Angst J: Switch from depression to mania: A record study over decades between 1920 and 1982. Psychopathology 18:140–154, 1985
12. Bartalena L, Pellegrini L, Meschi M, et al: Evaluation of thyroid function in patients with rapid-cycling and non-rapid-cycling bipolar disorder. Psychiatr Res 34:13–17, 1990
13. Bauer MS, Calabrese J, Dunner DL, et al: Multisite data reanalysis of the validity of rapid cycling as a course modifier for bipolar disorder in DSM-IV. Am J Psychiatry 151:506–515, 1994
14. Bauer MS, Wybrow PC: Rapid cycling bipolar affective disorder: II. Treatment of refractory rapid cycling with high-dose levothyroxine. Arch Gen Psychiatry 47:435–440, 1990
15. Bauer MS, Wybrow PC, Winokur A: Rapid cycling bipolar affective disorder: I. Association with grade I hypothyroidism. Arch Gen Psychiatry 47:427–432, 1990
16. Baxter LR, Schwartz JM, Phelps ME, et al: Reduction of prefrontal cortex glucose metabolism common to three types of depression. Arch Gen Psychiatry 46:243–250, 1989
17. Berman E, Wolpert EA: Intractable manic-depressive psychosis with rapid cycling in an 18-year-old woman successfully treated with electroconvulsive therapy. J Nerv Ment Dis 175:236–239, 1987
18. Bowden CL, Brugger AM, Swann AC, et al: Efficacy of divalproex vs lithium and placebo in the treatment of mania. JAMA 271:918–924, 1994
19. Bunney WE, Goodwin FK, Murphy DL, et al: The "switch process" in manic-depressive illness: II. Relationship to catecholamines, REM sleep, and drugs. Arch Gen Psychiatry 27:304–309, 1972
20. Bunney WE, Murphy D, Goodwin FK, et al: The switch process from depression to mania: Relationship to drugs which alter brain amines. Lancet 1:1022–1027, 1970
21. Calabrese JR, Delucchi G: Spectrum of efficacy of valproate in 55 patients with rapid cycling bipolar disorder. Am J Psychiatry 147:431–434, 1990
22. Calabrese JR, Markovitz PJ, Kimmel SE, et al: Predictors of valproate response in bipolar rapid cycling. J Clin Psychiatry 13:280–283, 1993
23. Calabrese JR, Meltzer HY, Markovitz PJ: Clozapine prophylaxis in rapid cycling bipolar disorder. J Clin Psychopharmacol 11:396–397, 1991
24. Calabrese JR, Rapport DJ, Kimmel SE, et al: Rapid cycling bipolar disorder and its treatment with valproate. Can J Psychiatry 38(suppl 2):S57–S61, 1993
25. Calabrese JR, Woyshville MJ: A medication algorithm for treatment of bipolar rapid cycling. J Clin Psychiatry 56(suppl 3):11–18, 1995
26. Camus V, Lima CAM, Antonioli D, et al: Rapid-cycling affective disorder in the elderly: Clinical subtype or specific course of manic-depressive illness? J Geriatr Psychiatry Neurol 10:105–110, 1997

27. Cassano GB, Akiskal HS, Musetti L, et al: Psychopathology, temperament, and past course in primary major depressions: 2. Toward a redefinition of bipolarity with a new semistructured interview for depression. Psychopathology 22:278–288, 1989
28. Cho JT, Bone S, Dunner DL, et al: The effect of lithium treatment on thyroid function in patients with primary affective disorder. Am J Psychiatry 136:115–116, 1979
29. Chouinard G, Beauclair L, Geiser R, et al: A pilot study of magnesium aspartate hydrochloride (magneiocard) as a mood stabilizer for rapid cycling bipolar affective disorder patients. Prog Neuropsychopharmacol Biol Psychiatry 14:171–180, 1990
30. Conlon P: Rapid cycling mood disorder in the elderly. J Geriatr Psychiatry Neurol 2:106–108, 1989
31. Coryell W, Endicott J, Keller M: Rapid cycling affective disorder: Demographics, family history and course. Arch Gen Psychiatry 49:126–131, 1992
32. Cowdry RW, Wehr TA, Zis AP, et al: Thyroid abnormalities associated with rapid-cycling bipolar illness. Arch Gen Psychiatry 40:414–420, 1983
33. Deltito J, Martin L, Riefkohl J, et al: Do patients with borderline personality disorder belong to the bipolar spectrum? J Affect Disord (in press)
34. Di Costanzo E, Schifano F: Lithium alone or in combination with carbamazepine for the treatment of rapid-cycling bipolar affective disorder. Acta Psychiatr Scand 83:456–459, 1991
35. Dilsaver SC, Greden JF: Antidepressant withdrawal-induced activation (hypomania and mania): Mechanism and theoretical significance. Brain Res 319:29–48, 1984
36. Dunner DL, Fieve RR: Clinical factors in lithium carbonate prophylaxis failure. Arch Gen Psychiatry 30:229–233, 1974
37. Dunner DL, Hensel BM, Fieve RR: Bipolar illness: Factors in drinking behavior. Am J Psychiatry 136:583–585, 1979
38. Dunner DL, Patrick V, Fieve RR: Rapid cycling manic depressive patients. Compr Psychiatry 18:561–566, 1977
39. Endicott J, Nee J, Andreasen N, et al: Bipolar II: Combine or keep separate. J Affect Disord 8:17–28, 1985
40. Expert Consensus Guideline Series: Treatment of bipolar disorder. J Clin Psychiatry 57(suppl 12A):1–89, 1996
41. Faedda GL, Baldessarini RJ, Tohen M, et al: Episode sequence in bipolar disorder and response to lithium treatment. Am J Psychiatry 148:1237–1239, 1991
42. Fatemi SH, Rapport DJ, Calabrese JR, et al: Lamotrigine in rapid-cycling bipolar disorder. J Clin Psychiatry 58:522–527, 1997
43. Feighner JP, Robins E, Guze SB, et al: Diagnostic criteria for use in psychiatric research. Arch Gen Psychiatry 26:57–63, 1972
44. Feldman-Naim S, Turner EH, Leibenluft E: Diurnal variation in the direction of mood switches in patients with rapid-cycling bipolar disorder. J Clin Psychiatry 58:79–84, 1997
45. Fujiwara Y, Honda T, Tanaka Y, et al: Comparison of early and late-onset rapid cycling affective disorders: Clinical course and response to pharmacotherapy. J Clin Psychopharmacol 18:282–288, 1998
46. Geller B, Sun K, Zimerman B, et al: Complex and rapid-cycling in bipolar children and adolescents: A preliminary study. J Affect Disord 34:259–268, 1995
47. Glue P: Rapid cycling affective disorders in the mentally retarded. Biol Psychiatry 26:250–256, 1989
48. Gold MS, Herridge P, Hapworth WE: Depression and "symptomless" autoimmune thyroiditis. Psychiatr Ann 17:750–757, 1987
49. Goodwin FK, Jamison KR: Manic-Depressive Illness. New York, Oxford University Press, 1990
49a. Gottschalk A, Bauer MS, Whybrow PC: Evidence of chaotic mood variation in bipolar disorder. Arch Gen Psychiatry 52:947–959, 1995
49b. Gyulai L, Jaggi J, Bauer MS, et al: Bone mineral density and L-thyroxine treatment in rapidly cycling bipolar disorder. Biolog Psychiatry 41:503–506, 1997
50. Hantouche EG, Akiskal HS, Lancrenon S, et al: Systematic clinical methodology for validating bipolar-II disorder: Data in mid-stream from a French national multisite study (EPIDEP). J Affect Disord 50:163–173, 1998

51. Hayes SG: Long-term use of valproic acid in primary psychiatric disorders. J Clin Psychiatry 50(suppl 3):35–39, 1989
52. Haykal RF, Akiskal HS: Buproprion as a promising approach to rapid cycling bipolar II patients. J Clin Psychiatry 51:450–455, 1990
53. Hendrick V, Altshuler L, Wybrow P: Psychoneuroendocrinology of mood disorders: The hypothalamic-pituitary-thyroid axis. Psychiatr Clin North Am 21:277–292, 1998
54. Himmelhoch JM, Mulla D, Neil JF, et al: Incidence and significance of mixed affective states in a bipolar population. Arch Gen Psychiatry 33:1062–1066, 1976
55. Jan JE, Abroms IF, Freeman RD, et al: Rapid cycling in severely multidisabled children: A form of bipolar affective disorder? Pediatr Neurol 10:34–39, 1994
56. Joffe RT: Carbamazepine, lithium, and life course of bipolar affective disorder. Am J Psychiatry 148:1270–1271, 1991
57. Joffe RT, Kutcher S, MacDonald C: Thyroid function and bipolar affective disorder. Psychiatr Res 25:117–121, 1988
58. Joyce PR, Fergusson DM, Woollard G, et al: Urinary catecholamines and plasma hormones predict mood state in rapid cycling bipolar affective disorder. J Affect Disord 33:233–243, 1995
59. Kirov G, Murphy KC, Arranz MJ, et al: Low activity allele catechol-O-methyltransferase gene associated with rapid cycling bipolar disorder. Mol Psychiatry 3:342–345, 1998
60. Koukopoulos A, Calliari B, Minnai G, et al: Rapid cyclers, temperament, and antidepressants. Compr Psychiatry 24:249–258, 1983
61. Koukopoulos A, Reginaldi D, Laddomada P, et al: Course of the manic-depressive cycle and changes caused by treatments. Pharmacopsychiatry 13:156–167, 1980
62. Kraepelin E: Manic Depressive Insanity and Paranoia. Edinburgh, Livingstone, 1921
63. Kramlinger KG, Post RM: Ultra-rapid and ultradian cycling in bipolar affective illness. Br J Psychiatry 168:314–323, 1996
64. Kruger S, Braunid P, Young LT: Biological treatment of rapid-cycling bipolar disorder. Pharmacopsychiatry 29:167–175, 1996
65. Kupfer DJ, Carpenter LL, Frank E: Possible role of antidepressants in precipitating mania and hypomania in recurrent depression. Am J Psychiatry 145:804–808, 1988
66. Kusumakar V, Yatham LN, Haslam DRS, et al: Treatment of mania, mixed state, and rapid cycling. Can J Psychiatry 42(suppl 2):79S–86S, 1997
67. Lazarus JH, John R, Bennie EH: Lithium therapy and thyroid function: A long-term study. Psychol Med 11:85–92, 1981
68. Leibenluft E, Clark CH, Myers FS: The reproducibility of depressive and hypomanic symptoms across repeated episodes in patients with rapid-cycling bipolar disorder. J Affect Disord 33:83–88, 1995
69. Leibenluft E, Turner EH, Feldman-Naim S, et al: Light therapy in patients with rapid cycling bipolar disorder: Preliminary results. Psychopharmacol Bull 31:705–710, 1995
70. Levit AJ, Joffe RT, Ennis J, et al: The prevalence of cyclothymia in borderline personality disorder. J Clin Psychiatry 51:335–339, 1990
71. Levy AB, Drake ME, Shy KE: EEG evidence of epileptiform paroxysms in rapid cycling bipolar patients. J Clin Psychiatry 49:232–234, 1988
72. Lish JD, Gyulai L, Resnick SM, et al: A family history study of rapid-cycling bipolar disorder. Psychiatry Res 48:37–45, 1993
73. Lowry MA, Sovner R: Severe behavior problems associated with rapid cycling bipolar disorder in two adults with profound mental retardation. J Intellect Disabil Res 36:269–281, 1992
74. Maj M, Magliano L, Pirozzi R, et al: Validity of rapid cycling as a course specifier for bipolar disorder. Am J Psychiatry 151:1015–1019, 1994
75. Nakamura J, Kinoshita S: The late-onset rapid cycling affective disorder. Jpn J Clin Med 52:1297–1301, 1994
76. Novac A: Atypical antipsychotics as enhancement therapy in rapid cycling mood states: A case study. Ann Clin Psychiatry 10:107–111, 1998
77. Nurnberger J, Guroff JJ, Hamovit J, et al: A family study of rapid-cycling bipolar illness. J Affect Disord 15:87–91, 1988
78. Okuma T: Effects of carbamazepine and lithium on affective disorders. Neuropsychobiology 27:138–145, 1993

79. Oomen HA, Schipperijn AJ, Drexhage HA: The prevalence of affective disorder and in particular of a rapid cycling of bipolar disorder in patients with abnormal thyroid function tests. Clin Endocrinol 45:215–223, 1996
80. O'Shanick GJ, Ellinwood EH: Persistent elevation of thyroid-stimulating hormone in women with bipolar affective disorder. Am J Psychiatry 139:513–514, 1982
81. Papolos DF, Veit S, Faedda GL, et al: Ultra-ultra rapid cycling bipolar disorder is associated with the low activity catecholamine-O-methyltransferase allele. Mol Psychiatry 3:346–349, 1998
82. Pazzaglia PJ, Post RM, Ketter TA, et al: Preliminary controlled trial of nimodipine in ultra-rapid cycling affective dysregulation. Psychiatr Res 49:257–272, 1993
83. Peet M: Induction of mania with selected serotonin-reuptake inhibitors and tricyclic antidepressants. Br J Psychiatry 164:549–550, 1994
84. Perugi G, Musetti L, Simonini E, et al: Gender-mediated clinical features of depressive illness: The importance of temperamental differences. Br J Psychiatry 157:835–841, 1990
85. Placidi GF, Signoretta S, Liguori A, et al: The semistructured affective temperament interview (TEMPS-I): Reliability and psychometric properties in 1010 14–26 year students. J Affect Disord 47:1–10, 1998
86. Post RM, Kramlinger KG, Altshuler LL, et al: Rapid cycling bipolar disorder: Treatment of rapid cycling bipolar illness. Psychopharmacol Bull 26:37–47, 1990
87. Post RM, Kramlinger KG, Joffe RT, et al: Rapid cycling bipolar affective disorder: Lack of relation to hypothyroidism. Psychiatr Res 72:1–7, 1997
88. Prien RF, Gelenberg AJ: Alternatives to lithium for preventive treatment of bipolar disorder. Am J Psychiatry 146:840–848, 1989
89. Reus VI: Behavioral aspects of thyroid disease in women. Psychiatr Clin North Am 12:153–165, 1989
90. Robins LN, Helzer JE, Weissman MM, et al: Lifetime prevalence of specific psychiatric disorders in three sites. Arch Gen Psychiatry 41:949–958, 1984
91. Roy-Byrne PP, Joffe RT, Uhde TW, et al: Approaches to the evaluation and treatment of rapid-cycling affective illness. Br J Psychiatry 145:543–550, 1984
92. Roy-Byrne PP, Post RM, Uhde TW, et al: The longitudinal course of recurrent affective illness: Life chart data from research patients at the NIMH. Acta Psychiatr Scand 71(suppl 317):1–34, 1985
92a. Sachs GS: Bipolar mood disorder: practical strategies for acute and maintenance phase treatment. J Clin Psychopharm 16:32S–47S, 1996
93. Schou M: Prophylactic lithium maintenance treatment in recurrent endogenous affective disorders. *In* Gershon S, Shopsin B (eds): Lithium: Its Role in Psychiatric Research and Treatment. New York, Plenum, 1973, pp 269–295
94. Sharma V, Persad E, Mazmanian D, et al: Treatment of rapid cycling bipolar disorder with combination therapy of valproate and lithium. Can J Psychiatry 38:137–139, 1993
95. Shen Q: A comparative study of rapid and non-rapid cycling types in bipolar affective disorder. Chung-Hua Shen Ching Ching Shen Ko Tsa Chih 25:199–202, 1992
96. Simpson HB, Hurowitz GI, Liebowitz MR: General principles in the pharmacotherapy of antidepressant-induced rapid cycling: A case series. J Clin Psychopharmacol 17:460–466, 1997
97. Stancer HC, Persad E: Treatment of intractable rapid-cycling manic-depressive disorder with levothyroxine: Clinical observations. Arch Gen Psychiatry 39:311–312, 1982
98. Stoll AL, Sachs GS, Cohen BM, et al: Choline in the treatment of rapid cycling bipolar disorders: Clinical and neurochemical findings in lithium-treated patients. Biol Psychiatry 40:382–388, 1996
99. Tay LK, Dunner DL: A report on three patients with "rapid cycling" unipolar depression. Compr Psychiatry 33:253–255, 1992
100. Tondo L, Laddomada P, Serra G, et al: Rapid cyclers and antidepressants. Int Pharmacopsychiatry 16:119–123, 1981
100a. Tondo L, Baldessarini RJ: Rapid cycling in women and men with bipolar manic-depressive disorders. Am J Psychiatry 155:1434–1436, 1998
100b. Tohen M, Sanger TM, McElroy SL, et al: Olanzapine versus placebo in the treatment of acute mania. Am J Psychiatry 156:702–709, 1999

101. Wehr TA: Can antidepressants induce rapid cycling? Arch Gen Psychiatry 50:495–496, 1993
102. Wehr TA, Goodwin FK: Rapid cycling in manic-depressives induced by tricyclic antidepressants. Arch Gen Psychiatry 36:555–559, 1979
103. Wehr TA, Sack DA, Rosenthal NE, et al: Rapid cycling affective disorder: Contributing factors and treatment responses in 51 patients. Am J Psychiatry 145:179–184, 1988
104. Weissman MM, Leaf PJ, Tischler GL, et al: Affective disorders in five United States communities. Psychol Med 18:141–153, 1988
105. Wolpert EA, Goldberg JF, Harrow M: Rapid cycling unipolar and bipolar affective disorders. Am J Psychiatry 147:725–728, 1990

Address reprint requests to

Nael Kilzieh, MD
VA Puget Sound HCS (116–MHC)
American Lake Division
Tacoma, WA 98493

Antidepressant-Induced Mania and Cycle Acceleration: A Controversy Revisited

Lori L. Altshuler, M.D., Robert M. Post, M.D., Gabriele S. Leverich, M.S.W., Kirstin Mikalauskas, B.S., Ann Rosoff, M.A., and Laura Ackerman, B.A.

Objective: The longitudinal course of 51 patients with treatment-refractory bipolar disorder was examined to assess possible effects of heterocyclic antidepressants on occurrence of manic episodes and cycle acceleration. Method: Using criteria established from life charts, investigators rated the patients' episodes of mania or cycle acceleration as likely or unlikely to have been induced by antidepressant therapy. Discriminant function analyses were performed to assess predictors of vulnerability to antidepressant-induced mania or cycle acceleration. Further, the likelihood of future antidepressant-induced episodes in persons who had had one such episode was assessed. Results: Thirty-five percent of the patients had a manic episode rated as likely to have been antidepressant-induced. No variable was a predictor of vulnerability to antidepressant-induced mania. Cycle acceleration was likely to be associated with antidepressant treatment in 26% of the patients assessed. Younger age at first treatment was a predictor of vulnerability to antidepressant-induced cycle acceleration. Forty-six percent of patients with antidepressant-induced mania, but only 14% of those without, also showed antidepressant-induced cycle acceleration at some point in their illness. Conclusions: Mania is likely to be antidepressant-induced and not attributable to the expected course of illness in one-third of treatment-refractory bipolar patients, and rapid cycling is induced in one-fourth. Antidepressant-induced mania may be a marker for increased vulnerability to antidepressant-induced cycle acceleration. Antidepressant-induced cycle acceleration (but not antidepressant-induced mania) is associated with younger age at first treatment and may be more likely to occur in women and in bipolar II patients.

(Am J Psychiatry 1995; 152:1130–1138)

Antidepressant medications are the main pharmacologic treatment for acute severe depression. The efficacy of these medications in patients with unipolar disorder is well established, and the benefit of continued treatment for prevention of future relapse is well documented (1–17). These medications, however, have been associated with the onset of mania (4, 5, 8, 10, 11, 13–15, 18–47) or cycle acceleration (22, 36, 37, 48–61) in some, but not all (62–67), reports. Because many patients with bipolar disorder have episodes of depression that are naturally followed by episodes of mania (22, 66, 68–70) or an illness characterized by increasing frequency of episodes over time (22, 68–71), determining whether switches to mania and cycle acceleration occur secondary to medication effects or to the disease process itself can be difficult. An ideal study design to assess this question might involve a randomized longitudinal investigation of antidepressant-exposed and antidepressant-naive bipolar groups. However, the potential ethical and logistical problems of such a prospective randomized study are substantial. Another approach might be a longitudinal open-label study in which bipolar patients represent their own controls. A modification of this study design, as reported in this article, allows for the retrospective assessment of the interplay between the natural illness and medication intervention.

Using the life charting method (72–74) to represent graphically the patient's illness over time, one can view the pattern of illness and assess the impact of medications on this pattern. It has previously been demonstrated that this approach both yields information regarding the prophylactic efficacy of medications and helps determine whether an apparent response to an acute depressive episode is driven by medication or is

Received Aug. 2, 1993; revision received Jan. 20, 1995; accepted March 14, 1995. From the Brentwood VA Medical Center, Los Angeles, and the Biological Psychiatry Branch, NIMH. Address reprint requests to Dr. Post, Biological Psychiatry Branch, Bldg. 10, Rm. 3N212, National Institute of Mental Health, 9000 Rockville Pike, Bethesda, MD 20892.

The authors thank Jim Mintz, Ph.D., for statistical consultation.

an expected remission given the patient's prior course of illness (75–78). Since the pattern and severity of illness are graphed in relation to medication interventions, the life chart (albeit retrospective) allows for much more precise categorization of a possible relation between a drug intervention and change in the course of the illness than does chart review, which has been the basis of most prior attempts to examine this issue. In this study we used life charts to assess whether antidepressants had an impact on the patient's course of illness or the changes that occurred in association with antidepressants were more likely part of the pattern inherent in the patient's course over time.

METHOD

The study subjects consisted of patients consecutively admitted to a clinical research ward of the Biological Psychiatry Branch, National Institute of Mental Health (NIMH), in a designated period of time, who met the Research Diagnostic Criteria (RDC) (79) or the DSM-III criteria for bipolar disorder and who had life charts constructed during their hospital stay. Most patients had a history of lithium-refractory illness. None had chronic medical illnesses requiring ongoing medical treatment, with the exception of thyroid replacement therapy in one instance and intermittent periods of thyroid replacement in five other cases. Demographic characteristics of the study group are shown in table 1.

Life Charting

After a detailed explanation of the life charting procedure, all subjects gave informed consent. The construction of the life chart and its validity have been described in detail elsewhere (72–74). Briefly, at the patient's admission to NIMH, all previous inpatient and outpatient records throughout the patient's illness were obtained. In some cases, charts from hospitalizations up to 30 years prior to admission were acquired, including information regarding medication treatment and response. This and all additional information provided to the physician and social worker by the patient and family members were used to construct a schematic and pictorial representation of the patient's entire course of illness. The number, type, duration, and severity of affective episodes, as indicated by the degree of accompanying functional incapacity, were recorded. Consistent with the life charting method, subsyndromal hypomanic and depressive symptoms were also noted. Medication interventions for each episode and continued medication treatments during euthymic periods were recorded. Furthermore, significant events that may have had an impact on the illness, such as anniversaries, birthdays, and holidays, were included but are not systematically analyzed in this report. The life chart was drawn by the treating physician and then reviewed at discharge with the social worker and patient to ensure that the information was correct and complete. Episodes of mania and depression were rated as mild, moderate, or severe on the basis of the degree of incapacitation with which they were associated (72–74). On graph paper, hypomania was scored at 2.5 or 5 boxes and mania at 10 boxes above the baseline.

Categorization of Data

To prevent investigator bias, only life charts constructed in a *time period prior to the concept and design of this study* were used. Thus, no life chart was constructed with the knowledge or purpose of the present study specifically in mind. All life charts and each antidepressant trial were reviewed by the authors. Criteria were established a priori to determine whether the patient's antidepressant trial was likely associated with either a switch to mania or an increase in cycle frequency. To categorize patients as having a manic episode or

TABLE 1. Gender and Diagnoses of the Total Study Group With Bipolar Disorder and the Patients With Likely Antidepressant-Induced Mania

Item	Total Study Group (N=51)		Patients With Likely Antidepressant-Induced Mania (N=18)[a]		
	N	%	N	%	% of N in Total Group
Gender					
Male	17	33	6	33	35
Female	34	67	12	67	35
Diagnosis					
Bipolar I disorder	38	75	12	67	32
Bipolar II disorder	13	25	6	33	46

[a]Percent of total study group=18/51=35%.

cycle induction/acceleration that was likely or unlikely to have been associated with antidepressant therapy, the following criteria were used.

1. *Proximity.* If an episode of mania or increased cycling occurred within 8 weeks of the initiation of antidepressant therapy, the episode was considered for further evaluation in the "likely" category.

2. *Change in pattern.* If, given the patient's previous and future illness pattern, the episode that occurred during an antidepressant trial would not have been expected from observing the patient's pattern after the trial, the patient was further considered for the likely category. For example, if there was a change in the order or occurrence of episodes of hypomania or mania and depression, the patient was further considered a candidate for the likely category. Subsyndromal symptoms, while on the life charts, were not recorded as events.

3. *Change in severity.* If the patient had a first episode of severe mania, or mania that for the first time required hospitalization in the setting of an antidepressant trial, and there was no evidence of such kinds of episodes in the patient's prior or future course when not taking antidepressants, the patient was further considered to be in the likely category. If cycling (that is, the time from one episode of mania or depression to the next episode of mania or depression) was accelerated compared with when the patient was not taking an antidepressant, the person was further considered for the likely category.

Statistical Analyses

Each antidepressant trial was independently reviewed by three raters (L.L.A., L.A., A.R.) and was assigned, with the use of the parameters just described, to one of three groups based on the perceived role that medications played in inducing the event: 1) likely: mania or cycle acceleration occurred during the trial and seemed, on the basis of the factors described, to be associated with the use of antidepressants; 2) unlikely: mania or cycle acceleration occurred during an antidepressant trial but, in accordance with our criteria, was probably related not to medications but to the expected or natural course of the illness; 3) no occurrence: antidepressants were used, but no mania or cycle acceleration occurred during the trial.

Each patient was assigned a category independently by the three investigators, and the three ratings were then reviewed together by the team to reach one consensus rating. When there was disagreement about the relation between medication and a manic or cycling event, the bias was to choose the more conservative category, that is, to decide that medication was not likely to be related to the event. To test the reliability of this categorization, a fourth person who was unaware of the study design or the hypotheses was trained in the method. Nine randomly chosen cases were then categorized by this rater. The overall kappa between the consensus ratings and those of the trained rater was 0.67 ($z=3.0$, $p=0.003$); the kappas for the three separate category ratings ranged from 0.57 to 0.73.

FIGURE 1. Life Chart of a Patient Rated as Likely to Have Had an Antidepressant-Induced Switch to Mania[a]

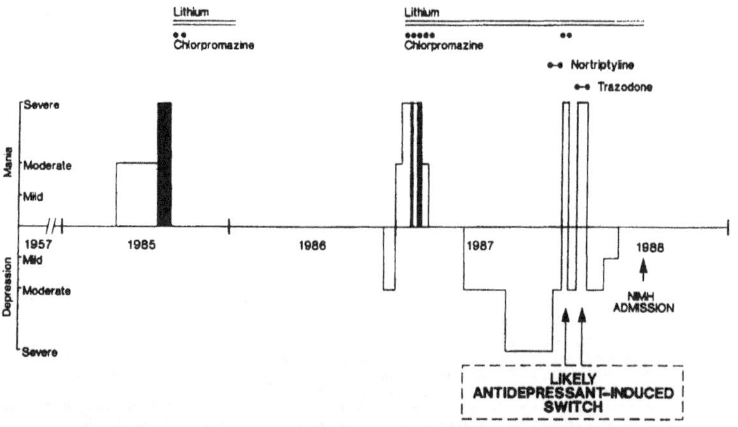

[a]Solid black shading indicates patient was hospitalized.

A stepwise discriminant function analysis was used to evaluate predictors of the likelihood of experiencing an antidepressant-induced switch to mania. The variables that were considered included age at first exposure to a heterocyclic antidepressant, age at first symptom of illness, age at first treatment, and age at first hospitalization. This analysis was repeated with the cycle acceleration data as well, with the entry of the additional variable of interepisode duration before the index trial. The F value for entry into the analysis was set at 4.0 for both analyses.

Conditional probabilities were calculated to examine 1) the likelihood that the subjects who had an antidepressant-induced switch to mania would have another switch upon subsequent exposure to a heterocyclic antidepressant, and 2) the likelihood that the subjects who had an antidepressant-induced switch to mania would have an antidepressant-induced cycle acceleration (during the same trial in which the switch occurred or during a later exposure to a heterocyclic antidepressant). An odds ratio was used to examine 3) whether those who had an antidepressant-induced switch to mania were more likely to experience an antidepressant-induced cycle acceleration than those who did not have an antidepressant-induced switch to mania. For both antidepressant-induced mania and cycle acceleration, chi-square analyses were used investigate associations with diagnosis and gender and to test the significance of the odds ratios. All chi-square tests were two-tailed.

RESULTS

Fifty-one patients with an RDC diagnosis of bipolar affective disorder had complete life charts and were included in the study. Sixty-seven percent of the group were female and 33% were male. Seventy-five percent had a diagnosis of bipolar I disorder, and the rest had a diagnosis of bipolar II disorder (table 1). Twenty-eight (55%) of our patients were rated as rapid cyclers on the basis of four or more episodes in 1 year before admission to NIMH. In both the bipolar I and bipolar II subgroups, the gender distribution was similar to that of the group as a whole (table 1).

Antidepressants and Switch to Mania

Heterocyclic antidepressants. During periods of antidepressant medication, episodes of mania occurred in 42 (82%) of the 51 patients. However, according to the stringent criteria we used, the majority of these manic episodes were judged unlikely to be directly attributable to the use of antidepressants. Nine (18%) of the 51 bipolar patients had no mania while taking antidepressants. Eighteen (35%) of the 51 were judged to be in the likely category for an antidepressant-induced manic episode. An example of a patient's life chart from the likely category is shown in figure 1. There were no statistically significant differences in the percentage of overall bipolarity (Fisher's exact test, p=0.50) or gender (χ^2=0.00, df=1, p=1.00) in this subgroup compared with the group as a whole (table 1).

The patients categorized as likely and those judged as unlikely to have had an episode of antidepressant-induced mania in association with an antidepressant trial were compared (table 2). None of the variables considered in the stepwise discriminant function analysis emerged as predictors of an antidepressant-induced switch to mania. However, of the 18 patients who had a likely antidepressant-induced manic episode, 15 had subsequent trials of heterocyclic antidepressants. Of these 15 patients, eight (53%) had at least one more trial in which a heterocyclic antidepressant was also judged likely to be associated with the mania. During the first likely antidepressant-induced episode, five (28%) of the 18 patients were taking lithium and 13 (72%) were taking no antimanic agents (none was taking carbamazepine). Five (63%) of the eight who on a subsequent antidepressant trial had a likely antidepres-

TABLE 2. Characteristics of Bipolar Patients With Likely and Unlikely Antidepressant-Induced Mania

Variable	Patients With Likely Antidepressant-Induced Mania (N=18)		Patients With Unlikely Antidepressant-Induced Mania (N=33)	
	Mean	SD	Mean	SD
Age at first symptom of bipolar disorder (years)	24.7	7.9	24.2	10.9
Age at first treatment for bipolar disorder (years)	27.8	7.6	26.6	10.5
Age at first hospitalization for bipolar disorder (years)	29.3	7.8	28.1	10.4
Age at first exposure to heterocyclic antidepressant (years)	34.0	9.8	34.2	11.8

TABLE 3. Gender and Diagnoses of Bipolar Patients With Likely Antidepressant-Induced Mania and the Subgroup With Likely Antidepressant-Induced Cycle Acceleration

Item	Total Group Assessed (N=35)		Patients With Likely Antidepressant-Induced Cycle Acceleration (N=9)[a]		
	N	%	N	%	% of N in Total Group
Gender					
Male	9	26	1	11	11
Female	26	74	8	89	31
Diagnosis					
Bipolar I disorder	26	74	5	56	19
Bipolar II disorder	9	26	4	44	44

[a]Percent of total group=9/35=26%.

sant-induced mania were taking antimanic agents during that trial: four were taking lithium and one was taking lithium and carbamazepine.

Monoamine oxidase inhibitors (MAOIs). Fourteen patients in the study group were exposed to MAOIs prior to their NIMH admission. Three (21%) of the 14 had manic episodes that were likely associated with their MAOI trials. Two of these three patients were also in the likely category for antidepressant-induced mania at some point in their course of illness. Of the 18 patients with antidepressant-induced mania, eight were exposed to MAOIs. Two of these eight also switched to mania while taking MAOIs.

Antidepressants and Cycle Acceleration

To assess effects on cycle length, only the patients with heterocyclic antidepressant trials of 6 months or longer were evaluated. Of the original 51 patients, 35 met this criterion (table 3). Nine (26%) of the 35 patients were judged to have had a heterocyclic antidepressant trial in the likely category for cycle acceleration. Eight of these nine were female. Further, while only 26% of the 35 had bipolar II disorder, 44% of the subgroup with likely antidepressant-induced cycle acceleration had bipolar II disorder. Thus, while no statistically significant demographic differences were discerned, female patients and patients with a diagnosis of bipolar II disorder appeared to be overrepresented in the antidepressant-induced cycle acceleration group. Of the nine patients, four were taking a mood stabilizer (lithium) and five were not taking a mood stabilizer at the time of increased cycling. In four cases, cycle acceleration was associated with the first exposure to a heterocyclic antidepressant. In eight of the nine cases, cycle acceleration occurred within 2 months of the initiation of the antidepressant trial. In all nine cases, the antidepressant trial was discontinued; eight patients demonstrated a cycle deceleration within 2 months of the discontinuation of medication and one within 5 months of discontinuation (table 4). An example of a patient in the likely category for antidepressant-induced cycle acceleration is shown in figure 2.

TABLE 4. Data on Bipolar Patients With Likely Antidepressant-Induced Cycle Acceleration

Patient Number	Duration of Illness at Time of Cycle Acceleration (years)	Number of Antidepressant Trial in Which Cycle Acceleration Occurred	Time Taking Antidepressant Before Index Cycle Acceleration (months)[a]
1	35	1	2
2	25	2	1.5
3	18	3	0
4	3	1	1
5	5	1	2
6	10	2	0
7	19	4	2
8	18	4	5
9	5	1	1

[a]All nine patients had a decrease in cycling when their antidepressant was discontinued.

Data on demographic variables are shown in table 5. Stepwise discriminant function analysis revealed that age at first treatment was the only statistically significant predictor of antidepressant-induced cycle acceleration.

Of the 35 patients rated for cycle acceleration, 13 were rated as likely to have had an antidepressant-induced episode of mania and 22 were rated as unlikely. Six (46%) of the 13 with antidepressant-induced mania had antidepressant-induced cycle acceleration, while only three (14%) of the 22 with no antidepressant-induced mania had cycle acceleration induction at some point in their illness (χ^2=4.52, df=1, p=0.03). The odds that patients with an antidepressant-induced manic episode would have an antidepressant-induced cycle acceleration later in their illness were 4.6 times greater than the odds for those who were rated not likely to have had an antidepressant-induced switch to mania (χ^2=2.18, df=1, p=0.14).

Thirteen patients taking MAOIs were rated for cycle acceleration. Of these, five (38%) fell into the category

FIGURE 2. Life Chart of a Patient Rated as Likely to Have Had an Antidepressant-Induced Cycle Acceleration[a]

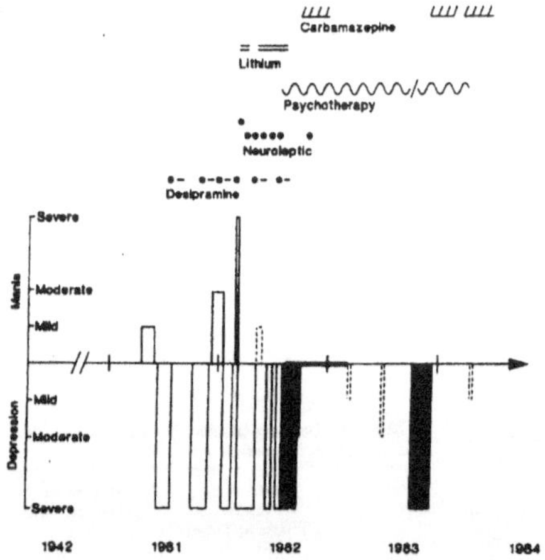

[a]Solid black shading indicates patient was hospitalized.

TABLE 5. Characteristics of Bipolar Patients With Likely and Unlikely Antidepressant-Induced Cycle Acceleration

Variable	Patients With Likely Antidepressant-Induced Cycle Acceleration (N=9)		Patients With Unlikely Antidepressant-Induced Cycle Acceleration (N=26)	
	Mean	SD	Mean	SD
Age at first symptom of bipolar disorder (years)	19.2	6.6	26.5	8.8
Age at first treatment for bipolar disorder (years)[a]	21.8	6.5	29.7	8.2
Age at first hospitalization for bipolar disorder (years)	24.3	8.8	31.0	8.1
Age at first exposure to heterocyclic antidepressant (years)	31.6	8.6	36.7	10.3
Duration of interval between last two episodes prior to antidepressant trial (weeks)	24.3	57.7	6.5	19.2

[a]Significant discriminator between groups (F=6.81, df=1, 33, p=0.02, discriminant function analysis).

of likely MAOI-related increase in cycling, with four (80%) of these five also experiencing cycle acceleration while taking a tricyclic antidepressant. Of the nine patients who showed antidepressant-induced cycle acceleration, only four were exposed to MAOIs, and all four were also likely MAOI-induced accelerated cyclers.

DISCUSSION

Heterocyclic Antidepressants and Mania

The difficulty in distinguishing manic episodes that are probably attributable to antidepressants versus those related to the natural course of illness may account for some of the controversy in the literature regarding incidence of mania after initiation of antidepressant treatment. In this retrospective nonblind study, the number of patients who switched from depression to mania during heterocyclic antidepressant treatment was very high (82%), suggesting that depression is often followed by mania in treatment-refractory bipolar patients regardless of cause. This rate is higher than that reported in nonrefractory populations (19, 64, 80) and may reflect the greater proportion in our study group of rapid-cycling and lithium-nonresponsive patients, who are more likely to have a pattern of depression/mania/euthymic interval rather than mania/depression/euthymic interval (81, 82). However, despite the high rate of switching from depression to mania during antidepressant treatment, in only 35% of patients were the manic episodes judged to be attributable to the antidepressants. Thus, in the remaining 47% of our subjects who had switches from depression to mania, these switches were judged more likely to be related to the natural course of their illness. This corresponds well with results reported by Lewis and Winokur (66), who found a switch rate from depression to mania of 41% in bipolar patients taking no medications.

Our study suggests that antidepressants can precipitate mania in roughly one-third of treatment-refractory patients at some point in their illness. No demographic factors or illness variables studied were able to predict the group who would be vulnerable to the antidepressant-induced switch phenomenon. Switch rates of patients taking heterocyclic antidepressants have been reported to occur at about double the rate of that seen in patients taking nonheterocyclic antidepressant medications or placebo (5, 44, 80). Quitkin et al. (44) found a rate of relapse into mania of 24% for bipolar I depressed patients treated with lithium and imipramine, compared with a relapse rate of 10.5% for those taking lithium and placebo; while the difference was not significant, it was suggestive of an association of imipramine with an increasing rate of switch from depression to mania. Prien et al. (5), in a double-blind, long-term follow-up study, found the incidence of mania to be 53% for bipolar patients taking imipramine alone and only 26% for those taking lithium and 28% for those taking lithium and imipramine. As there was no placebo group in that study, it is difficult to distinguish between the rate of natural switch from depression to mania and the rate of switch which might be drug-induced. However, that study implicates antidepressants in precipitating mania.

In the most recent comprehensive review, Rouillon et

al. (80) provided an overview of 15 placebo-controlled studies. In a total of 1,231 unipolar patients treated with antidepressants, the incidence of mania was 1.5% (N=19). Among those taking placebo, five (0.9%) of 555 developed mania or hypomania. Of patients specifically diagnosed as bipolar (N=158), the incidence of hypomania/mania was 51% (N=25) in the 49 patients treated with imipramine alone, 21% (N=13) in the 60 patients treated with lithium alone, 28% (N=10) in the 36 treated with lithium and imipramine, and 23% (N=3) in the 13 taking only placebo. These data, taken in conjunction with those of Prien et al. (5) as noted above, suggest that approximately one-half of the total switch rate for patients taking tricyclic antidepressants is attributable to the direct effects of tricyclic antidepressants, while natural course accounts for the other half of the observed switch rate during antidepressant treatment.

Whether mood stabilizers can block the induction of mania by heterocyclic antidepressants is a question that requires further study. While one study suggested a lack of protection against the mania-inducing properties of these antidepressants (44), two others found a protective prophylactic effect (5, 80). In our naturalistic study, while the majority of the bipolar patients were not taking a mood stabilizer at the time of the first likely antidepressant-induced switch to mania or cycle acceleration, the majority of those who had a switch to mania likely associated with another instance of exposure to an antidepressant were concurrently taking a mood stabilizer during this next switch. Thus, no clear evidence of a prophylactic effect of mood stabilizers against the antidepressant-induced switch phenomenon was noted in our study group.

Our data suggest that the existence of an antidepressant-induced mania in a given individual appears to increase the likelihood that it will occur again and may increase the risk for antidepressant-induced cycle acceleration at some point in that person's course of illness. It is possible that heterocyclic antidepressant "induction" of mania may sensitize a person to future such occurrences (83) as well as increase the likelihood of a future antidepressant-induced cycle acceleration. Alternatively, the occurrence of these may mark an underlying vulnerability or sensitivity to heterocyclic antidepressants that can manifest itself with either process.

Heterocyclic Antidepressants and Cycle Acceleration

While cycle acceleration occurred during a period of heterocyclic antidepressant administration in many of the subjects, it was judged to have been likely attributable to the antidepressant in just 26% of the study group. Thus, the speeding up of cycles during antidepressant treatment was related to the antidepressant itself and not to the natural course of illness in one-quarter of the patients. The antidepressant cycle acceleration group was statistically significantly younger at the first treatment intervention. Whether this suggests that these patients are sicker at an earlier age and this is a vulnerability to cycle acceleration, or that patients treated earlier may become "primed" to have cycle acceleration due to medication, remains to be determined. Further, the antidepressant-induced cycle accelerated group contained a greater proportion of bipolar II patients and female patients. These differences were not significant, perhaps because the group was small. The notion that bipolar II disorder and female gender may be phenotypic demographic risk factors for antidepressant-induced cycling acceleration is interesting in light of data showing that rapid cyclers are most likely to have bipolar II illness and to be female (59, 67, 84–86).

In the group likely to have had antidepressant-induced cycle acceleration, evidence of acceleration started within the first several months of a trial of a heterocyclic antidepressant. The occurrence of cycle acceleration within the first year of initiation of an antidepressant trial is consistent with the work of others (22, 60), who have observed that the development of rapid cycling is most likely to occur in the first year after initiation of antidepressant treatment. In some (48, 49, 59) but not all (67) controlled on-off-on drug studies, it has been demonstrated that cycling in some patients regularly increases when they are taking the drug and decreases when they are not, and that the rapid cycling can be significantly associated with antidepressants (59). Since only four reports of studies with large samples but extremely different methods currently exist in the literature exploring the relation of medications to cycling (22, 59, 60, 67), we add our observations to this important clinical question. Our study suggests—as do three of the four studies (22, 59, 60)—that antidepressants can induce cycle acceleration in a subpopulation of bipolar patients.

MAOIs

Our preliminary data suggest that MAOIs may also induce mania and cycle acceleration at rates similar to those for the heterocyclic antidepressants. Furthermore, there may be a cross-sensitivity to the two classes of drugs, as two (67%) of three patients who switched while taking an MAOI had previously switched while taking heterocyclic antidepressants. Similarly, four (80%) of five of those who had MAOI-induced cycle acceleration had had a previous antidepressant-induced cycle acceleration. Given that our study group was small, the MAOI findings are reported as highly preliminary data that need to be further explored, in relation both to the traditional MAOIs observed in this study (phenelzine, tranylcypromine, and isocarboxazid) and to newer agents, such as MAOI-A selective medications (87) or the reversible inhibitors now available in Europe. However, as MAOIs have recently been found to be significantly more effective than classic tricyclic antidepressants in the treatment of anergic bipolar depression (88), with less evidence of risk of switching, and are highly effective in tricyclic-antidepressant-resistant bipolar depression (89, 90), the ability of these drugs to induce mania and cycle acceleration warrants further study.

CONCLUSIONS

Our exploratory study suggests that heterocyclic antidepressants may contribute to the induction or exacerbation of episodes of mania in one-third of treatment-refractory bipolar patients at some point in their illness. Heterocyclic antidepressants may contribute to cycle acceleration in one-quarter of these patients. While there are limitations to a retrospective study, this naturalistic study represents treatment given in actual clinical practice and assesses the relationship of mania or cycle acceleration to antidepressant treatment in a systematic longitudinal fashion. Our data suggest that some treatment-refractory bipolar patients with antidepressant-induced mania may be more vulnerable to future episodes of antidepressant-induced mania and to antidepressant-induced cycle acceleration. Patients with clear evidence of antidepressant-induced cycle acceleration (confirmed by a decrease in cycling rate upon drug discontinuation) are younger at first treatment intervention and tend to be female. How these findings 1) generalize to less treatment-refractory patient populations or to the newer second-generation antidepressants (such as the selective serotonin reuptake inhibitors, bupropion, and venlafaxine) and 2) are affected by concurrent use of a mood stabilizer (lithium, carbamazepine, or valproic acid) requires further study and more rigorous prospective designs.

REFERENCES

1. Seager CP, Bird RL: Imipramine with ECT in depression: a controlled trial. J Ment Sci 1962; 108:704–707
2. Kay DW, Fahy T, Garside RF: A seven-month double-blind trial of amitriptyline and diazepam in ECT-treated depressed patients. Br J Psychiatry 1970; 117:667–671
3. Mindham RHS, Howland DC, Shepherd M: Continuation therapy with tricyclic antidepressants in depressive illness. Lancet 1972; 2:854–855
4. Prien RF, Klett CJ, Caffey EM Jr: Lithium carbonate and imipramine in prevention of affective episodes: a comparison in recurrent affective illness. Arch Gen Psychiatry 1973; 29:420–425
5. Prien RF, Kupfer DJ, Mansky PA, Small JG, Tuason VB, Voss CB, Johnson WE: Drug therapy in the prevention of recurrences in unipolar and bipolar affective disorders. Arch Gen Psychiatry 1984; 41:1096–1104
6. Klerman GL, DiMascio A, Weissman MM, Prusoff B, Paykel ES: Treatment of depression by drugs and psychotherapy. Am J Psychiatry 1974; 131:186–191
7. Coppen A, Ghose K, Montgomery S, Rama-Rao VA, Bailey J, Jorgensen A: Continuation therapy with amitriptyline in depression. Br J Psychiatry 1978; 133:28–33
8. van Praag H, de Hann S: Depression vulnerability and 5-hydroxytryptophan prophylaxis. Psychiatry Res 1980; 3:75–83
9. Stein MK, Rickels K, Weise CC: Maintenance therapy with amitriptyline: a controlled trial. Am J Psychiatry 1980; 137:370–371
10. Rouillon F, Phillips R, Serrurier D, Amsart E, Gerard MJ: Rechutes des dépressions unipolaires et efficacité de la maprotiline. L'Encéphale 1989; 15:527–534
11. Kane JM, Quitkin PM, Rifkin A, Ramos-Lorenz JR, Noyak HA: Lithium carbonate and imipramine in the prophylaxis of unipolar and bipolar II illness. Arch Gen Psychiatry 1982; 39:1065–1069
12. Bialos D, Giller E, Jatlow P, Docherty J, Harkness L: Recurrence of depression after discontinuation of long-term amitriptyline treatment. Am J Psychiatry 1982; 139:325–329
13. Glen AIM, Johnson AI, Shepherd M: Continuation therapy with lithium and amitriptyline in unipolar depressive illness: a randomized double-blind controlled trial. Psychol Med 1984; 14: 37–50
14. Montgomery SA, Dufour M, Brion S, Gailledreau J, Laqueille X, Ferrey G, Moron P, Parant-Lucena N, Singer L, Danion JN, Beuzen JN, Pierredon MA: The prophylactic efficacy of fluoxetine in unipolar depression. Br J Psychiatry 1988; 193(Sept suppl):69–76
15. Lendresse P, Cren MC, Lemarie JC: Traitement prolongé par nomifensine 75 mg dans les états dépressifs névrotiques et réactionnels. Psychiatrie Française 1984; 16(suppl):156–158
16. Frank E, Kupfer DJ, Perel JM, Cornes C, Jarrett DB, Mallinger AG, Thase ME, McEachran AB, Grochocinski VJ: Three-year outcomes for maintenance therapies in recurrent depression. Arch Gen Psychiatry 1990; 47:1093–1099
17. Kupfer DJ, Frank E, Perel JM, Cornes C, Jarrett DB, Mallinger AG, Thase ME, McEachran AB, Grochocinski VJ: Five-year outcome for maintenance therapies in recurrent depression. Arch Gen Psychiatry 1992; 49:769–773
18. Henry EW, Chandler LP, Rasmussen JGC: Assessment of manic reactions during treatment with the SSRI sertraline. Clin Neuropharmacol 1992; 15(suppl 1):317
19. Angst J, Dittrich A, Grof P: Course of endogenous affective psychoses and its modification by prophylactic administration of imipramine and lithium. Int Pharmacopsychiatry 1969; 2:1–11
20. Crane GE: The psychiatric side-effects of iproniazid. Am J Psychiatry 1956; 112:494–501
21. Siegel D: Bulimia, tricyclic antidepressants, and mania. Clinical Pediatr (Phila) 1989; 28:123–126
22. Kukopulos A, Reginaldi D, Laddomada P, Floris G, Serra G, Tondo L: Course of the manic-depressive cycle and changes caused by treatment. Pharmakopsychiatrie Neuro-Psychopharmakologie 1980; 13:156–167
23. Ball JR, Kiloh LG: A controlled trial of imipramine in treatment of depressive states. Br Med J 1959; 2:1052–1055
24. Leyberg JT, Denmark JC: The treatment of depressive states with imipramine hydrochloride (Tofranil). J Ment Sci 1959; 105: 1123–1126
25. Kiloh LG, Child JP, Latner G: Controlled trial of iproniazid in the treatment of endogenous depression. J Ment Sci 1960; 106: 1139–1144
26. Klein DF: Chlorpromazine-procyclidine combination, imipramine and placebo in depressive disorders. Can Psychiatr Assoc J 1966; 11(Suppl):146–149
27. Bartholomew AA: Evaluation of tranylcypromine ("Parnate") in the treatment of depression. Med J Aust 1962; 49:655–662
28. Rees L, Davies B: A controlled trial of phenelzine ("Nardil") in the treatment of severe depressive illness. J Ment Sci 1961; 107: 560–566
29. Hohn R, Gross GM, Gross M, Lasagna L: A double-blind comparison of placebo and imipramine in the treatment of depressed patients in a state hospital. J Psychiatr Res 1961; 1:76–91
30. Miller A, Baker EFW, Lewis D, Jones A: Imipramine: a clinical evaluation in a variety of settings. Can Psychiatr Assoc J 1960; 5:150–160
31. Freyhan FA: Zur modernen psychiatrischen Behandlung der Depressionen. Nervenarzt 1960; 31:112–118
32. Browne MW, Kreeger LC, Kazamias NG: A clinical trial of amitriptyline in depressive patients. Br J Psychiatry 1963; 109:692–694
33. Gottfries CG: Clinical trial with the monoamine oxidase inhibitor tranylcypromine on a psychiatric clientele. Acta Psychiatr Scand 1963; 39:463–472

34. Skarbek A: Trial of amitriptyline in chronic depression. Dis Nerv Syst 1963; 24:115–119
35. Vahia NS, Bagadia VCN, Doongaji DR: Value of some antidepressants. Hospital Reports by the Medical and Professorial Staff of the Jamsetji Jijibhai Hospital and Grant Medical College 1964; 9:199–203
36. Arnold OH, Kryspin-Exner K: Zur Frage der Beeinflussung des Verlaufes des manisch-depressiven Krankheitgeschehens durch Antidepressive (On the question of the influence of antidepressants on the course of manic-depressive illness). Wien Med Wochenschr 1965; 45/46:929–934
37. Till E, Vukovic S: Uber den Einfluss der thymoleptischen Behandlung auf den Verlauf endogener Depressionen (On the influences of thymoleptic treatment on the course of endogenous depression). Int Pharmacopsychiatry 1970; 4:210–219
38. Murphy DL: The behavioral toxicity of monoamine oxidase-inhibiting antidepressants. Adv Pharmacol Chemother 1977; 14: 71–105
39. Murphy DL, Brand E, Baker M, van Kammen D, Gordon E: Phenelzine effects in hospitalized unipolar and bipolar depressed patients: behavioral and biochemical relationships, in Neuropsychopharmacology: Proceedings of the IX Congress of the CINP, 7–12 July, 1974. Edited by Bossier JR, Hippius H, Pichot P. New York, American Elsevier, 1975
40. Bunney WE Jr: Psychopharmacology of the switch process in affective illness, in Psychopharmacology: A Generation of Progress. Edited by Lipton MA, DiMascio A, Killiam KF. New York, Raven Press, 1978
41. Van Schenyen JC, van Kammen DP: Clomipramine-induced mania in unipolar depression. Arch Gen Psychiatry 1979; 36:560–565
42. Akiskal HS: External validating criteria for psychiatric diagnosis: their application in affective disorders. J Clin Psychiatry 1980; 41:6–15
43. Wehr TA, Goodwin FK: Do antidepressants cause mania? Psychopharmacol Bull 1987; 23:61–65
44. Quitkin FM, Kane J, Rifkin A, Lorenzi-Ramos JR, Nayak DV: Prophylactic lithium carbonate with and without imipramine for bipolar I patients. Arch Gen Psychiatry 1981; 38:902–907
45. Wehr TA, Goodwin FK: Can antidepressants cause mania and worsen the course of affective illness? Am J Psychiatry 1987; 144:1403–1411
46. Zis AP, Cowdry RW, Wehr TA, Muscetolla G, Goodwin FK: Tricyclic-induced mania and MHPG excretion. Psychiatry Res 1979; 1:93–99
47. Geller B, Fox L, Fletcher M: Effect of tricyclic antidepressants on switching to mania and on the onset of bipolarity in depressed 6–12 year olds. J Am Acad Child Adolesc Psychiatry 1993; 32: 43–50
48. Wehr TA, Goodwin FK: Tricyclics modulate frequency of mood cycles. Chronobiologia 1979; 6:377–385
49. Wehr TA, Goodwin FK: Rapid cycling in manic-depressives induced by tricyclic antidepressants. Arch Gen Psychiatry 1979; 36:555–559
50. Wehr TA, Goodwin FK: Rapid cycling between mania and depression caused by maintenance tricyclics. Psychopharmacol Bull 1979; 15:17–21
51. Ghadirian AM, Kusalic M: Rapid cycling following antidepressant in an adolescent. Biol Psychiatry 1990; 27:1183–1184
52. Extein I, Pottash ALC, Gold MS: Does subclinical hypothyroidism predispose to tricyclic-induced rapid mood cycles? J Clin Psychiatry 1982; 43:290–293
53. Oppenheim G: Drug-induced rapid cycling: possible outcomes and management. Am J Psychiatry 1982; 139:939–941
54. Siris SG, Chertoff HR, Perel JM: Rapid-cycling affective disorder during imipramine treatment: a case report. Am J Psychiatry 1979; 136:341–342
55. Lerer B, Birmacher B, Ebstein RP, Belmaker RH: 48-hour depressive cycling induced by antidepressant. Br J Psychiatry 1980; 137: 183–185
56. Kukopulos A, Caliari B, Tundo A, Minnai G, Floris G, Reginaldi D, Tondo L: Rapid cyclers, temperament, and antidepressants. Compr Psychiatry 1983; 24:249–258
57. Ko GN, Leckman JF, Heninger GR: Induction of rapid mood cycling during L-dopa treatment in a bipolar patient. Am J Psychiatry 1981; 138:1624–1625
58. Mattsson A, Seltzer RL: MAOI-induced rapid cycling bipolar affective disorder in an adolescent. Am J Psychiatry 1981; 138: 677–679
59. Wehr TA, Sack DA, Rosenthal NE, Cowdry RW: Rapid cycling affective disorder: contributing factors and treatment responses in 51 patients. Am J Psychiatry 1988; 145:179–184
60. Tondo L, Laddomada P, Serra G, Minnai G, Kukopulos A: Rapid cyclers and antidepressants. Int Pharmacopsychiatry 1981; 16:119–123
61. Tondo L, Burrai C, Scamonatti L, Rudas N: Effect of lithium discontinuation on rapid cycling course. Lithium 1990; 1:221–226
62. Solomon RL, Rich CL, Darko DF: Antidepressant treatment and the occurrence of mania in bipolar patients admitted for depression. J Affect Disord 1990; 18:253–257
63. Angst J: Switch from depression to mania, or from mania to depression: role of psychotropic drugs. Psychopharmacol Bull 1987; 23:66–67
64. Angst J: Switch from depression to mania—a record study over decades between 1920 and 1982. Psychopathology 1985; 18: 140–154
65. Kupfer DJ, Carpenter LL, Frank E: Possible role of antidepressants in precipitating mania and hypomania in recurrent depression. Am J Psychiatry 1988; 145:804–808
66. Lewis JL, Winokur G: The induction of mania: a natural history study with controls. Arch Gen Psychiatry 1982; 39:303–306
67. Coryell W, Endicott J, Keller M: Rapid cycling affective disorder: demographics, diagnosis, family history, and course. Arch Gen Psychiatry 1992; 49:126–131
68. Angst J: The course of affective disorders. Psychopathology 1986; 19:47–52
69. Kraepelin E: Manic-Depressive Insanity and Paranoia. Translated by Barclay RM, edited by Robertson GM. Edinburgh, E & S Livingstone, 1921
70. Goodwin FK, Jamison KR: Manic-Depressive Illness. New York, Oxford University Press, 1990
71. Post RM, Rubinow DR, Ballenger JC: Conditioning and sensitization in the longitudinal course of affective illness. Br J Psychiatry 1986; 149:191–201
72. Squillace K, Post RM, Savard R, Erwin-Gorman M: Life charting of the longitudinal course of recurrent affective illness, in Neurobiology of Mood Disorders. Edited by Post RM, Ballenger JC. Baltimore, Williams & Wilkins, 1984
73. Roy-Byrne PP, Post RM, Uhde TW, Porcu T, Davis DD: The longitudinal course of recurrent affective illness: life chart data from research patients at the NIMH. Acta Psychiatr Scand Suppl 1985; 317:5–34
74. Post RM, Roy-Byrne PP, Uhde TW: Graphic representation of the life course of illness in patients with affective disorder. Am J Psychiatry 1988; 145:844–848
75. Baastrup PC, Schou M: Lithium as a prophylactic agent: its effect against recurrent depressions and manic-depressive psychosis. Arch Gen Psychiatry 1967; 16:162–172
76. Calabrese JR, Delucchi GA: Spectrum of efficacy of valproate in 55 patients with rapid-cycling bipolar disorder. Am J Psychiatry 1990; 147:431–434
77. Grof P, Angst J, Haines T: The clinical course of depression: practical issues, in Medica Hoechst 8: Classification and Prediction of Outcome of Depression. Edited by Angst J. Stuttgart, Germany, Schattauer Verlag, 1974
78. Post RM, Leverich GS, Rosoff AS, Altshuler LL: Carbamazepine prophylaxis in refractory affective disorders: a focus on long-term followup. J Clin Psychopharmacol 1990; 10:318–327
79. Spitzer RL, Endicott J, Robins E: Research Diagnostic Criteria: rationale and reliability. Arch Gen Psychiatary 1978; 35:773–782
80. Rouillon F, Lejoyeux M, Filteau MJ: Unwanted effects of long term treatment, in Long Term Treatment of Depression. Edited by Montgomery SA, Rouillon FA. New York, John Wiley & Sons, 1992
81. Maj M: Clinical prediction of response to lithium prophylaxis in

bipolar patients: the importance of the previous pattern of course of illness. Clin Neuropharmacol 1990; 13(suppl 1):S66–S70
82. Faedda GL, Baldessarini RJ, Tohen M, Strakowski SM, Waternaux C: Episode sequence in bipolar disorder and response to lithium treatment. Am J Psychiatry 1991; 148:1237–1239
83. Pickar D, Cowdry RW, Zis AP, Cohen RM, Murphy DL: Mania and hypomania during antidepressant pharmacotherapy: clinical and research implications, in Neurobiology of Mood Disorders. Edited by Post RM, Ballenger J. Baltimore, Williams & Wilkins, 1984
84. Dunner DL, Patric V, Fieve RR: Rapid cycling manic depressive patients. Compr Psychiatry 1977; 18:561–566
85. Wolpert EA, Goldberg JF, Harrow M: Rapid cycling in unipolar and bipolar affective disorders. Am J Psychiatry 1990; 147:725–728
86. Dunner DL: Rapid cycling bipolar manic depressive illness. Psychiatr Clin North Am 1979; 2:461–467
87. Potter WZ, Murphy DL, Wehr TA, Linnoila M, Goodwin FK: Clorgyline: a new treatment for patients with refractory rapid cycling disorder. Arch Gen Psychiatry 1982; 39:505–510
88. Himmelhoch JM, Thase ME, Mallinger AG, Houck P: Tranylcypromine versus imipramine in anergic bipolar depression. Am J Psychiatry 1991; 148:910–916
89. McGrath PJ, Stewart JW, Harrison W, Quitkin FM: Treatment of tricyclic refractory depression with a monoamine oxidase inhibitor antidepressant. Psychopharmacol Bull 1987; 23:169–172
90. Thase ME, Mallinger AG, McKnight D, Himmelhoch JM: Treatment of imipramine-resistant depression, IV: a double-blind crossover study of tranylcypromine for anergic bipolar depression. Am J Psychiatry 1992; 149:195–198

Suicide and Bipolar Disorder

Kay Redfield Jamison, Ph.D.

Suicide, which is both a stereotypic yet highly individualized act, is a common endpoint for many patients with severe psychiatric illness. The mood disorders (depression and bipolar manic-depression) are by far the most common psychiatric conditions associated with suicide. At least 25% to 50% of patients with bipolar disorder also attempt suicide at least once. With the exception of lithium—which is the most demonstrably effective treatment against suicide—remarkably little is known about specific contributions of mood-altering treatments to minimizing mortality rates in persons with major mood disorders in general and bipolar depression in particular. Suicide is usually a manifestation of severe psychiatric distress that is often associated with a diagnosable and treatable form of depression or other mental illness. In a clinical setting, an assessment of suicidal risk must precede any attempt to treat psychiatric illness. *(J Clin Psychiatry 2000;61[suppl 9]:47–51)*

Unless someone lives an unthinkably boring life, has no hopes that can be shattered, no love that can be lost, or transits from birth to death in a bubble above the frays of earth, he or she experiences the same griefs or strains that, for a few, become the 'cause' of death.[1]

The relationship between the events of life, stress, and psychiatric illness is not always straightforward. Psychological pain or stress alone—however profound the loss, disappointment, shame, or rejection—is rarely sufficient cause for suicide. Much of the decision to die lies in the construing of events, and most people, when healthy, do not construe any event as devastating enough to warrant killing themselves. Nonetheless, more than 30,000 Americans commit suicide every year and nearly half a million others make a suicide attempt that is serious enough to warrant medical treatment in a hospital emergency room.[1]

Suicide is the anchor point on a continuum of suicidal thoughts and behaviors. This continuum is one that ranges from risk-taking behaviors at one end, extends through different degrees and types of suicidal thinking, and ends with suicide attempts and suicide. For some people, suicide is a sudden act; for others, it is a long-considered decision based on cumulative despair or dire circumstances. For many, it is both—a brash moment of action taken during a span of settled and suicidal hopelessness. The suffering of the suicidal person is private and inexpressible, which leaves family members, friends, and colleagues to deal with an almost unfathomable kind of loss as well as guilt. The aftermath of a suicidal act is at a level of confusion and devastation that is, for the most part, beyond description.

Suicide, which is both a stereotypic yet highly individualized act, is a common endpoint for many patients with severe psychiatric illness. While no single illness or set of circumstances can predict suicide, certain vulnerabilities, illnesses, and events make some individuals far more likely than others to kill themselves. The most common element in suicide and serious suicide attempts is psychopathology. Of the numerous mental illnesses, a relative few are particularly and powerfully bound to self-inflicted death: these are the mood disorders (depression and bipolar manic-depression), schizophrenia, borderline and antisocial personality disorders, alcoholism, and drug abuse. Mood disorders, especially when comorbid with alcohol and drug abuse, are by far the most common psychiatric conditions associated with suicide.

SUICIDE AND MOOD DISORDERS

Understanding the origins of suicide is the first step in preventing it. Mann and colleagues[2] at the New York State Psychiatric Institute have proposed a stress-diathesis model to explain the relationship between the underlying biological predisposition to suicide and the precipitants that trigger it. Several factors influence the predisposition to commit suicide, and together they act to establish a threshold for suicidal behavior. These factors include genetic vulnerabilities such as family history and compromised serotonergic functioning in the brain; temperamen-

From the Department of Psychiatry and Behavioral Sciences, Johns Hopkins University School of Medicine, Baltimore, Md.

Excerpted in part from Night Falls Fast: Understanding Suicide. *Jamison KR. New York, NY: Knopf; 1999.*

Supported by an unrestricted educational grant from Solvay Pharmaceuticals, Inc.

Reprint requests to: Kay Redfield Jamison, Ph.D., Department of Psychiatry, The Johns Hopkins School of Medicine. Meyer 3–181, 600 North Wolfe St., Baltimore, MD 21287.

tal variables such as aggressiveness and impulsivity; chronic alcohol and drug abuse; chronic medical conditions; and certain social factors such as the early death of a parent, social isolation, or a childhood history of physical or sexual abuse. One factor, brain serotonergic functioning, is particularly important in setting an individual's threshold for acting on suicidal impulses.[3] Researchers have shown that serotonin function is lower in suicide attempters than in controls by measuring serotonin metabolites in cerebrospinal fluid and prolactin response to fenfluramine.[4] Postmortem studies of suicide victims also reveal decreased serotonin activity in the ventrolateral prefrontal cortex.[5]

Alcohol and drugs can precipitate acute episodes of psychosis, worsen the overall course of the underlying illness, and undermine the individual's willingness to seek clinical treatment. In a review of 504 patients with mood disorders who were hospitalized in 4 psychiatric units in Sardinia, there was a significant association of substance use disorders with suicide attempts.[6] Substance use disorders were diagnosed in 28% of the subjects: substance abuse was found in 26% and dependence in 2%. The most frequent substance abused was alcohol (15%) followed by cannabis (4%) and heroin (3%). Substance abuse was most commonly found in patients with bipolar I disorder, whereas the presence and annual rate of suicide attempts were much higher in patients with bipolar II and major depressive disorders. The mood state associated with suicide attempts was more commonly dysphoric-mixed or depressive than manic.

Substance use disorders typically start in adolescence and thus may play a particularly ominous role in the 3-fold increase in adolescent suicides in the last 30 years. In this age group, substance abuse may be associated with high rates of depression and bipolar disorder as well as the common tendency toward youthful risk-taking. A study of suicides in adolescents under the age of 20 years revealed that 90% of the suicide victims had a diagnosable psychiatric disorder at the time of their death, and more than half of these individuals had experienced significant symptoms for longer than 2 years.[7] In a Swedish retrospective investigation of 58 consecutive suicides by adolescents and young adults (15–29 years of age), a psychoactive substance use disorder—primarily alcohol dependence—was present in 47% of the youth suicides.[8]

SUICIDE AND BIPOLAR DISORDER

Patients with bipolar disorder have a higher risk of committing suicide than patients with other psychiatric or medical disorders, but determining the exact risk of suicide is difficult for several reasons.[9] First, suicide attempts and completed suicides are easier to identify than suicidal thoughts, which may range from fleeting to intrusive and persistent. The relationship of suicidal ideation to completed suicide has not been well documented in patients with bipolar disorder. Second, interpreting suicide rates is complicated. Most cohort studies are of an untreated or partially compliant population, and ethical considerations preclude a clinical study of suicidality in medicated versus nonmedicated patients. Third, few, if any, studies of suicide separate patients by severity of illness. Most studies are done with hospitalized patients, which slants the data toward severely ill patients. Fourth, changes in suicide rates are difficult to decipher since diagnostic criteria vary across time and treatments change. Finally, methodological problems confound interpretation; for example, the distinctions between bipolar and unipolar disorder became standard in the literature in the past decade only. Therefore, the enormous variability across follow-up studies has resulted in uncertainty concerning suicide risk.

For many years, the lifetime suicide risk in bipolar disorder was accepted as 15%. However, because of sampling bias (e.g., severely depressed inpatients), the actual lifetime suicide risk may be somewhat lower. Inskip et al.[10] used mathematical modeling techniques to reassess the lifetime risk of suicide in individuals with mood disorders and concluded that the overall suicide risk in mood disorders is lower (6%) than generally accepted but is particularly high around the time of diagnosis. A meta-analysis of the suicide risk among patients with bipolar disorder was performed by Harris and Barraclough[11] and was based on a combined population of 3700 bipolar patients from 14 studies in 7 countries. The population was treated between 1900 and 1985, and some patients had been followed for 60 to 70 years. Expected values were either given in the articles studied or were estimated using World Health Organization statistical reports. Combining the studies gave a total suicide risk 15 times the expected value; the wide range (0–133 times) indicated the variability across studies. The meta-analysis also showed that increased suicide risks were associated with past suicide attempts, alcohol abuse, and the amount of time elapsed after discharge from hospital—from recent discharge to 5 years prior to suicide.

The Epidemiologic Catchment Area study[12] revealed a much higher rate of suicide attempts in individuals with bipolar disorder or major depression than in those without a lifetime history of psychiatric illness. Despite often using nonviolent methods, such as drug overdoses, patients with bipolar disorder who attempted suicide showed detailed planning and a resolute intent to die. At least 25% to 50% of patients with bipolar disorder attempt suicide at one or more times in their lifetime, but the epidemiology of a suicide attempt, or parasuicide, is quite distinct from that of suicide.[1] Suicide attempters are more likely to be women than men; they generally use less lethal means, often act in the presence of others, and typically notify others of their intent. Women attempt suicide 2 to 3 times more often than men. However, women may be more willing than men to admit previous suicide attempts, and men may be more prone to disguise suicide attempts by choosing risk-taking behavior or car accidents, which are seldom explored in surveys of suicide attempts.

Suicide as a consequence of depressive episodes is one of the primary causes of increased mortality in patients with mood disorders.[13] Rapid changes in mood states at the beginning and toward the end of a depressive episode constitute an increased risk for suicide, especially in the 6 to 12 months after discharge from hospital. Although suicide appears to be slightly more common in patients with major depression than in those with bipolar disorder, many individuals who are diagnosed with depression may also have mild forms of mania.[1] These so-called hypomanias generally go unreported by the patients and may fail to be detected by clinicians or ascertained through psychological autopsies. Individuals who experience mild periods of mania—usually characterized by high energy, little sleep, and marked irritability—often have coexisting alcohol or drug problems, have chaotic lifestyles, and are frequently noncompliant with medication. When irritability and substance abuse are part of the prolonged depressive phase of bipolar illness, the volatile elements may prove to be a particularly deadly combination.

Anyone who suggests that coming back from suicidal despair is a straightforward journey has never taken it. The violent agitation of some suicidal patients is impossible to comprehend unless it is intimately observed or personally experienced. These high-voltage, perturbed, yet morbid conditions are particularly common in bipolar illness during mixed states. Broadly conceptualized as the simultaneous occurrence of both depressive and manic symptoms, mixed states may exist as independent clinical forms (as mania or depression), or they may occur as transitional conditions, bridging and blending one phase of the illness with another. They are particularly common when depression escalates into mania, mania ratchets down into depression, or depression clears into normal functioning. Of 31 bipolar individuals in a Finnish postmortem suicide study,[14] the final manifestation of illness occurred during major depressive episodes in 79%, mixed states in 11%, and during or immediately after remission of psychotic mania in another 11%.

LITHIUM AND OTHER MEDICATIONS AS PROPHYLAXIS AGAINST SUICIDE

Major mood disorders, including bipolar disorder, are highly treatable across the spectrum of different ages, but only a minority of affected persons are diagnosed and adequately treated for these disorders.[15] Psychiatric treatment rates are also low for persons with mood disorders who commit suicide, which suggests low levels of detection and lack of appropriate medical interventions among those at risk for suicide. Moreover, with the exception of lithium, remarkably little is known about specific contributions of mood-altering treatments to minimizing mortality rates in persons with major mood disorders in general, and bipolar depression in particular.

The most demonstrably effective and extensively studied treatment against suicide is lithium. It has been used since 1949 to stabilize the dangerous mood swings and erratic behavior associated with bipolar manic-depressive illness and—by Europeans particularly—to prevent recurrent depression. Convincing evidence exists that appropriate long-term lithium prophylaxis reduces the suicide risk and can possibly normalize the excess mortality of patients with unipolar, bipolar, and schizoaffective mood disorders.[15] The antisuicidal effect of lithium may be related to the serotonergic and antiaggressive properties of lithium and may be independent of its episode-preventing efficacy. Notwithstanding its benefits, lithium is an effective antisuicidal medication only if patients are willing to take the drug and if they respond to it. Some patients cannot tolerate the side effects, and many others are noncompliant.

The selective serotonin reuptake inhibitors (SSRIs) are antidepressants that not only alleviate and prevent depression but also appear to decrease angry, aggressive, and impulsive behavior, and their effects on such dangerous suicide risk factors are important.[1] The SSRIs may also be easy to administer by general practitioners, internists, and psychiatrists. However, the ease of SSRI administration can also increase the likelihood that they may be given to patients who would show more benefit from a mood-stabilizing drug. Some bipolar patients may actually get worse when taking antidepressant monotherapy; that is, their episodes may increase in frequency and intensity, and they may experience severely agitated or mixed states.

The ability of anticonvulsant medications to prevent suicide is unproved, although some anticonvulsants stabilize moods and have a beneficial impact on agitated and aggressive states. Open studies indicate that the types of mood disorders that correlate with a better response to anticonvulsants than to lithium are bipolar rapid cycling, mixed episodes, a previous poor response to lithium, secondary mania, and concurrent substance abuse.[16] Antipsychotics, particularly the newer agents, share some of the same problems and promise in preventing suicide as the antidepressants.[1] Akathisia can result, but the atypical antipsychotics given in moderate doses may reduce the suicide rates in psychotically ill patients. Clearly, some of the newer agents provide a real and important alternative to lithium. Ultimately, the best course of treatment for many bipolar patients may be a combination of lithium with another mood stabilizer or with an antipsychotic, antidepressant, or antianxiety agent.

Medications are often remarkably effective in preventing or diminishing the pain and suffering of the major psychiatric illnesses most closely linked to suicide. However,

Table 1. Evaluation of Major Suicide Risk Factors[a]

Acknowledged plans for suicide
Presence or absence of severe anxiety, agitation, or perturbation
Pervasiveness, type, and severity of psychopathology
Extent of hopelessness
Presence of severe sleep disturbances or mixed states
Current alcohol or drug abuse
Ease of access to a lethal means, especially firearms
Lack of access to medical and psychological treatment
Recent severe stress events, eg, divorce, job loss, or death in family
Family history of suicidal or violent behavior
Social isolation or lack of friends and family
Close proximity to a first episode of depression, mania, or schizophrenia
Recent release from a psychiatric hospital
History of previous suicide attempts

[a]Adapted from reference 1.

Table 2. Medical Interventions to Prevent Suicide[a]

Improve public and professional awareness of risk factors for suicide
Limit access to firearms and alcohol
Enhance access to appropriate clinical assessment and safe, effective treatments for mood and psychotic disorders
Support additional research to clarify specific benefits and risks of medical and social interventions aimed at preventing suicide

[a]From refererence 17, with permission.

whether they actually lessen the chances of suicidal individuals killing themselves is less clear. The very success of psychopharmacology in treating serious mental illness has had the unfortunate effect of minimizing the importance of psychotherapy in healing patients and keeping them alive. Psychotherapy can be extremely helpful, not only in sustaining patients through times of terrible psychological suffering and encouraging them to learn better ways of handling suicidal impulses, but also in helping patients to deal with the critical and gnarly problem of medication noncompliance.

CLINICAL CONSIDERATIONS

In a clinical setting, an assessment of suicidal risk must precede any attempt to treat psychiatric illness, and asking a patient directly about suicidal thoughts or plans is an essential part of history taking. Many patients, especially women, are reluctant to acknowledge violent and impulsive behavior, either in themselves or in relationships with others. However, it is vitally important to obtain an accurate and comprehensive history of violence and impulsivity, because these two risk factors in conjunction with psychiatric illness can create a flash point for suicide.

In addition to an individual's suicidal thoughts or plans, other risk factors that should be evaluated include the presence or absence of severe anxiety, agitation, or perturbation; pervasiveness, type, and severity of psychopathology; extent of hopelessness; presence of a severe sleep disturbance or of mixed states; current alcohol or drug abuse; ease of access to a lethal means of suicide, especially firearms; lack of access to good medical and psychological treatment; recent severe stress events, such as a divorce, job loss, or death in the family; family history of suicidal or violent behavior; social isolation or a lack of friends and family; close proximity to a first episode of depression, mania, or schizophrenia; recent release from a psychiatric facility; and a history of previous suicide attempts (Table 1).[1]

Attitudes about suicide are changing.[1] Suicide is increasingly perceived as a manifestation of severe psychiatric distress that is often associated with a diagnosable and treatable form of depression or other mental illness. In 1997, Senator Harry Reid of Nevada—whose father committed suicide and whose home state has consistently had the highest suicide rate in the nation—introduced a resolution in the U.S. Senate that proposed a coherent and comprehensive national strategy to prevent suicide. The resolution acted as a catalyst for government health agencies, suicide prevention groups, mental health advocacy groups, and active grassroots organizations to begin to network with each other and to respond to and promote safe and effective treatment for people at risk for suicide. Leading the effort is David Satcher, M.D., Ph.D., Surgeon General of the United States and former director of the Centers for Disease Control and Prevention. His 1999 *Surgeon General's Report on Suicide* is the first official report published on the subject of suicide in the 200 years of his office.

At a recent symposium on suicide, the participants formulated a consensus statement on suggested medical interventions in preventing suicide (Table 2).[17] Proposed interventions included (1) improving public and professional awareness of risk factors for suicide, (2) limiting access to firearms and alcohol, (3) enhancing access to appropriate clinical assessment and promoting increasingly safe and effective treatments for mood and psychotic disorders, and (4) supporting additional research to clarify the specific benefits and risks of medical and social interventions aimed at preventing suicide.

Disclosure of off-label usage: The author has determined that, to the best of her knowledge, no investigational information about pharmaceutical agents has been presented in this article that is outside U.S. Food and Drug Administration–approved labeling.

REFERENCES

1. Jamison KR. Night Falls Fast: Understanding Suicide. New York, NY: Knopf; 1999
2. Mann JJ, Waternaux C, Haas GL, et al. Toward a clinical model of suicidal behavior in psychiatric patients. Am J Psychiatry 1999;156:181–189
3. Mann JJ, Oquendo M, Underwood MD, et al. The neurobiology of suicide risk: a review for the clinician. J Clin Psychiatry 1999;60(suppl 2):7–11
4. Asberg M, Nordstrom P, Traskman-Bendz L. Cerebrospinal fluid in suicide: an overview. Ann N Y Acad Sci 1986;487:243–255
5. Arango V, Underwood MD, Gubbi AV, et al. Localized alterations in pre- and postsynaptic serotonin binding sites in the ventrolateral prefrontal cortex of suicide victims. Brain Res 1995;688:121–133

6. Tondo L, Baldessarini RJ, Hennen J, et al. Suicide attempts in major affective disorder patients with comorbid substance use disorders. J Clin Psychiatry 1999;60(suppl 2):63–69
7. Shaffer D, Craft L. Methods of adolescent suicide prevention. J Clin Psychiatry 1999;60(suppl 2):70–74
8. Runeson B. Psychoactive substance use disorder in youth suicide. Alcohol 1990:25:561–568
9. Simpson SG, Jamison KR. The risk of suicide in patients with bipolar disorder. J Clin Psychiatry 1999;60(suppl 2):53–56
10. Inskip HM, Harris EC, Barraclough B. Lifetime risk of suicide for affective disorder, alcoholism, and schizophrenia. Br J Psychiatry 1998;172:35–37
11. Harris EC, Barraclough B. Suicide as an outcome for mental disorders: a meta-analysis. Br J Psychiatry 1997;170:205–208
12. Eaton WW, Kessler RG, eds. Epidemiologic Field Methods in Psychiatry: The NIMH Epidemiologic Catchment Area Program. Orlando, Fla: Academic Press; 1985
13. Angst J, Angst F, Stassen HH. Suicide risk in patients with major depressive disorder. J Clin Psychiatry 1999;60(suppl 2):57–62
14. Isometsä ET, Henriksson MM, Aro HM, et al. Suicide in bipolar disorder in Finland. Am J Psychiatry 1994;151:1020–1024
15. Baldessarini RJ, Tondo L, Hennen J. Effects of lithium treatment and its discontinuation on suicidal behavior in bipolar manic-depressive disorders. J Clin Psychiatry 1999;60(suppl 2):77–84
16. Thies-Flechtner K, Müller-Oerlinghausen B, Seibert W, et al. Effect of prophylactic treatment on suicide risk in patients with major affective disorders: data from a randomized prospective trial. Pharmacopsychiatry 1996;29:103–107
17. Baldessarini RJ, Jamison KR. Effects of medical interventions on suicidal behavior [Summary and Conclusions]. J Clin Psychiatry 1999;60(suppl 2):117–122

This is the 10th in a series of 10-year updates in child and adolescent psychiatry. Topics are selected in consultation with the AACAP Committee on Recertification, both for the importance of new research and its clinical or developmental significance. The authors have been asked to place an asterisk before the five or six most seminal references.

J. McD.

Child and Adolescent Bipolar Disorder: A Review of the Past 10 Years

BARBARA GELLER, M.D., AND JOAN LUBY, M.D.

ABSTRACT

Objective: To provide a review of the epidemiology, phenomenology, natural course, comorbidity, neurobiology, and treatment of child and adolescent bipolar disorder (BP) for the past 10 years. This review is provided to prepare applicants for recertification by the American Board of Psychiatry and Neurology. **Method:** Literature from *Medline* and other searches for the past 10 years, earlier relevant articles, and the authors' experience and ongoing National Institute of Mental Health–funded project "Phenomenology and Course of Pediatric Bipolarity" were used. **Results:** Age-specific, developmental (child, adolescent, and adult) *DSM-IV* criteria manifestations; comorbidity and differential diagnoses; and episode and course features are provided. Included are age-specific examples of childhood grandiosity, hypersexuality, and delusions. Differential diagnoses (e.g., specific language disorders, sexual abuse, conduct disorder [CD], schizophrenia, substance abuse), suicidality, and BP-II are discussed. **Conclusion:** Available data strongly suggest that prepubertal-onset BP is a nonepisodic, chronic, rapid-cycling, mixed manic state that may be comorbid with attention-deficit hyperactivity disorder (ADHD) and CD or have features of ADHD and/or CD as initial manifestations. Systematic research on pediatric BP is in its infancy and will require ongoing and future studies to provide developmentally relevant diagnostic methods and treatment. *J. Am. Acad. Child Adolesc. Psychiatry,* 1997, 36(9):1168–1176. **Key Words:** child, adolescent, bipolar disorder, mania, hypomania, delusions, grandiosity, hypersexuality.

As noted in a recent letter by Schneider et al. (1996), if one looks to fit children and adolescents into adult criteria for manic-depressive illness, it will be difficult except for those adolescents who have adult-type onset, i.e., individuals with good functioning until the abrupt onset of marked manic symptomatology that often requires hospitalization, is responsive to treatment, and is succeeded by interepisode well being (McGlashan, 1988). Thus, a developmental, age specific viewpoint needs to be considered for pediatric patients who do not have the adult-type onset.

Analogies to two other occurrences in bioscience are useful to understand the developmental perspective. The first occurrence is that different illnesses may have different neurobiological (e.g., genetic, neurotransmitter) mechanisms and thus have differences in severity with earlier age of onset (Childs and Scriver, 1986). A classic example is the comparison of juvenile to adult onset diabetes in which genetic mechanisms and severity differ. The second situation occurs when the same causative agent can have different clinical manifestations at different times in the life cycle. An example of the second situation is when 6-OH dopamine is given to infant versus adult rats. Infant rats given this compound develop hyperactivity, whereas geriatric rats develop parkinsonian symptomatology.

On the basis of the occurrence of either (or both) of the neurobiological mechanisms noted above, it is developmentally possible for childhood onset manic-

Accepted January 31, 1997.

Dr. Geller is Professor of Psychiatry and Dr. Luby is Assistant Professor of Psychiatry, Department of Psychiatry, Washington University School of Medicine, St. Louis.

This work was supported by NIMH grant R01 MH53063, "Phenomenology and Course of Pediatric Bipolarity," to Dr. Geller.

Reprint requests to Dr. Geller, Washington University School of Medicine, 4940 Children's Place, St. Louis, MO 63110.

0890-8567/97/3609-1168$0.300/0

depressive illness to be more severe; to have a chronic, nonepisodic course; and to have mixed, rapid-cycling features similar to the clinical picture reported for severely ill, treatment resistant adults (Geller et al., 1995; Himmelhoch and Garfinkel, 1986; Hsu, 1986; Hsu and Starzynski, 1986; Stancer and Persad, 1982). A possibility also exists that only the most severe manic-depressive children receive clinical attention because manic episodes that last a few weeks might be tolerated by parents as a phase of growing up, especially if these do not interfere with school performance. Our experience of colleagues requesting "hallway" consultations suggests that this may be the case.

The following review assumes that future data will support continuities across the age span.

Epidemiology

As yet, no national or international epidemiological study of bipolar disorder (BP) during the pediatric years is available. However, data from Carlson and Kashani (1988) and Lewinsohn et al. (1995) suggest that prevalence during the adolescent years is at least that of the adult population.

These reports and those below taken together—i.e., epidemiological data, secular trends, high switch rates, data from inpatient services, and reports from chart reviews—support that the prevalence of child and adolescent manic-depressive illness is at least that in the adult population and may be increasing. A secular trend, i.e., earlier age of onset of BP with successively later years of birth, has also been reported (Rice et al., 1987).

Underdiagnosis of childhood bipolarity has been noted by several authors who have described a high prevalence on inpatient services (Gammon et al., 1983; Isaac, 1995) and a high prevalence of both diagnosed and undiagnosed cases on chart reviews (Weller et al., 1986; Wozniak et al., 1995). Another source of underdiagnosis during childhood and adolescence is that many parents who are bipolar, and thus at higher risk of having bipolar offspring, remain underdiagnosed themselves (Geller, 1996). These parents may not recognize the pathological implications of their children's manic behaviors.

Literature on adult samples has noted that 20% to 40% of adults report that their onset was during childhood (Joyce, 1984; Lish et al., 1994). Adults with childhood onset by history often also report that the initial episode was depressive (Lish et al., 1994). The latter is consistent with the high rate of switching of prepubertal depression to prepubertal mania (32%) reported by Geller et al. (1994b) and of depressed adolescents switching to adolescent-onset mania (20%) (Strober and Carlson, 1982). These rates of switching may be conservative because of the probable underdiagnosis of childhood mania discussed above.

Clinical Characteristics

At all ages, manic subjects in the cross-section appear to be the happiest of people because of their infectious, amusing, elated affect. This is also true of children, and it can be very misleading to see a happy child laughing in the office in the context of a miserable history (e.g., school suspensions, family fights). This contrasts with sad, depressed children who everyone thinks are ill because it is more difficult to acknowledge conceptually that happy children have serious psychopathology. Thus, it is important to evaluate children's affect in relationship to historical features in exactly the way one evaluates the incongruity between the infectious elation of manic adult patients in the context of histories that include loss of family, unemployment, and jail sentences.

Across the life span, grandiose delusions must be judged by failure to follow the laws of logic and by a firm belief (often to an extent that action is taken). A common presentation for bipolar children is to harass teachers about how to teach the class; this harassment is often so intense that teachers telephone parents, begging them to ask their children to desist. These children may fail subjects intentionally because they believe the courses are taught incorrectly. Therefore, their thinking bypasses laws of logic (i.e., that children can choose what to fail or pass), and the beliefs are acted upon by purposely failing courses. Another common grandiose manifestation in children as young as seven is to steal expensive items and be impervious to police officers who attempt to make them understand that what they have done is wrong and illegal. Similar to grandiose adults, grandiose children believe that stealing may be illegal for other people but not for them. Unlike patients with pure conduct disorder, manic children and adolescents, similar to bipolar adults, frequently know that stealing is a bad thing to do, but they believe that they are "above" the law. Common adolescent grandiose delusions are that they will achieve a prominent profession (e.g., lawyer) even though they are failing at school, i.e., the belief that they can have a high attainment when they have failing school grades bypasses the laws of logic. Asked how he or she will become a lawyer, an adolescent will answer, "I just know I will." Similarly, a manic adolescent, even in the absence of musical talent or ability to carry a tune, might practice all day with the belief that he or she can become a rock star.

Dissimilar to depressed patients who have trouble falling asleep and lie in bed brooding, manic children have high activity levels in the bedroom prior to sleep, e.g., rearranging furniture for several hours. Manic adolescents will wait until parents are asleep and then go out "partying," whereas manic adults will party and work around the clock.

Pressured speech is relatively similar at all ages in that the individual can be difficult or impossible to interrupt. Racing thoughts are frequently described by children and adolescents in very concrete terms. For example, children state that they are not able to get anything done because their thoughts keep interrupting. An adolescent wished she had a button on her forehead to turn off her thoughts. Flight of ideas in children is similar to that in adults except for age-specific content, e.g., "Do you live in Nashville? Some people have hogs for Thanksgiving. Do you have a key to that door?"

Also at all ages, minor perturbations in the environment can produce marked amounts of distractibility. Increased motor activity and goal-directed behaviors in children and adolescents frequently look like normal activities done in a profuse amount. The manic child may in a brief period of time make curtains, begin an illustrated book, rearrange furniture, and make multiple phone calls, compared with the manic adult, who may start many businesses and join many social groups.

Involvement in pleasurable activities with a high level of danger is manifested in age-specific behaviors. Hypersexuality in children frequently begins when a child brought up in a conservative home without any history of sexual abuse or excessive exposure to sexual situations begins to use profanity and may tell a teacher to "f— herself" and "gives her the finger." Children may masturbate frequently, initially openly, and then when told not to do it publicly will simply make frequent trips to the bathroom to continue the stimulation. Children will begin to proposition teachers and make overt sexual comments to classmates. Adolescents develop romantic fantasies and delusions about teachers (see vignette in Geller et al., 1995). Older children and adolescents will call the 1-900 sex telephone lines, which the family discovers when the telephone bill arrives. Older adolescents and adults will have multiple partners with unprotected sexual behaviors and frequently will feel an urgency to have sex, e.g., an adolescent wrote to her boyfriend, starting the letter with the sentence, "When are we going to f—?" Adults will have multiple partners; males may be womanizers; and often there are multiple marriages.

Interest in money appears in young children when they start their own businesses in school and when they begin to order multiple items, trips, and plane tickets from advertised 1-800 and 1-900 telephone numbers. Again, the family frequently does not discover this until items arrive at the house and telephone bills arrive. Adults may overdraw on bank accounts and "top out" on multiple credit cards.

Across the age span, taking more dares is common. In older adolescents and adults, this frequently appears as wild driving, eventuating in many speed and "driving under the influence" tickets. In children it manifests as grandiose delusions that they can fly out the window because they believe that they have that ability or in exaggerations of usual childhood hopping around on trees or between rooftops, based on beliefs that they are above the possibility of danger.

To further exemplify pediatric features, characteristic vignettes of children and adolescents with BP can be reviewed in Geller et al. (1995). Characterization of preschool age BP is an important avenue for future investigation.

Differential Diagnosis and Comorbidity

Table 1 provides a list of differential diagnoses and/or comorbid conditions by age group.

Sexual abuse is especially important as a differential diagnosis during the childhood years because manic hypersexuality is often manifested in children by self-stimulatory behaviors including frequent masturbation. Thus, it is useful to obtain a careful history of whether the child could have been abused or exposed to adult sexual behaviors.

Specific language disorders need to be differentiated from flight of ideas because children and adolescents with language disabilities can sound as though they have a thought disorder when they partake in conversation without actual comprehension of the content and/or the ability to find the appropriate words to use.

At present, data suggest that for some prepubertal onset bipolar children, hyperactivity manifestations begin at preschool age and are followed by a full manic syndrome during the early grade school years (Geller, 1997b). In these children, it is possible that hyperactivity is the first developmentally age-specific manifestation of prepubertal onset BP. This hypothesis is consistent with the higher prevalence of attention deficit hyperactivity disorder (ADHD) in prepubertal versus adolescent onset BP. For other bipolar children, ADHD and BP may be comorbid, i.e., hyperactivity is a separate disorder that coexists. Numerous authors (Biederman et al., 1995; Borchardt and Bernstein, 1995; Fristad et al., 1992; Geller et al., 1995; Strober et al., 1988; West et al., 1995) have noted the high prevalence of symptoms of hyperactivity among children and adolescents with bipolarity. When subjects are seen initially because of bipolar symptomatology, approximately 90% of prepubertal and 30% of adolescent bipolar subjects have ADHD (Geller et al., 1995). Manifestations of ADHD overlap with those of multiple other *DSM-IV* diagnoses (e.g., BP, major depressive disorder [MDD]). Thus, validation of the distinctness of coexistent ADHD versus similar symptom clusters but dissimilar pathogenesis must await future naturalistic course, family genetic, and other neurobiological studies (Biederman et al., 1991; Geller, 1997b).

Even with the relatively conservative *DSM-IV* criteria, conduct disorder occurs in approximately 22% of bipolar children and 18% of bipolar adolescents (Geller et al., 1995). Conduct disorder, similar to ADHD, may be an initial manifestation of prepubertal-onset BP (Geller, 1997b; Kovacs and Pollock, 1995). These comorbid conduct disorders appear related to poor judgment and grandiosity. As an example, a 7-year-old child stole a go-cart, an item that costs several hundred dollars, and was completely unphased when the police appeared and tried to admonish him, thus demonstrating the grandiosity of stealing such a large object and of being impervious to legal intervention. Conduct disorders during adolescence (which may include driving under the influence, running away for sexual adventures, and stealing large amounts of jewelry) frequently lead to placement of these youngsters in juvenile facilities. Adult antisocial equivalents are well known (e.g., buying new television sets for every room in the hospital; obtaining real estate that the individual cannot afford).

During the teenage years, because of greater perceptual distortions seen in bipolar illness during adolescence, schizophrenia is a major differential (Horowitz, 1975). Differentiation is greatly aided by a family history of mania, which is more probable for BP than schizophrenic adolescents (Strober et al., 1988).

Substance abuse begins to be an important comorbid condition during the teenage years and is an important differential (Horowitz, 1975, 1977). For example, laughing fits may be due to smoking marijuana as a differential from the laughing fits that occur during the pediatric years as a manifestation of elation. Furthermore, very rapid cycling (Table 2) that is a hallmark of child and adolescent bipolarity (Geller et al., 1995) can easily be mimicked by amphetamine highs followed by withdrawal "crashes." Hallucinogens can mimic bipolar perceptual distortions (Horowitz, 1975, 1977).

Similar to the multiple comorbid anxiety conditions seen with MDD, bipolar patients also manifest multiple comorbid anxiety conditions (approximately 33% of bipolar prepubertal patients and 12% of bipolar adolescent patients) (Geller et al., 1995).

Naturalistic Course

Table 2 provides a comparison between pubertal-onset versus adult-onset episode and course features.

TABLE 1
Differential Diagnoses and/or Comorbid Conditions

	Child	Adolescent	Adult
Specific language disorders	X		
Attention-deficit hyperactivity disorder	X	X	
Oppositional defiant disorder	X	X	
Conduct disorder	X	X	
Sexual abuse	X	X	
Schizophrenia		X	X
Substance abuse		X	X
Antisocial personality			X

TABLE 2
Hypothesized Clinical Course by Age of Onset

	Prepubertal and Young Adolescent	Older Adolescent and Adult
Initial episode	Major depressive disorder	Mania
Episode type	Rapid-cycling, mixed	Discrete with sudden onsets and clear offsets
Duration	Chronic, continuous cycling	Weeks
Interepisode functioning	Nonepisodic	Improved functioning

As noted in the beginning of this article, prepubertal-onset manic-depressive disorder may not present with the sudden or acute onset and improved interepisode functioning characteristic of the disorder in older adolescents and adults. Rather, it may present with a picture of continuous, mixed manic, rapid cycling of multiple brief episodes described in detail by Geller et al. (1995). Thus, children may be having a laughing fit and happily doing an arts and crafts project when, without any environmental prompt, they will suddenly become miserable and acutely suicidal, talking about wanting to shoot themselves. Parents frequently describe their frustration at not being able to convince practitioners that their children rapidly cycle, sometimes numerous times in each day. Because this history has been given independently by parents (including those from many parts of the United States who have received Dr. Geller's name from the National Institutes of Health) who have no idea that this cycling pattern has been described by other parents, there is no reason to disbelieve these parental observations. Adults with mixed manic, rapid-cycling BP have a poorer prognosis than those with discrete episodes (Keller et al., 1993). Therefore, future studies of the adult course of BP children will be crucial for developing long-term, prophylactic treatments for implementation during the prepubertal years. Naturalistic follow-up of bipolar adolescent inpatients has evidenced a poor prognosis (Strober et al., 1995).

One of the issues that arises for child and adolescent manic-depressive individuals is whether or not BP-II disorder has the same implications as it does in the adult population (Coryell et al., 1995; Geller et al., 1994b). The switch rate from BP-II to BP-I in adults has been estimated by Coryell et al. (1989, 1995) to be similar to the low rate reported by Geller et al. (1994b) for switching from BP-II to BP-I among prepubertal subjects who switched during the prepubertal period. However, it remains possible that BP-II in children and adolescents may be an age-specific, developmental precursor to BP-I (Geller et al., 1994b). If the latter were established, then treatment for BP children might differ from that for BP adults, in whom BP-II is often treated with the same regimen as is used to treat MDD (Frank and Kupfer, 1985). Treatment for MDD in potentially BP pediatric patients may be contraindicated because there is evidence, albeit controversial, that antidepressant therapy may precipitate or worsen rapid cycling (Akiskal et al., 1985, 1995; Geller et al., 1993; Wehr and Goodwin, 1979; Wehr et al., 1988).

Further research will also be needed to provide better differentiation of whether the Akiskal et al. (1995) concept of temperamental issues (i.e., that there is essentially a constant temperamental modulation in some patients) is only semantically different from the mixed manic picture of BP-I and BP-II children, adolescents, and adults (Geller et al., 1995; Keller et al., 1993).

The role of comorbid personality disorders as prognostic and course features of adolescent BP remains a poorly studied but important area based on reported interepisode personality trait impairments in BP adults (Solomon et al., 1996). Johnson et al. (1995) have noted cluster II personality disorders were more prominent among BP adolescents. Other work in the area of personality disorders among pediatric BP individuals is not yet available, in part because of the need for further work on instrumentation (Brent et al., 1990).

Data support a higher risk of suicidality among BP adolescents compared with adolescents with other diagnoses (Brent et al., 1988, 1993). In addition, comorbidity of mood and substance use disorders has been correlated with higher suicide risk in older adolescents and young adults (Rich et al., 1986, 1990). The well-known high rate of comorbidity of substance dependency and BP in adults is especially notable because data suggest that "secondary" substance use is more amenable to treatment and has a better prognosis (Geller, 1997a; Winokur et al., 1995).

Neurobiology

In their classic 1986 paper, Childs and Scriver describe different genetic mechanisms for medical illnesses that have both an early- and late-onset form, e.g., diabetes mellitus. In 1988 and 1992, Strober et al. described this phenomenon for pediatric bipolarity, noting that prepubertal-onset bipolarity was more likely to be associated with early aggressive hyperactivity, lithium resistance, and greater familial loading. Thus, clinically it is useful to identify parents who may have undiagnosed bipolarity (Geller, 1996). This is best done by asking way-of-life questions (e.g., how relatives manage money, driving histories, relatives with more than four marriages) because patients with undiagnosed mania are unlikely to think of themselves as ill. Vignettes of relatives with undiagnosed mania appear in Geller (1996). Also, possible relationships of genomic imprinting (preferential maternal or parental transmission) and mitochondrial inheritance (maternal transmission) to pediatric age of onset of BP remain intriguing issues for future research (Grigoroiu-Serbanescu et al., 1995; McMahon et al., 1995).

Familial aggregation of alcoholism among bipolar adults has been noted to be greater than among subjects with other diagnoses (Winokur et al., 1995, 1996). A similar high prevalence of alcoholism among first-degree relatives of prepubertal and adolescent subjects with mood disorders has been reported (Geller, 1997a; Geller et al., 1990, 1992; Puig-Antich et al., 1989; Todd et al., 1996). Further research on prognostic implications of familial alcoholism among pediatric BP cases is warranted. Another promising line of investigation includes genetically based malformation syndromes that include BP behavioral manifestations (Papolos et al., 1996).

The few available neurobiological studies include a single case study of a hypomanic child who had a significantly different urinary methoxyhydroxyphenylglycol level from those of normal controls (McKnew et al., 1974), a report of enlarged ventricles and increased number of hyperintensities in a small open pilot study of bipolar children and adolescents (Botteron et al., 1995), and a report comparing sleep and neuroendocrine parameters in depressed adolescents with BP outcomes and those who remained depressed (Rao, 1994).

Available work on cognitive characteristics of child and adolescent bipolarity is sparse but includes the work of Decina et al. (1983). That report noted a significant discrepancy between Verbal and Performance IQ scores in offspring of bipolar parents but not in the normal control group. This is consistent with neurobiological data in adult samples that support right-sided brain impairments in manic individuals (Sackeim and Decina, 1983). Fristad (personal communication, November 1993) noted that bipolar subjects had higher IQs than an ADHD control group. Also, Kutcher (1993) reported a decrease in math performance based on school records among prebipolar adolescents. This finding may be consistent with the Decina et al. (1983) findings on lower Performance IQ. It is clear that further work on cognitive impairments and their prognostic and treatment implications is needed.

Psychopharmacological Treatment

Treatment of childhood bipolarity remains a remarkably understudied area in spite of voluminous literature comprising more than 400 case reports, studies with small numbers, and investigations with populations that were not diagnosed with *DSM-III* or higher criteria (Botteron and Geller, 1995; Fetner and Geller, 1992; Kafantaris, 1995; Youngerman and Canino, 1978). Thus, unless there is an expectation that childhood bipolarity completely mimics the adult treatment considerations, separate study is warranted. Compelling arguments, however, against the similarity of treatment of bipolarity across age groups can be constructed by analogy to the treatment differences between childhood and adult MDD (Geller et al., 1996). Because there is as yet only one completed double-blind, placebo-controlled study of any medication for child or adolescent mania using rigorous methodology and design (Geller, 1997a), the clinician will be tempted to extrapolate from studies of adults. However, extrapolation from treatment of MDD in adults did not prove useful, i.e., tricyclic antidepressants have never been shown to work better than placebo in any study of a child and adolescent population (Geller et al., 1996).

The pharmacokinetics of lithium in children has been studied (Vitiello et al., 1988), and, as expected, lithium has a shorter half-life in children than in adults. The latter is expected because of the more efficient renal system of children. More recently, in a completed double-blind, placebo-controlled study of lithium for adolescents who were bipolar and substance-dependent, lithium was significantly more effective than placebo by both completer and intent-to-treat analyses (Geller, 1997a). Literature on lithium suggests that it can be given to children with the same safety precautions used in adults and with similar monitoring at 6-month intervals for renal, thyroid, calcium, and phosphorus indices (Fetner and Geller, 1992; Khandelwal et al., 1984). Furthermore, a double-blind, placebo-controlled study of lithium for aggressive children has highlighted that there may be some children who will develop cognitive impairment at low plasma levels (Silva et al., 1992). This was also noted in a double-blind, placebo-controlled study of lithium for depressed children who had predictors of future bipolarity (Geller et al., 1994a).

The safest, most rapid method of prescribing lithium is to do so pharmacokinetically using a nomogram (Cooper et al., 1973; Fetner and Geller, 1992; Geller and Fetner, 1989). Alternately, if obtaining a serum lithium level 24 hours after a single dose is impractical, a 300-mg total daily dose can be administered until steady state is reached (Fetner and Geller, 1992). If the lithium level at the 300-mg daily dose is not between 0.8 and 1.2 mEq/L, then a linear proportion can be made to estimate the dose needed to reach the desired level (Geller and Fetner, 1989). Because of genetic variation in rate of elimination of lithium, slow eliminators can develop unacceptably high serum lithium levels and adverse effects if nonpharmacokinetic administration such as milligram-per-kilogram dosing is used (Hagino et al., 1995). Tactical problems and side effects with lithium are discussed in detail by Fetner and Geller (1992).

Lithium, however, is not a drug that can be given either to chaotic families or families who are unable to keep multiple appointments for monitoring of lithium levels and renal and thyroid functioning. Many young bipolar patients have at least one bipolar parent, and some (Gaensbauer et al., 1984; Grigoroiu-Serbanescu et al., 1989), but not all (Anderson and Hammen, 1993), offspring studies attest to the negative impact bipolar parenting can produce. Therefore, it is imperative to have choices of medications that can safely and effectively be given in chaotic environments. Furthermore, because of the cycling and abrupt onset of suicidality, it is also important to have medications that would be safer than lithium if taken in overdose.

There are a few open, uncontrolled studies addressing anticonvulsant treatment of BP. Papatheodorou and Kutcher (1993) reported that valproate showed promising results. Himmelhoch and Garfinkel (1986) reported on the use of carbamazepine for lithium-resistant adolescents. A report by Isojarvi et al. (1993) in the *New England Journal of Medicine* showed that polycystic ovarian disease developed in 80% of young females receiving valproic acid for epilepsy compared with 27% of epileptic females who were not receiving this preparation. In a 1996 article, Isojarvi et al. noted that valproate was associated with onset of obesity in more than half of the women and that polycystic ovarian disease developed in these individuals as well. Obviously, these would be prohibitive side effects for most female children with manic-depressive illness. Further work on whether or not this side effect appears only when the medication is given for epilepsy and independent replication of these findings are warranted. Details of valproate and carbamazepine administration are provided by Botteron and Geller (1995). Low-dose chlorpromazine may be another alternative (Botteron and Geller, 1995).

Methylphenidate has been reported, in case studies, both to worsen (Koehler-Troy et al., 1986) and to be a first line of medication (Max et al., 1995) for bipolar children and adolescents. At present, there is a need to use trial and error to judge which patients benefit and which might be made worse by stimulant medication.

Because of the chronic course of childhood manic-depressive illness and because of rapid-cycling, mixed features that are known to predict poor response in older populations (Geller et al., 1995; Himmelhoch and Garfinkel, 1986; Hsu, 1986; Keller et al., 1993), duration of antimanic treatments is complex. Furthermore, literature on adults suggests that intermittent lithium therapy is worse for outcome than continuous, noninterrupted therapy and that it can be difficult to restabilize patients on lithium after interruptions (Ahrens et al., 1995; Muller-Oerlinghausen et al., 1992, 1994; Schou, 1995; Schou et al., 1989). Of note, Strober et al. (1990, 1995) keep adolescents on antimanic treatments throughout the teenage years. Strober et al. (1990) have also reported an open, uncontrolled naturalistic follow-up study of adolescents taking lithium. These data strongly support long-term maintenance lithium because subjects who discontinued lithium had a significantly higher relapse rate.

Psychosocial Treatment

As yet, this area has not been investigated for children and adolescents with BP. It may, however, be especially important because of the known increased significance of nonshared environmental factors during the early childhood years (Pike and Plomin, 1996). Studies showing the relationship of negative expressed emotion to poorer outcome among bipolar adults argue for similar investigation of nonshared environmental factors among childhood populations (Miklowitz et al., 1988).

Among adults, impairment in psychosocial functioning between BP episodes has been reported (Coryell et al., 1993; Gitlin et al., 1995). The latter is relevant to an ongoing controlled study of adults who, after stabilization on medication, are randomly assigned to either a family-focused or a combined interpersonal and social rhythm (e.g., sleep) intervention (Miklowitz et al., 1996). It is clear that similar studies of psychosocial therapies among younger populations will be warranted when medication maintenance studies for pediatric BP become available.

National Institute of Mental Health Research Roundtable on Prepubertal Bipolar Disorder

ABSTRACT

Objective: A research roundtable meeting was convened at the National Institute of Mental Health on April 27, 2000, to discuss the existing controversial areas in the diagnosis of bipolar disorder in prepubertal children. **Method:** Invited clinicians and researchers with expertise on bipolar disorder in children were asked to share and discuss their perspectives on diagnostic issues for bipolar disorder in prepubertal children. **Results:** The group reached agreement that diagnosis of bipolar disorder in prepubertal children is possible with currently available psychiatric assessment instruments. In addition to phenotypes that fit *DSM-IV* criteria for bipolar I and bipolar II, participants agreed on the existence of other phenotypic possibilities that do not meet diagnostic criteria. Bipolar not otherwise specified (NOS) was recommended as a "working diagnosis" for the non-*DSM-IV* phenotype. **Conclusions:** Bipolar disorder exists and can be diagnosed in prepubertal children. In children who present with both the *DSM-IV* and non-*DSM-IV* phenotypes (i.e., those given a diagnosis of bipolar-NOS), assessment should include careful evaluation of all behaviors that are impairing. Moreover, these children should be monitored systematically to explore stability and change over time in diagnosis and impairment. *J. Am. Acad. Child Adolesc. Psychiatry*, 2001, 40(8):871–878. **Key Words:** bipolar disorder, prepubertal, assessment, diagnosis.

On April 27, 2000, the National Institute of Mental Health (NIMH) Developmental Psychopathology and Prevention Research Branch, in collaboration with the Child and Adolescent Treatment and Preventive Intervention Research Branch, convened a small roundtable meeting for open-ended discussion of possible approaches to outstanding issues for research on the diagnosis of prepubertal bipolar disorder. The participants are listed at the end of the text.

Discussion centered on two interrelated issues: (1) clinical assessment for treatment disposition and (2) definition of phenotype for resolving questions of nosology. Relevant to both is ascertainment (whether clinic-based, school-based, or community- or population-based) with specification of inclusion and exclusion criteria.

There was general agreement that a diagnosis of bipolar disorder, using *DSM* criteria, is possible in prepubertal children. Children seen in clinics fall into two categories: (1) those who clearly have a bipolar disorder (because they meet *DSM-IV* criteria for bipolar I or II) and (2) those who *may have* bipolar disorder but do not meet *DSM-IV* criteria. That is, some children meet full criteria for bipolar I (BP-I) or bipolar II (BP-II), as currently defined; other children do not meet full criteria but suffer from mood disturbances and symptoms of bipolar disorder and are severely impaired. The latter group currently receives a diagnosis of bipolar not otherwise specified (BP-NOS).

Discussion resulted in agreement on two basic definitions:

- Phenotypes that fit *DSM-IV* BP-I and BP-II criteria.
- Phenotypes that encompass more heterogeneity, basically BP-NOS, and include children who do not meet *DSM-IV* criteria but who are still severely impaired by symptoms of mood instability.

Relationship of Prepubertal Phenotypes to Adult Phenotypes. The modal adult-onset of bipolar disorder with discrete episodes of mania or depression lasting 2 to 9 months, with clear onset and offset (Goodwin and Jamison, 1990), was not reported as a common child-onset mania presentation by any of the participants. Investigators studying BP-I and BP-II phenotypes that fit *DSM-IV* criteria in prepubertal children noted that the most frequent course is a long-duration episode with rapid cycling (ultradian or continuous cycling as the predominant type) and mixed mania (i.e., co-occurring mania and depression) (e.g., Geller et al., 2000a, 2001a). The children who meet *DSM-IV* criteria are similar to the <20% of adults who have continuous psychopathology with few well periods (Geller et al., 2000a,b, 2001a). Investigators studying the BP-NOS

Accepted April 3, 2001.

Participants are listed at the end of the text.

Reprint requests to Dr. Editha Nottelmann, NIMH, 6001 Executive Boulevard, Room 6200-MSC 9617, Bethesda, MD 20892-9617; e-mail: enottelm@nih.gov.

phenotypes have also reported chronic, continuous pathology (Biederman et al., 2000a,b).

Assessment of Prepubertal Mania Symptoms. Eight of the nine studies of prepubertal children currently funded by the NIMH are using one of three versions of the Schedule for Affective Disorders and Schizophrenia for School-Age Children (K-SADS) (Table 1). Six of the studies use either the Washington University in St. Louis K-SADS (WASH-U-KSADS) in its entirety or the K-SADS-Present and Lifetime (PL) (Kaufman et al., 1997) with the WASH-U-KSADS mood disorders and rapid cycling sections. Characteristics of the three versions of the K-SADS are compared in Table 2. All sites use these diagnostic instruments to assess BP-I, BP-II, and BP-NOS. The WASH-U-KSADS (Geller et al., 1996, 1998b, 2001b) was modified from the K-SADS-1986 (Puig-Antich and Ryan, 1986) to include items specific to prepubertal mania and rapid cycling, attention-deficit hyperactivity disorder (ADHD) and all other *DSM-IV* diagnoses, and items for the onset and offset of each symptom and syndrome for both current and lifetime diagnoses. Thus it is useful for longitudinal-course studies that require precise onset and offset data as well as for assessment of psychopathology. The WASH-U-KSADS has good reliability and has been validated against parent and teacher reports (Geller et al., 1998a, 2001b). It should be useful also for establishing thresholds for boundaries between bipolar disorder subtypes (BP-I, BP-II, cyclothymia), which is important for defining phenotypically homogeneous samples that are useful to biological and genetic research.

Stability and Longitudinal Diagnostic Validation of a DSM-IV Phenotype. One study reported high 6-month stability and 1-year diagnostic validation of a *DSM-IV* prepubertal and early adolescent bipolar disorder phenotype (PEA-BP) defined by elation and/or grandiosity as one criterion (Geller et al., 2000a, 2001a). Follow-up of this PEA-BP sample (which frequently manifested mixed mania, rapid cycling, and long episode duration) will be important to determine whether these subjects become modal late-teenage/adult-onset types (episodic course with well periods) or continue to have chronic, mixed/cycling pathology. The naturalistic treatment data from this longitudinal study (Geller et al., 2000a, 2001a) also are informative for the ongoing development of prevention and intervention strategies.

BP-NOS Phenotype. Several investigators have reported extensively on severely impaired children with mood disturbance who do not meet full *DSM-IV* criteria for BP-I or BP-II (Biederman et al., 2000a,b; Carlson et al., 1998; Carlson and Kelly, 1998; Wozniak et al., 1995), characterized mainly as irritable and aggressive. To advance research on this non-*DSM-IV* phenotype, it was agreed in general that BP-NOS could be used as a "working diagnosis," as long as the children are well described (with particular attention to symptoms of ADHD, but also to symptoms of anxiety, oppositional defiant disorder [ODD], and prepubertal onset of substance use). It was recommended

TABLE 1
Studies of Prepubertal Mania by Investigator, Site, Study Domain, and Main Diagnostic Instrument

Study	Investigator	Institution	Study Domain	Main Diagnostic Instrument
1	Axelson, D.	WPIC, Pittsburgh	Pharmacotherapy	K-SADS-PL with WASH-U-KSADS mood and rapid cycling sections
2	Birmaher, B.	WPIC, Pittsburgh	Offspring	K-SADS-PL with WASH-U-KSADS mood and rapid cycling sections
3	Davanzo, P.	UCLA	Neuroimaging	WASH-U-SADS
4	Frazier, J.	Harvard Medical School	Neuroimaging	K-SADS-E
5	Geller, B.	Washington U. in St. Louis	Phenomenology and longitudinal course	WASH-U-KSADS
6	Geller, B.	Washington U. in St. Louis	Family psychopathology	WASH-U-KSADS
7	Kowatch, R.	U. Texas, Dallas	Pharmacotherapy	WASH-U-KSADS
	Findling, R., et al.	Case Western, U. Cincinnati		
8	Wozniak, J.	Harvard Medical School	Phenomenology	K-SADS-E
9	Sanchez, S.	U. Pennsylvania	Pre- and perinatal risk factors	ChIPS

Note: Some of these studies include adolescents. These instruments do not assess comprehensively the possible impact of factors such as pervasive developmental disorder, seizure disorders, head injury, or other medical conditions. To overcome this limitation, other assessment of such medical conditions should be considered. K-SADS-PL = Schedule for Affective Disorders and Schizophrenia for School-Age Children—Present and Lifetime version; K-SADS-E = K-SADS Epidemiologic version; WASH-U-KSADS = Washington University in St. Louis K-SADS; ChIPS = Children's Interview for Psychiatric Syndromes.

TABLE 2
Comparison of K-SADS Versions Used in NIMH-Funded Studies of Prepubertal Mania

Characteristic	K-SADS-E (Orvaschel et al., 1982)	K-SADS-PL (Kaufman et al., 1997)	WASH-U-KSADS (Geller et al., 1996, 1998b, 2001b)
Semistructured	Yes	Yes	Yes
Experienced clinicians	Yes	Yes	Yes
Mother and child separately	Yes	Yes	Yes
Lifetime and present	Yes	Yes	Yes
DSM-IV diagnoses	Yes	Yes	Yes
Dichotomous scales	Yes	No	No
Trichotomous scales	No	Yes	No
Multilevel rating scales (e.g., 1–4, 1–6)	No	No	Yes
Developed for clinical studies	No	Yes	Yes
Developed for epidemiological studies	Yes	No	No
Screening	Yes	Yes	No
Skip-outs	Yes	Yes	No
Symptom onset and offset items	No	No	Yes
Rapid cycling section	No	No	Yes
Expanded prepubertal mania section	No	No	Yes

Note: NIMH = National Institute of Mental Health; K-SADS-E = Schedule for Affective Disorders and Schizophrenia for School-Age Children-Epidemiologic Version; K-SADS-PL = K-SADS-Present and Lifetime Version; WASH-U-KSADS = Washington University in St. Louis K-SADS.

that careful assessment include all impairing behaviors, giving consideration, as relevant, to the frequency with which they occur as well as to severity (e.g., aggressiveness, agitation, explosiveness, irritability, excessive mood lability [fluctuation out of proportion to stimulus], thought disorder [paranoia, misinterpretation of social cues], communication disorder [pragmatic language disorder that can look like flight of ideas; receptive and expressive language disorder than can interfere with the accurate performance and interpretation of structured interviews], and cognitive ability/cognitive impairment [significantly low IQ, reading disabilities]). One approach suggested for building a communication platform among researchers was to operationalize in a more refined way dimensions of the various behavior problems seen in these children who may or may not meet specific criteria for disorders. This could be accomplished by collecting instruments for each dimension, preparatory to obtaining general agreement on the assessment of the various dimensions and developing a common battery for multi-informant assessments. Alternatively, it was suggested that these dimensions could be assessed with measures of individual choice and that the Child Behavior Checklist (CBCL), less likely to be affected by measurement and diagnostic differences, could then be used for calibration across sites. The CBCL should be a useful addition to the assessment battery in either case.

Role of Comorbid Disruptive Disorders. All investigators report a very high prevalence of comorbid ADHD and ODD for *DSM-IV* and non-*DSM-IV* phenotypes (e.g., Biederman, 1995; Biederman et al., 1995, 2000a,b; Fristad et al., 1992; Geller et al., 1995, 1998b, 2000a,b, 2001a). There was agreement that more work should be done to define and map comorbid conditions. It was recommended that assessment not rely strictly on *DSM* criteria to determine absence or presence of co-occurring disorders. It is important to track both number and type of specific as well as nonspecific symptoms, because nonspecific symptoms, such as hyperactivity, irritability, temper tantrums, etc., may be symptoms of co-occurring disorders, prodromal signs of an impending bipolar disorder, or part of the clinical presentation of bipolar disorders in young children.

Ancillary Instruments. Ancillary instruments used for additional quantification of comorbid conditions in the NIMH-funded studies listed in Table 1, such as ADHD, ODD, and conduct disorder, include the CBCL (Achenbach, 1991); the K-SADS Mania Rating Scale (Axelson et al., 1999), developed to monitor weekly treatments; and the Children's Global Assessment Scale (CGAS) (Shaffer et al., 1983). Several sites have reported data on CBCL profiles of children with mania (diagnoses were independent of the CBCL) (Biederman et al., 1995; Geller et al., 1998a). One site also reported Teacher's Report Form (Achenbach, 1991) profiles (Geller et al.,

1998a). Multiple sites use the CGAS for global severity assessment. Several investigators use consensus conferences to bring such additional information to bear on diagnoses (e.g., Biederman et al., 2000b; Geller et al., 2001a); other sites may be using them as well.

Etiological Relationships. With further agreement on exclusion criteria (i.e., certain comorbid disorders and/or physical disease) as well as inclusion criteria for the BP-NOS phenotype, it should be possible to address questions about etiological relationships among the disorders, e.g., whether BP-NOS or subtypes of BP-NOS are precursors of BP-I and/or BP-II or have a different course; also, whether BP-II in children may be an anlage of BP-I (Geller et al., 1998b). As noted above, adult-onset modal manic-depressive course includes an episodic course with well periods, while childhood-onset *DSM-IV* BP-I and BP-II are more likely to resemble nonepisodic adult-onset bipolar disorder (Geller et al., 2000a, 2001a). Follow-up should tell us whether these children will have an episodic adult course. Moreover, it should be possible to identify and fully characterize children with BP-NOS who are severely impaired and to monitor them prospectively, with attention to developmental stages and transitions, to resolve whether they have a childhood-onset variant of bipolar disorder.

Offspring Studies. Validation studies also should take developmental manifestations into consideration. Reconstruction of the history of adults with early-onset bipolar illness may be useful as well. For example, in studies of offspring of bipolar parents, in which all of their children should be included, parents should be asked also about their own age at onset. In an ongoing study of family psychopathology, Geller et al. (personal communication, 2000) are administering the WASH-U-KSADS mania and rapid cycling sections to parents and adult siblings to elicit information about their own childhood. In studies of both children who have bipolar illness and children who *may* have bipolar illness, the children as well as their parents should be interviewed with developmentally appropriate measures. For distinguishing between hypomania and mania, in fact, information across settings (home and school) as well as across informants (child, parent, and teacher) should be useful. A novel approach to antecedent factors by Sanchez is to examine the predictability of adult BP-I disorder in a birth cohort studied as part of the National Collaborative Perinatal Project (National Institutes of Health [NIH] Computer Retrieval of Information on Scientific Projects [CRISP] database).

Preschool Samples. It was suggested that studies could include children as young as 4 years of age. For children in the 4- to 6-year age range, additional assessments at a developmentally appropriate level should be especially important, as evaluation of these younger children needs to be heavily based on observations, ideally supplemented by (videotaped) observations in the home and other settings. Instrumentation developed by Luby et al. (unpublished data) to examine *DSM-IV* criteria of depressive disorders in preschool children could serve as a model for similar developmentally appropriate tools for investigating preschool mania. A new scale developed by Egger et al. (1999, 2000) has a preschool mania module that is currently undergoing field testing for reliability and validity.

Mood Variability. Unresolved assessment areas include mood variability. Across the postpubertal age span (i.e., later adolescence and adulthood), evidenced by the voluminous literature on the topic, "mood lability" (and its numerous synonyms) and BP-II microsubtypes have been contentious areas of assessment and categorization. Thus the difficulties involved in categorizing "mood lability" microsyndromes in children parallel the contentious issues reported for older adolescents and adults with "mood lability." That is, across the entire age span, "mood lability" is an ambiguous area and a challenge. Although there was wide consensus that BP-NOS (including subthreshold bipolar syndromes) can also be assessed with the various versions of the K-SADS, it may be premature to propose criteria for "mood lability" syndromes in children until data from ongoing funded investigations become available.

Comorbidity With Pervasive Developmental Disorders. Several reports in the literature include observations of co-occurrence of bipolar and autism type symptoms (e.g., Wozniak et al., 1997). There also are widespread clinical observations of this entity (the Research Units for Pediatric Psychopharmacology [RUPP] sites are considering a drug study of this patient population). The recently available Social Reciprocity Scale is a reliable screening tool for autism spectrum disorders (Constantino et al., 2000) and is being used for siblings of bipolar children in an ongoing study of family psychopathology (Geller et al., personal communication, 2000).

Outstanding Issues. Outstanding issues for the study of bipolar disorder in prepubertal children include the following:

- Describing the course of BP-I, BP-II, cyclothymia, and BP-NOS, with attention to possible developmental changes in symptom expression, with the goal of establishing the predictive validity of various BP-I, BP-II, and BP NOS subtypes.

- Defining thresholds for and boundaries between BP-I, BP-II, and cyclothymia.
- Defining occasions for combining versus separating BP-I and BP-II. (For instance, in treatment studies of mania, where severity is an issue, it is not clear whether combining manic with hypomanic patients is appropriate. However, combining should be appropriate when the focus of treatment is on decreasing number of cycles. Data from genetic studies suggest similarities as well as differences between BP-I and BP-II in adult onset BP, but the possibility that BP-II and hypomania are anlage of mania in children needs to be investigated.)
- Establishing inclusion and exclusion criteria for BP-NOS (and identifying subtypes?).

According to the Robins and Guze model as expanded by Cantwell (1996), the stages for establishing the validity of disorders includes studies of:

- Clinical phenomenology of the disorder: the core clinical picture and its common associated features, subtypes, and comorbid conditions.
- Demographic factors (incidence, prevalence, morbidity risk, and lifetime expectancy) and documentation of age, gender, social class, ethnicity, and culture.
- Biological factors correlated with a particular clinical picture (presence of damage and/or brain dysfunction, physical handicaps and disorders, neurological disorders) and laboratory studies in the areas of neurophysiology, neuroendocrinology, biochemistry, neuropharmacology, brain imaging, and neuropsychology.
- Family environmental factors (e.g., discipline styles and other aspects of parent–child interaction).
- Family genetics, including family aggregation, adoption, twin, linkage, segregation, gene mapping, etc.
- Natural history of the disorder, including true prospective, true retrospective, catch-up prospective, and anterospective studies to explore continuities and discontinuities between childhood, adolescent, and adult disorders and the mechanism for these continuities and discontinuities.
- Response to intervention.

This model can serve as a touchstone to set goals and mark progress. Some of the work is ongoing. To date, most research in prepubertal bipolar disorder has been conducted at the level of exploring clinical phenomenology, associated features, and co-occurring conditions, such as ADHD and ODD. While these studies appear to support the existence of one or more identifiable syndromes, further study across domains of genetics, natural history, and treatment response are required to establish more firmly the validity and utility of these putative diagnostic entities.

The major questions on the table at this meeting were the following:

- How early can bipolar disorder be diagnosed?
- What is the predictive value of the early manifestations of bipolar illness in children (before puberty) in adolescents?
- If "prodromal" symptoms are found, what is the risk/benefit ratio of treating children and adolescents with prodromal symptoms? Which treatments should be considered? For how long?
- What is the potential impact of early treatment on course of illness?

Although discussion did not go beyond basic diagnostic issues for bipolar disorder in prepubertal children, the general agreement that was reached on these issues should be helpful in further efforts to address these questions.

Roundtable Participants

Joseph Biederman, M.D.
Pediatric Psychopharmacology Unit of the Child Psychiatry Service
Massachusetts General Hospital

Boris Birmaher, M.D.
Department of Psychiatry
University of Pittsburgh Medical Center

Gabrielle A. Carlson, M.D.
Department of Psychiatry and Behavioral Sciences
State University of New York at Stony Brook

Kiki D. Chang, M.D.
Division of Child and Adolescent Psychiatry
Stanford University School of Medicine

Wayne S. Fenton, M.D.
National Institute of Mental Health

Barbara Geller, M.D.
Washington University School of Medicine

Kimberly E. Hoagwood, Ph.D.
National Institute of Mental Health

Steven E. Hyman, M.D.
National Institute of Mental Health

Kenneth S. Kendler, M.D.
Virginia Institute for Psychiatric and Behavioral Genetics
Virginia Commonwealth University

Doreen S. Koretz, Ph.D.
Developmental Psychopathology and Prevention Research Branch
National Institute of Mental Health

Robert A. Kowatch, M.D.
Department of Psychiatry
University of Cincinnati Medical Center

David J. Kupfer, M.D.
Department of Psychiatry
University of Pittsburgh School of Medicine

Ellen Leibenluft, M.D.
Pediatric and Developmental Neuropsychiatry Branch
National Institute of Mental Health

Richard K. Nakamura, Ph.D.
National Institute of Mental Health

Editha D. Nottelmann, Ph.D.
Developmental Psychopathology and Prevention Research Branch
National Institute of Mental Health

Ellen Stover, Ph.D.
National Institute of Mental Health

Benedetto Vitiello, M.D.
Child and Adolescent Treatment and Preventive Intervention Research Branch
National Institute of Mental Health

Gemma Weiblinger
National Institute of Mental Health

Elizabeth Weller, M.D.
Department of Psychiatry
University of Pennsylvania School of Medicine

REFERENCES

Achenbach TM (1991), *Manual for the Child Behavior Checklist/4–18 and 1991 Profile*. Burlington: University of Vermont Department of Psychiatry

Axelson DA, Birmaher B, Brent DA, Ryan N (1999), The KSADS Mania Rating Scale for Pediatric Bipolar Disorder. Presented at the 46th Annual Meeting of the American Academy of Child and Adolescent Psychiatry, October

Biederman J (1998), Developmental subtypes of juvenile bipolar disorder. *Harv Rev Psychiatry* 3:227–230

Biederman J, Faraone SV, Wozniak J, Monuteaux MC (2000a), Parsing the association between bipolar, conduct, and substance use disorders: a familial risk analysis. *Biol Psychiatry* 48:1037–1044

Biederman J, Mick E, Faraone SV, Spencer T, Wilens TE, Wozniak J (2000b), Pediatric mania: a developmental subtype of bipolar disorder? *Biol Psychiatry* 48:458–466

Biederman J, Wozniak J, Kiely K et al. (1995), CBCL clinical scales discriminate prepubertal children with structured interview–derived diagnosis of mania from those with ADHD. *J Am Acad Child Adolesc Psychiatry* 34:464–471

Cantwell DP (1996), Classification of child and adolescent psychopathology. *J Child Psychol Psychiatry* 37:[illegible]3–12

Carlson GA, Kelly KL (1998), Manic symptoms in psychiatrically hospitalized children: what do they mean? *J Affect Disord* 51:123–135

Carlson GA, Loney J, Salisbury H, Volpe RJ (1998), Young referred boys with DICA-R-P manic symptoms vs. two comparison groups. *J Affect Disord* 51:113–121

Constantino JN, Przybeck T, Friesen D, Todd RD (2000), Reciprocal social behavior in children with and without pervasive developmental disorders. *J Dev Behav Pediatr* 21:[illegible]2–11

Egger HL, Ascher BH, Angold AA (1999, 2000), *The Preschool Age Psychiatric Assessment (PAPA)*. Durham, NC: Duke University Medical Center

Fristad MA, Weller EB, Weller RA (1992), The Mania Rating Scale: can it be used in children? A preliminary report. *J Am Acad Child Adolesc Psychiatry* 31:252–257

Geller B, Craney JL, Bolhofner K, DelBello MP, Williams M, Zimerman B (2001a), One-year recovery and relapse rates of children with a prepubertal and early adolescent bipolar disorder phenotype. *Am J Psychiatry* 158:303–305

Geller B, Sun K, Zimerman B, Luby J, Frazier J, Williams M (1995), Complex and rapid-cycling in bipolar children and adolescents: a preliminary study. *J Affect Disord* 34:259–268

Geller B, Warner K, Williams M, Zimerman B (1998a), Prepubertal and young adolescent bipolarity versus ADHD: assessment and validity using the WASH-U-KSADS, CBCL and TRF. *J Affect Disord* 51:93–100

Geller B, Williams M, Zimerman B, Frazier J (1996), *Washington University in St. Louis Kiddie Schedule for Affective Disorders and Schizophrenia (WASH-U-KSADS)*. St Louis: Washington University

Geller B, Williams M, Zimerman B, Frazier J, Beringer L, Warner KL (1998b), Prepubertal and early adolescent bipolarity differentiate from ADHD by manic symptoms, grandiose delusions, ultra-rapid or ultradian cycling. *J Affect Disord* 51:81–91

Geller B, Zimerman B, Williams M et al. (2001b), Reliability of the Washington University in St. Louis Kiddie Schedule for Affective Disorders and Schizophrenia (WASH-U-KSADS) mania and rapid cycling sections. *J Am Acad Child Adolesc Psychiatry* 40:450–455

Geller B, Zimerman B, Williams M et al. (2000a), Six-month stability and outcome of a prepubertal and early adolescent bipolar disorder phenotype. *J Child Adolesc Psychopharmacol* 10:165–173

Geller B, Zimerman B, Williams M et al. (2000b), Diagnostic characteristics of 93 cases of a prepubertal and early adolescent bipolar disorder phenotype by gender, puberty and comorbid attention deficit hyperactivity disorder. *J Child Adolesc Psychopharmacol* 10:157–164

Goodwin FK, Jamison KR, eds (1990), *Manic-Depressive Illness*. New York: Oxford University Press, pp 22–55, 127–1[illegible]

Kaufman J, Birmaher B, Brent D et al. (1997), Schedule for Affective Disorders and Schizophrenia for School-Age Children–Present and Lifetime Version (K-SADS-PL): initial reliability and validity data. *J Am Acad Child Adolesc Psychiatry* 36:980–988

Orvaschel H, Puig-Antich J, Chambers WJ, Tabrizi MA, Johnson R (1982), Retrospective assessment of prepubertal major depression with the Kiddie-SADS-E. *J Am Acad Child Psychiatry* 21:392–397

Puig-Antich J, Ryan N (1986), *The Schedule for Affective Disorders and Schizophrenia for School-Age Children (Kiddie-SADS)–1986*. Pittsburgh: Western Psychiatric Institute and Clinic

Shaffer D, Gould MS, Brasic J et al. (1983), A children's global assessment scale (CGAS). *Arch Gen Psychiatry* 40:1228–1231

Wozniak J, Biederman J, Faraone SV et al. (1997), Mania in children with pervasive developmental disorder revisited. *J Am Acad Child Adolesc Psychiatry* 36:1552–1559; discussion 1559–1560

Wozniak J, Biederman J, Kiely K et al. (1995), Mania-like symptoms suggestive of childhood-onset bipolar disorder in clinically referred children. *J Am Acad Child Adolesc Psychiatry* 34:867–876

SUPPORTING LITERATURE

Akiskal HS (1995), Developmental pathways to bipolarity: are juvenile-onset depressions pre-bipolar? *J Am Acad Child Adolesc Psychiatry* 34:754–763

Alexander PJ, Raghavan R (1997), Childhood mania in India (letter). *J Am Acad Child Adolesc Psychiatry* 36:1650–1651

Biederman J (1995), Developmental subtypes of juvenile bipolar disorder. *Harv Rev Psychiatry* 3:227–230

Biederman J (1998), Resolved: mania is mistaken for ADHD in prepubertal children (debate forum)—affirmative. *J Am Acad Child Adolesc Psychiatry* 37:1091–1093

Biederman J (1998), Resolved: mania is mistaken for ADHD in prepubertal children (debate forum)—affirmative rebuttal. *J Am Acad Child Adolesc Psychiatry* 37:1096–1098

Biederman J, Mick E, Prince J et al. (1999), Systematic chart review of the pharmacologic treatment of comorbid attention deficit hyperactivity disorder in youth with bipolar disorder. *J Child Adolesc Psychopharmacol* 9:247–256

Biederman J, Russell R, Soriano J, Wozniak J, Faraone SV (1998), Clinical features of children with both ADHD and mania: does ascertainment source make a difference? *J Affect Disord* 51:101–112

Biederman J, Rivinus T, Kemper K, Hamilton D, MacFadyen J, Harmatz J (1985), Depressive disorders in relatives of anorexia nervosa patients with and without a current episode of nonbipolar major depression. *Am J Psychiatry* 142:1495–1497

Burke MG (1997), Atypical bipolar symptoms (letter). *J Am Acad Child Adolesc Psychiatry* 36:1319

Carlson GA (1995), Identifying prepubertal mania. *J Am Acad Child Adolesc Psychiatry* 34:750–754

Carlson GA (1998), Mania and ADHD: comorbidity or confusion. *J Affect Disord* 51:177–187

Carlson GA, Fahim F (1998), "George" (case report #2). *J Affect Disord* 51:195–198

Chang KD (2000), Psychiatric phenomenology of child and adolescent bipolar offspring. *J Am Acad Child Adolesc Psychiatry* 39:453–460

Faraone SV, Biederman J, Mennin D, Russell R (1998), Bipolar and antisocial disorders among relatives of ADHD children: parsing familial subtypes of illness. *Neuropsychiatr Genet* 81:108–116

Faraone SV, Biederman J, Mennin D, Wozniak J, Spencer T (1997), Attention-deficit hyperactivity disorder with bipolar disorder: a familial subtype? *J Am Acad Child Adolesc Psychiatry* 36:1378–1387

Faraone SV, Biederman J, Monuteaux MC (2001), Attention deficit hyperactivity disorder with bipolar disorder in girls: further evidence for a familial subtype? *J Affect Disord* 64:19–26

Frazier JA, Meyer MC, Biederman J et al. (1999), Risperidone treatment for juvenile bipolar disorder: a retrospective chart review. *J Am Acad Child Adolesc Psychiatry* 38:960–965

Fristad MA, Cummins J, Verducci JS, Teare M, Weller EB, Weller RA (1998), Study IV: concurrent validity of the *DSM-IV* revised Children's Interview for Psychiatric Syndromes (ChIPS). *J Child Adolesc Psychopharmacol* 8:227–236

Fristad MA, Glickman AR, Verducci JS, Teare M, Weller EB, Weller RA (1998), Study V: Children's Interview for Psychiatric Syndromes (ChIPS): psychometrics in two community samples. *J Child Adolesc Psychopharmacol* 8:237–245

Fristad MA, Teare M, Weller EB, Weller RA, Salmon P (1998), Study III: development and concurrent validity of the Children's Interview for Psychiatric Syndromes-parent version (P-ChIPS). *J Child Adolesc Psychopharmacol* 8:221–226

Fristad MA, Weller RA, Weller EB (1997), Atypical bipolar symptoms (letter). *J Am Acad Child Adolesc Psychiatry* 38:1320

Geller B (1997), BPD and ADHD (letter). *J Am Acad Child Adolesc Psychiatry* 36:720

Geller B (1997), Commentary on "Attention-deficit hyperactivity disorder with bipolar disorder: a familial subtype?" (discussion). *J Am Acad Child Adolesc Psychiatry* 36:1387–1388

Geller B, Bolhofner K, Craney JL, Williams M, DelBello MP, Gundersen K (2000), Psychosocial functioning in a prepubertal and early adolescent bipolar disorder phenotype. *J Am Acad Child Adolesc Psychiatry* 39:1543–1548

Geller B, Cook EH (1999), Serotonin transporter gene (HTTLPR) is not in linkage disequilibrium with prepubertal and early adolescent bipolarity. *Biol Psychiatry* 45:1230–1233

Geller B, Cook EH (2000), Ultradian rapid cycling in prepubertal and early adolescent bipolarity is not in transmission disequilibrium with Val/Met COMT alleles. *Biol Psychiatry* 47:605–609

Geller B, Cooper TB, Sun K et al. (1998), Double-blind placebo controlled study of lithium for adolescent bipolar disorders with secondary substance dependency. *J Am Acad Child Adolesc Psychiatry* 37:171–178

Geller B, Cooper TB, Zimerman B et al. (1998), Lithium for prepubertal depressed children with family history predictors of future bipolarity: a double blind, placebo-controlled study. *J Affect Disord* 51:165–175

Geller B, Luby J (1997), Child and adolescent bipolar disorder: review of the past 10 years. *J Am Acad Child Adolesc Psychiatry* 36:1168–1176

Geller B, Luby J (1998), Mania in young children (letter). *J Am Acad Child Adolesc Psychiatry* 37:347–348

Geller B, Luby J (1998), Mania in young children (letter). *J Am Acad Child Adolesc Psychiatry* 37:1005

Geller B, Zimerman B, Williams M, Bolhofner K, Craney JL (2001), Bipolar disorder at prospective follow up of adults who had prepubertal major depressive disorder. *Am J Psychiatry* 158:125–127

Hellander ME, Burke T (1999), Children with bipolar disorder (letter). *J Am Acad Child Adolesc Psychiatry* 38:495

Kafantaris V, Coletti DJ, Dicker R, Padula G, Pollack S (1998), Are childhood psychiatric histories of bipolar adolescents associated with family history, psychosis, and response to lithium treatment? *J Affect Disord* 51:153–164

Klein RG, Pine DS, Klein DF (1998), Resolved: mania is mistaken for ADHD in prepubertal children (debate forum)—negative. *J Am Acad Child Adolesc Psychiatry* 37:1093–1096

Klein RG, Pine DS, Klein DF (1998), Resolved: mania is mistaken for ADHD in prepubertal children (debate forum)—negative rebuttal. *J Am Acad Child Adolesc Psychiatry* 37:1098–1099

Klein RG, Pine DS, Klein DF (1999), Children with bipolar disorder (letter). *J Am Acad Child Adolesc Psychiatry* 38:496

Kovacs M, Pollock M (1995), Bipolar disorder and comorbid conduct disorder in childhood and adolescence. *J Am Acad Child Adolesc Psychiatry* 34:715–723

Kowatch RA (1998), Mania in young children (letter). *J Am Acad Child Adolesc Psychiatry* 37:1003

Kutcher S, Robertson HA, Bird D (1998), Premorbid functioning in adolescent onset bipolar I disorder: a preliminary report from an ongoing study. *J Affect Disord* 51:137–144

Lombardo GT (1997), BPD and ADHD (letter). *J Am Acad Child Adolesc Psychiatry* 36:719

McClellan J (1998), Mania in young children (letter). *J Am Acad Child Adolesc Psychiatry* 37:346–347

McClellan J (1998), Mania in young children (letter). *J Am Acad Child Adolesc Psychiatry* 37:1004

McDermott J (1994), Listening to psychotherapy (editor's note). *J Am Acad Child Adolesc Psychiatry* 33:1079

Nottelmann ED, Jensen PS (1995), Bipolar affective disorder in children and adolescents: Introduction to Special Section. *J Am Acad Child Adolesc Psychiatry* 34:705–708

Nottelmann ED, Jensen PS (1998), Current issues in childhood bipolarity: Introduction to Special Issue. *J Affect Disord* 51:77–80

Staton D, Lysne D (1999), Children with bipolar disorder (letter). *J Am Acad Child Adolesc Psychiatry* 38:495–496

Strober M, DeAntonio M, Schmidt-Lackner S, Freeman R, Lampert C, Diamond J (1998), Early childhood attention deficit hyperactivity disorders predicts poorer response to acute lithium therapy in adolescent mania. *J Affect Disord* 51:145–151

Teare M, Fristad MA, Weller EB, Weller RA, Salmon P (1998), Study I: development and criterion validity of the Children's Interview for Psychiatric Syndromes (ChIPS). *J Child Adolesc Psychopharmacol* 8:205–211

Teare M, Fristad MA, Weller EB, Weller RA, Salmon P (1998), Study II: concurrent validity of the *DSM-III-R* Children's Interview for Psychiatric Syndromes (ChIPS). *J Child Adolesc Psychopharmacol* 8:213–219

Weller E, Weller RA, Dogin JW (1998), A rose is a rose is a rose (case report #1). *J Affect Disord* 51:189–193

Weller E, Weller RA, Fristad M (1995), Bipolar disorder in children: misdiagnosis, underdiagnosis, and future directions. *J Am Acad Child Adolesc Psychiatry* 34:709–714

Weller EB, Weller RA, Fristad AE, Rooney MT (1999), *Administrative Manual for the ChIPS*. Washington, DC: American Psychiatric Press

Weller EB, Weller RA, Fristad MA, Teare M, Schechter J (2000), Children's Interview for Psychiatric Syndromes (ChIPS). *J Am Acad Child Adolesc Psychiatry* 39:76–84

Weller EB, Weller RA, Teare M, Fristad MA (1999), *Children's Interview for Psychiatric Syndromes (ChIPS)*. Washington, DC: American Psychiatric Press

Weller EB, Weller RA, Teare M, Fristad MA (1999), *Parent Version Children's Interview for Psychiatric Syndromes (P-ChIPS)*. Washington, DC: American Psychiatric Press

Werry JS (1997), Attention deficit hyperactivity disorder with bipolar disorder: a familial subtype? (discussion). *J Am Acad Child Adolesc Psychiatry* 36:1388–1390

Wilens T, Biederman J, Millstein R, Wozniak J, Hahsey A, Spencer T (1999), Risk for substance use disorders in youths with child- and adolescent-onset bipolar disorder. *J Am Acad Child Adolesc Psychiatry* 36:680–685

Wilens TE, Biederman J, Milberger S et al. (2000), Is bipolar disorder a risk for cigarette smoking in ADHD youth? *Am J Addict* 9:187–195

Wozniak J, Biederman J (1996), A pharmacological approach to the quagmire of comorbidity in juvenile mania. *J Am Acad Child Adolesc Psychiatry* 35:826–828

Wozniak J, Biederman J (1997), Atypical bipolar symptoms (letter). *J Am Acad Child Adolesc Psychiatry* 36:1319–1320

Time Trends in Autism and in MMR Immunization Coverage in California. Loring Dales, MD, Sandra Jo Hammer, RN, PHN, Natalie J Smith, MD, MPH

Context: Considerable concern has been generated in the lay and medical communities by a theory that increased measles-mumps-rubella (MMR) immunization among young children may be the cause of an apparent marked increase in autism occurrence. *Objective:* To determine if a correlation exists in secular trends of MMR immunization coverage among young children and autism occurrence. *Design, Setting, and Participants:* Retrospective analyses of MMR immunization coverage rates among children born in 1980–1994 who were enrolled in California kindergartens (survey samples of 600–1900 children each year) and whose school immunization records were reviewed to retrospectively determine the age at which they first received MMR immunization; and of autism caseloads among children born in these years who were diagnosed with autism and were enrolled in the California Department of Developmental Services regional service center system. *Main Outcome Measures:* Measles-mumps-rubella immunization coverage rates as of ages 17 months and 24 months and numbers of Department of Developmental Services system enrollees diagnosed with autism, grouped by year of birth. *Results:* Essentially no correlation was observed between the secular trend of early childhood MMR immunization rates in California and the secular trend in numbers of children with autism enrolled in California's regional service system. For the 1980–1994 birth cohorts, a marked, sustained increase in autism case numbers was noted, from 44 cases per 100000 live births in the 1980 cohort to 208 cases per 100000 live births in the 1994 cohort (a 373% relative increase), but changes in early childhood MMR immunization coverage over the same time period were much smaller and of shorter duration. Immunization coverage by the age of 24 months increased from 72% to 82%, a relative increase of only 14%, over the same time period. *Conclusions:* These data do not suggest an association between MMR immunization among young children and an increase in autism occurrence. **JAMA** 2001;285:1183–1185. Copyright 2001, American Medical Association.

Abstracts selected by Michael J. Maloney, M.D., Assistant Editor

BIPOLARITY IN CHILDREN

Laura Sanchez, MD, Owen Hagino, MD, Elizabeth Weller, MD, and Ronald Weller, MD

Bipolar disorders in children and adolescents have been less studied than adult-onset bipolar illness. The incidence and validity of the diagnosis of mania in this age group, particularly in prepubertal children, remain unsettled. Most reports on mania in childhood have small samples, lack control groups, do not use standardized assessments, or are retrospective in design. Existing reports suggest that mania in childhood (1) is often misdiagnosed or underdiagnosed; (2) is a severe illness frequently associated with mixed or rapid-cycling features, psychotic features, and comorbid disruptive disorders; and (3) is associated with greater familial loading for affective illnesses than adult-onset bipolar disorder.

HISTORICAL OVERVIEW

Case reports of mania in preschool and prepubertal school-age children date to the mid-nineteenth century.[12, 15, 23, 38, 62, 68, 88] Kraepelin[68] believed mania was rare in prepubertal children. Of 900 patients with mania studied by Kraepelin, only 0.4% had an onset before the age of 10 years; however, he believed the incidence did increase after the onset of puberty.

Anthony and Scott[8] also believed mania in childhood to be rare. Of 60 children reported to have manic-depressive psychosis, they concluded that only 3 (5%) met their strict diagnostic criteria for mania; this in-

From the Department of Psychiatry, University of Pennsylvania School of Medicine (LS, OH, EW, RW); and Hospital of the University of Pennsylvania (RW), and Children's Hospital of Philadelphia (EW), Philadelphia, Pennsylvania

cluded one subject who met criteria both at age 12 and when followed up as an adult. Their criteria were restrictive. A diagnosis of mania required all of the following: (1) an abnormal psychiatric state approximating the descriptions of mania provided by Kraepelin,[68] Bleuler,[15] Meyer,[86] and others; (2) a positive family history for mania; (3) a history of either cyclothymia or sporadic manic or depressive outbursts during fevers; (4) a history of recurrence—at least two episodes; (5) a biphasic pattern; (6) an endogenous origin; (7) treatment in an inpatient setting and use of heavy sedation or electroconvulsive therapy; (8) an extroverted personality; (9) an absence of schizophrenia or organic states; and (10) a current assessment of symptoms (i.e., diagnosis could not be based on history). Thus, most children who clearly meet *Diagnostic and Statistical Manual of Mental Disorders*, third edition (DSM-III)[6] or DSM-IV[7] criteria for mania fail to meet the criteria of Anthony and Scott. In fact, many adults with bipolar illness would not meet their criteria.

A second set of criteria to diagnose mania in children was proposed by Weinberg and Brumback[120] in 1976. They adjusted the criteria by Feighner et al[40] (which formed the basis for the DSM-III[5] diagnostic system) for use in children. Their criteria included euphoria, irritable mood, or both and three or more of the following symptoms, which must constitute a change from the child's normal behavior: (1) hyperactivity, (2) push of speech, (3) flight of ideas, (4) grandiosity, (5) sleep disturbance, and (6) distractibility. Symptom duration of 1 month was required to diagnose mania in children.

In 1979, Davis[34] proposed that mania in children be diagnosed using broader and *softer* criteria than those proposed for adults, a concept somewhat comparable to the idea of *depressive equivalents* in the diagnosis of depression in childhood. Mania in childhood required all of the following primary criteria: (1) affective storms, (2) positive family history for mania, (3) hyperactivity, (4) chronically disturbed personal relationships, and (5) absence of psychotic thought disorder. One or more of the following secondary criteria were required as well: (1) sleep disturbance, (2) minimal brain dysfunction, (3) abnormal electroencephalogram (EEG), (4) enuresis, and (5) neuropathology.

Since 1980, the DSM-III,[5] DSM-III-R,[6] and DSM-IV[7] have applied adult criteria to diagnose mania in children, with some modifications to take into account differences in age and developmental stage. Despite these improvements in criterion-based diagnostic systems, mania in childhood is frequently underdiagnosed or misdiagnosed.[123]

Several factors work against accurate diagnosis of bipolar disorder in pediatric populations. These include (1) a clinical bias against the diagnosis of mania in childhood[61]; (2) the low base rate of bipolar disorder relative to other psychiatric illnesses in children; (3) symptom overlap between bipolar disorder and other more prevalent childhood psychiatric illnesses, such as attention deficit hyperactivity disorder (ADHD) and conduct disorder; and (4) developmental constraints and variability in symptom expression and clinical presentation. In their review of the English-language psychiatric literature from 1809 to 1984,

Weller et al[123] reported that 33 children met modified DSM-III-R[6] criteria for mania. In this study, the symptom "involvement in activities with a high potential for painful consequences" was not counted toward the diagnosis of mania because of concerns regarding its prevalence among children with attention deficit and conduct disorder. Of the 33 children diagnosed by the investigators as manic, 52% had originally been assigned some other diagnosis, including obsessive-compulsive disorder, loss reaction, *psychopathic* personality, borderline personality, immature personality, and schizophrenia.

EPIDEMIOLOGY

To date, no comprehensive epidemiologic study to determine the prevalence of bipolar disorder in childhood has been completed. Thus, current estimates of the prevalence of bipolar disorder in childhood are based on relatively small community surveys or retrospective data.

Prepubertal onset of mania is estimated to be rare. In a retrospective study involving adult patients with well-established diagnoses of bipolar disorder, only 0.5% reported the age of onset of their illness to have been between 5 and 9 years; only 7.5% reported onset between ages 10 and 14 years.[76] Furthermore, although bipolar disorder in adulthood affects both sexes equally, reports of mania in childhood suggest that prepubertal-onset mania may be more common in boys than in girls.[48, 118]

The incidence of mania appears to increase after onset of puberty, and the prevalence of mania during late adolescence is estimated to approximate that in adulthood. A community-based school survey reported a lifetime prevalence rate of bipolar disorder of approximately 1% in adolescents ages 14 to 18 years. Most of these patients, however, had bipolar II disorder.[73] The lifetime prevalence of mania in another epidemiologic survey of adolescents ages 14 to 16 years varied from 0.6% to 13.3% depending on whether duration and severity criteria were applied.[29] The effects of duration and severity on prevalence should be considered when reviewing the literature on childhood mania. DSM-III-R[6] removed the 7-day minimal duration criterion for mania required by DSM-III.[5] Thus, reports based on DSM-III-R[6] criteria may overdiagnose mania in childhood. In DSM-IV,[7] the 7-day duration criterion was reinstated, and a severity requirement was added.

Evidence suggests that the prevalence of childhood-onset mania may be increasing. Earlier age of onset of bipolar disorder in successive birth cohorts has been reported.[100] Anticipation, a tendency for a disease phenotype to worsen (e.g., to be expressed at an earlier age and to run a more severe course) in consecutive generations, is one proposed explanation of this phenomenon.[78]

CLINICAL CHARACTERISTICS

Children with mania frequently present with symptoms that are considered *atypical* in adults.[18] Mixed features; rapid-cycling features;

psychotic features; high rates of comorbidity, especially with externalizing disorders; and significant psychosocial impairment are common.[26, 48, 67, 84] Mania in childhood may be a more serious form of the adult illness. Some suggest that the clinical presentation of mania in prepubertal children resembles that of treatment-resistant, chronically ill adults.[45, 127] Furthermore, early-onset bipolar illness has been associated with greater familial loading than adult-onset illness. Lifetime rates of bipolar illness are higher among families of children than among families of adults with bipolar disorder.[91, 100, 109, 112, 115, 116]

Whether the phenotypic differences reported between childhood-onset and adult-onset bipolar disorder result from developmental variations of the same genotype or genotypic differences remains to be determined. Furthermore, the role that early exposure to psychotropic agents, in particular psychostimulants, may contribute to the presentation of mania in children has not been adequately addressed. Psychotropic medications have been reported to induce rapid cycling and mixed episodes in adults.[96]

In young children, it is often difficult to identify discrete episodes. Common symptoms include a worsening of disruptive behavior, moodiness, difficulty sleeping at night, impulsiveness, overactivity, and an inability to concentrate. Episodic short attention span, low frustration tolerance, explosive anger followed by guilt, sulkiness, depression, and poor school performance are described. There are also case reports of *model* children who dramatically change and become *wild*.[26]

Few reports have focused on preschool children. Pathologically prolonged states of emotional arousal in response to minimal stimuli, episodic frenzied activity with minor symptoms of depression, explosive temper tantrums, sexual joking, and nightmares have all been reported.[27, 93] Poznanski et al[95] described a 4 year old with hypomania who when followed up as an adolescent manifested full-blown manic episodes. Six preschool children admitted to the child inpatient unit at Ohio State University Hospitals between October 1992 and April 1998 met DSM-III-R[6] criteria for mania or hypomania. The clinical presentation of these children was not substantially different from that of older children.[121]

Symptoms of mania were reported for 10 hospitalized prepubertal children who met DSM-III[5] criteria for bipolar disorder and responded to lithium therapy.[118] Each of these children had a mood disturbance. Five reported a primarily elated mood, and five reported a primarily irritable mood. All were restless, and nine reported decreased sleep associated with the onset of the mood disturbance. Six children exhibited sexual preoccupation and sexual *acting out*. All exhibited speech disturbances, including pressured speech, increased talkativeness, or rhyming. Racing thoughts were reported by six children, five children had flight of ideas, and five had increased distractibility. All 10 children had onset of psychosis with the onset of the mood disturbance; 6 children reported persecutory delusions, 5 reported auditory hallucinations, 7 reported visual hallucinations, and 2 reported grandiose delusions. Almost all the children in this study had previously been diagnosed as *hyperactive* despite the fact that their symptoms represented a distinct change from their previous behavior. A gradual rather than abrupt onset of symptoms was reported. Two children reported a positive family history of mania.

The clinical presentation of 43 children aged 12 years or younger who met DSM-III-R[6] criteria for mania on a semistructured diagnostic interview was not typical of adult-onset mania.[127] Severe irritability rather than euphoria; a chronic, noncyclical course; and mixed symptoms of depression and mania characterized this sample. Of these children, 98% also met DSM-III-R[6] criteria for ADHD. Other comorbid conditions included anxiety disorder, conduct disorder, and oppositional defiant disorder. Significant psychosocial impairment and repeated hospitalizations were reported. Similar findings were reported in 29 prepubertal children with ADHD who met DSM-III-R[6] criteria for bipolar disorder on a semistructured interview.[13] Methodologic limitations of both of these studies include failure to interview children directly and the relative lack of clinical experience among the interviewers.

A preliminary account of 60 children from the first controlled phenomenologic study of bipolar disorder in childhood reports that children with bipolar disorder are significantly and substantially more likely than children with ADHD to endorse cardinal symptoms of mania, including elated mood, grandiosity, hypersexuality (in the absence of abuse or overstimulation), decreased need for sleep, flight of ideas, racing thoughts, social intrusiveness, and increased goal-directed activity.[48] Hyperactivity and distractibility did not differ substantially between the two groups. Furthermore, high rates of mixed mania, rapid cycling, and psychosis characterized this young outpatient bipolar sample. The authors of this study applied the term *mixed mania* to episodes in which there was temporal overlap in the onset and offset of mania or hypomania with major depression or dysthymia; 86.7% of the sample reported having this type of mixed manic episode. Furthermore, 83.3% of the children were rapid cyclers, reporting four or more episodes of mood disturbance a year. Of the rapid cyclers, 8.3% reported ultrarapid cycling, with mood disturbances lasting a few days to a few weeks, and 75% reported ultradian cycling, with mood disturbances occurring within a 24-hour period. Sixty percent of the sample reported psychotic symptoms; of this 60%, 92% reported grandiose delusions. Of the sample, 26.7% endorsed suicidality with plan and intent. It is not yet known whether the cycling patterns of these youths will evolve into more classic descriptions as they enter adulthood.

The phenomenology of mania in adolescents has been reported to be more similar to adult-onset mania than to prepubertal-onset mania.[17, 30, 32, 125] Furthermore, follow-up studies have confirmed the diagnosis in most cases.[63, 69] Marked mood lability, mixed manic features, and psychotic symptoms, including mood-incongruent hallucinations, paranoid delusions, and thought disorder, complicate the clinical presentation of mania in adolescence.[1, 10, 11, 52, 111] Only one study has prospectively compared adolescent-onset and adult-onset bipolar disorder.[83] Mixed mania was more prevalent and psychotic symptoms less prevalent among the younger cohort, but there was significant overlap of symptoms reported between the two groups.

Bipolar illness may first manifest itself in childhood as depression.[75] Of youth with major depression, 20% to 30% go on to develop mania.[44, 97, 110] Risk factors associated with developing mania after an episode of depression include (1) a depression characterized by rapid onset, psychotic features, and psychomotor retardation; (2) a *loaded* family history for mood disorders, especially bipolar disorder; and (3) a history of antidepressant-induced hypomania or mania.[2, 110]

DIFFERENTIAL DIAGNOSIS AND COMORBIDITY

The differential diagnosis of mania includes both medical and psychiatric conditions. Symptoms of mania can result from a variety of medical conditions, including (1) prescription drug use (i.e., steroids, antidepressants, stimulants), (2) neurologic disorders (i.e., head trauma, multiple sclerosis, temporal lobe seizures), (3) systemic disorders (i.e., hyperthyroidism, porphyria), and (4) substances of abuse (e.g., amphetamines, cocaine). Children presenting with symptoms of mania require a thorough physical examination and neurologic assessment to rule out these conditions.[4]

Symptoms of mania must also be distinguished from normal childhood phenomena, including bragging, reckless behavior, overactivity, and imaginary play. Furthermore, the hypersexuality associated with mania can mimic the self-stimulatory and sexual *acting out* behaviors associated with children who have been abused or have witnessed adult sexual behavior. Obtaining a careful history regarding these issues is important.

The psychiatric differential diagnosis for children with mania can be complex. Symptom overlap between mania and childhood disruptive disorders and schizophrenia is particularly troublesome. Many symptoms associated with childhood disruptive disorders overlap with presenting symptoms of mania, including psychomotor agitation, distractibility, aggression, poor school performance, restless sleep, and sexually inappropriate behavior. Adding to this confusion is the fact that youths with bipolar disorder may have comorbid ADHD,[46, 127] conduct disorder, or both.[46, 67] ADHD and conduct disorder differ from mania in several respects, however. Onset of ADHD is typically in the preschool or early elementary school years (i.e., before age 7), whereas mania is much more common after puberty. The sleep disturbance and overactivation associated with ADHD are chronic and part of the child's baseline behavior. The sleep disturbance in mania is associated with the onset of the mood disturbance. Although both children with conduct disorder and children with mania often become involved in dangerous acts with painful consequences, children with mania are mischievous rather than vindictive and calculating. Their conflicts with authority usually result from poor judgment and grandiosity. Neither conduct disorder nor ADHD is typically associated with psychosis, flight of ideas, euphoria, or grandiosity, which are common symptoms in mania. In fact, children with disruptive disorders usually display low self-esteem. Most importantly, ADHD and conduct disorder are chronic, persistent conditions. Mania is an episodic illness associated with affective, mental, and behavioral excitement. Onset of mania involves a discernible change from baseline functioning.

Adolescents with bipolar disorder are frequently misdiagnosed with schizophrenia.[26, 28, 81, 124] Mood-incongruent hallucinations, paranoia, and thought disorders have been reported. Children with schizophrenia usually have an insidious onset of illness, lack the engaging quality associated with mania, and are less likely to have a family history of mania.

ASSESSMENT

A longitudinal history, including psychiatric symptoms, treatment, response to treatment, and psychosocial stressors, needs to be obtained.[4] The child should be interviewed alone and with the family. Family members should also be interviewed separately. Input from teachers and other school personnel is necessary. Parents of manic children frequently have psychopathology themselves. Information provided by school staff may help clarify whether parents are accurately reporting the child's symptoms.

Reports suggest that diagnostic accuracy improves when DSM criteria are applied.[28] Both structured and semistructured interviews may aid in the assessment of mania in children. Structured interviews include the Diagnostic Interview for Children and Adolescents–Revised (DICA-R),[98] the Diagnostic Interview Schedule for Children (DISC),[33] and the Children's Interview for Psychiatric Syndromes (ChIPS).[122] Semistructured interviews include the Interview Schedule for Children (ISC),[66] the Schedule for Affective Disorders and Schizophrenia for School-Age Children (KSADS),[31] and the Washington University Kiddie and Young Adult Schedule for Affective Disorders and Schizophrenia–Lifetime and Present Episode Version for DSM-IV[7] (WASH-U-KSADS).[47] All of these diagnostic tools provide thorough coverage of DSM-defined disorders. An advantage of structured interviews is that many can be satisfactorily conducted by trained psychometricians. Semistructured instruments usually require an experienced clinician to be the interviewer. Even with standardized assessment instruments, there is a risk of overdiagnosis of bipolar disorder in children with conduct disorder and ADHD.

Clinical rating scales can be used to document severity and track changes in target symptoms. The Mania Rating Scale[129] has acceptable validity and reliability and can distinguish manic and hyperactive children,[41, 42] whereas the Connors Teacher and Parent Scales have not been reported to distinguish these two groups.[41] The Child Behavior Checklist (CBCL) has also been reported to distinguish manic children from those with ADHD.[14, 47] It is not a diagnostically derived instrument, however, and it has not been validated in bipolar disorder. Differences in scores may reflect severity of illness rather than diagnostic differences.

COURSE AND PROGNOSIS

There are no systematic follow-up data on preschool or prepubertal school-age children with bipolar disorder. Anecdotal reports suggest that children with mania *do not grow out of it*.[94] The only naturalistic prospective follow-up study involved 54 children with adolescent-onset bipolar disorder. All but two children recovered from their initial episode over a 5-year period.[113] Of the 54 children, however, 44% had a relapsing course and 21% experienced two or more episodes during the 5-year follow-up. Furthermore, rate of recovery was influenced by the polarity of the index episode. Subjects with depression took longer to recover (median 26 weeks) than subjects with cycling (median 15 weeks), mixed (median 11 weeks), or pure manic (median 9 weeks) episodes.

Reports suggest that compared to adults, adolescents with bipolar disorder have a more prolonged early course and are less responsive to treatment.[84, 113] Long-term outcome, however, is reported to be similar to that of adult-onset bipolar disorder. Approximately half are significantly impaired compared to their premorbid state.[81, 84, 124] Adolescents with bipolar disorder are at increased risk for suicide relative to children with other psychiatric illnesses.[19, 20] Eleven of 54 bipolar adolescents made suicide attempts that required medical attention during 5-year follow-up.[113] Comorbid substance abuse further increases an adolescent's risk for suicide.[101, 102]

TREATMENT STUDIES

Advances in the treatment of bipolar disorder in children and adolescents have lagged behind those in adults. Between 1993 and 1998, there has been only one published, randomized clinical trial of a drug therapy (lithium carbonate) for adolescents with bipolar disorder.[43] By contrast, during the same period, the literature on the treatment of bipolar disorder in adults has included a large-scale double-blind, placebo-controlled trial of valproic acid[16]; a smaller double-blind, placebo-controlled study of verapamil[58]; randomized comparisons of risperidone to lithium and haloperidol[103]; and a lithium versus carbamazepine versus combined treatment study.[36] Preliminary studies and case reports have also included the use of two other anticonvulsants, gabapentin[82] and lamotrigine,[70, 71, 108] as pharmacotherapy for adults with treatment-resistant bipolar disorder. Research on pharmacotherapies for children and adolescents with bipolar disorder has been limited. A U.S. Food and Drug Administration (FDA) regulation requires that "new drugs or biologics that are therapeutically important for children, or will be commonly used in children, have labeling information on safe pediatric use" (FDA press release P98-37, 27 November 1998). This regulation should stimulate additional research in this area.

Lithium

A large body of literature suggests that lithium is a potentially efficacious treatment for mania in children and adolescents.[3, 45, 59] This evidence consists primarily of case reports, open-label trials, and small placebo-controlled studies of its use in children and adolescents with a variety of conditions. The most recently published randomized clinical trial of lithium for the treatment of bipolar illness in adolescents included 25 adolescents who met criteria for DSM-III-R[6] bipolar I disorder (n = 12), bipolar II disorder (n = 5), or major depressive disorder with *adolescent predictors of future bipolar disorder* (n = 8).[43] These youths also had secondary substance abuse. No difference was seen between active drug and placebo on measures of affective symptoms. Furthermore, no study has addressed efficacy of lithium in prepubertal mania, although safety[25, 55, 104] and dosing[54, 80] have been examined.

Divalproex

In May 1995, the FDA approved divalproex sodium (Depakote) for the acute treatment of mania in bipolar disorder in adults. There is a substantial body of evidence from randomized clinical trials[16, 35, 92] that supports the efficacy of divalproex in adults with bipolar illness. Presently the evidence for its use for children and adolescents is limited to case reports and small open-label trials.[89, 90] Papatheodorou et al[90] treated 15 adolescents and young adults with acute mania for 7 weeks with divalproex sodium in an open-label trial. Nine subjects showed some improvement on a clinical severity scale for mania after 6 to 26 days of treatment. In addition to reports of fatal hepatotoxicity associated with valproic acid use in children[65] and the teratogenic risk for neural tube defects,[74] there have been more recent concerns about a possible association between childhood valproic acid use and later risk for polycystic ovarian disease in women.[56, 57] Although these serious adverse effects have been reported in patients treated for epilepsy, not bipolar disorder, caution should be advised when prescribing divalproex to any adolescent girl.

Carbamazepine

In several studies in adults, the anticonvulsant carbamazepine has been shown to have equal efficacy with lithium in reducing symptoms of acute mania.[105, 106] The comparative efficacy of carbamazepine versus lithium in maintenance treatment in adult bipolar disorder appears to favor lithium.[53] To date, there have been *no* published studies examining the effect of carbamazepine on mania in children and adolescents, either as an acute or as a maintenance treatment. Two small studies found minimal to no therapeutic effect of carbamazepine on reducing aggression in children with conduct disorder.[24, 60] Furthermore, mania has been described as a potential side effect of carbamazepine in children.[87, 99]

Lamotrigine

To date, the literature on the anticonvulsant lamotrigine for the treatment of bipolar disorder has been limited to case series[21, 108, 119] and open-label trials in adults.[39, 70, 71] The usefulness of lamotrigine as an antimanic (as well as an anticonvulsant) for children and adolescents is limited by its age-related association with the potentially life-threatening Stevens-Johnson syndrome.[37, 77, 85] As in the treatment of epilepsy, its use in the treatment of juvenile bipolar disorder should be limited to patients 16 years old and older who have failed other therapies.

Gabapentin

Gabapentin as an adjunctive treatment for acute mania in adults has been suggested by a series of case reports, case series, and open-label studies.[49, 64, 82, 128] Soutullo et al[107] report a favorable response to gabapentin plus carbamazepine in a 13-year-old boy with bipolar disorder. The pediatric neurology literature, however, suggests that gabapentin has potential for inducing disruptive and aggressive behavior in children treated for seizure control.[72, 114, 126] Investigation into its efficacy in pediatric bipolar disorder is clearly needed.

Atypical Antipsychotics

As with the newer anticonvulsants, the literature supporting use of the newer antipsychotics in the treatment of bipolar disorder is still limited. There have been reports of adults with treatment-refractory mania being treated with two novel antipsychotics: clozapine[9, 22, 79] and risperidone.[50, 51, 117] These medications have not been studied in children.

SUMMARY

Childhood and adolescent bipolar disorder have been less studied than adult onset bipolar illness. However, case reports of mania in childhood can be found as early as the mid 19th century. Historically, several factors have made the accurate diagnosis of bipolar disorder in childhood difficult: clinical bias against the diagnosis of mania in children; low base rate of disorder; symptom overlap between bipolar disorder and other more prevalent childhood-onset psychiatric disorders; and developmental constraints and variability in clinical presentation. The epidemiology of juvenile–onset bipolar disorder remains an open topic for research. The disorder appears to increase in prevalence with advancing age until young adulthood. Reported phenomenology of bipolar disorder in children and adolescents indicates a highly variable presentation with a developmental trend towards increased resemblance to the adult phenotype with increasing age of onset. Diagnostic accuracy for the disorder is improved by adherence to diagnostic and statistical manual of mental disorders (DSM) criteria and may be aided by structured or semistructured diagnostic interviews. The course of bipolar disorder in children and adolescents has also received limited systematic study. However, research to date supports a clinical picture of a relapsing, recurrent illness with substantial morbidity. Systematic studies of pharmacologic treatments of acute mania in children and adolescents are limited in number and scope. Clinical justification for the use of acute antimanic treatments such as lithium and valproic acid is still based upon studies conducted in adults. There remains an immediate and significant need for additional research into all aspects of juvenile-onset bipolar disorder.

ACKNOWLEDGMENTS

The authors thank Kathleen Hoffman and Charles Keller for their contributions in the preparation of this article.

References

1. Akiskal HS: The bipolar spectrum: Research and clinical perspectives. Encephale 21:3–11, 1995
2. Akiskal HS, Walker P, Puzantian VR: Bipolar outcome in the course of depressive illness: Phenomenologic, familial, and pharmacologic predictors. J Affect Disord 5:115–128, 1983
3. Alessi N, Naylor MW, Ghaziuddin M, et al: Update on lithium carbonate therapy in children and adolescents [see comments]. J Am Acad Child Adolesc Psychiatry 33:291–304, 1994
4. American Academy of Child and Adolescent Psychiatry: Practice Parameters for the Assessment and Treatment of Children and Adolescents With Bipolar Disorder. J Am Acad Child Adolesc Psychiatry 36(suppl):157S–176S, 1997
5. American Psychiatric Association: Diagnostic and Statistical Manual of Mental Disorders, ed 3. Washington, DC, American Psychiatric Association, 1980
6. American Psychiatric Association: Diagnostic and Statistical Manual of Mental Disorders, ed 3, rev. Washington, DC: American Psychiatric Association, 1987
7. American Psychiatric Association: Diagnostic and Statistical Manual of Mental Disorders, ed 4. Washington, DC, American Psychiatric Association, 1994
8. Anthony J, Scott P: Manic-depressive psychosis in childhood. Child Psychol Psychiatry 4:53–72, 1960

9. Antonacci DJ, Swartz CM: Clozapine treatment of euphoric mania. Ann Clin Psychiatry 7:203–206, 1995
10. Ballenger JC, Reus VI, Post RM: The "atypical" clinical picture of adolescent mania. Am J Psychiatry 139:602–606, 1982
11. Bashir M, Russell J, Johnson G: Bipolar affective disorder in adolescence: A ten year study. Aust NZ J Psychiatry 21:36–43, 1987
12. Barrett AM: Manic-depressive psychosis in childhood. Int Clin 3:41, 205–217, 1931
13. Biederman J, Faraone S, Mick E, et al: Attention deficit hyperactivity disorder and juvenile mania: An overlooked comorbidity. J Am Acad Child Adolesc Psychiatry 35:997–1008, 1996
14. Biederman J, Wozniak J, Kiely K, et al: CBCL scales discriminate prepubertal children with structured interview-derived diagnosis of mania from those with ADHD. J Am Acad Child Adolesc Psychiatry 34:464–471, 1995
15. Bleuler E: Textbook of Psychiatry. New York, Macmillan, 1934
16. Bowden CL, Brugger AM, Swann AC, et al: Efficacy of divalproex vs. lithium and placebo in the treatment of mania. The Depakote Mania Study Group [published erratum appears in JAMA 271:1830, 1994] [see comments]. JAMA 271:918–924, 1994
17. Bowden CL, Sarabia F: Diagnosing manic-depressive illness in adolescents. Compr Psychiatry 21:263–269, 1980
18. Bowring MA, Kovacs M: Difficulties in diagnosing manic disorders among children and adolescents. J Am Acad Child Adolesc Psychiatry 31:611–614, 1992
19. Brent DA, Perper JA, Goldstein CE, et al: Risk factors for adolescent suicide: A comparison of adolescent suicide victims with suicidal inpatients. Arch Gen Psychiatry 45:581–588, 1988
20. Brent DA, Perper JA, Moritz G, et al: Psychiatric risk factors for adolescent suicide: A case-control study. J Am Acad Child Adolesc Psychiatry 32:521–529, 1993
21. Calabrese JR, Fatemi SH, Woyshville MJ: Antidepressant effects of lamotrigine in rapid cycling bipolar disorder [letter] [see comments]. Am J Psychiatry 153:1236, 1996
22. Calabrese JR, Kimmel SE, Woyshville MJ, et al: Clozapine for treatment-refractory mania. Am J Psychiatry 153:759–764, 1996
23. Campbell J: Manic-depressive psychoses in children. J Nerv Ment Dis 116:424–439, 1952
24. Campbell M, Kafantaris V, Cueva JE: An update on the use of lithium carbonate in aggressive children and adolescents with conduct disorder. Psychopharmacol Bull 31:93–102, 1995
25. Campbell M, Silva RR, Kafantaris V, et al: Predictors of side effects associated with lithium administration in children. Psychopharmacol Bull 27:373–380, 1991
26. Carlson GA: Child and adolescent mania—diagnostic considerations. J Child Psychol Psychiatry 31:331–341, 1990
27. Carlson GA: Bipolar affective disorders in childhood and adolescence. *In* Cantwell DP, Carlson G (eds): Affective Disorders in Childhood and Adolescence: An Update. New York, Spectrum Publications, 1983
28. Carlson GA, Fennig S, Bromet EJ: The confusion between bipolar disorder and schizophrenia in youth: Where does it stand in the 1990s? J Am Acad Child Adolesc Psychiatry 33:453–460, 1994
29. Carlson GA, Kashani JH: Manic symptoms in a non-referred adolescent population. J Affect Disord 15:219–226, 1988
30. Carlson GA, Strober M: Manic-depressive illness in early adolescence: A study of clinical and diagnostic characteristics in six cases. J Am Acad Child Adolesc Psychiatry 17:138–153, 1978
31. Chambers WJ, Puig-Antich J, Hirsch M, et al: The assessment of affective disorders in children and adolescents by semistructured interview. Arch Gen Psychiatry 42:696–702, 1985
32. Coryell W, Norten SG: Mania during adolescence: The pathoplastic significance of age. J Nerv Ment Dis 168:611–613, 1980
33. Costello AJ, Edelbrook C, Kalas R, et al: The NIMH Diagnostic Interview Schedule for Children (DISC). Pittsburgh, Pergamon Press, 1982

34. Davis RE: Manic-depressive variant syndrome in childhood: A preliminary report. Am J Psychiatry 136:702–706, 1979
35. Denicoff KD, Smith-Jackson EE, Bryan AL, et al: Valproate prophylaxis in a prospective clinical trial of refractory bipolar disorder. Am J Psychiatry 154:1456–1458, 1997
36. Denicoff KD, Smith-Jackson EE, Disney ER, et al: Comparative prophylactic efficacy of lithium, carbamazepine, and the combination in bipolar disorder. J Clin Psychiatry 58:470–478, 1997
37. Dooley J, Camfield P, Gordon K, et al: Lamotrigine-induced rash in children. Neurology 46:240–242, 1996
38. Esquirol E: Mental Maladies: A Treatise on Insanity. Philadelphia, Lea & Blanchard, 1845
39. Fatemi SH, Rapport DJ, Calabrese JR, et al: Lamotrigine in rapid-cycling bipolar disorder. J Clin Psychiatry 58:522–527, 1997
40. Feighner JP, Robins E, Guze SB, et al: Diagnostic criteria for use in psychiatric research. Arch Gen Psychiatry 26:57–63, 1972
41. Fristad M, Weller E, Weller RA: The Mania Rating Scale: Can it be used in children? A preliminary report. J Am Acad Child Adolesc Psychiatry 31:252–257, 1992
42. Fristad MA, Weller RA, Weller EB: The Mania Rating Scale (MRS): Further reliability and validity studies with children. Ann Clin Psychiatry 7:127–132, 1995
43. Geller B, Cooper TB, Sun K, et al: Double-blind and placebo-controlled study of lithium for adolescent bipolar disorders with secondary substance dependency. J Am Acad Child Adolesc Psychiatry 37:171–178, 1998
44. Geller B, Fox LW, Clark KA: Rate and predictors of prepubertal bipolarity during follow-up of 6- to 12-year-old depressed children. J Am Acad Child Adolesc Psychiatry 33:461–468, 1994
45. Geller B, Luby J: Child and adolescent bipolar disorder: A review of the past 10 years [see comments] [published erratum appears in J Am Acad Child Adolesc Psychiatry 36:1642, 1997]. J Am Acad Child Adolesc Psychiatry 36:1168–1176, 1997
46. Geller B, Sun K, Zimerman B, et al: Complex and rapid-cycling in bipolar children and adolescents: A preliminary study. J Affect Disord 34:259–268, 1995
47. Geller B, Warner K, Williams M, et al: Prepubertal and young adolescent bipolarity versus ADHD: Assessment and validity using the WASH-U-KSADS, CBCL, and TRF. J Affect Disord 51:93–100, 1998
48. Geller B, Williams M, Zimerman B, et al: Prepubertal and early adolescent bipolarity differentiate from ADHD by manic symptoms; grandiose delusions; ultra-rapid or ultradian cycling. J Affect Disord 51:81–91, 1998
49. Ghaemi SN, Katzow JJ, Desai SP, et al: Gabapentin treatment of mood disorders: A preliminary study. J Clin Psychiatry 59:426–429, 1998
50. Ghaemi SN, Sachs GS: Long-term risperidone treatment in bipolar disorder: 6-month follow up. Int Clin Psychopharmacol 12:333–338, 1997
51. Ghaemi SN, Sachs GS, Baldassano CF, et al: Acute treatment of bipolar disorder with adjunctive risperidone in outpatients. Can J Psychiatry 42:196–199, 1997
52. Goodwin FK, Jamison KR: Manic-Depressive Illness. New York, Oxford University Press, 1990
53. Greil W, Ludwig-Mayerhoffer W, Erazo N, et al: Lithium versus carbamazepine in the maintenance treatment of bipolar disorders—a randomized study. J Affect Disord 43:151–161, 1997
54. Hagino OR, Weller EB, Weller RA, et al: Comparison of lithium dosage methods for preschool- and early school-age children. J Am Acad Child Adolesc Psychiatry 37:60–65, 1998
55. Hagino OR, Weller EB, Weller RA, et al: Untoward effects of lithium treatment in children aged four through six years. J Am Acad Child Adolesc Psychiatry 34:1584–1590, 1995
56. Irwin M, Masand P: Valproate and polycystic ovaries [letter, comment]. J Am Acad Child Adolesc Psychiatry 37:9–10, 1998
57. Isojarvi JI, Laatikainen TJ, Pakarinen AJ, et al: Polycystic ovaries and hyperandrogenism in women taking valproate for epilepsy. N Engl J Med 329:1383–1388, 1993

58. Janicak PG, Sharma RP, Pandey G, et al: Verapamil for the treatment of acute mania: A double blind, placebo-controlled trial. Am J Psychiatry 155:972–973, 1998
59. Kafantaris V: Treatment of bipolar disorder in children and adolescents. J Am Acad Child Adolesc Psychiatry 34:732–741, 1995
60. Kafantaris V, Campbell M, Padron-Gayol MV, et al: Carbamazepine in hospitalized aggressive conduct disorder children: An open pilot study [published erratum appears in Psychopharmacol Bull 28:220, 1992]. Psychopharmacol Bull 28:193–199, 1992
61. Kanner L: The development and present status of psychiatry in pediatrics. J Pediatr 11:418–435, 1937
62. Kasanin J: The affective psychoses in children. Am J Psychiatry 10:897–926, 1931
63. Kimura S, Fujito T, Wakabayashi T: On adolescent manic-depressive psychosis: Long-term observation and follow-up study. Folia Psychiatr Neurol Jpn 34:433–450, 1980
64. Knoll J, Stegman K, Suppes T: Clinical experience using gabapentin adjunctively in patients with a history of mania or hypomania. J Affect Disord 49:229–233, 1998
65. Konig SA, Siemes H, Blaker F, et al: Severe hepatotoxicity during valproate therapy: An update and report of eight new fatalities. Epilepsia 35:1005–1015, 1994
66. Kovacs M: The Interview Schedule for Children. Psychopharmacol Bull 21:991–994, 1978
67. Kovacs M, Pollock M: Bipolar disorder and comorbid conduct disorder in childhood and adolescence. J Am Acad Child Adolesc Psychiatry 34:715–723, 1995
68. Kraepelin E: Mixed states. *In* Manic-Depressive Insanity and Paranoia. Edinburgh, E & S Livingston Ltd, 1921
69. Krasa NR, Tolbert HA: Adolescent bipolar disorder: A nine-year experience. J Affect Disord 30:175–184, 1994
70. Kusumakar V, Yatham LN: An open study of lamotrigine in refractory bipolar depression. Psychiatry Res 72:145–148, 1997
71. Kusumakar V, Yatham LN: Lamotrigine treatment of rapid cycling bipolar disorder [letter, comment]. Am J Psychiatry 154:1171–1172, 1997
72. Lee DO, Steingard RJ, Cesena M, et al: Behavioral side effects of gabapentin in children. Epilepsia 37:87–90, 1996
73. Lewinsohn PM, Klein DN, Seeley JR: Bipolar disorders in a community sample of older adolescents: Prevalence, phenomenology, comorbidity, and course. J Am Acad Child Adolesc Psychiatry 34:454–463, 1995
74. Lindhout D, Omtzigt JG, Cornel MC: Spectrum of neural-tube defects in 34 infants prenatally exposed to antiepileptic drugs. Neurology 42:111–118, 1992
75. Lish JD, Dime-Meenan S, Whybrow PC, et al: The National Depressive and Manic-Depressive Association (DMDA) survey of bipolar members. J Affect Disord 31:281–294, 1994
76. Loranger A, Levine P: Age at onset of bipolar affective illness. Arch Gen Psychiatry 35:1345–1348, 1978
77. Mackay FJ, Wilton LV, Pearce GL, et al: Safety of long-term lamotrigine in epilepsy. Epilepsia 38:881–886, 1997
78. MacKinnon DF, Jamison KR, DePaulo JR: Genetics of manic depressive illness. Annu Rev Neurosci 20:355–373, 1997
79. Mahmood T, Devlin M, Silverstone T: Clozapine in the management of bipolar and schizoaffective manic episodes resistant to standard treatment. Aust NZ J Psychiatry 31:424–426, 1997
80. Malone RP, Delaney MA, Luebbert JF, et al: The lithium test dose prediction method in aggressive children. Psychopharmacol Bull 31:379–382, 1995
81. McClellan JM, Werry JS, Ham M: A follow-up study of early onset psychosis: Comparison between outcome diagnoses of schizophrenia, mood disorders, and personality disorders. J Autism Dev Disord 23:243–262, 1993
82. McElroy SL, Soutullo CA, Keck PE Jr, et al: A pilot trial of adjunctive gabapentin in the treatment of bipolar disorder. Ann Clin Psychiatry 9:99–103, 1997
83. McElroy SL, Strakowski SM, West SA, et al: Phenomonology of adolescent and adult mania in hospitalized patients with bipolar disorder. Am J Psychiatry 154:44–49, 1997
84. McGlashan TH: Adolescent versus adult onset of mania. Am J Psychiatry 145:221–223, 1988

85. Messenheimer J, Mullens EL, Giorgi L, et al: Safety review of adult clinical trial experience with lamotrigine. Drug Saf 18:281–296, 1998
86. Meyer A: Collected Papers of Adolf Meyer. Baltimore, Johns Hopkins Press, 1952
87. Myers WC, Carrera F 3rd: Carbamazepine-induced mania with hypersexuality in a 9-year-old boy [letter]. Am J Psychiatry 146:400, 1989
88. Olsen T: Follow-up study of manic-depressive patients whose first attack occurred before the age of 19. Acta Psychiatr Scand 162(suppl):45–51, 1961
89. Papatheodorou G, Kutcher SP: Divalproex sodium treatment in late adolescent and young adult acute mania. Psychopharmacol Bull 29:213–219, 1993
90. Papatheodorou G, Kutcher SP, Katic M, et al: The efficacy and safety of divalproex sodium in the treatment of acute mania in adolescents and young adults: An open clinical trial. J Clin Psychopharmacol 15:110–116, 1995
91. Pauls DL, Morton LA, Egeland JA: Risks of affective illness among first degree relatives of bipolar I old-order Amish probands. Arch Gen Psychiatry 49:703–708, 1992
92. Pope HG Jr, McElroy SL, Keck PE Jr, et al: Valproate in the treatment of acute mania: A placebo-controlled study. Arch Gen Psychiatry 48:62–68, 1991
93. Popper C: Biological cyclicity in two preschool children. Paper presented at the 137th Annual Meeting of the American Psychiatric Association, Los Angeles, 1984
94. Poznanski EO: Mania in preschool children with case vignette and videotape: Questions and answers. Presented at American Psychiatric Association 146th annual meeting, San Francisco, May 22–27, 1993
95. Poznanski EO, Israel MC, Grossman J: Hypomania in a four-year-old. J Am Acad Child Psychiatry 23:105–110, 1984
96. Prien RF, Potter WZ: NIMH workshop report on treatment of bipolar disorder. Psychopharmacol Bull 26:409–427, 1990
97. Rao U, Ryan ND, Birmaher B, et al: Unipolar depression in adolescents: Clinical outcome in adulthood. J Am Acad Child Adolesc Psychiatry 34:566–578, 1995
98. Reich W, Weiner Z: Diagnostic Interview for Children and Adolescents (DICA-R-C), DSMIII III-R Version. St. Louis, Washington University, Division of Child Psychiatry (unpublished)
99. Reiss AL, O'Donnell DJ: Carbamazepine-induced mania in two children: Case report. J Clin Psychiatry 45:272–274, 1984
100. Rice J, Reich T, Andreasen NC, et al: The familial transmission of bipolar illness. Arch Gen Psychiatry 44:441–447, 1987
101. Rich CL, Sherman M, Fowler RC: San Diego suicide study: The adolescents. Adolescence 25:856–865, 1990
102. Rich CL, Young D, Fowler RC: San Diego Suicide Study: I. Young vs. old subjects. Arch Gen Psychiatry 43:577–582, 1986
103. Segal J, Berk M, Brook S: Risperidone compared with both lithium and haloperidol in mania: A double-blind randomized controlled trial. Clin Neuropharmacol 21:176–180, 1998
104. Silva RR, Campbell M, Golden RR, et al: Side effects associated with lithium and placebo administration in aggressive children. Psychopharmacol Bull 28:319–326, 1992
105. Simhandl C, Denk E, Thau K: The comparative efficacy of carbamazepine low and high serum level and lithium carbonate in the prophylaxis of affective disorders. J Affect Disord 28:221–231, 1993
106. Small JG, Klapper MH, Milstein V, et al: Carbamazepine compared with lithium in the treatment of mania. Arch Gen Psychiatry 48:915–921, 1991
107. Soutullo CA, Casuto LS, Keck PE Jr: Gabapentin in the treatment of adolescent mania: a case report. J Child Adolesc Psychopharmacol 8:81–85, 1998
108. Sporn J, Sachs G: The anticonvulsant lamotrigine in treatment-resistant manic-depressive illness. J Clin Psychopharmacol 17:185–189, 1997
109. Strober M: Relevance of early age-of-onset in genetic studies of bipolar affective disorder. J Am Acad Child Adolesc Psychiatry 31:606–610, 1992
110. Strober M, Carlson G: Bipolar illness in adolescents with major depression: Clinical, genetic, and psychopharmacologic predictors in a 3- to 4-year prospective follow-up. Arch Gen Psychiatry 39:549–555, 1982
111. Strober M, Hanna G, McCracken J: Bipolar disorder. *In* Last CG, Hersen M (eds):

Handbook of Child Psychiatric Diagnoses. New York, John Wiley & Sons, 1989, pp 229–316
112. Strober M, Morrell W, Burroughs J, et al: A family study of bipolar I disorder in adolescence: Early onset of symptoms linked to increased familial loading and lithium resistance. J Affect Disord 15:255–268, 1988
113. Strober M, Schmidt-Lackner S, Freeman R, et al: Recovery and relapse in adolescents with bipolar affective illness: A five-year naturalistic, prospective follow-up. J Am Acad Child Adolesc Psychiatry 34:724–731, 1995
114. Tallian KB, Nahata MC, Lo W, et al: Gabapentin associated with aggressive behavior in pediatric patients with seizures. Epilepsia 37:501–502, 1996
115. Todd RD, Neuman R, Geller B, et al: Genetic studies of affective disorders: Should we be starting with childhood onset probands? J Am Acad Child Adolesc Psychiatry 32:1164–1171, 1993
116. Todd RD, Reich W, Reich T: Prevalence of affective disorders in the child and adolescent offspring of a single kindred: A pilot study. J Am Acad Child Adolesc Psychiatry 33:198–207, 1994
117. Tohen M, Zarate CA Jr, Centorrino F, et al: Risperidone in the treatment of mania. J Clin Psychiatry 57:249–253, 1996
118. Varanka TM, Weller RA, Weller EB, et al: Lithium treatment of manic episodes with psychotic features in prepubertal children. Am J Psychiatry 145:1557–1559, 1988
119. Walden J, Hesslinger B, van Calker D, et al: Addition of lamotrigine to valproate may enhance efficacy in the treatment of bipolar affective disorder. Pharmacopsychiatry 29:193–195, 1996
120. Weinberg WA, Brumback RA: Mania in childhood: Case studies and literature review. Am J Dis Child 130:380–385, 1976
121. Weller EB, Weller RA, Fristad MA: Bipolar disorder in children: Misdiagnosis, underdiagnosis, and future directions. J Am Acad Child Adolesc Psychiatry 34:709–714, 1995
122. Weller EB, Weller RA, Teare M, et al: Children's Interview for Psychiatric Syndromes (ChIPS). Washington, DC, American Psychiatric Press 1999
123. Weller RA, Weller EB, Tucker SG, et al: Mania in prepubertal children: Has it been underdiagnosed? J Affect Disord 11:151–154, 1986
124. Werry JS, McClellan JM, Chard L: Childhood and adolescent schizophrenic, bipolar, and schizoaffective disorders: A clinical and outcome study. J Am Acad Child Adolesc Psychiatry 30:457–465, 1991
125. White JH, O'Shanick G: Juvenile manic-depressive illness. Am J Psychiatry 134:1035–1036, 1977
126. Wolf SM, Shinnar S, Kang H, et al: Gabapentin toxicity in children manifesting as behavioral changes. Epilepsia 36:1203–1205, 1995
127. Wozniak J, Biederman J, Kiely K, et al: Mania-like symptoms suggestive of childhood-onset bipolar disorder in clinically referred children. J Am Acad Child Adolesc Psychiatry 34:867–876, 1995
128. Young LT, Robb JC, Patelis-Siotis I, et al: Acute treatment of bipolar depression with gabapentin. Biol Psychiatry 42:851–853, 1997
129. Young RC, Biggs JT, Ziegler VE, et al: A rating scale for mania: Reliability, validity, and sensitivity. Br J Psychiatry 133:434, 1978

Address reprint requests to

Laura Sanchez, MD
The Children's Hospital of Philadelphia
Department of Child & Adolescent Psychiatry
34th Street and Civic Center Boulevard
Philadelphia, PA 19104

APPENDIX 1

Clinical Case Summary

The following case report highlights some of the clinical characteristics of bipolar disorder in childhood.

CHIEF COMPLAINT AND HISTORY OF PRESENT ILLNESS

This was the second psychiatric evaluation for a 6 year-9 month-old Caucasian boy who was brought by his mother for a diagnostic evaluation because of "mood swings," "erratic behavior" at home and at school, and anxiety. According to his mother, the child had been experiencing almost "continuous, drastic mood swings" for the past 1½ years. His mother expressed concern about his frequent crying, "clinginess" towards her, initial insomnia, and prolonged temper tantrums over minor incidents. In addition, he worried that he was going to die and he displayed checking behaviors. He would check on his mother to make sure she was all right, and repeatedly checked to make sure he had closed doors and covered his sandbox. His mother reported that he was "negative about everything." He felt everything was someone else's fault and that no one liked him. Over the past several months his behavior in school had become more problematic. Although he was doing well academically, he was reported to have "periods" during which he had difficulty focusing, sitting still, and was defiant. He was not getting along with peers at school because he was loud, demanding, "annoying" and would "tease them to get their attention." His mother complained that behavioral modification had been ineffective in changing his behavior and that the family was at a loss as to what to do.

PAST PSYCHIATRIC HISTORY

At the age of 3 years-3 months, the child's mother returned to work and the child was placed two days a week with a baby sitter. Initially everything was fine, but when the baby-sitter began to care for a 5-week old infant, the child developed behavioral problems. He began to "act out." He was unhappy, stopped napping and ran around uncontrollably. The baby-sitter asked that he be removed from her home. The child was subsequently placed 5 days a week in a private nursery school. There were 18 other children in his class. In this setting his behavior was not reported to be problematic. Although the child continued to resist napping, he slept well at night. His teacher reportedly described him as well-focused, outgoing, and well-liked by peers. He was reported to have difficulty at times "gaining control of himself after an exciting activity." Furthermore, he was reported to be overly afraid of fire alarms and elevators. His parents sought consultation from a pediatric neurologist who reassured them that the child's behavior was within normal limits for a 3½-year-old child and that since he was doing well in his new school setting, there was no need for further intervention.

At the age of 5½ years, the child had a "nervous breakdown." His mother reports a "dramatic change" in his behavior, which she feels was brought on by his maternal grandfather's moving away. The child could not stop talking. He became very distractible, loud and "speedy." He could not sit still. He could not sleep; he would go to bed at 1 a.m. and get up by 6:00 a.m. His energy level was high. "He had to be in control and became very demanding." He became physically aggressive towards his mother and she needed to physically restrain him to prevent him from hurting her. His mood was very labile; he would alternate between crying and laughing inappropriately. He was convinced his grandfather no longer loved him. These symptoms persisted for approximately 6 weeks and then improved but have never completely subsided. He was evaluated by a psychologist who diagnosed the child with an *adjustment disorder* with mixed features of emotions and conduct. He was treated in play therapy for 6 months but his behavior never returned to baseline. He was subsequently evaluated by a psychiatrist and diagnosed with Anxiety Disorder NOS. As part of this evaluation he was seen by a psychologist who conducted psychoeducational testing. In his report the psychologist commented that the child appeared anxious, needed to be in control, and was easily frustrated. He displayed disinhibition, for example asking the psychologist personal questions. He attempted to impress the psychologist with his competence, becoming defensive if he felt threatened. His full-scale IQ score on the WISC-R was 108 (verbal IQ 111; performance IQ 104). He was reported to perform better than average on tests of attention and concentration. The psychologist recommended intensive twice weekly psychotherapy.

At 6½ years, the child was evaluated by a pediatric neurologist who diagnosed him with ADHD and mild oppositionality and initiated a trial of Ritalin. The child had a paradoxical reaction to his first dose of Ritalin. He became more hostile and hyperactive. His mother complained, "It magnified all his behaviors." He "hyperverbalized," and "ran around the room screaming, 'I'm going crazy, I'm going crazy, please make it stop.' " The medicine was discontinued and no other medications were initiated.

MEDICAL HISTORY AND REVIEW OF SYMPTOMS

Past medical history was significant for chronic ear infections as an infant and asthma. Review of symptoms was negative.

DEVELOPMENTAL HISTORY

The child was the product of a full-term, uncomplicated pregnancy and vaginal delivery. He weighed 7 lb 4 oz at birth. He had difficulty with jaundice perinatally and was treated with phototherapy. He was described as an average baby; he ate and slept well. He reached his developmental milestones on time. His behavior was reported to be more difficult after the age of 3 years.

SOCIAL HISTORY

He lives with his mother and father. Both parents are employed in the field of special education. He is an only child. He has no good friends. His mother reported that he would like to make friends and can engage children but has difficulty maintaining friendships because of his controlling manner: "He is annoying and loud." There was no history of physical or sexual abuse.

FAMILY PSYCHIATRIC HISTORY

The child's paternal grandfather has been diagnosed with bipolar disorder and is treated with lithium. His paternal grandmother was described as a worrier and highly anxious. His father has a history of depression and panic attacks, for which he has received treatment with Zoloft; he was described as moody and irritable.

MENTAL STATUS EXAMINATION

This child was alert and oriented to time, place, and person. He displayed no abnormal movements but was mildly psychomotorically activated. He was loud and extremely talkative. He interrupted conversations but was not interruptible himself. He initially was not cooperative with the interview. He did not believe the doctor had a right to interview him. He claimed his uncle owned the hospital and the university and had given it to him. The doctor therefore worked for him. He later consented to an interview: "Okay, ask me your questions" and began to change the doctor's name to words that rhymed with the doctor's real name. He was easily distracted. He denied that he had any problems and became irritable when challenged, stating, "I'm finished now". He commented several times on how attractive the receptionists were, as well as the women in the billing department. He said he would like to get to know them all better. He denied hallucinations, thought insertion, thought broadcasting and ideas of reference. His insight and judgement were fair. He was above average in intelligence.

SUMMARY

This child presented with a history of irritability, dysphoria, impulsivity, hyperactivity, anxiety, grandiosity, push of speech, sleep disturbance, and "out-of-control" behavior. These symptoms occurred with disabling intensity at ages 5 and 6½ years. Although he had symptoms of ADHD before age 7, these were present episodically and only occurred in the context of significant mood disturbance and behavior disruption. His oppositionality had a grandiose quality to it. His attention and comments on the physical attractiveness of women is unusual behavior for a young child who has not been sexually abused or overstimulated. He had a paradoxical reaction to low dose Ritalin that exacerbated rather than helped his symptomatology. This patient's symptoms in the face of significant family history of mood disorder are much more characteristic of a mood disorder than ADHD.

British Journal of Medical Psychology (1998), 71, 375–395 *Printed in Great Britain* 375

Evolutionary epidemiology and manic depression

Daniel R. Wilson
The Lewis Centre, 1101 Summit Road, Cincinnati, OH 45237, USA

The reformulation of epidemiological prevalence rates as evolutionary frequency rates puts medical genetics within an explicit framework of Darwinian theory. Yet an enduring and still current assumption of genomic medicine is that genes associated with disease are necessarily maladapted. Indeed, it seems it could hardly be otherwise. However, evolutionary epidemiology has begun to uncover important and surprising counter-exemplary case-studies. Thus, the present aim is to first outline this emerging sub-discipline of 'evolutionary epidemiology'. Then, a major psychopathological syndrome—manic-depression—is examined in some detail within the purview of evolutionary epidemiology. Its medical genetics are those of an adaptive polymorphism in the human genome. Hence, genes associated with what is now a major public health problem accrued as they conferred selective advantage in phylogeny. Why should manic-depressive etiogenes have been selected? A preliminary anatomic–functional model, assembled from facts of human paleoneuropsychiatry, more adequately contextualises manic-depressive genomics and phenotypy. In this model, manic-depression finds its heuristic origins in a hierarchy of behavioural strategies stabilised in phylogeny and embedded at serial levels in the brain (Hawk–Dove ESS). A proportion of the population has variant genotypy which appears to have been favoured in social competition phylogenetically but express more pathogenic phenotypy in the current environment. The paper closes with a brief consideration of clinical practices and ethical issues as alternative considerations emerge with the syndrome recast in a more positive Darwinian light.

The paucity of evolutionary genetical analysis in medical and psychiatric research despite its probable utility

The current state of scientific and philosophical orientation for most biomedical theory and practice is not adequate to even ask, much less answer, deep questions of phylogenetic aetiology. Much biomedical science lacks a coherence to be adduced from its mongering of study design, outcome curves and other enthusiasms of the currently reigning, largely inductive philosophy. Conventional wisdom holds that deep concerns are to be pursued only by persons without practical things to say. It is perhaps better to make a minor inductive advance than risk a crashing deductive error. Theory, when robust, can be of sufficient coherence to yield quantitative data or, at least, crisp qualitative incongruencies. These, in turn, can lead to insights which, being both counter-intuitive and non-obvious, would never be appreciated by mere experiment, no matter how clever.

Within psychiatric research these problems are only magnified. Psychiatry, lacking as

* Requests for reprints (e-mail: wilson@fuse.net).

it does, both a foundations theory and cogently integrated intellectual aims, in certain respects has become a pastiche of arid facts, abstruse ideological claims and grandiose speculations. This leads, ineluctably, to the trap in which psychiatry all too often trips up: its surfeit of plausible but contradictory explanations which cannot be properly sorted out for lack of any encompassing framework. Yet psychiatrists have long had available one such framework beginning with Darwin's elegantly reasoned theory of evolution. It is particularly difficult to sort out historical questions (such as the past function of phenotypes and the selection of their genes in the environment of their evolution) since experimental observation is constrained, largely, to modern environmental circumstances.

Empirical studies of course would be quite valuable. Unfortunately, ambitious cross-cultural epidemiology of rigorous reliability and validity might constitute a robust database. These are nigh non-existent. It is, moreover, unlikely the few remaining foraging cultures shall be compared with industrial ones before the former are either extinct or grossly contaminated with diffusionist phenomena (Galton, 1884). It would be useful to enlarge the comparisons to include cross-genus studies of the primated as well as other relevant ethology. The prospect for such inductive studies is limited. Induction is, in any event, a dubious approach in the sphere of comprehensive biology, which is nowhere yet systematized as a science (Kendrew, 1978). Darwinism is, therefore, of probable utility in psychiatric research. At the very least it is otherwise quite difficult to experiment with, much less prove, that evolutionarily useful features of major disorders exist since these illnesses are viewed with respect to modern environs and cultural circumstances.

One place to begin is with the sure Darwinian deduction that common, genetically simple pathological syndromes must be the residua of positive adaptation. Such lineages were adaptive at least before the rise of civilization since spontaneous maladaptations cannot surpass thresholds of surprisingly low prevalence. This seems especially true in the realm of disorders that arose phylogenetically from genes expressing a variety of neurobiological sensitivities and talents. The modern environment may sometimes induce among individuals newer, more vulnerable and less adaptive phenotypes.

A method of evolutionary epidemiological analysis

Disorders that are clinically well-validated, nosologically reliable, epigenetic and common are amenable to reanalysis within the framework of evolutionary epidemiology (Wilson, 1992, 1993, 1994). Indeed, it would seem that any epigenetic medical or psychiatric disorder which attains prevalence higher than basic theorems of evolutionary genetics predict thereby satisfies the two prime conditions of hypothetico-deductive inference at the heart of evolutionary epidemiology. That is, common genes can be generally inferred to have been selected on the basis of advantageous characteristics. The strengthening of such inferences is a major application of evolutionary epidemiology. One such strong inference is the almost inescapable deduction that some syndromes of biomedical pathology held benefits in the course of evolution (and may yet confer advantage).

Epidemiology is, one recalls, a science of disease which specifies rates (illness prevalences, incidences, distributions, etc.). Evolution is a science of life which specifies changes (gene frequencies, generations, forms, functions, etc.). Evolutionary epidemiology is a deductive synthesis of these two sciences which combines the empirical power of classical observations in genetical epidemiology with the interpretive capacities of neo-Darwinian evolutionary genetics. Novel conclusions are thus derived from primary data integrated from these two sciences. In particular, prevalence rates of genetical disease are important data points when reformulated for the purpose of analysis in terms of their evolutionary frequencies. Traits which exceed prevalences beyond frequency of mutation (in Hardy–Weinberg or biometrical calculations are even more complex mixed models) or evidence an unusual range of phenotype reaction are also of special interest.

The 'algebra' of evolutionary epidemiological analysis

The integration of evolutionary (population) genetics theory with epidemiology consitutes a new subdiscipline which, in turn, extends basic tools of Darwinian genetics towards an ultimate biological explantion of some 'diseases' as expressions of much more normative biological mechanisms. From all this directly follows the hypothesis that much illness is caused by phenotypic 'friction' arising as abiding hominoid genes react with the more recent and brisk rise of human civilization. This appears true because only traits which conferred advantages in the environment of evolutionary adaptation accede to significant rates of genomic prevalence. These deductive methods can be used to test the hypothesis that some 'diseases' have been promoted in the course of natural selection due to intrinsic, if obscure, advantages.

The relative irrelevance of modes of transmission

The assumption may arise that evolutionary epidemiological analysis can only be used for similarly Mendelian syndromes. This is not the case. Whether pathological predispositions are coded as Mendelian dominant, recessive or even multigene systems is not in itself crucial to deductive analysis. Traits need only to be epigenetic and common to be made amenable to the analytical tools of evolutionary epidemiology.

Clearly, Mendelian dominance with strong penetrance is the most crisp mechanism of putative transmission. Therefore it would also be the most amenable to analyses deducing that positive selection was a needed condition to establish prevalence beyond an estimable threshold. Necessary threshold rates of genetic prevalence are the lowest. Most technical studies are simpler than is the case with other modes of transmission. Implications are the most striking: genes coding for disease vulnerability evolved via selective advantage of other as yet underappreciated traits. A spectrum of trait expression in various phenotypes is largely a function of the degree of penetrance.

Recessive transmission is somewhat more complex and requires higher prevalence to substantiate past positive selective advantage. Recessivity also requires modifications of the hypothesis to account for heterosis. An example of such hybrid vigour occurs in the classic phenomenon of high sickle cell anaemia with the selective scenario being that a single recessive trait was adaptive (whereas homozygosity was unfortunate maldaptive genetic loading). Trait expression is on a spectrum at two levels and dependent on zygosity as well as phenotypic variation.

More complex polygenic models of transmission are not implausible. However, they do become increasingly cumbersome and less likely relevant in hypothetical positive evolutionary scenarios. The more genes, alleles and complex interactions, the higher the threshold of prevalence needed to establish that positive and non-random selection was responsible. For example, syndromes with complex and weak genetic roots, such as the senile diabetes or dementias, appear to have not accrued through positive evolution. Several evolutionary scenarios by which newly diseased phenotypes may emerge can be modelled. These include (1) discrete Mendelian traits, whether dominant or heterozygotic, (2) continuous polygenic traits, and (3) more complex mixed, composite or multifactorial systems. These models all presuppose that prevalence rates in epidemiological studies are, with minor adjustments, equivalent to frequency rates for evolutionary calculations.

Therefore, *the frequency threshold which a genetic locus can surpass only via selection* equals the net *prevalence divided by equilibrium*. Rarely, non-Darwinian or other factors may have prevailed, e.g. drift, neutral linkage selection, mutability, phenocopy, assortative mating, etc. Otherwise, genes which attain such thresholds were not pathological in the environment of evolutionary adaptation:

$$(\mathrm{Pdg})/(\mathrm{Egf}) = (\mathrm{Sgt}): \qquad (1)$$

(disease gene prevalence)/(equilibrium frequency) = (gene selection threshold)

With the redundant genetical terms deleted this yields

(prevalence of disease)/(equilibrium frequency) = (selection threshold)

Or more generally:

$$P/E = S$$

Of course, evolutionary mechanisms typically require aeons of favourable selections for new mutations or simple gene systems to obtain epidemiology prevalence at rates much above one-half per cent. The precise rate of prevalence involves technical adjustments for rates of such things as mutation, back-mutation, fertility, drift, and assumes broadly stable environmental conditions. Similarly, epidemiological prevalence rates must be adjusted by such factors as the degree of identical twin concordance, phenocopy events and so on. Still, as noted above, if a simple gene system occurs to such a degree it was (though not necessarily, is) abidingly adaptive, *ipso facto* spontaneous maladaptations cannot achieve such prevalence (Fisher, 1930; Wilson & Bossert, 1971).

In a classic Darwinian system, evolutionary selective value must be presumed to have existed at the genomic population level where genetic alleles of high prevalence covary with the manifestation of individual disease. This if the case in the absence of drift due to linkage or similar random non-Darwinian events. An important deduction follows in consequence of this fact—any common, epigenetic pathology had a likely 'silver-lining' to be best appreciated in the context of ancestral environs. The task of establishing a proper phylogenetic perspective, though daunting, is as central to genomic analysis as are the vantages of molecular or cellular biology.

To reveal any such Darwinian advantages, attention must first focus on how genes now expressing pathology operated in the natural environment of past evolutionary adaptation. Subsequently the phylogenetic 'how', 'why', 'when' and 'what' can be considered. All this is difficult to do. Certainly, it is not easy to recalibrate views formed in the contemporary world to the conditions which prevailed in prehistory. Clinicians, in particular, suffer an ethnocentrism of time. It is quite difficult to imagine phenotypes as they would have emerged in the environment of evolutionary adaptation when one knows little about that environment. This is a crucial step before attention can then focus on whether any salutary features of these genes are expressed in the current environment. This must be considered in any enlightened clinical practice or public policy (viz. genetic counselling including selective abortion).

Clinicians, in particular, often cannot separate evolutionary epidemiological insights from the interesting but separate and far more complex question as to whether genes find adaptive, maladaptive or neutral phenotypic expression in the environs of contemporary development. If genes are rather common and simple then there is little question they were positively selected. This is, however, an entirely different matter than how they are now being selected, much less when, where, why, what and how such selection took place. Anthropologists and geneticists commonly are inclined to something of an evolutionary perspective. Physicians rarely are. Having been taught about disease, they cannot readily reorient to the notion that certain syndromes may be more precisely regarded as stories of Darwinian success.

Of course, questions of current selection, if any, are to be answered only by long and painstaking research. Indeed, some of the best validated and reliably diagnosed medical and psychiatric disorders may satisfy the requisite conditions of genetic mediation and high prevalence. So, hypotheses about certain disorders can be posited wherever there exists substantive data on the genetics and epidemiology of a given disease. At this juncture the evolutionary epidemiology of sickle cell anaemia is instructive.

A prototype in medicine: Sickle cell anaemia

An illustrative case might more directly sustain the idea that what is today thought of as disease can have been advantageous. Sickle cell anaemia is a benchmark example in which, counter-intuitive thought it seems, genes expressing a pathological medical syndrome attained a high population frequency due to the Darwinian selection of advantages sustained in the environment of their evolutionary adaptation.

Such a point of reference as this, simple enough to state, has profound consequences. Not the least of these consequences is the way in which the definition of disease itself becomes context dependent and subject to significant reappraisals within evolutionary perspective. A thorough going review of this as it relates to sickle cell anaemia, neither necessary nor feasible within the present aims, is otherwise available (Kettlewell, 1958). What is here notable is that research concerning human haemoglobin polymorphisms and related anaemia syndromes is now more widely seen as the first and surely the most well-known example of what is here termed evolutionary epidemiology.

Reliable and valid epidemiology, when coupled with theorems of population genetics, permits a meaningful reconstruction of the evolutionary scenario by which positive selective forces in the past account for the contemporary distribution of alleles. In all of medicine, the investigations concerning sickle cell haemoglobinopathy exemplifies the materials and methods by which evolutionary epidemiological analysis proceeds. For the present discussion, it is sufficient to briefly outline relevant research on sickle cell anaemia to conclude that, *in toto*, the syndrome demonstrates much of the increased allelic frequency of anomalous haemoglobins served to counterbalance the selective pressure of malaria.

With the widespread use of modern haematological screening over the past 40 years, the populational features of haemoglobin anomalies have become one of the most intensively studied elements of human biochemistry (Livingstone, 1958, 1964, 1967, 1969). By the early 1950s it was clear a variety of anomalous haemoglobins existed in high frequencies in specific human populations. These high frequencies were found almost exclusively in tropical and subtropical climes. Neel (1950) first noted how such high frequencies must be due to either high rates of mutation or conditions favouring heterozygotes.

Allison (1954 *a,b,c*) provided the first case evidence that such haemoglobinopathies covaried with population areas in which malaria was endemic. Allison's original work is useful despite the fact that selective advantage is not definitely proven. While there are residual problems with this model, these are of a technical nature and do not grossly undermine the point that genetic traits regarded as pathological by medical researchers may be the residua of what, in evolutionary terms, were successful products of Darwinian selection. As it happens, work on haemoglobinopathies has advanced well beyond Allison's early reports.

Subsequently, investigations confirmed that sickle cell heterozygosity is associated with improved resistance to malaria. In tandem with this haemotological research has emerged an appreciation for the Darwinian consequences of this resistance. The high frequency of alleles for anomalous haemoglobins is consistent with a selective advantage to carriers which outweighs the disadvantage to homozygote recessives. It is widely assumed there exists a casual connection; however, the mechanism is not known.

This body of work on sickle cell anaemia is relevant as it underscores that contemporary illnesses may be due to genes which were advantageous in evolutionary selection. By this example the further question is raised as to how much of human 'disease' genetics may have been promoted by natural selection of factors conferring Darwinian fitness in the environment of evolutionary adaptation. The evolutionary perspective—so crucial for the full understanding of the coevolution of haemoglobin polymorphisms and parasitical diseases endemic in the environment of evolutionary selection—may well be informative in connection with other disorders, notably manic depression.

Other 'diseases genes' may come to be seen as not intrinsically pathological or even as expressions of phylogenetic vigour. With this approach, a clearer picture of evolutionary adaptation is possible. A window on the past can be opened. The corpus of medical epidemiology can be readily reformulated as substantive data for reanalysis in evolutionary and palaeoanthropological terms. Only recently has this corpus begun to attract the interests of pathologists in a wide variety of clinical fields (Wilson, 1992). Of course, the vast majority of anomalous alleles in a population are either neutral or deleterious. They are not promoted in genomic frequency but are selected against or, in the case of neutral traits, 'ignored'. It is, therefore, crucial that the incidence of a trait be high and, further, that it be clearly epigenetic to a great degree (it need not be a Mendelian character, although such traits are more amenable to evolutionary epidemiological analysis). Only in such circumstances of significant genetic causality and prevalence can Darwinian selection by adduced, particularly that of the heterozygotic type.

There are, likewise other less common yet possible non-selectionist causes of sustained polymorphism but heterosis is the primary mechanism in natural systems (Wilson & Bossert, 1971). Certainly a given gene locus may be (for whatever reasons) highly mutable. Phenomenal mutability, though rare, is a possible cause of high frequency for traits which otherwise appear deleterious. Likewise, drift or other non-Darwinian phenomena must be considered. Heterosis *ala'* sickle cell anaemia is not the sole model, it is merely the first and most simple. Much detailed knowledge was marshalled from genetics, medicine, anthropology and other fields to arrive at a sensible explanation of these anomalies. Unfortunately, the genetics of much biomedical pathology are not known in such detail. This is especially true of many major psychiatric disorders. Nonetheless, more definitive answers as to which 'disease' genes positively evolved appear at hand as the human genome is progressively mapped.

Evolutionary epidemiological assessment of the operations of natural selection upon the phenotypic spectrum of clinical traits

The clinical and theoretical importance of evolutionary epidemiology extends to not just the physical aspect of medicine, but to the psychological realm as well. As noted above, the body of psychiatric genetic epidemiology accumulated over the past century is large and cogent. Indeed, this indirect genetic analysis has had a long and prosperous, if unpresupposing, role in psychiatric research (Goodwin & Jamison, 1990). For a variety of reasons this is especially true with respect to manic depression (Winokur, 1980).

The body of primary data deriving from psychiatric epidemiology is quite amenable to reformulation into terms appropriate for reanalysis with the theorems of population genetics. Of special interest in this body of data are the many genetic polymorphisms with significant population prevalence. Careful examination of these variant alleles may demonstrate some have been sustained by the operations of natural selection rather than transient or even random events.

Indeed, evolutionary epidemiology may require a refinement in the notion of disease itself, at least as such a label might be attached to several of the most common and genetical syndromes in medicine and especially psychiatry. Several important psychiatric conditions (manic depression, sociopathy, obsessive–compulsivity, anxiety and even drug abuse and some disorders of personality) are so common and so strongly epigenetic that their epidemiological frequencies surpass even quite conservative thresholds of evolutionary selection.

The deduction follows that such frequency thresholds were surpassed due to the Darwinian selection of genes advantageous over the course of evolution. Features inherent to these syndromes most certainly served, and perhaps still serve, useful functions in human society. This is not, necessarily, to aver that such genes now express entirely healthy phenotypes. Such would be something of a naturalistic fallacy in reverse. The current environments to which young humans are exposed and in which their phenotypes develop are, by and large, different from those in which much relevant human, primate, mammalian and reptilian ancestry achieved increasing optimal and evolutionarily stable strategies (Wilson, Stanton & Wilson, in press).

This underscores the point that the same genes which conferred advantages in the environment of evolution might, upon ontogenic exposure to new biosocial ecology, lead to deleterious phenotypes. Developmental and social forces become important aetiological factors by which the ecological cues of the modern environment *nurture nature* in emergent, not evolved, ways. The deleterious expressions of such genes are not 'genetic *qua* genetic' but only the product of gene–environment interactions. Thus, even a disease phenotype which is a 100 per cent penetrant, twin concordant and Mendelian dominant retains a component of environmental expression. This component is a function of the differences between the ideal and the real phenotypes (Wilson, 1975). These two phenotypes arise, respectively, in the environment of evolutionary adaptation (to which genome and ideal phenotype are, at equilibrium, adapted) and the environment of ontogenic adjustment (in which the genome is evoked to express the real phenotype).

All this is of importance both for palaeoanthropology and the full appreciation of continuing advantages, if any, of these 'disease' genes. Clinically, there must be potential, if latent, benefits of the ideal phenotype residual in genes now more typically expressive of diseased real phenotypes. There are, of course, further ethical, legal, social and even theological consequences to be explored with respect to these latencies and potential.

But the main objective here is to explain a method by which standard epidemiological data concerning genetical disease rates can be reanalysed from an evolutionary point of view. Again, the point of such reanalysis is to establish whether such genetical systems have accumulated over the course of evolution due to the effects of Darwinian natural selection. With the business of 'how' specified, attention can be turned in earnest to questions as to who, when, where and why all this happened (Mayr, 1963).

With this comprehensive view of genetic processes by which is expressed the modern extended phenotype (Dawkins, 1976), certain major epigenetic diseases—most notably mental illness—can be better appreciated as atavisms of previously adaptive hominoid biopatterns. An improved grasp of the adaptive essence of mental illness may well lead to their destigmatization while, also, giving rise to improved methods of rehabilitation.

Evolutionary mechanisms, generally, require aeons of favourable selections for new mutations to obtain epidemiological prevalence at substantial rates. The threshold rate is not precisely known for specific genes and involves high technical adjustments for rates of such things as mutation, back-mutation, fertility, penetrance and dominance. The calculation of threshold rates also assumes broadly stable environmental conditions, i.e. an environment of evolutionary adaptedness.

The mathematical clarification of such evolutionary dynamics is the aim of population genetics. The Hardy–Weinberg equilibrium is perhaps the fundamental theorem of population genetics as every student of evolution may remember. The equation summates genetical fluctuations across generations in a precise way to specify the net effects of evolution via natural selection (Cavalli-Sforza & Bodmer, 1976). Genes arise by mutation and are selected for or against over time. If a new gene is helpful enough for long enough, it will accumulate. Genes at prevalences well beyond frequency of spontaneous mutation, except in decidedly unusual circumstances, were selected into the genome on the basis of positive characteristics expressed in the phenotype. They evolved.

As a rule, prevalence above the mutation rate is likely when a gene occurs in the frequency range of 1/10 000 to 1/1000 members of a population (Wilson, 1975). Therefore, in mammalian systems rates beyond 0.001 per cent are suggestive of past positive natural selection and rates beyond 0.01 per cent highly suggestive. Given average mutation rates and neutral fertility effects it is unlikely that a deleterious gene should attain a frequency of much more than 0.01 per cent. Moreover, to secrete even this random level in the genome might take many generations—up to 10 000. If a simple gene system occurs to such a degree it was, though not necessarily is, abidingly adaptive.

On the other hand, deleterious mutations cannot achieve high prevalences spontaneously nor even via neutral selection (Kimura, 1955). Consequently, the majority of inherited abnormalities should be rare as a function, more or less, of mutation rate divided by fertility and penetrance. Genetic disease should be, by definition, of very low prevalence (e.g. achondroplasia) and are often enclosed within sporadic idioethnic lines (e.g. Tay-Sachs disease). Prevalence of even a deleterious gene will equilibrate over generations at a rate balancing new mutations against the selective pressure, e.g. in achondroplasia the equilibrium frequency is one in 8000 births for what is a classical autosomal dominant condition. Tay-Sachs is seen only rarely and in certain lineages: some Ashkenazi Jews have it, Laplanders do not (Dobzhansky, 1962). Neither of these conditions evidence past positive selection and, indeed, such positive attributes are not to be predicted in the established tests of evolutionary epidemiology. Though strongly genetic, they are too rare to have been promoted by natural selection: they are counter-exemplary evolutionary 'noise' existing, more or less, at equilibrium rates.

As noted earlier, there is a limit to the range of phenotypic reactive adjustment to ecological change or novel environs. This is true whether the genes concerned were adaptive, neutral or deleterious. Beyond these limits, environmental fluctuations extrude genes which are less flexible in expressing a reproducible phenotype. Heredity does not predict the future but rather transmits the past. While future environments are presupposed to be similar to past ones, they cannot be exactly anticipated by the genome. Some genes are, however, more supple in achieving a phenotype fit to new circumstances. These tensions played out across generations is what natural selection is all about: heredity is specific to population and environs, especially the environment of past evolution. Still, any archetype (including specifically, evolutionary stable strategies of behaviour) was abidingly adapted to life in a past ecosystem.

Indeed, in some cases, elements of the environment were so stable as to have been phylogenetically interiorized into the genome. Given time and stability, diversity converges upon the normative which converges upon the ideal. It is in this frame of thought that the example of the essential amino acids in the human diet comes to mind (Wilson, 1993), We have lost the capacity to construct certain of these molecules even though our lives depend upon them. They have been so consistently available as foodstuffs for so long in the environment of our ancestry that our lineage has lost the capacity to anabolize them *de novo*. These features of the environment of our evolutionary adaptedness are—by means of evolutionary dialectics—now interiorized into our genome. Perhaps the best evidence of such curious interiorization lies in the fact that such deletion mutations induce little evolutionary consequence. The selection which accounts for most current gene prevalences took place in the past environment of evolution. This environment has substantially changed—in the blink of a Darwinian eye—with the rise of complex culture which constrains the genome in ways not anticipated in the Pleistocene environment of human evolution.

Therefore, studies of human behaviour which do not vigorously consider these evolutionary parameters are comparable to Zuckerman's (1932) early and elegant but erroneous assessments of 'normal' primate behaviour as derived from his observations of creatures in captivity (Wilson, 1975). One need not invoke the spirit of Rousseau to acknowledge the parallels between primates in a zoo and the enclosures of human nature brought about by contemporary society. Evolved tendencies are distorted in each. Behaviour in the zoo is a property emergent from past selection in evolution. But, selection in the past environment accounts for much persistent human genomic structure and function. Yet the once predominant conditions of this past environment have changed rapidly with the rise of complex culture which increasingly encloses human nature (Weber, 1947).

In any case, if current phenotypes can be identified as the robust expressions of genes which themselves have population prevalences higher than predicted by Hardy–Weinberg calculations, then the genes evolved via the past natural selection of inherently favourable characteristics. This is true, with only technical exception, no matter how pathological may be the phenotypes now unfolding from the genes nor how elusive or subtle may be the appreciation of the advantages.

Still, if and when the thresholds of epigenetic vigour and high frequency are simultaneously surpassed, then the two major conditions of the deductive premises upon which evolutionary epidemiological reasoning is based are satisfied. Consequently, the gene locus must have evolved by virtue of beneficial characteristics expressed, at least, in the course of natural selection. This approach, inchoate in Allison's work in sickle cell anaemia, has been recently formalized as a more general system (Wilson, 1992). Genetic loci of 'disease', both somatic and behavioural, can be assessed as to the likelihood of their having been evolved in the environment of their evolution on the basis of their advantageous characteristics in the struggle for existence.

A prototype in psychiatry: Manic depression

(A) The importance of value, reliable and common diagnostic categories. For all the scientific and especially the popular disdain to which psychiatric theory and practice is sometimes subjected, its backbone of epidemiological research is surprisingly strong. Some of the most common, well-validated and reliably diagnosed disorders of the human genome have been established within the field of psychiatry. In passing, it is useful to recall that validity and reliability are basic, if technical, terms widely used in epidemiology. The former expresses the meaningfulness of a given category and the latter expresses the degree to which such descriptions are made by independent observers.

Again, the high prevalence (as population polymorphisms) of such abiding genomic traits points to intrinsic, if overlooked, positive characteristics that caused them to be so avidly retained by long-term and widespread natural selection. These genes and their phenotypic expressions can be said to be highly canalized (Wimsatt, 1989).

So far, only indirect, phenotypic descriptions of psychopathology have been firmly established. The era of direct, genotypic description is at hand. This era should prove interesting since some diagnostic categories thought to denote discrete diseases may ultimately prove to be mere phenotypic variants of the same aetiological genes. Such genomic equivalent through phenotypic 'co-morbidity' can only mask much higher aggregate genetic prevalence rates (Akiskal, 1989; Hudson & Pope, 1990; Kendler, Neale, Kessler, Heath & Eaves, 1993; Wilson, 1996). If so, the indices of their twin concordance, prevalence and natural selection will be all the higher.

Indeed, on closer examination it appears that several of the variant genes most common in the entire human genome express psychopathology (e.g. manic depression, sociopathy and obsessive–compulsive disorder). Thus they have been marked Darwinian successes. Moreover, these same diagnoses are universal features of the human genome which evidence little, if any, ontogenic idiosyncrasies of epidemiology due to geographical ethnic, cultural, racial or other influences on the phenotype. Therefore, their Darwinian success was an enduring and universal feature of the evolutionary history of the structure and function of the genome of the entire species.

Still much important psychopathology can already be regarded as the product of natural selection. This is true even without recourse to the greater genetic frequencies which are necessarily involved in concepts of a broader spectrum of extended phenotypes. It is likewise true even without recourse to direct gene analysis. In the era of modem science it is easy to forget that gene characteristics and behaviour can be quite usefully scrutinized without direct biochemical technology as the ingenuity of both Darwin and Mendel demonstrated so remarkably. In any case, indirect methods of epidemiology will remain the most useful approach to research in psychiatric research until techniques of direct gene studies are better validated (Hyman & Nestler, 1993).

A recent, well-designed program has generated indirect population genetics data highly (if unintentionally) amenable to reanalysis in the genetic terms of evolutionary epidemiology. The National Institute of Mental Health Epidemiological Catchment Area Program (US-NIMH-ECA) is an excellent example of highly reliable and valid multi-centre data on mental disorders derived from a comprehensive, community-based US sample (Eaton, Regier, Locke & Taube, 1981). The program analyses data derived from structured interviews utilizing highly systematic diagnostic criteria in the best descriptive tradition established by Kraepelin (1904).

A strong example of how evolutionary epidemiological analysis belies any simplistic notions of 'disease' status can be appreciated with the reconsideration of bipolar disorder, i.e. manic depression. Prevalence has been estimated at 0.6 to 6.0 per cent depending on the rigour with which the phenotype is defined. In the benchmark ECA it was noted as carrying a lifetime risk of 1.2 per cent (Eaton *et al.*, 1981). More inclusive diagnostic schemes raise the frequency to some 6 per cent (Akiskal, 1995). The former figure is widely accepted as reliable, although the latter estimate may have greater genomic validity.

(B) The quasi-Mendelian character of manic depression. Twin concordance rates, adoptee studies and family risk studies have long suggested a strong genetic contribution in the manic depressive phenotype (Mollica, 1988). Even a highly conservative concordance estimate is that at least 65 per cent of the phenotype of identical twins is due to direct genetic expression; moreover, concordance may well exceed 90 per cent (Hyman & Nestler, 1993). The consensus view from non-molecular studies has emphasized the essentially Mendelian character of manic depression (Cadoret, 1978).

More recent direct gene studies have begun to trace the chromosomal locale of operative genotypy. Such direct studies initially identified pedigrees consistent with autosomal dominance as the mode of inheritance (Egelund *et al.*, 1987; Hodgkinson *et al.*, 1987). The interpretation of these findings remains somewhat obscured by inconsistencies arising from the application of gene analytic techniques to categories of psychiatric diagnosis (Hyman & Nestler, 1992). These studies are complicated by terminological problems of 'lod-scoring' but are most promising. Moreover, initial linkage findings have not been sustained (J. Kelsoe, personal communication, 1996).

Nevertheless, more recent direct genomic analyses of bipolar pedigrees appear more promising (S. Barondes, personal communication, 1996; Berretini & Pekkarinen, 1996; R. DePaulo, personal communication, 1996). While it is not yet clear how many genes are involved in manic depressive phenotypy, evidence is consistent with an essentially Mendelian (oligogenic) mode of transmission (R. DePaulo, personal communication, 1996). There is little support for the notion it is a highly complex, multifactorial or additive trait (S. Barondes, personal communication, 1996).

(C) Implausibility of highly complex inheritance. Quite apart from the question as to whether manic depression is a Mendelian or even quasi-Mendelian trait, it is sometimes assumed to be a highly complex character which is a continuous or additive factor in genomic terms (Risch & Botstein, 1996). There is exceedingly little evidence this is the case (R. DePaulo, personal communication, 1996; Winokur, 1980). It is true manic depressive phenotypy constitutes a complex spectrum of phenomenology in a clinical sense. This is not at all the same idea that the trait is an additive trait continuous in the population (Rosenthal, 1974).

Moreover, this issue has long been a matter settled by the indirect analyses of family risk, adoptees and twins; the trait 'breeds true' along family lines independent of much environmental effect (Winokur, 1980). At the population genomic level, manic depressive phenotypy is not evident as an additive factor as is, for example, height (Winokur, 1980). It is more consistent with oligogenic—quasi-Mendelian—models of transmission than with continuously variable traits. This is particularly clear where the phenotypes observed by degrees of relatedness have been mapped to Mendelian ratios (Akiskal, 1995).

Further, continuous traits are evident in the population as a gaussian single modal variation, or bell-curve, whereas polymorphisms are at least bimodal (Fisher, 1930). The human genome does not exhibit an obvious bell-curve smoothly linking manic depressive phenotypy to modal norms. Instead, a strong *J*-curve is noted. The vast majority of individuals and families are free of manic depressive phenomena but there are a few lineages which genetially transmit manic depressive traits (Akiskal, 1995).

Finally, it is possible that ongoing direct genetic studies may alter this picture with new and convincing demonstrations of a highly complex mode of transmission of manic depressive genes. At this juncture there is no such critical mass of findings and available evidence supports the strong inference that manic depressive phenotypy is the quasi-Mendelian expression of a few genes.

(D) Implausibility of non-Darwinian mechanisms as a primary factor. With the inference manic depressive phenotypy is broadly Mendelian in nature, questions next arise as to why these genes accrued well beyond putative mutation rate prevalence. That is, what may explain the preponderance of evidence which suggests manic depressive genotypy is a population polymorphism with selective advantage?

Population genetics offers several possibilities which can explain genomic polymorphisms beginning with the basic Hardy–Weinberg postulate that gene frequencies are stable in the absence of selective forces. The Hardy–Weinberg postulate is useful as a basis to determine aspects of the magnitude and directionality of changes even though assumptions intrinsic to it are not realistic. More realistic extensions of this postulate have been made: the classic selection model and the balanced polymorphism model, which each include some elements of evolutionary change.

The standard selection-mutation equilibrium model assumes mutations come and go in a stochastic manner. This is largely the realm of evolutionary error and inefficiency rather than innovation. Harmful mutations are removed by natural selection at some equilibrium with the occurrence of new mutations. Most traits of this type are not true polymorphisms as they are rare. The presence of mutant forms near the rate of mutation–selection equilibrium is an important way by which genetic diversity is maintained. Such diverse forms may gain advantage in the event of environmental fluctuations as exaptations, but are otherwise merely unfortunate medical liabilities.

Mutation–selection is the default explanation for almost any medical condition linked to genetic aetiology. Often rightly but sometimes quite wrongly, an epigenetic disease is presumed to be a non-adaptive, random mistake until proven otherwise. Generally, epigenetic medical conditions due to this driving force exist in the population at low levels approximating the mutation rate itself. Still, equilibrium explains a wide range of rare medical–genetic ailments which occur near mutation rate prevalence, e.g. many deleterious conditions such as albinism, dwarfism and the like. These syndromes are of narrow biomedical or anthropological interest. They do not cast much light on evolutionary process in any but a stochastic sense.

The balanced polymorphism model posits that differential selective advantages exist between individuals as a function of alternative alleles and zygotic condition. Here certain variant alleles are maintained in the genome at frequencies above mutation rate due to heterozygotic advantage, viz. sickle cell anaemia. Epigenetic medical conditions due to this driving force can attain prevalence well above mutation rate frequency but, thus far, have been demonstrated for only a few traits. Apart from these examples, of Darwinian selection, other deterministic or stochastic forces can account for polymorphism.

Neutral selection. It has been noted many genetic variations accrue not due to intrinsic Darwinian advantage but because they are proximal to highly advantageous genetic loci. They are, hence, far less likely to be shuffled randomly by the action of polymerases in meiosis (Hyman & Nestler, 1993). Thus such genetic variants quite simply defy the Mendelian principle of independent segregation. A gene proximal to such an advantageous locus can be swept along in the selective success of the heuristic trait. This accumulation is incidental but can be particularly significant if the selected locus is highly advantageous, the incidental locus carries little net selective load, and the molecular distance separating the two is small. This has been termed 'neutral selection' insofar as the incidental locus is typically neither of much benefit or liability (Kimura, 1955). Neutral selection is difficult to delineate in the absence of detailed knowledge of molecular physiology. It is, however, less likely a casual factor in the persistence of conditions which are clearly deleterious. Should manic depression be even a classically Mendelian single major locus effect, it might yet have accrued randomly.

It is remotely possible that, were such a deleterious gene adjacent to a locus encoding for a major foetal induction (e.g. the notochord or heart), it could attain high, even universal genomic prevalence (E. M. Hundert, personal communication, 1990). Currently, there is insufficient evidence to prove or disprove the role, if any, of neutral selection in the maintenance of manic depression at a high level of worldwide population prevalence. However, no empirical evidence demonstrates that manic depressive genotypy is sustained by neutral selective events.

Genetic drift and founder effects. Non-random events can produce non-Darwinian results. Small populations can, upon adaptive radiation within new environs, account for high prevalences of genes. The relatively low selective force operative in an unexploited ecosystem coupled with aspects of subsequent inbreeding of the founding stock can induce non-Darwinian fluctuation in genetic frequencies. Likewise, analysis of non-probabilistic genetic samples can misrepresent the total population. Early medical–anthropological research often relied on non-random opportunistic or judgment sampling. Such sampling renders invalid any statistical analysis based on an assumption of random distributions. If for convenience one were to sample the blood of volunteers at a sickle cell clinic the prevalence rate obtained could not be usefully ascribed to the universal population. Such events have been advanced in the explanation of rare, idioethnic syndromes (e.g. Tay-Sachs disease or glucose-6-phosphate dehydrogenase).

Again, it is difficult to disprove the possibility of this as a factor contributing to the prevalence of manic depressive genotypy. However, the manic depressive genetic spectrum has little variation in prevalence worldwide and in no sense appears as an idioethnic entity (Kleinman, 1988). As a universal feature of the human genome, it is thus implausible to attribute manic depressive phenomena to genetic drift or related processes.

Phenocopies. Phenocopies of manic depression acquired in the course of ontogenic development may confound genomic analyses. This is a particular problem when the environmentally mediated form is clinically homologous with the classical epigenetic syndrome. Such environmentally engendered clinical equivalents are rare as is evident from studies of twin concordance and adoption outcome. The vast majority of cases of manic depression are due to familial genetic risk rather than environmental acquisition (Goodwin & Jamison, 1990).

In practical terms, manic depressive phenocopies are limited to a small set of neuromental dysfunctions in the brain. These dysfunctions, in turn, typically arise as organic impairments in centres which modulate affective neurology (Benton, 1979; Demasio, 1994). Here there is a predictable complement of aetiogenic factors ranging from trauma, toxicity, infection, neoplasia, inflammation and the like (Robins, 1978).

However, in clinical terms organic–affective syndromes are relatively uncommon. Traumatic brain injuries specifically those involving the frontolimbic cortices, are the most frequent source of non-genetic syndromes which are readily mistaken for epigenetic manic depression (Lishman, 1978). These constitute less that 1 per cent of the total population prevalence of manic depressive phenomena (Hales & Yodofsky, 1987). Thus, syndromes acquired in the course of development are not, in evolutionary terms, a significant factor in the population prevalence of manic depression.

Mutability. Excessive mutability is a further source of high population prevalence for deleterious genetic traits, as an extreme form of the mutation–selection equilibrium. Genes differ as to their intrinsic propensity to mutate, largely as a function of chromosomal conformations, some of which render loci susceptible to disruption by electromagnetic radiation or other factors such as oncoviruses (Hyman & Nestler, 1993). A genetic locus which is prone to unusually frequent mutation will exist at a relatively high equilibrium rate.

With the paucity of current data as to mutation rates of specific human loci, it is difficult to exclude the possibility that manic depression is sustained at a high population prevalence due to intrinsically common aetiologic mutation. On the other hand, there is no available evidence that genes aetiogenic of manic depression lie at loci prone to high rates of mutagenesis. Here again a non-Darwinian causal factor remains possible, if unlikely.

Assortative mating. The non-random matings of similar parental stocks is not, strictly speaking, an extra-Darwinian mechanism. It is instead simply a departure from the Mendelian and Hardy–Weinberg postulates of random breeding. However, clinicians sometimes offer assortative mating towards an explanation for the high prevalence of certain disease traits (Rosenthal, 1974). In fact, the non-random breeding by similar types does not alter population rates of genes, *per se* (Fisher, 1930). More precisely, assortative mating can account for variations from expected ratios for some Mendelian characteristics, e.g. recessive homozygotes. This can be further complicated by sampling errors.

Assortative mating does not alter the totally genomic alleles. Rather, as more recessives are sequestered amongst themselves, there are fewer phenotypically obscured by dominants. The population is phenotypically partitioned but the overall genotypic ratios are retained. When blue-eyed parents breed preferentially, there are more evidently blue-eyed children but not more genes for blue eyes in the population as a whole. Recessive traits can thus achieve greater degrees of phenotypic expression without increasing genomic proportion.

Affective disorders, including manic depression, subsume considerable assortative mating (Goodwin & Jamison, 1990). This is a significant clinical and research fact and one which has not been exhaustively researched. Clearly, both direct and indirect epidemiological studies must carefully control for assortative matings to maintain valid statistical power (Hyman & Nestler, 1993). Likewise, clinicians must often contend with complex pedigree dynamics (K. R. Jamison, personal communication, 1996). However, assortative mating cannot account for the prevalence of a genetic trait well beyond its mutation rate threshold. Therefore, it is not a causal factor in the frequency of genes in the manic depressive spectrum.

There are reasons, then, any search for the causal factors for the high frequency of genes expressive of the manic depressive phenotypic spectrum moves beyond non-Darwinian explanations. It is possible, indeed likely, these genes accumulated in the environment of evolutionary adaptation due to selective advantage.

Calculation of an estimated index of selection for manic depression

The manic depressive phenotype is strongly genetic in a fundamentally Mendelian sense and very common at the population level. By the most conservative estimates its degree of twin concordance of at least 65 per cent with prevalence is at least 0.5 per cent of the human genome worldwide. *Taken together, these facts lead to the highly conservative deduction that bipolar disorder is some 300 times more common than might be calculated from Hardy–Weinberg equilibrium predictions alone:*

Calculation 1:

$$(P/E = S) = [0.325]/(0.001] = 325$$

(where P is prevalence [adjusted by concordance, oligozygosity, etc., $0.5 \times 65\%$] and where E is the frequency [known or estimated by Hardy–Weinberg law] then S is the coefficient of natural selection). Oligozygosity [Z] reduces the selection index by a factor of S/Z where Z is the total constituent loci.

Moreover, with the higher prevalence figures emerging from the ECA (1.2 per cent) and with an extended clinical spectrum (and the higher rates of twin concordance such a spectrum denotes, i.e. 90 per cent), a more realistic estimate is that the manic depressive phenotype is beyond 1000 times more common than it would be in the absence of the sustained operations of natural selection.

Calculation 2:

$$(P/E = S) = [1.2]/[0.001] = 1200$$

If a broader range of psychiatric conditions are, indeed, phenotypic variants of manic depressive genotypy then frequency may be as high as 6 per cent. This, with a high concordance rate, would sustain a genetic prevalence some 6000 times mutation rate levels alone:

Calculation 3:

$$(P/E = S) + [6]/[0.001] = 6000$$

In any case, these genes so greatly exceed their predicted rate prevalence as to be best explained with reference to their promotion in the operations of natural selection sustained in the environment of evolutionary adaptation (Wilson, 1992).

The deductive imperative: If so, then what, when, where, why and how

Clearly, evolutionary epidemiology is a simple but powerful instrument of medical anthropological investigation. It derives from understanding that the term 'prevalence', as used by epidemiological geneticists, is in essential ways equivalent to the concept of 'frequency' as used by evolutionary geneticists (Wilson, 1992). Given the importance of these terms it is useful to review their technical meanings. Prevalence refers to the rate of existence of a disease (gene) within a population. Frequency similarly refers to the rate of existence of a gene (disease) within a population. These two concepts can be melded in a rigorous fashion to deduce a number of remarkable insights concerning the ultimate origin of genes now predisposing to phenotypic pathologies of body and mind.

Darwinian evolution is, after all, a reflection of past intergenerational increases in the demographic representation of healthy reproductive lines and reductions in unhealthy ones. Darwinism offers a rare longitudinal rather than a common cross-sectional perspective.

As noted earlier, Allison's (1954*a,b,c*) work on sickle cell anaemia is the founding contribution to what is now emerging as a more systematic approach to diverse questions regarding the evolved basis of epidemiologically prevalent genetic illness. But sickle cell anaemia is not a universal morbidity of the human genome. It is, rather, a special gene system which arose in special environments. It is, to some extent, thought of as an idioethnic curiosity of limited medical interest as, again, Africans have it, Laplanders do not. Moreover, it is essentially a disease of somatic, as opposed to behavioural, pathophysiology. Still, sickle cell anaemia provides the conceptual foundation on which might be built a more considerable research programme (Cavalli-Sforza & Bodmer, 1976).

Though the full theoretical and practical implications of such evolutionary epidemiological analyses are only now gaining the attention of medical researchers, the work concerning sickle cell anaemia was the first demonstration that carriers of 'disease' genes were endowed with superior Darwinian fitness in certain ecosystems. The prevalence of what had been thought of as simply 'bad' genes was inexplicably high in such ecosystems. Carriers were, it was soon learned, resistant to the ravages of malaria. The malarial organism and the human blood system had coevolved in the environment of evolutionary adaptation. Sickle cell anaemia, however, pathological as it is today, was selected into the human genome. More simply and generally, genes common enough to have evolved by means of natural selection can have done so only by virtue of advantages conferred to lineages which carried such genes even if such genes now express a degree of phenotypic disease.

So it is that techniques of evolutionary epidemiological analysis elucidate whether genes which now express pathological phenotypes nevertheless surpass both their rates of mutation and evolutionary equilibrium and, if so, were promoted by natural selection. In some cases they appear to exceed these expected rates by orders of magnitude. Yet often such genes now seem clearly and rather tightly linked to pathological expression. This seeming paradox that something so 'bad' can have been adaptive in the past disappears in the light of what we know about the genotypic and phenotypic aspects of genomes in changing environs. Selective parameters shift when an evolutionarily stable genomic strategy experiences a new or changed environment. This is why the *range of phenotypic reaction* emerges as a critical factor in selection as phenotypic capacities are stretched to adapt in the new ecology.

There is, of course, a limit to the amount of genetic stretch in individuals and populations. Less flexible genes are selected against. What was healthy can be made ill. Only such a phenomenon might explain the worldwide excess prevalence of 'disease'genes noted in biomedical pathology. Just as sickled blood cells are no longer needed for resistance to malaria in environs with effective antimalarial agents, culture can also marginalize the value of other somatic and behavioural gene polymorphisms. It has become harder—in complex, large-scale cultures—to healthfully express some genes which were rather sublime in the more intimate kinship foraging bands and low population density of the paleaolithic. The range of phenotypic reaction intrinsic to a genome cannot always or readily adapt to new developmental demands.

Within this framework, much epidemiological data can be reconsidered from an evolutionary genetics standpoint. Such reconsideration will lead to fresh implications about the ancient origins, ongoing processes and current phenotypic modulation of 'disease' genes. There is, then, a vast amount of extant and high quality genetic epidemiological data which will yield new clinical knowledge upon consideration from an explicitly evolutionary point of view. The body of genetic epidemiology accumulated over the past century of medical studies is quite amenable to reformulation into terms appropriate for analysis by the theorems of population genetics. Of special interest in this considerable body of primary data are the many genetic polymorphisms which evidence significant population prevalence. Studies which synthesize evolution and epidemiology will repay any careful analysis to clarify how natural selection works on these variant alleles. Such studies may not only demonstrate some clinical syndromes to be epiphenomena of highly evolved forms, but will also, necessarily, stimulate new ideas and insights in palaeoanthropology.

In any case, such a programme of research will eventually expand medical understanding of the theoretical and clinical consequences of evolutionary epidemiology. Central to this expansion is the fact that several important gene systems now expressing 'pathological' phenotypes had—in a Darwinian sense—intrinsic positive qualities that account for the frequency at the high rates observed today. More immediately, several essential tasks are to demonstrate whether a variety of 'disease' genes:

(1) accrued, via natural selection, as advantageous population polymorphisms;
(2) retain a normative essence which conferred selective advantage in the past;
(3) may respond to novel treatments which evoke healthy if latent phenotypies or reduce developmental reactions aetiologic of pathological phenotypy.

Further possibilities

The deduction follows that Darwinian advantages inhered to conditions which surpass specific thresholds of epigenesis and prevalence. Initial attention in general medicine has already turned towards the reassessment of common 'inborn errors of metabolism' (whether Mendelian dominant, recessive, polygenic or mixed). In some cases, Garrod's fine turn of phrase may need to be amended with respect to other highly evolved gene systems which, as has been noted with sickle cell, cannot be said to be truly erroneous. Cystic fibrosis and the anomalies of alpha-1-proteases are obvious candidate genes in that they are not only common, but that it can be readily postulated that they conferred resistance to infectious diseases in prehistory (Wilson, 1993). Similarly, further examples are emerging from a range of medical specialities. To name but a few, one notes rheumatology (Human Leucocyte Antigen (HLA) type mediating various health liabilities), ophthalmology (myopia, presbyopia), neurology (innate 'wiring' syndromes such as dyslexia and autism) and endocrinology (humoral anomalies, notably certain thyroidities) are all specialties now keening on the possibility that some genetic diseases must have definite, if still obscure, advantages.

The clinical and theoretical importance of evolutionary epidemiology extends to not just the physical aspect of medicine, but also to the psychological. The psychiatric genetic epidemiology, collated from indirect studies of the genome as well as from newer direct studies, points to a robust genetic basis for and significant, species-general expression of manic depression. Thus several important psychiatric syndromes, notably manic depression, are likely to surpass thresholds of epigenetic frequency.

Meanwhile, radical shifts in sociodevelopmental ecology at the genomic level can induce extensive phenotypic reactivity, e.g. epochal events such as the agricultural or industrial revolution. Radical shifts from the environment of evolutionary adaptation predispose to conditions of mismatch with the new selective milieu. Reactivity to such shifts can be a factor important in the aetiology of epigenetic disease. Thus, deleterious phenotypes now expressed by genes linked to manic depression may primarily derive from new mismatches between ancestral and current environments rather than an intrinsic 'inborn error of metabolism'. Clinical applications of evolutionary epidemiology therefore provide an opportunity to better understand and treat disease states recently emergent from genes that had long been adaptive.

The phylogenetic accumulation of what now constitutes aetiogenes will be much clarified as the Human Genome Project moves forward (Lander & Botstein, 1986). Likewise, such a project shall clarify much more the epidemiology of diseases (both genotypic and phenotypic). The time is nearly at hand when it will be feasible to routinely assess whether a wide range of genes linked to contemporary pathophenotypes were, by the criteria of evolutionary epidemiology, selected into the human genome. Already, it is clear that at least some contemporary pathological syndromes are expressions not of genetic error but of past advantageous selection stretched by the current environment beyond the plasticity of their healthy range of phenotypic reaction. Such knowledge will constitute an unavoidable temptation to therapeutic adventurism and misadventurism. It is important that any genetic therapies do not assume disease is simply disease. Certain polymorphisms of at least possible utility are at risk of misguided 'therapy'. Surely other gene systems now notable only as causes of individual disease will come to be seen, in the full light of evolutionary epidemiological analysis, as fundamentally salubrious characteristics.

Inferences from evolutionary epidemiology will further revise psychopathological theory and practice as pertains to other syndromes, as well. The deductive methods of evolutionary epidemiology suggest that natural selection promoted genetic lineages now expressing (1) sociopathy, (2) depression, (3) anxiety–panic disorder, (4) obsessive–compulsive disorder, (5) dyslexia, as well as the biological underpinnings of some (6) personality disorders, (7) substance abuse syndromes, (8) psychodynamic conflicts and (9) various isolated traits of cognition, personality or temperament.

References

Akiskal, H. S. (1989). Psychopathology, temperament and past course in primary major depressions. 1. Review of evidence for a bipolar spectrum. *Psychopathology*, 22, 268–277.

Akiskal, H. S. (1995). The bipolar spectrum: Research and clinical perspectives. *Encephale*, 21 (Spec 6), 3–11.

Allison, A. C. (1954*a*). The distribution of the sickle-cell trait in East Africa and elsewhere and its apparent relationship to the incidence of subtertian malaria. *Transactions of the Royal Society of Tropical Medicine and Hygiene*, 48, 312.

Allison, A. C. (1954*b*). Protection by the sickle-cell trait against subtertian malarial infection. *British Medical Journal*, 2, 290.

Allison, A. C. (1954*c*). Notes on sickle-cell polymorphism. *Annals of Human Genetics*, 13, 39.

Benton, A. (1979). *Visuoperceptive, visuospatial and visuoconstructive disorders.* In K. Heilman & E. Valenstein (Eds), *Clinical Neuropsychology.* New York: Oxford University Press.

Berretini, W. H. & Pekkarinen, P. H. (1996). Molecular genetics of bipolar disorder. *Annals of Medicine,* 28, 191–194.

Cavalli-Sforza, L. & Bodmer, W. F. (1976). *The Genetics of Human Populations.* San Francisco, CA: Freeman.

Cadoret, R. J. (1978). Psychopathology of adopted-away offspring of biological parents with antisocial personality. *Archives of General Psychiatry,* 35, 176–184.

Dawkins, R. (1976). *The Selfish Gene.* p. 74. Oxford: Oxford University Press.

Demasio, A. (1994). *Descartes' Error: Emotion, Reason and the Human Brain.* New York: Putnam.

Dobzhansky, T. (1962). *Mankind Evolving.* New Haven, CT: Yale University Press.

Eaton, W. W., Regier, D. A., Locke, B. Z. & Taube, C. A. (1981). The epidemiological catchment area program of the National Institute of Mental Health. *Public Health Reports,* 96, 319–325.

Egelund, J. A., Gerhard, D. S., Pauls, D. L., Sussex, J. N., Kidd, K. K., Allen, C. R., Hostetter, A. M. & Housman, D. E. (1987). Bipolar affective disorders linked to DNA markers on chromosome 11. *Nature,* 325, 783–787.

Fisher, R. A. (1930). *The Genetical Theory of Natural Selection.* Oxford: Clarendon Press.

Galton, F. (1884). Measurement of character. *Fortnightly Review,* 42, 179–185.

Goodwin, D. & Jamison, K. R. (1990). *Manic Depressive Illness.* Oxford: Oxford University Press.

Hales, R. E. & Yodofsky, S. C. (1987). *Textbook of Neuropsychiatry.* Washington, DC: American Psychiatric Press.

Hodgkinson, S., Sherrington, R., Gurling, H., Marchbanks, R., Reeders, S., Mallet, J., McInnes, M., Petursson, H., & Brynjolfson, J. (1987). Molecular evidence for heterogeneity in manic-depression. *Nature,* 325, 805–806.

Hudson, J. & Pope, H. (1990). Affective spectrum disorder. *American Journal of Psychiatry, 47,* 552–564.

Hyman, S. E. & Nestler, E. J. (1993). *The Molecular Foundation of Psychiatry.* Washington DC: American Psychiatric Press.

Kendler, K. S., Neale, M., Kessler, R., Heath, A. C. & Eaves, L. (1993). Major depression and generalized anxiety disorder: Same genes, (partly) different environments? *Archives of General Psychiatry,* 49, 716–722.

Kendrew, J. (1978). *Introduction.* In R. Duncan & M. Smith (Eds), *The Encyclopedia of Ignorance.* New York: Pocket Books.

Kettlewell, H. B. D. (1958). A survey of frequencies of *Biston betalaria* and its melanic forms in Great Britain. *Heredity,* 12, 51–72.

Kimura, M. (1955). Stochastic processes and distribution of gene frequencies in natural selection. *Cold Spring Harbor Symposia on Quantitative Biology,* 22, 33–53.

Kleinman, A. (1988). *Rethinking Psychiatry.* London: Collier Macmillan.

Kraepelin, E. (1904). *Lectures on Clinical Psychiatry.* London: Baillière.

Lander, E. & Botstein, D. (1986). Strategies for studying heterogeneous genetic traits in humans using a linkage map of restriction fragment polymorphisms. *Proceedings of the National Academy of Sciences, USA,* 83, 7353–7357.

Lishman, W. A. (1978). *Organic Psychiatry.* Oxford: Blackwell.

Livingstone, F. B. (1958). Anthropological implications of sickle cell gene distribution in West Africa. *American Anthropologist,* 60, 533–562.

Livingstone, F. B. (1964). The distribution of the abnormal hemoglobin genes and their significance for human evolution. *Evolution,* 18, 685–699.

Livingstone, F. B. (1967). *Abnormal Hemoglobins in Human Populations.* Chicago, IL: Aldine.

Livingstone, F. B. (1969). An analysis of the ABO blood group clines in Europe. *American Journal of Physical Anthropology,* 31, 1–10.

Mayr, E. (1963). *Populations, Species and Evolution.* Cambridge, MA: Belknap/Harvard University Press.

Mollica, R. F. (1988). Mood disorders: Epidemiology. In H. Kaplan & B. Sadock (Eds), *Comprehensive Textbook of Psychiatry.* 5th ed. Baltimore, MD: Williams & Wilkins.

Neel, J. V. (1950). The population genetics of two inherited blood dyscrasias in man. *Cold Spring Harbor Symposia on Quantitatve Biology,* 13, 141–158.

Risch, N. & Botstein, D. (1996). Editorial. *Nature Genetics,* 12, 351–353.

Robins, L. N. (1978). Psychiatric epidemiology. *Archives of General Psychiatry,* 35, 697–702.

Rosenthal, D. (1974). *Genetic Theory and Abnormal Behavior.* New York: McGraw-Hill.

Weber, M. (1947). *The theory of social and economic organization.* In H. H. Gerth & C. W. Mills (Eds), *Max Weber.* Oxford: Oxford University Press.

Wilson, D. R. (1992). Evolutionary epidemiology. *Acta Biotheoretica,* 40, 87–90.

Wilson, D. R. (1993). Evolutionary epidemiology: Darwinian theory in the service of medicine and psychiatry. *Acta Biotheoretica,* 41, 205–218.

Wilson, D. R. (1994). The Darwinian roots of human neurosis. *Acta Biotheoretica,* 42, 49–62.

Wilson, D. R. (1996). Darwinian psychiatry. *Proceedings of the Xth Congress, World Psychiatric Association.* Madrid: World Psychiatric Association.

Wilson, D. R., Stanton, S. & Wilson, S. L. (in press). Serotonin and dopamine in the service of kinship selection. In *Darwin and the Sociobiological Heritage.* New York: Praeger.

Wilson, E. O. (1975). *Sociobiology: The New Synthesis.* Cambridge, MA: Belknap/Harvard University Press.

Wilson, E. O. & Bossert, W. (1971). *A Primer of Population Biology.* Sunderland, MA: Sinauer Associates.

Wimsatt, W. (1989). Evolutionary entrenchment (Proceedings of the Human Behavior and Evolution Society Second Annual Meeting). *Ethology and Sociobiology.* 10, 5.

Winokur, G. (1980). Is there a common genetic factor in bipolar disorder and unipolar affective disorder? *Comprehensive Psychiatry,* 21, 460–468.

Zuckerman, S. (1932). *The Social Life of Monkeys and Apes.* London: Butler & Tanner.

Increased Anterior Cingulate and Caudate Activity in Bipolar Mania

Hilary P. Blumberg, Emily Stern, Diana Martinez, Sally Ricketts, Jose de Asis, Thomas White, Jane Epstein, P. Anne McBride, David Eidelberg, James H. Kocsis, and David A. Silbersweig

Background: *Executive control of cognition, emotion, and behavior are disrupted in the manic state of bipolar disorder. Whereas frontal systems are implicated in such dysfunction, the localization of functional brain abnormalities in the manic state is not well understood.*

Methods: *We utilized a high-sensitivity $H_2{}^{15}O$ positron emission tomography technique to investigate regions of increased brain activity in mania, compared to euthymia, in bipolar disorder.*

Results: *The principal findings were manic state-related increased activity in left dorsal anterior cingulate, and left head of caudate.*

Conclusions: *The findings suggest that the manic state of bipolar disorder may be associated with heightened activity in a frontal cortical–subcortical neural system that includes the anterior cingulate and caudate.* Biol Psychiatry 2000;48:1045–1052 © *2000 Society of Biological Psychiatry*

Key Words: Bipolar disorder, mania, affective disorders, tomography emission-computed, gyrus cinguli, caudate nucleus

Introduction

Classic manic symptoms include sustained heightened mood, as well as associated abnormalities in attentional and executive functions, such as distractibility and excessive maladaptive behaviors. There are a number of nonimaging studies suggesting that manic states are associated with greater right than left hemisphere prefrontal and subcortical impairment, and greater ventral than dorsal cortical impairment (reviewed in Bear 1986; Sackeim et al 1982; Starkstein and Robinson 1997; Wexler 1980). Although human brain lesion studies can help to localize regions of decreased functioning, post-lesion compensation and reorganization can complicate the interpretation of findings. Furthermore, the elucidation of dysregulated or heightened activity in associated brain regions, which might also underlie manic symptoms, has been limited by available experimental methods. Functional neuroimaging techniques allow for the investigation, in vivo, of such possible manic state-related abnormalities in regional brain function.

Functional neuroimaging techniques have been applied to a greater extent to the study of depression, than of mania, in mood disorders. Positron emission tomography (PET) studies of depression have demonstrated abnormalities in ventral, rostral and dorsal anterior cingulate cortex (AC), dorsolateral prefrontal cortex, as well as caudate, which receives significant projections from these cortical structures (Baxter et al 1989; Bench et al 1993; DeAsis et al 1999; Drevets et al 1997; George et al 1997; Mayberg et al 1997).

The regional brain involvement in mania is less clear. There are findings that support possible frontal lobe, temporal lobe, and basal ganglia involvement in primary mania, although the associated studies differ in the imaging techniques and normalization procedures used, the delineation of the frontal lobe regions examined, and whether increases or decreases were found in these regions (Table 1).

Decreased anterior–posterior gradients and general frontal activity have been reported in mania (al-Mousawi et al 1996; O'Connell et al 1995; Rubin et al 1995). More specifically, mania-associated increased activity has been reported in dorsal and ventral AC (Drevets et al 1995, 1997; Goodwin et al 1997), and increased activity has been reported in more lateral prefrontal cortices (Baxter et al 1989).

There has been evidence to suggest possible involvement of the temporal polar cortex in mania; however; there have been conflicting findings in this area. Decreased right basotemporal activity has been reported, with a trend toward a negative correlation between mania ratings and

From the Functional Neuroimaging Laboratory, Department of Psychiatry, The Weill Medical College of Cornell University, New York (HPB, ES, DM, SR, JdA, TW, JE, PAM, DE, JHK, DAS) and the Department of Neurology, North Shore University Hospital–New York University School of Medicine, Manhassett (DE).

Address reprint requests to Hilary P. Blumberg, M.D., Veterans Administration Connecticut Healthcare System, Department of Psychiatry 116A, 950 Campbell Avenue, West Haven CT 06516.

Received November 24, 1999; revised May 23, 2000; accepted June 14, 2000.

0006-3223/00/$20.00
PII S0006-3223(00)00962-8

Table 1. Results of Regional Functional Neuroimaging Studies of Primary Mania in Resting States

Group	Technique	n^a	Frontal findings	Temporal findings	Basal ganglia findings	Correlation to mania scores	Comments
Baxter et al 1989	FDG PET	6 (6)	Increased left anterolateral compared to depression				Differences may be accounted for by the metabolic reduction in the depressed phase
Migliorelli et al 1993	HMPAO SPECT	5 (5)		Decreased right basotemporal		Negative trend with right basotemporal	All subjects female, normalized to cerebellum
Drevets et al 1995	FDG PET	3 (3)	Increased right ventral AC		Increased right ventral striatum		
O'Connell et al 1995	IMP SPECT	11	Decreased frontal (in four of 11 subjects)	Increased temporal (in 11/11)	Increased right > left basal ganglia (in 5/11)	Positive with right temporal	Abnormalities on visual inspection
Rubin et al 1995	rCBF	11	Decreased anterior cortical rCBF in depression and mania				Preliminary suggestion of left > right rCBF in mania compared to depression in inferior prefrontal cortex
al-Mousawi et al 1996	FDG PET	15 (2)	Decreased anterior-posterior gradient	Increased right temporal and decreased left amygdala			Normalized to the area-weighted mean of all regions of interest
Drevets et al 1997	FDG PET	4 (3)	Increased ventral AC				
Goodwin et al 1997	EMZ SPECT	7 (7)	Increased dorsal AC				Subjects manic after lithium discontinuation
Gyulai et al 1997	IMP SPECT	3		Increased right > left anterior temporal (in 2/3)			
Blumberg et al 1999	$H_2{}^{15}O$ PET	5	Decreased orbitofrontal				

FDG, 18 fluorodeoxyglucose; PET, positron emission tomography; HMPAO, 99mTchexamethylpropyleneamine oxime; SPECT, single photon emission computed tomography; AC, anterior cingulate; IMP, isopropyliodoamphetamine; rCBF, regional cerebral blood flow; EMZ, 99mTc-exametazime.

[a]Numbers in parentheses represent the number of unmedicated subjects.

Table 2. Brain Regions of Increased Activity in the Manic State of Bipolar Disorder

Brain area (Brodmann area)	x	y	z	Z	Mania rCBF	Euthymia rCBF
Left, dorsal AC (24/32)	−18	12	34	4.69[a]	60.54 ± 0.33	54.61 ± 0.66
Left caudate head	−16	20	0	4.20[a]	75.76 ± 1.32	67.52 ± 0.66
Right, dorsal AC (24/32)	24	6	38	3.32	60.49 ± 0.89	57.10 ± 0.49
Right ventral AC (32)	10	26	−8	3.13	77.29 ± 0.63	74.22 ± 0.76

The brain areas represent regions of increased activity in the manic state, compared to the euthymic state, above significance thresholds of $p < .001$, uncorrected for multiple comparisons. Coordinates of the maxima within a region of increased regional cerebral blood flow (rCBF) are in millimeters relative to the anterior commissure in standardized stereotactic space (Talairach and Tournoux 1988); x is the lateral distance from the midline (positive, right), y is the anteroposterior distance from the anterior commissure (positive, anterior), and z is the height relative to the anterior commissure–posterior commissure plane (positive, dorsal). Z is the significance level converted to the unit normal distribution. rCBF, mean adjusted rCBF ± SD in mL/100 g/min. AC, anterior cingulate.

[a] $p < .05$, corrected for multiple comparisons.

right basotemporal cerebral blood flow (CBF) (Migliorelli et al 1993); however, increased right temporal activity (al-Mousawi et al 1996; Gyulai et al 1997; O'Connell et al 1995) and decreased left amygdala activity (al-Mousawi et al 1996) have also been reported, and right temporal increases have been shown to positively correlate with mania scores (O'Connell et al 1995).

Abnormalities have been reported in bipolar mania in the basal ganglia. There was a report of increased uptake in the basal ganglia, greater in the right hemisphere (O'Connell et al 1995). Another preliminary report suggests that there may be increased right ventral striatal activity (Drevets et al 1995).

We previously reported manic state-related decreased orbitofrontal activity (Blumberg et al 1999). We suggested that dysfunction in ventral cortices might be associated with increased activity in associated cortical and subcortical structures with significant connectivity to these regions. As noted above, the nonimaging literature suggests that an imbalance with right more than left, and ventral more than dorsal, frontal lesions are associated with mania. It is plausible that, conversely, increased left dorsal frontal activity may contribute to a similar regional imbalance, in the absence of gross lesions. The small functional neuroimaging literature of mania to date has not resolved these issues. In this article we describe analyses performed to examine increases in brain activity in mania compared to euthymia with particular interest in lateralized frontal systems.

Methods and Materials

Subjects with Bipolar I Disorder, non–rapid-cycling, established by Structured Clinical Interview (First et al 1995) included five manic subjects (M; four female, one male; mean age 34.2 years, SD = 12.2), and six euthymic subjects (E; four female, two male; 32.5 years, SD = 11.0). Manic subjects met DSM-IV criteria for a current manic episode. Euthymic subjects did not meet DSM-IV criteria for a current manic or depressive episode and had a score of <6 on the 29-item Hamilton Depression Rating Scale (Hamilton 1960). Subjects were without comorbid Axis I or II Disorders, except distant substance abuse (>5 years in 3 M, 3 E). All subjects were right-handed (Oldfield 1971), spoke English as a first language, and were without neurologic or medical illness. Patient groups did not differ significantly in estimated premorbid verbal intelligence quotient (Grober and Sliwinski 1991): M = 111.6 ± 6.0, E = 118.7 ± 7.6. The manic and euthymic groups also did not differ significantly in illness duration: M = 14.2 years ± 14.9, E = 12.0 ± 5.6. Subjects denied family history of psychotic or anxiety disorder. Medications included mood stabilizers (lithium [4 M, 5 E], valproic acid [2 M, 2 E], and carbamazepine [1 M, 2 E]), antipsychotic agents (3 M), benzodiazepines (4 M, 1 E), and antidepressants (2 E). No subject required acute sedation for scanning. After complete description of the study to the subjects, written informed consent was obtained in accordance with hospital institutional review board protocols.

A General Electric ADVANCE Positron Emission Tomograph was operated in three-dimensional mode (Lewellen et al 1996). Four scans, in one study session, were performed in the resting condition with eyes closed, lights dimmed, and low levels of ambient noise. Regional cerebral blood flow (rCBF) was measured as an index of local neuronal activity (Raichle 1987). $H_2{}^{15}O$ delivery and data acquisition were performed according to a previously published technique (Silbersweig et al 1993). Realignment of images across runs within subject was performed to correct for slight head movement, and spatial smoothing (15 mm full-width-at-half-maximum) was performed. Head movement was significantly less than the resolution of smoothing for all subjects. Regional CBF was normalized to a mean of 50 mL/100 gm/min. Group effects were identified with multiple linear regression analysis. Image processing and analyses were performed with statistical parametric mapping (SPM '96, Wellcome Department of Cognitive Neurology, University College London, UK) according to the General Linear Model, and probability estimates were determined according to the Theory of Random Fields (Friston et al 1995).

Results

Mean mania scores (Altman et al 1994) for the manic group and the euthymic group were 21.8 ± SD 6.7 and 2.5 ± 4.5, respectively. The groups differed significantly on 7 of the 10 mania items ($p < .05$; Student's t test, two

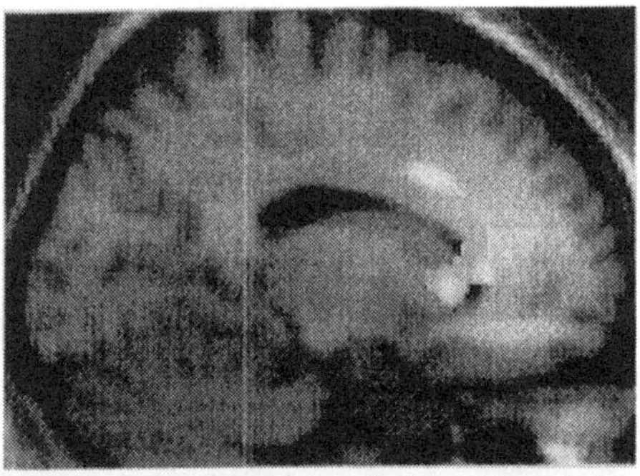

Figure 1. Sagittal section 16 mm left of the midsagittal plane demonstrating increased activity in the head of the caudate, and in left dorsal anterior cingulate in mania, compared to euthymia. Regional cerebral blood flow functional results ($p < .001$) are displayed in color and superimposed on a structural T_1-weighted magnetic resonance imaging template.

tailed), including measures of mood elevation, irritability, pressured speech, racing thoughts, distractibility, grandiosity, and sleep disturbance. Although there were trends toward increases in mania, there were no significant differences on measures of hyperactivity, increased energy, and impaired judgment. The lack of difference between groups on these items may reflect a bias in selecting manic subjects without psychomotor agitation that would render them unable to complete scanning, and in choosing only those subjects judged by an attending physician to have capacity to make an informed decision to participate in the study.

Increased mania-associated rCBF was detected in the bilateral dorsal AC, the right ventral AC, and in the left head of the caudate at a threshold of $p < .001$, uncorrected (Table 2). Applying correction for multiple comparisons, significant findings were restricted to the left dorsal AC and left head of caudate ($p < .05$, corrected for multiple comparisons; Figures 1 and 2).

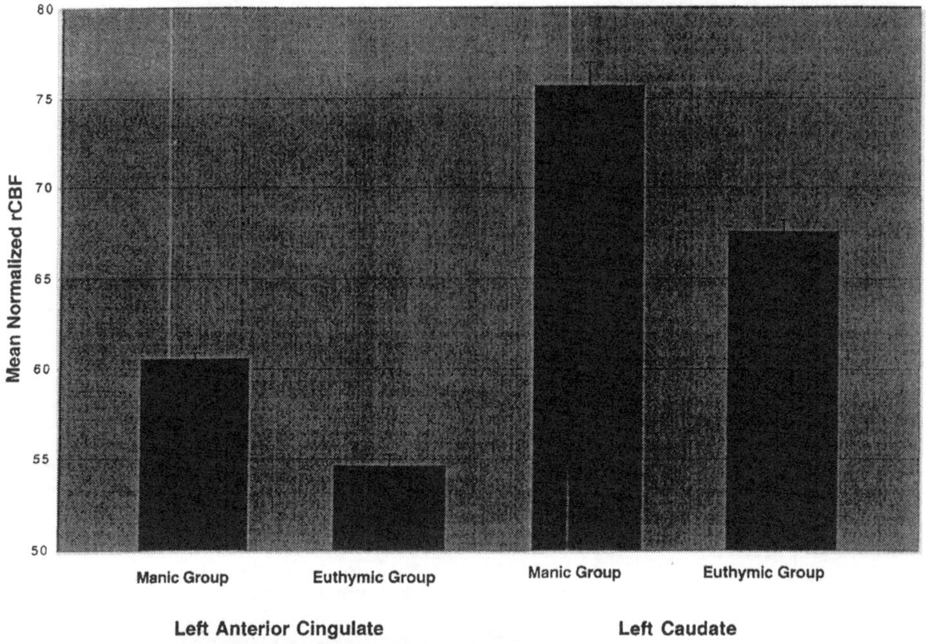

Figure 2. Mean normalized regional cerebral blood flow (rCBF) for the manic and the euthymic groups in the left dorsal anterior cingulate and caudate. Regional cerebral blood flow values (the Y axis) were normalized to a mean of 50 mL/100 g/min for the manic and euthymic subject groups. Each column corresponds to the mean (±SD) rCBF for a group of subjects. Results for subjects in the manic state are represented in blue, and results for subjects in the euthymic state are represented in red. The two columns on the left are values for the left dorsal anterior cingulate at the statistical parametric mapping (SPM) regional maximum. The two columns on the right are values for the left head of caudate at the SPM regional maximum.

Discussion

DSM-IV criteria for a manic episode include a sustained heightened emotional state, as well as accompanying symptoms of distractibility, rapid loosely connected thoughts, and behaviors associated with increased motivational drives (American Psychiatric Association 1994). We report here greater manic, versus euthymic, state-related activity in the AC and caudate. The greater activity in these structures may relate to behavioral abnormalities observed in mania.

The AC is associated with attentional, emotional, and cognitive functions. The AC has significant reciprocal connections to the amygdala (Vogt et al 1992), a brain structure thought to be central to emotional processing. Stimulation of AC can lead to euphoria and a sense of well-being, as well as alterations in rate, volume, and degree of perseveration in speech (reviewed in Devinsky et al 1995). Cingulate seizures have been associated with ictal emotional changes, and interictal irritability, emotional lability, and sexual behaviors (Devinsky et al 1995). Rats will self-stimulate in this brain region in a manner enhanced over time and thought to be associated with kindling (Corbett and Stellar 1983), a process theorized to develop in limbic brain regions in bipolar disorder. Anticonvulsant agents, also used as mood stabilizing agents in bipolar disorder, have been demonstrated to interfere with this process (Post et al 1982).

The principal finding of this study was in the dorsal region of the AC. This region of the AC has relatively organized and granular cytoarchitecture, and the related behavioral functions are of higher order (Devinsky et al 1995), than the ventral AC. The dorsal AC has been associated with cognitive functions, such as the appropriate directing of attention, conflict monitoring, and response selection (Botvinick et al 1999; Carter et al 1998; Peterson et al 1999; Posner and Rothbart 1998). Decreased activity in the left dorsal AC has been described in association with depressive cognitive abnormalities (Bench et al 1993; DeAsis et al 1999; George et al 1997).

The more ventral regions of the AC region have a more agranular cytoarchitecture and the related functions are more primitive. The ventral AC has efferent connections to autonomic, endocrine, and visceral effectors (Nauta 1971), and is thought to regulate the associated functions. The rostral AC has also been associated with the expression of internal states, including vocalizations and social behaviors (Devinsky et al 1995). The ventral AC region has been demonstrated to activate more to emotional stimuli, in contrast to the dorsal AC, which may activate more during cognitive tasks (Whalen et al 1998). One region of increased activity in this study, the ventral AC, is a region that overlaps that previously reported to have increased activity in mania (Drevets et al 1997), representing a possible convergence of findings.

This study also demonstrated increased activity in the left head of the caudate in mania, ipsilateral to the increased activity in the dorsal AC. The AC has excitatory efferent input to the head of the caudate (Eblen and Graybiel 1995; Yeterian and van Hoesen 1978). The modulatory caudate input back to the AC has intervening connections via the globus pallidus and thalamus (Alexander et al 1986). The known structural connectivity between the cingulate and caudate suggests that the increased activity occurs within the context of this cortical–subcortical neural system. Increased activity has previously been reported in mania in the basal ganglia (Drevets et al 1995; O'Connell et al 1995) and warrants further investigation.

We speculate that increased AC activity could relate to heightened, dysregulated attentive and cognitive processes, such as manic-type distractibility and maladaptive excessive behaviors. An alternative possible interpretation for increased left AC activity in the manic state relates to the behavioral constraint required during scanning. The scanning requirement of decreasing inappropriate behavioral outputs, such as psychomotor movements and speaking, may require additional efforts on the part of manic subjects. Heightened AC and caudate activity could be associated with this demand.

The findings here are preliminary and require replication, as this study is limited by the relatively small number of subjects and their medication status. More manic subjects were receiving both antipsychotic and benzodiazepine medications, and more euthymics were receiving antidepressants. In each group all but one subject was on lithium at the time of study. Goodwin et al (1997) reported decreases in anterior cingulate and right caudate CBF after lithium withdrawal, whereas development of mania on lithium withdrawal was associated with increased AC CBF. There have been reports of increased caudate activity and basal ganglia size associated with antipsychotic medication (Buchsbaum et al 1987; Chakos et al 1994; Holcomb et al 1996), and decreased rostral AC activity with antidepressant treatment (Mayberg et al 1997); however, there is not clear evidence to suggest a contribution to the lateralized effects seen in this study. Both antipsychotic and benzodiazepine medication have been reported to be associated with decreased AC activity (Holcomb et al 1996; Veselis et al 1997), which would have predicted the opposite outcome in the AC in the manic group. Findings in ventral AC and striatum have previously been reported in three unmedicated manic subjects, although the results were lateralized to the right hemisphere (Drevets et al 1995).

Increased anterior cingulate activity is not specific to

bipolar manic states. Elevated emotional states in healthy subjects have been reported in association with increased AC activity. For example, Ketter et al (1997) demonstrated increased rCBF in AC associated with procaine-induced euphoria in healthy subjects. In a study of transient psychologically induced emotional states (via emotional memory and face presentation) also in healthy subjects, AC rCBF has been demonstrated to increase significantly in sad states, and there was a trend toward an increase in happy states (George et al 1995). Increased anterior cingulate activity is also not specific to the bipolar diagnosis, and has also been demonstrated in symptomatic states of anxiety disorders, such as obsessive-compulsive disorder and phobias (Rauch et al 1994, 1995). These and our findings, seen in the light of the behavioral neuroscientific literature, suggest that the AC is a vulnerable part of an important final common pathway of emotional regulation.

As this study was designed to examine relative regional changes in CBF, mean CBF measures were normalized for each subject, and global changes were not assessed. There has been a previous report to suggest possible global brain changes in mania. Kishimoto et al (1987), reported generalized increases in 11C-glucose uptake in three medication-free manic patients compared to control subjects. Other groups have not found an increase in global activity (Rubin et al 1995; Schwartz et al 1987; Silfverskiold and Risberg 1989).

Concurrent volumetric measurements were not performed in this study. A possible contribution of dorsal AC volume change across mood states can be a subject for further study. There have been reports of volumetric differences in ventral AC grey matter (Drevets et al 1997), and a conflicting literature on the possibility of caudate volume abnormalities in mood disorders (Aylward et al 1994; Dupont et al 1995; Krishnan et al 1992; Lenze and Sheline 1999). This literature suggests possible trait abnormalities; however, volumetric state abnormalities that would have greater implications for the current work are less clear.

The most significant areas of increased manic state-related activity were in the left dorsal AC and head of caudate. This finding, and our previously reported finding of decreased orbitofrontal activity in mania (Blumberg et al 1999), are consistent with theories that relative right lower than left, and ventral less than dorsal, prefrontal activity is associated with manic states (Bear 1986; Sackeim et al 1982; Starkstein and Robinson 1997; Wexler 1980). This has been theorized to extend to relative impairment in activity in related right hemisphere subcortical structures, including caudate, thalamus, and medial diencephalon (Mega et al 1997; Starkstein and Robinson 1997). Much of the reasoning for these theories is based upon manic behavior described in association with brain lesions. The data in this functional neuroimaging study suggest that greater left dorsal AC and caudate activity may contribute to an equivalent net imbalance in brain function associated with the manic state in bipolar disorder.

Supported by the DeWitt-Wallace Fund in the New York Community Trust.

The authors thank the volunteers for their participation, and Vijay Dhawan, PhD, Abdelfatihe Belakhlef, PhD, and Claude Marguleff, MA for their expert technical assistance, and Hong Pan, PhD for his statistical input.

The findings of this study were presented at the 53rd annual meeting of the Society of Biological Psychiatry, May 27–31, 1998, Toronto.

References

Alexander GE, DeLong MR, Strick PL (1986): Parallel organization of functionally segregated circuits linking basal ganglia and cortex. *Annu Rev Neurosci* 9:357–381.

al-Mousawi AH, Evans N, Ebmeier KP, Roeda D, Chaloner F, Ashcroft GW (1996): Limbic dysfunction in schizophrenia and mania. A study using 18F-labelled fluorodeoxyglucose and positron emission tomography. *Br J Psychiatry* 169:509–516.

Altman EG, Hedeker DR, Janicak PG, Peterson JL, Davis JM (1994): The clinician-administered rating scale for mania (CARS-M): Development, reliability and validity. *Biol Psychiatry* 36:124–134.

American Psychiatric Association. (1994): *Diagnostic and Statistical Manual of Mental Disorders*, 4th ed. Washington, DC: American Psychiatric Press.

Aylward EH, Roberts-Twillie JV, Barta PE, Kumar AJ, Harris GJ, Geer M, et al (1994): Basal ganglia volumes and white matter hyperintensities in patients with bipolar disorder. *Am J Psychiatry* 151:687–693.

Baxter LR Jr, Schwartz JM, Phelps ME, Mazziotta JC, Guze BH, Selin CE, et al (1989): Reduction of prefrontal cortex glucose metabolism common to three types of depression. *Arch Gen Psychiatry* 46:243–250.

Bear DM (1986): Hemispheric asymmetries in emotional function: A reflection of lateral specialization in cortical-limbic connections. In: Doane BK, Livingston KE, editors. *The Limbic System: Functional Organization and Clinical Disorders.* New York: Raven, 29–42.

Bench CJ, Friston KJ, Brown RG, Frackowiak RSJ, Dolan RJ (1993): Regional cerebral blood flow in depression measured by positron emission tomography: The relationship with clinical dimensions. *Psychol Med* 23:579–590.

Blumberg H, Stern E, Ricketts S, Martinez D, de Asis J, McBride A, et al (1999): Rostral and orbital prefrontal cortex dysfunction in the manic state of bipolar disorder. *Am J Psychiatry* 156:1986–1988.

Botvinick M, Nystrom LE, Fissell K, Carter CS, Cohen JD (1999): Conflict monitoring versus selection-for-action in anterior cingulate cortex. *Nature* 402:179–181.

Buchsbaum MS, Wu JC, DeLisi LE, Holcomb HH, Hazlett E,

Cooper-Langston K, Kessler R (1987): Positron emission tomography studies of basal ganglia and somatosensory cortex neuroleptic drug effects: Differences between normal controls and schizophrenic patients. *Biol Psychiatry* 22:479–494.

Carter CS, Braver TS, Barch DM, Botvinick MM, Noll D, Cohen JD (1998): Anterior cingulate cortex, error detection, and the online monitoring of performance. *Science* 280:747–749.

Chakos MH, Lieberman JA, Bilder RM, Borenstein M, Lerner G, Bogerts B, et al (1994): Increase in caudate nuclei volumes of first-episode schizophrenic patients taking antipsychotic drugs. *Am J Psychiatry* 151:1430–1436.

Corbett D, Stellar JR (1983): Neurological reactivity during medial prefrontal cortex stimulation: Effects of self-stimulation experience. *Physiol Behav* 31:771–776.

DeAsis J, Silbersweig D, Alexopoulos G, Blumberg H, Kalayam B, Eidelberg D, Stern E (1999): Decreased hippocampal and anterior cingulate activation in geriatric depression. *Biol Psychiatry* 45:5115–5116.

Devinsky O, Morrell MJ, Vogt BA (1995): Contributions of anterior cingulate cortex to behaviour. *Brain* 118:279–306.

Drevets WC, Price JL, Simpson JR Jr, Todd RD, Reich T, Vannier M, Raichle ME (1997): Subgenual prefrontal cortex abnormalities in mood disorders. *Nature* 386:824–827.

Drevets WC, Price JL, Videen TO, Todd RD, Raichle ME (1995): Metabolic abnormalities in the subgenual prefrontal cortex and ventral striatum in mood disorders. *Neurosci Abstr* 21:260.

Dupont RM, Jernigan TL, Heindel W (1995): Magnetic resonance imaging and mood disorders—localization of white matter and other subcortical abnormalities. *Arch Gen Psychiatry* 52:747–755.

Eblen F, Graybiel (1995): Highly restricted origins of prefrontal cortical inputs to striosomes in the macaque monkey. *J Neurosci* 15:5999–6013.

First MB, Spitzer RL, Gibbon M, Williams JBW (1995): *Structured Clinical Interview for DSM-IV Axis I & II Disorders (Version 2.0)*. New York: New York State Psychiatric Institute, Biometrics Research.

Friston KJ, Holmes A, Worsley K, Poline J, Frith C, Heather J, Frackowiak RSJ (1995): Statistical parametric maps in functional imaging: A general linear approach. *Hum Brain Mapp* 2:189–210.

George MS, Ketter TA, Parekh PI, Horwitz B, Herscovitch P, et al (1995): Brain activity during transient sadness and happiness in healthy women. *Am J Psychiatry* 152:341–351.

George MS, Ketter TA, Parekh PI, Rosinsky N, Ring HA, Pazzaglia PJ, et al (1997): Blunted left cingulate activation in mood disorder subjects during a response interference task (the Stroop). *J Neuropsychiatry Clin Neurosci* 9:55–63.

Goodwin GM, Cavanagh JTO, Glabus MF, Kehoe RF, O'Carroll RE, Ebmeier KP, et al (1997): Uptake of 99mTc-exametazime shown by single photon emission computed tomography before and after lithium withdrawal in bipolar patients: associations with mania. *Br J Psychiatry* 170:426–430.

Grober E, Sliwinski M (1991): Development and validation of a model for estimating premorbid verbal intelligence in the elderly. *J Clin Exp Neuropsychol* 13:933–949.

Gyulai L, Alavi A, Broich K, Reilly J, Ball WB, Whybrow PC (1997): I-123 Iofetamine single-photon emission tomography in rapid cycling bipolar disorder: A clinical study. *Biol Psychiatry* 41:152–161.

Hamilton M (1960): A rating scale for depression. *J Neurol Neurosurg Psychiatry* 23:56–62.

Holcomb HH, Cascella NG, Thaker GK, Medoff DR, Dannals RF, Tamminga CA (1996): Functional sites of neuroleptic drug action in the human brain: PET/FDG studies with and without haloperidol. *Am J Psychiatry* 153:41–49.

Ketter TA, Andreason PJ, George MS, Lee C, Gill DS, Parekh PI, et al (1997): Anterior paralimbic mediation of procaine-induced emotional and psychosensory experiences. *Arch Gen Psychiatry* 53:59–69.

Kishimoto H, Takazu O, Ohno S, Yamaguchi T, Fujita H, Kuwahara H, et al (1987): 11C-glucose metabolism in manic and depressed patients. *Psychiatry Res* 22:81–88.

Krishnan KR, McDonald WM, Escalona PR, Doraiswamy PM, Na C, Husain MM, et al (1992): Magnetic resonance imaging of the caudate nuclei in depression: Preliminary observations. *Arch Gen Psychiatry* 49:553–557.

Lenze EJ, Sheline YI (1999): Absence of striatal volume differences between depressed subjects with no comorbid medical illness and matched comparison subjects. *Am J Psychiatry* 156:1989–1991.

Lewellen TK, Kohlmyer RS, Miyaoka RS, Kaplan MS, Stearns CW, Schubert SF (1996): Investigation of the performance of the General Electric ADVANCE positron emission tomograph in 3D mode. *IEEE Trans Nucl Sci* 43:2199–2207.

Mayberg HS, Brannan SK, Mahurin RK, Jerabek PA, Brickman JS, Tekell JL, et al (1997): Cingulate function in depression: A potential predictor of treatment response. *Neuroreport* 8:1057–1061.

Mega MS, Cummings JL, Salloway S, Malloy P (1997): The limbic system: An anatomic, phylogenetic, and clinical perspective. *J Neuropsychiatry Clin Neurosci* 9:315–330.

Migliorelli R, Starkstein SE, Teson A, de Quiros G, Vazquez S, Leiguarda R, et al (1993): SPECT findings in patients with primary mania. *J Neuropsychiatry Clin Neurosci* 5:379–383.

Nauta WJH (1971): The problem of the frontal lobe: A reinterpretation. *J Psychiatr Res* 8:167–187.

O'Connell RA, van Heertum RL, Luck D, Yudd AP, Cueva JE, Billick SB, et al (1995): Single-photon emission computed tomography of the brain in acute mania and schizophrenia. *J Neuroimaging* 5:101–104.

Oldfield RC (1971): The assessment and analysis of handedness: The Edinburgh Handedness Inventory. *Neuropsychologia* 9:97–113.

Peterson BS, Skudlarski P, Gatenby C, Zhang H, Anderson AW, Gore JC (1999): An fMRI study of Stroop word-color interference: Evidence for cingulate subregions subserving multiple distributed attentional systems. *Biol Psychiatry* 45:1237–1258.

Posner MI, Rothbart MK (1998): Attention, self-regulation and consciousness. *Philos Trans R Soc Lond B Biol Sci* 353:1915–1927.

Post RM, Uhde TW, Putnam FW, Ballenger JC, Berrettini WH (1982): Kindling and carbamazepine in affective illness. *J Nerv Ment Dis* 170:717–731.

Raichle ME (1987): The nervous system. In: Mountcastle VB, editor. *Handbook of Physiology*, Sec 1, Vol V. Bethesda, MD: American Physiological Society, 643–674.

Rauch SL, Jenike MA, Alpert NM, Baer L, Breiter HC, Savage CR, et al (1994): Regional cerebral blood flow measured during symptom provocation in obsessive-compulsive disorder using oxygen 15-labeled carbon dioxide and positron emission tomography. *Arch Gen Psychiatry* 51:62–70.

Rauch SL, Savage CR, Alpert NM, Miguel EC, Baer L, Breiter HC, et al (1995): A positron emission tomographic study of simple phobic symptom provocation. *Arch Gen Psychiatry* 52:20–28.

Rubin E, Sackeim HA, Prohovnik I, Moeller JR, Schnur DB, Mukherjee S (1995): Regional cerebral blood flow in mood disorders: IV. Comparison of mania and depression. *Psychiatry Res* 61:1–10.

Sackeim HA, Greenberg MS, Weiman AL, Gur RC, Hungerbuhler JP, Geschwind N (1982): Hemisphere asymmetry in the expression of positive and negative emotions. *Arch Neurol* 39:210–218.

Schwartz JM, Baxter LR, Mazziotta JC, Gerner RH, Phelps ME (1987): The differential diagnosis of depression. Relevance of positron emission tomography studies of cerebral glucose metabolism to the bipolar-unipolar dichotomy. *JAMA* 258: 1368–1374.

Silbersweig DA, Stern E, Frith CD, Cahill C, Schnorr L, Grootoonk S, et al (1993): Detection of thirty-second cognitive activations in single subjects with positron emission tomography: A new low-dose $H_2{}^{15}0$ regional cerebral blood flow three-dimensional imaging technique. *J Cereb Blood Flow Metab* 13:617–629.

Silfverskiold P, Risberg J (1989): Regional cerebral blood flow in depression and mania. *Arch Gen Psychiatry* 46:253–259.

Starkstein SE, Robinson RG (1997): Mechanisms of disinhibition after brain lesions. *J Nerv Ment Dis* 182:108–114.

Talairach J, Tournoux P (1988): *Co-Planar Stereotaxic Atlas of the Human Brain.* New York: Thieme.

Veselis RA, Reinsel RA, Beattie BJ, Mawlawi OR, Feshchenko VA, DiResta GR, et al (1997): Midazolam changes cerebral blood flow in discrete brain regions: An H2(15)O positron emission tomography study. *Anesthesiology* 87: 1106–1117.

Vogt BA, Finch DM, Olson CR (1992): Functional heterogeneity in cingulate cortex: The anterior executive and posterior evaluative regions. *Cereb Cortex* 2:435–443.

Wexler BE (1980): Cerebral laterality and psychiatry: A review of the literature. *Am J Psychiatry* 137:279–291.

Whalen PJ, Bush G, McNally RJ, Wilhelm S, McInerney SC, Jenike MA, Rauch SL (1998): The emotional counting Stroop paradigm: A functional magnetic resonance imaging probe of the anterior cingulate affective division. *Biol Psychiatry* 44:1219–1228.

Yeterian EH, van Hoesen GW (1978): Cortico-striate projections in the rhesus monkey: The organization of certain cortico-caudate connections. *Brain Res* 139:43–63.

PSYCHIATRY RESEARCH

Psychiatry Research 63 (1996) 161-168

Relationship between sleep and mood in patients with rapid-cycling bipolar disorder

Ellen Leibenluft*[a], Paul S. Albert[b], Norman E. Rosenthal[a], Thomas A. Wehr[a]

[a]Clinical Psychobiology Branch, National Institute of Mental Health, 10/4S-239, 10 Center Drive, MSC 1390, Bethesda, MD 20892-1390, USA

[b]Office of Biostatistics Research, National Heart, Lung, Blood Institute, Bethesda, MD, USA

Received 12 June 1995; revised 4 December 1995; accepted 25 February 1996

Abstract

The relationship between sleep and mood was examined in a longitudinal, naturalistic data set derived from outpatients with rapid-cycling bipolar disorder. Eleven patients completed daily self-ratings of mood and sleep logs for 18 months. Using logistic regression with autoregressive terms, we examined the effect of prior sleep (sleep duration, time of sleep onset, and time of wake onset) on the probability of being in a depressed, manic, or hypomanic episode on one or more subsequent days. Of the three sleep parameters, decreased sleep duration was the best predictor of mania or hypomania the next day, followed by wake onset time. The association between sleep duration and subsequent mood was less consistent for depression than for mania or hypomania. Four of the patients showed no relationship between mood and any of the sleep variables measured. These results reinforce the importance of monitoring, and perhaps controlling, sleep duration and wake onset time in at least some patients with rapid-cycling bipolar disorder.

Keywords: Circadian rhythms; Hypomania; Mania; Depression; Wake onset

1. Introduction

The relationship between mood and sleep has important theoretical and clinical implications. Sleep can vary with mood state: mania and hypomania are associated with decreased sleep duration while depression in bipolar patients is generally associated with hypersomnia and/or psychomotor retardation (Winokur et al., 1969; Detre et al., 1972; Carlson and Strober, 1979; Casper et al., 1985). Conversely, sleep deprivation can precipitate remission (or induce a switch into mania) in approximately 60% of depressed patients, with most patients relapsing after a night of recovery sleep (Wehr, 1990). These sleep deprivation experiments suggest that changes in the sleep patterns of depressed or manic/hypomanic patients are not merely symptoms of the illness but have pathogenic significance; that is, that sleep is depressogenic while wakefulness has antidepressant properties (Wehr, 1989). Only one study, however, has examined the relationship between sleep and mood by following the two variables longitudinally in a sample of patients with mood disorders (Albert et al., 1991). In that study, changes in the sleep patterns of patients with

* Corresponding author.

PII S0165-1781(96)02854-5

seasonal affective disorder followed, rather than anticipated, changes in mood.

Patients with rapid-cycling bipolar disorder represent an interesting population in which to perform a longitudinal study of the relationship between mood and sleep. By definition, such patients experience four or more affective episodes per year (Dunner and Fieve, 1974). In a sample of rapid cyclers, data about the relationship between mood and sleep can be obtained for a number of episodes within a relatively short period of time.

In our research clinic for rapid-cycling bipolar disorder, patients complete daily mood ratings and sleep logs while they are followed longitudinally. Applying logistic regression with autoregressive terms to account for the correlation of mood measures across time, we used these sleep logs and mood ratings to examine the effect of prior sleep on the probability of being in a manic/hypomanic or depressive episode on one or more subsequent days. The specific sleep parameters that we examined included sleep duration, time of sleep onset, and time of wake onset. Sleep duration reflects the ratio between the activity phase and the rest phase; as noted above, this ratio varies with mood state, increasing during mania and hypomania and decreasing during bipolar depression. The times of sleep and wake onset reflect, among other things, circadian phase markers, knowledge of which might shed light on the various chronobiological theories of depression (Wehr et al., 1980; Linkowski et al., 1985; Souêtre et al., 1989; Sack et al., 1990). In addition to these theoretical considerations, knowledge of the relationship between sleep parameters and mood has direct clinical implications, since therapeutic interventions could be designed to affect sleep duration and/or the times of sleep and wake onset.

These longitudinal data also afforded us the opportunity to examine one measure of the variability of the patients' clinical course. Specifically, using intraclass correlations, we analyzed the degree to which the length of each patient's depressive, manic, hypomanic, and euthymic episodes remained relatively constant throughout the period of observation. These data may have clinical and theoretical implications, as well as providing some useful information for researchers designing clinical trials for patients with rapid-cycling bipolar disorder.

2. Methods

Data were obtained from an outpatient research clinic of the National Institute of Mental Health for patients with rapid-cycling bipolar disorder. To be enrolled in the clinic, patients had to meet *DSM-III-R* criteria for bipolar disorder, as established by the Structured Clinical Interview for *DSM-III-R* (American Psychiatric Association, 1987; Spitzer et al., 1987). Patients who met *DSM-III-R* criteria for borderline or antisocial personality disorder were excluded. In addition, each patient had to have had at least four affective episodes that met *DSM-III-R* criteria within the last year, including at least one episode of mania or hypomania and one episode of major depressive disorder. An affective episode was defined as an episode meeting *DSM-III-R* criteria (including the duration criterion) for major depressive disorder, hypomania, or mania.

Each patient in the clinic completes a sleep log with 15-min resolution every morning upon awakening. In addition, twice each day (shortly after awakening and just before going to bed), each patient rates his or her mood on a 100-mm line (1 = most depressed ever felt; 100 = most manic ever felt; 35–65 = 'well range') (Whybrow and Guylia, 1995). In this analysis, we treated the self-ratings as categorical variables (<35 as depressed and >65 as manic, consistent with the markings on the patients' mood rating forms) because we were interested in the predictive effect of various sleep variables on the occurrence of manic/hypomanic and depressive mood states. We used the morning ratings and included in the analysis all patients for whom ≥ 18 months of data were available.

We computed the mean and median duration of each patient's episodes. We then examined the similarity of the progression by computing intraclass correlations (Snedecor and Cochran, 1980) for the duration of each of the three mood states (depression, mania, and normal mood). Intraclass correlations were computed on the log scale; an intraclass correlation above 0.5 suggests more variation between subjects than within subjects. Episodes with missing data were excluded from the calculations of both the descriptive statistics and the intraclass correlations.

Since logistic regression allows one to examine the effect of a set of independent variables on a binary (0 or 1) outcome, we used logistic regression to examine the effect of prior sleep on both the probability of being in a depressive episode and the probability of being in a manic or hypomanic episode at day t. Logistic regressions with 7-day lagged (autoregressive) effects (Cox and Shell, 1972; Zeger and Qaqish, 1988) were fit on each of the 11 patients. The models were fit using a statistical software package called SPLUS (Version 3.2, 1993, Mathsoft, Inc., Seattle, WA). As an illustration, the logistic regression model

$$logit\ P(Y_{t=1}) = \beta_0 + \beta_1 S_t + \gamma_1 Y_{t-1} + \gamma_2 Y_{t-2} + \ldots + \gamma_7 Y_{t-7}$$

examines the effect of the prior night's sleep (S_t) on the probability of being depressed ($P(P_{t=1})$) after adjusting for a lagged effect of depression ($Y_t, Y_{t-1}, \ldots, Y_{t-7}$).

Multiple models were fit on each person's data to examine the effect of each of the three sleep variables (sleep duration, sleep onset, and wake onset) on the probability of being depressed and of being manic or hypomanic. We defined the three sleep variables of interest as follows: sleep duration = the number of hours asleep during a 24-h period, beginning at 12 noon; wake onset = the time at the start of the first run of three 15-min awake intervals from 03:00 h to noon; and sleep onset = the time at the start of the first run of three 15-min asleep intervals from 20:00 h to 06:00 h.

Models for predicting depression were fit on all 11 patients, but only 8 patients had a sufficient number of manic days for analysis. Models with a 1-day, 3-day, and 7-day lagged effect were fit to examine the delay in the effect of sleep in predicting mood state. A χ^2 (likelihood ratio) test was used to compare models. The average (over all the patients) effect of each of the prior night sleep variables in predicting depression and mania or hypomania was summarized by averaging the effects (β_1) over patients and using the Wilcoxon signed rank test to determine whether the mean was different from zero. Due to the many statistical comparisons inherent in the analysis of the individual data, we used $P < 0.01$ as the cutoff for statistical significance of the individual data. For the group data, $P < 0.05$ was used as the cutoff for statistical significance.

3. Results

Table 1 presents the clinical and demographic data for the 11 patients in the study. Table 2 shows

Table 1
Patient demographics and medications

Patient No.	Sex	Age (years)	Medications
1	Female	42	Chlorpromazine, haloperidol, hydroxyzine, symmetrel, trazodone, chloral hydrate[a], clozapine[a], sodium valproate[a]
2	Female	31	Bupropion, sodium valproate, alprazolam PRN, fluoxetine[a], thyroxine[a]
3	Female	50	Lithium, bupropion[a], doxepin[a]
4	Female	42	Lithium, clonazepam[a], phenelzine[a]
5	Male	47	Sodium valproate, nortriptyline[a], sertraline, tranylcypromine[a]
6	Female	47	Lithium, loxitane, sodium valproate, clonazepam[a]
7	Female	49	Clonazepam, sodium valproate, thyroxine, lithium[a], tranylcypromine[a]
8	Female	39	Fluoxetine, sodium valproate
9	Female	37	Doxepin, lithium, lorazepam, carbamazepine[a]
10	Male	43	Lithium, haloperidol[a]
11	Female	39	Fluoxetine, lithium, perphenazine[a]

[a]Patient took this medication for part of the period of observation.

Table 2
Effect of prior night's sleep (duration, time awake, and time asleep) on predicting the occurrence of either a depressed or a manic/hypomanic episode

Patient No.	Mania/hypomania						Depression					
	Duration		Time awake		Time asleep		Duration		Time awake		Time asleep	
	β_1[a]	P[b]	β_1	P	β_l	P	β_l	P	β_l	P	β_l	P
1	NA	NA	NA	NA	NA	NA	0.015	NS	−0.030	NS	0.065	NS
2	−0.281	$P < 0.001$	−0.290	$P = 0.009$	0.381	$P = 0.009$	0.168	$P < 0.001$	0.200	$P < 0.001$	−0.084	NS
3	NA	NA	NA	NA	NA	NA	−0.488	$P < 0.001$	−0.701	$P = 0.001$	0.323	NS
4	−0.270	NS	−0.881	$P < 0.001$	−0.128	NS	0.096	NS	0.364	NS	0.415	NS
5	−0.422	$P < 0.001$	−0.357	NS	−0.118	NS	0.500	$P < 0.001$	0.285	$P < 0.001$	0.334	NS
6	NA	NA	NA	NA	NA	NA	−0.206	NS	−0.240	NS	−0.254	NS
7	−0.219	NS	0.074	NS	−0.097	NS	0.103	NS	−0.019	NS	−0.013	NS
8	−0.605	$P = 0.001$	−0.536	$P = 0.003$	0.000	NS	0.249	NS	0.102	NS	−0.084	NS
9	−0.256	$P < 0.001$	−0.150	NS	0.066	NS	0.106	NS	0.084	NS	−0.104	NS
10	−0.423	$P < 0.001$	0.017	NS	−0.171	NS	0.294	$P < 0.001$	−0.113	$P = 0.01$	−0.045	NS
11	−0.149	NS	−0.238	NS	0.042	NS	−0.030	NS	−0.089	NS	−0.076	NS
Average***	−0.328	$P = 0.008$	−0.295	$P = 0.040$	−0.003	NS	0.074	NS	−0.014	NS	0.043	NS

Note. NS, not significant. NA, not analyzed because of insufficient data.
[a]The estimated effect (β_1) in the model: logit + $P(Y_{t=1}) = \beta_0 + \beta_1 S_t + \gamma_2 Y_{t-2} + \ldots + \gamma_7 Y_{t-7}$
[b]The P value based on a likelihood ratio test (χ^2 with $df = 1$) testing whether $\beta_1 = 0$ in the model

logit + $P(Y_{t=1}) = \beta_o + \beta_1 S_t + \gamma_1 Y_{t-1} + \gamma_2 Y_{t-2} + \ldots + \gamma_7 Y_{t-7}$

***A Wilcoxon signed rank test was used to test whether the overall effect was different from zero.

Table 3
Duration (days) in each of the three mood states

Patient No.	Depression				Euthymia				Mania/hypomania			
	Episodes[a]	Mean	Median	Range	Episodes[a]	Mean	Median	Range	Episodes[a]	Mean	Median	Range
1	5	113	111	59–157	1	1	1	1–1	4	5.8	6	4–7
2	47	2.9	2	1–17	88	4.7	2	1–46	60	2.2	1	1–23
3	15	2.5	1	1–11	20	17.3	4	1–163	1	1	1	1-1
4	23	10.3	10	2–34	32	9.2	7	1–50	8	5.9	6	1–11
5	37	6.5	5	1–19	48	6.0	2	1–24	16	3.5	2.5	1–10
6	23	4.7	3	1–33	28	7.5	4	1–24	3	1.3	1	1–6
7	41	3.6	2	1–23	48	8.1	3.5	1–48	11	1.3	1	1–7
8	34	4.3	2.5	1–22	39	2.1	2	1–5	21	1.7	1	1–8
9	77	2.9	2	1–16	119	2.3	2	1–15	80	1.9	1	1–10
10	31	6.5	4	1–25	49	14.3	5	1–185	22	2.8	2	1–8
11	20	17.2	8	1–71	27	5.8	3	1–27	17	5.5	4	1–11

[a]Number of complete episodes.

the β_1 P value and direction of the effect of sleep 1 day earlier as a predictor of mood in each of the 11 patients and the average effect for the group as a whole. Of the eight patients who had a sufficient number of manic or hypomanic days to permit analysis of their data, five showed a significant effect of the prior night's sleep duration on the next day's mood. In all cases, the direction of the effect was such that increased sleep duration lowered the subsequent probability of being in a manic or hypomanic episode, and the average effect was significant ($P = 0.008$). Compared with sleep duration, the two other sleep measures were less predictive of a manic or hypomanic mood state: three of eight showed a predictive effect of wake onset (later awakening lowered the probability of being in a manic or hypomanic state), and only one of eight showed a predictive effect of sleep onset (earlier time asleep lowered the probability of being in a manic or hypomanic state). The average effect was significant for time awake ($P = 0.04$) but was not significantly different from zero for time asleep.

The sleep variables were less able to predict depressive episodes than to predict manic or hypomanic episodes. Of the 11 patients in the study, four showed a predictive effect of sleep duration, four showed a predictive effect for wake onset, and none showed a predictive effect for sleep onset. In addition, the direction of the significant effects was inconsistent, with half showing that an increase in sleep duration or later wake onset increased the probability of becoming depressed, and half showing the opposite. The inconsistent direction of the significant effects is reflected in the fact that the average effect for the group is insignificant.

Models with 3- and 7-day lagged sleep terms were fit on each subject's data to assess whether sleep variables more than 1 day earlier had an additional predictive effect over the prior night's sleep in either mania/hypomania or depression. We found little statistical evidence for an additional predictive effect of any sleep variable in the prediction of mania/hypomania or depression. That is, sleep status 3 or 7 days earlier played no significant role in improving the prediction of mood state provided by the prior night's sleep alone.

Table 3 shows the mean, median, and range for the number of days in each patient's depressive, manic/hypomanic, and euthymic episodes. The intraclass correlations were 0.61, 0.39, and 0.14 for the length of the depressed, manic/hypomanic, and euthymic episodes, respectively. Thus, the intraindividual variation in the length of the depressive episodes was relatively low (compared with the interindividual variation). In contrast, the intraindividual variation in the length of euthymic episodes was relatively high (compared with the interindividual variation).

4. Discussion

In this sample of patients with rapid-cycling bipolar disorder, our data show that the most consistent relationship between sleep and mood is that between sleep duration and mania/hypomania. Specifically, decreased sleep duration predicts that the next morning's mood rating will be hypomanic. Since decreased sleep duration can be conceptualized as a form of partial sleep deprivation, these data provide prospective, naturalistic evidence of a possible association between sleep deprivation and mania or hypomania, similar to the association that has been demonstrated in experimental settings (Wehr, 1990). These findings reinforce the clinical importance of attending to bipolar patients' sleep patterns. Specifically, clinicians should ensure that patients with rapid-cycling bipolar disorder maintain a schedule that allows them to get adequate amounts of sleep. In addition, should the patient begin to experience decreased sleep duration, the clinician should treat the insomnia aggressively to interrupt the manic or hypomanic cycle (Wehr, 1989).

As with decreased sleep duration, on average there was a significant association between wake onset and mania or hypomania. Specifically, earlier wake onset was associated with an increased probability of mania or hypomania the next day. The direction of this effect is consistent with the reported antidepressant effects of advancing the times of both sleep onset and wake onset (Wehr et al, 1979) and with the association between delayed sleep phase syndrome (DSPS) and depression (Regestein and Monk, 1995). However, in both the study of Wehr et al. (1979) and in DSPS, the times of sleep onset and wake onset shifted in parallel, so that the separate contributions of each to mood changes could not be assessed. Here, we analyzed the predictive effects of the times of wake onset and sleep onset separately, and found that wake onset time was a better predictor of both mania/hypomania and depression than was sleep onset time. Clinically, these data indicate the potential importance of monitoring (and perhaps manipulating) patients' time of awakening. Wake-up time has received considerably less attention than sleep onset time, perhaps because wake-up time is more difficult to manipulate pharmacologically. Our data suggest that interventions designed to shift bipolar patients' wake onset time deserve further study.

The possible finding of increased predictive value for wake onset time (compared with sleep onset time) also has potential theoretical implications. In animals, seasonal changes in sleep duration are thought to be regulated by a photoperiodic pacemaker consisting of two oscillators, one tracking dusk (the E, or evening, oscillator) and one tracking dawn (the M, or morning, oscillator) (Illnerova and Vanecek, 1982). Recent data in humans are also consistent with such a model (Wehr et al., 1993). In terms of the two-oscillator model, data from this study indicate that the changes in sleep duration that occur in association with rapid cycling may be related to shifts in the phase (timing) of the M, but not the E, oscillator. Further studies of this question are warranted.

Both the association between sleep duration and depressed mood, and the direction of that association, are less consistent in depression than in (hypo)mania. Although a number of investigators have found that bipolar depression is generally characterized by hypersomnia (Winokur et al., 1969; Detre et al., 1972; Carlson and Strober, 1979; Casper et al., 1985), our data may reflect the fact that some bipolar patients (like some unipolar patients) may instead suffer from insomnia when they become depressed. Few studies compare the clinical characteristics and treatment response of bipolar patients with typical depressive symptoms (such as insomnia) to those with atypical depressive symptoms (such as hypersomnia) (Casper et al., 1985); this may be a fruitful area for further study.

For several reasons, these results should be viewed as preliminary. (1) The sample size was small, and 4 of the 11 patients showed no significant relationship between mood and the sleep variables measured. (2) Although we attempted to keep our patients' medication regimens stable, we were sometimes unable to do so because of their clinical instability. Medication changes were not considered in the data analysis, and their effects on the results are unknown. However, we have no reason to believe that they are systematically biased and would therefore skew our results in a specific direction. (3) Since all of the patients in our sample had a rapid-cycling pattern to their illness, we do not know if these results are generalizable to bipolar patients who are not rapid cyclers.

In addition, our data do not permit causal conclusions because they are derived from a naturalistic study rather than from an experiment. We cannot exclude the possibility that decreased sleep duration on a given night reflects a manic/hypomanic process that began sometime between the morning mood rating and the patient's bedtime; consequently, we cannot conclude that decreased sleep duration on a given night causes mania or hypomania the following day. In addition, we cannot exclude the possibility that a third, unknown variable affects mood and sleep and therefore creates the impression of a causal relationship when none exists.

In sum, we have examined the ability of sleep parameters to predict the mood of a patient with rapid-cycling bipolar disorder on the subsequent day. Decreased duration of sleep and, to a lesser extent, earlier wake onset time predicted mania or hypomania on the next day. For both depression and mania, wake onset time was a better predictor of mood than was sleep onset time, although the relationship between each of the sleep parameters and mood was less consistent for depression than for mania. Since the sleep parameters that we studied can all be manipulated therapeutically, further examination of these relationships is warranted to improve the treatment of patients with rapid-cycling bipolar disorder.

References

Albert, P.S., Rosen, L.N., Alexander, J.R. and Rosenthal N.E. (1991) Effect of daily variation in weather and sleep on patients with seasonal affective disorder. *Psychiatry Res* 36, 51–63.

American Psychiatric Association. (1987) *DSM-III-R: Diagnostic and Statistical Manual of Mental Disorders*. 3rd rev. edn. American Psychiatric Press, Washington, DC.

Carlson, G.A. and Strober, M. (1979) Affective disorders in adolescence. *Psychiatr Clin North Am* 2, 511–526.

Casper, R.C., Redmond, E., Jr., Katz, M.M., Schaffer, C.B., Davis, J.M. and Koslow, S.H. (1985) Somatic symptoms in primary affective disorder: presence and relationship to classification. *Arch Gen Psychiatry* 42, 1098–1104.

Cox, D. and Shell, E. (1989) *Analysis of Binary Data*. Chapman and Hall, London.

Detre, T., Himmelhoch, J., Swartzburg, M., Anderson, C.M., Byck, R. and Kupfer, D.J. (1972) Hypersomnia and manic-depressive disease. *Am J Psychiatry* 128, 1303–1305.

Dunner, D.L. and Fieve, R.R. (1974) Clinical factors in lithium carbonate prophylaxis failure. *Arch Gen Psychiatry* 30, 229–233.

Illnerova, H. and Vanecek, J. (1982) Two-oscillator structure of the pacemaker controlling the circadian rhythm of *N*-acetyltransferase in the rat pineal gland. *J Comp Physiol* 145, 539–548.

Linkowski, P., Mendlewicz, J., Kerkhofs, M., Leclercq, R., Brasseur, M., Hubain, P., Golstein, J., Copinschi, G. and Van Cauter, E. (1985) The 24-h profile of adrenocorticotropin and cortisol in major depressive illness. *J Clin Endocrinol Metab* 65, 141–150.

Regestein Q.R. and Monk T.H. (1995) Delayed sleep phase syndrome: a review of its clinical aspects. *Am J Psychiatry* 152, 602–608.

Sack, R.L., Lewy, A.J., White, D.M., Singer, C.M., Fireman, M.J. and Vandiver, R. (1990) Morning vs. evening light treatment for winter depression. *Arch Gen Psychiatry* 47, 343–351.

Snedecor; G. and Cochran, W. (1980) *Statistical Methods*. The Iowa State University Press, Ames, IA.

Souêtre, E., Salvatis, E., Belugou, J-L., Pringuey, D., Candito, M., Krebs, B., Ardisson, J.-L. and Darcourt, G. (1989) Circadian rhythms in depression and recovery: evidence for blunted amplitude as the main chronobiological abnormality. *Psychiatry Res* 28, 263–278.

Spitzer, R.L., Williams, J.B.W. and Gibbon, M. (1987) *Structured Clinical Interview for* DSM-III-R, *Patient Version*. New York State Psychiatric Institute, New York.

Wehr, T.A. (1989) Sleep loss: a preventable cause of mania and other excited states. *J Clin Psychiatry* 50, 8–16.

Wehr, T.A. (1990) Effects of sleep and wakefulness in depression and mania. In: Montplaisir, J. and Godbout, R. (Eds.), *Sleep and Biological Rhyhms*. Oxford University Press, London.

Wehr, T.A., Moul, D.E., Barbato, G., Giesen, H.A., Seidel, J.A., Barker, C. and Bender, C. (1993) Conservation of photoperiod-responsive mechanisms in humans. *Am J Physiol* 265 (Regulatory, Integrative, and Comparative Physiology, 34), R846–R857.

Wehr, T.A., Muscettola, G. and Goodwin, F.K. (1980) Urinary MHPG circadian rhythm: early timing (phase advance) in manic-depressives compared with normal subjects. *Arch Gen Psychiatry* 37, 257–263.

Wehr, T.A., Wirz-Justice, A., Goodwin, F.K., Duncan, W.C. and Gillin, J.C. (1979) Phase advance of the circadian sleep-wake cycle as an antidepressant. *Science* 206, 149–158.

Whybrow, P.C. and Guylia, L. (1995) The chronorecord: tracking bipolar patterns and treatment effects. In: *Abstracts for the 2nd International Conference on New Directions in Affective Disorders*, Jerusalem.

Winokur, G., Clayton, P.J. and Reich, T. (1969) *Manic-Depressive Illness*. C.V. Mosby, St. Louis, MO.

Zeger, S. and Qaqish, B. (1988) Markov regression models for time series: a quasi-likelihood approach. *Biometrics* 44, 1019–1031.

Molecular Mechanisms Underlying Mood Stabilization in Manic-Depressive Illness: The Phenotype Challenge

Ognian C. Ikonomov, M.D., Ph.D., and Husseini K. Manji, M.D.

Objective: The authors critically examine the evidence supporting the hypothesis that lithium's therapeutic effects in bipolar affective disorder are mediated by alterations in the expression of specific genes in critical neuronal circuits. **Method:** Using the heuristic "initiation and adaptation paradigm," the authors appraise the biological effects and underlying molecular and cellular mechanisms of lithium's action. The evidence is critically reviewed, with special attention to the reductive and integrative approaches necessary for identifying lithium's clinically relevant cellular and molecular targets. **Results:** Lithium's acute effects are mediated through inhibition of specific enzymes involved in two distinct but interacting signaling pathways—the protein kinase C and glycogen synthase kinase 3β signaling cascades—that converge at the level of gene transcriptional regulation. The expression of different genes, including transcription factors, is markedly altered by chronic lithium administration. Chronic lithium treatment also robustly increases the expression of the neuroprotective protein Bcl-2, raising the intriguing possibility that some of lithium's effects are mediated through underappreciated neurotrophic/neuroprotective effects. The importance of lithium's effect on circadian rhythms and the related methodological problems in validating the role of specific genes in lithium's therapeutic effects are discussed. **Conclusions:** Despite the plethora of lithium effects at the genomic level, direct evidence that the genes identified thus far are responsible for phenotypic changes associated with chronic lithium treatment is still lacking. The combination of sensitive molecular technologies, appropriately designed paradigms, better behavioral analysis, and a chronobiologic approach seems necessary for the future identification of one or more clinically relevant lithium-target genes.

(Am J Psychiatry 1999; 156:1506–1514)

Bipolar affective disorder (manic-depressive illness) is a common, severe, chronic, and often life-threatening illness (1). Despite the devastating impact of bipolar disorder on the lives of millions, there is still a dearth of knowledge concerning its etiology and pathophysiology. The discovery of lithium's efficacy as a mood-stabilizing agent revolutionized the treatment of patients with bipolar disorder, and after three decades of use in North America, lithium continues to be the mainstay of treatment for this disorder, both for the acute manic phase and as prophylaxis for recurrent manic and depressive episodes (1, 2). Adequate lithium treatment also reduces the excessive mortality observed in the illness (1, 2). However, the biochemical basis for lithium's antimanic and mood-stabilizing actions remains to be fully elucidated (3–6). Understanding the molecular and cellular mechanisms by which lithium stabilizes an underlying dysregulation in critical neuronal circuits not only offers the potential for the development of improved treatments but may also help to delineate the pathophysiology of bipolar disorder (4, 7).

A useful "initiation and adaptation" paradigm for understanding the long-term action of psychotropic drugs has been proposed (8). This paradigm posits that the effect of acute drug administration is medi-

Received Aug. 12, 1998; revision received March 29, 1999; accepted May 11, 1999. From the Laboratory of Molecular Pathophysiology, Department of Psychiatry and Behavioral Neurosciences, the Department of Pharmacology, and the Cellular and Clinical Neurobiology Program, Wayne State University School of Medicine. Address reprint requests to Dr. Ikonomov, Laboratory of Molecular Pathophysiology, Department of Psychiatry and Behavioral Neurosciences, Wayne State University School of Medicine, 2309 Scott Hall, 540 East Canfield Ave., Detroit, MI 48201; aa0970@wayne.edu (e-mail).

Supported by NIMH grant MH-57743, the Theodore and Vada Stanley Foundation, the National Alliance for Research on Schizophrenia and Depression, and the Joseph Young Senior Foundation.

The authors thank Ms. Celia Knobelsdorf for editorial assistance.

A complete list of the studies on which this article is based can be obtained on request.

ated through initial direct perturbation of one or more target proteins; repeated administration, by means of the same initial event, over time leads to enduring adaptive changes in critical neuronal networks, thereby resulting in stable long-term effects (8). Based on this model, two experimental approaches to understanding the molecular mechanisms of chronic lithium action can be envisioned. First, the identification of the initial lithium target(s) will facilitate the elucidation of the downstream events mediating its chronic effects. Second, and in a reverse direction, delayed "adaptations" occurring in the context of stable long-term lithium-induced phenotypes should be identified and their relationship with the initial events subsequently established.

Irrespective of the approach, the identification of lithium targets requires an initial reductive step and a subsequent integrative step. The reductive step isolates and characterizes candidate genes and proteins. In the integrative step, the importance of the protein is validated in the original experimental system. For example, if an acute lithium effect is associated with selective enzyme inhibition, the causal relationship between the two events may be established by specific inhibition of the same enzyme with another inhibitor. In the same vein, if a single gene is deemed responsible for some of the long-term lithium-induced changes, a selective manipulation of its protein level should mimic this facet of chronic lithium action. In this context, the search for targets of chronic lithium administration is similar to the task of identifying genes responsible for complex behavioral and physiological traits, such as obesity, hypertension, and circadian rhythms. In all these situations the role of an identified candidate protein is proven by its capacity to correct the abnormal phenotype (for reviews see references 9 and 10). Thus, it is critical to bear in mind that the analysis of the molecular basis of lithium action is meaningful only under conditions of a clear-cut lithium-induced phenotype. This is because the magnitude of the effect, the built-in "redundancy," and the degree to which the biochemical effect can be compensated for by other pathways all determine whether the molecular or cellular event actually has functional significance. Indeed, any observed biochemical phenomenon may, in fact, even represent a compensatory adaptation to the "true" therapeutic effect. Finally, as lithium targets are inevitably first identified in experimental systems, the identification of genes potentially responsible for lithium's therapeutic effects involves one additional step—the validation of the role of the gene product in lithium-induced mood stabilization in patients with bipolar disorder. Thus, although a surfeit of biochemical effects associated with lithium administration have been identified (3–5), attributing therapeutic relevance to these findings requires extensive validation. In this article we use the initiation-adaptation paradigm to critically assess our current understanding of lithium's acute and long-term actions.

PHENOTYPIC CHANGES WITH SHORT-TERM AND LONG-TERM LITHIUM APPLICATION

In addition to its beneficial mood-stabilizing effect in bipolar disorder, lithium treatment does produce significant phenotypic changes in a variety of experimental systems. Moreover, in addition to its direct functional effects, lithium treatment markedly modulates the effects of other stimuli. The biological effects of lithium can be divided into short-term effects (manifested soon after lithium's application and likely mediated through the available cellular machinery) and long-term effects (presumably based on selective changes in gene expression and appearing after a lag period of several days to weeks).

Many of lithium's short-term effects appear to be cell type or tissue specific. Examples of short-term stimulatory effects include lithium-induced corticotropin secretion by rat anterior pituitary cells (11) and acute glutamate release in lithium-treated brain slices (12). Inhibitory effects of short-term lithium treatment are documented in angiotensin-II-induced aldosterone secretion by adrenal glomerulosa cells (13) and in the relaxation rate following cholinergic induction of smooth muscle contraction (14). A separate group of effects includes the teratogenic effects of short-term lithium exposure in early development. Thus, a brief treatment at a stage of 32–64 cells in a *Xenopus* embryo leads to an embryo with two dorsal structures, an effect called "dorsalization." Profound developmental effects of lithium have also been documented in sea urchins, zebrafish, and *Dictyostelium* (15). It should be noted that many of these developmental effects are observed at concentrations that are considerably greater than those attained therapeutically.

Among the long-term phenotypic changes are lithium-induced alterations in circadian rhythmicity (16) and, of course, changes in mood in patients with bipolar disorder (1), appearing after 2–3 days or weeks, respectively. Chronic lithium treatment in the laboratory rat leads to a persistent performance deficit in some behavioral tests (active avoidance and visually cued maze), whereas the deficit in a spatial memory task is transient. A similar transient deficit is found in the ability of acetylcholine to potentiate N-methyl-D-aspartic acid (NMDA) responses in hippocampal neurons (17). Furthermore, chronic lithium treatment has been reported to inhibit the seizures in a kindling model of epilepsy in the rat (18), although similar treatment potentiates the seizure response to cholinergic agonists (19). Most recently, chronic lithium administration has been shown to exert neuroprotective effects against a variety of insults both in vitro and in vivo (discussed in references 20–22), effects that are likely mediated by lithium's robust increase in the expression of the neuroprotective protein Bcl-2 (discussed later in this article).

Finally, an important (but often overlooked) consideration is that, in addition to the beneficial effects on mood, chronic lithium treatment is associated with many side effects, including polyuria, polydipsia, and

FIGURE 1. Cellular and Molecular Mechanisms of Action of Lithium[a]

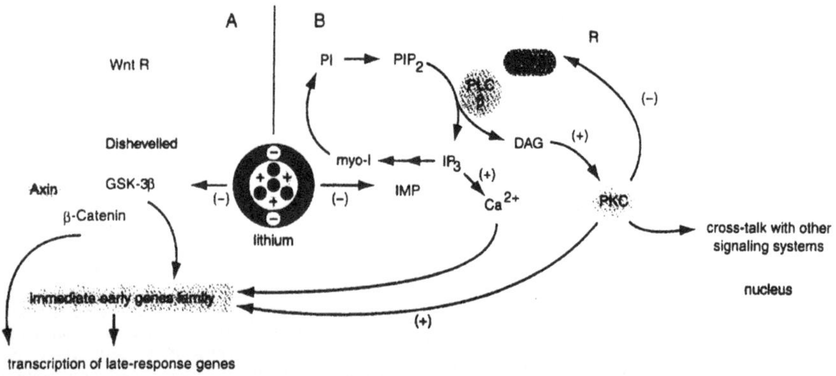

[a] At therapeutic concentrations lithium directly inhibits (arrows) two enzymes—glycogen synthase kinase 3β (GSK-3β) and inositol monophosphate phosphatase (IMP). In certain systems (see part A), GSK-3β is in a cytosolic complex with other proteins—Axin and β-Catenin. β-Catenin is a transcription factor and the effector of the Wnt signaling pathway, which also involves extracellular ligands (encoded by the *Wnt* gene family, not shown), Wnt membrane receptors (encoded by the *Frizzled* gene family), and Dishevelled proteins. The Wnt signaling activation leads to a nuclear translocation of β-Catenin and activation of c-Jun. Short lithium exposure blocks the tonic inhibitory action of GSK-3β and activates the Wnt signaling pathway, an effect that can be imitated by a dominant negative GSK-3β mutant. In the brain (see part B), lithium inhibits IMP, resulting in a lowering of myoinositol (myo-I). This acute effect has the potential to induce a cascade of effects in the DAG/PKC limb of the signal transduction pathway (DAG, diacylglycerol; PKC, protein kinase C). The effect of lithium is complex and involves biphasic changes—an initial activation of PKC followed by a decrease in PKC α and ε. Lithium, through its effects on PKC, also regulates the expression of the important neuronal phosphoprotein MARCKS (myristoylated alanine-rich C kinase substrate). Increased intracellular Ca^{2+} and PKC activate the transcription of immediate early genes, including the *fos* and *jun* families. Similar to the effects observed with PKC, lithium induces complex, biphasic effects on c-*fos* expression. Multiple late-response genes have been shown to be significantly affected by lithium treatment. Following are definitions of other terms appearing in the figure: PLC, phospholipase C; PIP_2, phosphatidylinositol-4,5-bisphosphate; IP_3, inositol-1,4,5-trisphosphate; PI, phosphoinositide; R, membrane receptor; $G_{q/11}$, G protein subtype.

clinical or subclinical impairment of thyroid function (1, 3). It is believed that these common side effects are due, at least in part, to lithium-induced inhibition of vasopressin- and thyrotropin-sensitive adenylate cyclase in kidney distal tubules and the thyroid gland, respectively (3). In addition, lithium toxicity in yeast is associated with inhibition of RNA-processing enzymes (23). Furthermore, the diabetes-insipidus-like status accompanying chronic administration of dietary lithium to the rat increases the vasopressin mRNA levels in paraventricular and supraoptic hypothalamic nuclei (24). Similarly, thyroid hormones are known to bring about a variety of changes in expression of genes in the central nervous system (CNS). These observations illustrate the multiple causes of differential regulation of gene expression that have to be carefully considered in the search for therapeutically relevant lithium-target genes.

CURRENT HYPOTHESES ABOUT LITHIUM'S INITIATING EFFECTS

Lithium, whose hydrated ionic radius is similar to that of magnesium, inhibits several enzymes in vitro (15, 25). Most notably, inositol monophosphatases (IMPases) and glycogen synthase kinase 3β (GSK-3β) play important roles in two distinct but interacting signal transduction pathways. The study of these pathways has led to the formulation of two major hypotheses for the cellular basis of lithium's acute action: the inositol depletion hypothesis (25) and the GSK-3β inhibition hypothesis (15, 26). Here we briefly present these hypotheses, focusing on observations that these acute cellular actions of lithium converge at the level of gene transcription regulation (figure 1).

LITHIUM AND THE PHOSPHOINOSITIDE CYCLE

Inositol phospholipids play a major role in receptor-mediated signal transduction pathways, and they are involved in diverse responses in the CNS (27). Many cell surface receptors interact with guanine nucleotide binding proteins (G proteins, generally $G_{q/11}$), resulting in the generation of two second messengers—inositol-1,4,5-trisphosphate (IP_3) and diacylglycerol (DAG) (figure 1B).

Maintaining sufficient myoinositol supplies is crucial to the resynthesis of phosphoinositides and the efficiency of signaling. Lithium, at therapeutic concentrations, inhibits inositol-1-phosphatase (K_i, 0.8 mM), thereby impairing a major "inositol recycling pathway." Lithium also inhibits inositol polyphosphate-1-phosphatase, which is involved in recycling inositol polyphosphates to inositol. Since the mode of enzyme inhibition is uncompetitive, lithium's effects have been postulated to be most pronounced in systems with high rates of phosphoinositide turnover (25, 28). Thus, it was proposed that lithium's action is mediated through a depletion of free inositol, and its selectivity was attributed to its preferential action on the most active receptor-mediated neuronal pathways (25, 29). Since several subtypes of neurotransmitter receptors are coupled to hydrolysis of phosphatidylinositol-4,5-bisphosphate (PIP_2) in the brain, the inositol depletion hypothesis offered a plausible explanation for lithium's therapeutic efficacy in bipolar disorder and gained wide acceptance.

There is indeed experimental evidence to show that inhibition of IMP does underlie some of lithium's acute effects. In yeast, for example, acute lithium administration induces a prolongation of the ultradian period (normally around 30 minutes) in a cellular variable called the "septation index." Overexpression of the human IMP markedly increases the lithium concentration necessary for this effect, suggesting that this lithium effect depends on IMP inhibition (30). However, numerous studies have examined lithium's effects on CNS-receptor-mediated phosphoinositide responses, and although some have shown a reduction in agonist-stimulated PIP_2 hydrolysis in rat brain slices following acute lithium administration, these changes have often been small, inconsistent, and subject to the studies' numerous methodological differences (see reference 31 for an excellent critique). Most recently, a magnetic resonance spectroscopy study (32) demonstrated that lithium-induced myoinositol reductions are observed in the frontal cortex of patients with bipolar disorder after only 5 days of lithium administration, at a time when the patients' clinical state is completely unchanged. Consequently, these and other studies suggest that while inhibition of IMP may be an initiating lithium effect, reduction of myoinositol levels itself does not underlie lithium's therapeutic effects. The hypothesis that these effects initiate a cascade of changes in PKC signaling and gene expression, effects that are ultimately responsible for lithium's therapeutic effects, is discussed later.

GSK-3β: THERAPEUTICALLY RELEVANT TARGET FOR LITHIUM'S ACTIONS?

In recent years a hitherto unexpected target for lithium's acute effects has been identified. Klein and Melton (15) were the first to demonstrate that lithium, at therapeutically relevant concentrations, is an inhibitor of GSK-3β in vitro (figure 1). GSK-3β is an evolutionary highly conserved kinase, originally identified as a regulator of glycogen synthesis. Overexpression of a negative GSK-3β mutant (a biologically inactive version of the enzyme inhibiting the endogenous protein) also induces dorsalization of the *Xenopus* embryo, indicating the important role of GSK-3β in this teratogenic lithium effect (26). It is now known that GSK-3β plays an important role in the CNS, by regulating various cytoskeletal processes through its effects on Tau and Synapsin I and by inducing long-term nuclear events through phosphorylation of c-Jun and nuclear translocation of β-Catenin (26, 33, 34). As discussed, lithium is known to bring about a variety of biochemical effects, and it is unclear whether inhibition of GSK-3β is a therapeutically relevant effect. We therefore investigated whether the structurally highly dissimilar antimanic (and likely mood-stabilizing) agent valproate also regulates GSK-3β. We found that both lithium and valproate significantly inhibited GSK-3β at therapeutically relevant concentrations (35). Consistent with GSK-3β inhibition, both lithium and valproate produced significant time-dependent increases in cytosolic and nuclear β-Catenin levels in human cells of neuronal origin. These data indicate that GSK-3β is a common initial target for both mood stabilizers and support its implication in lithium's beneficial long-term action. It is important for the present discussion that GSK-3β is known to phosphorylate the protein c-Jun at three sites adjacent to its DNA binding domain, thereby reducing binding of activator protein 1 (AP-1) (see later discussion) (36). Thus, the acute inhibition of GSK-3β by lithium and valproate has the potential to bring about long-term changes in the CNS through the transcriptional activity of both β-Catenin and AP-1.

LONG-TERM MEDIATORS OF LITHIUM'S THERAPEUTIC EFFECTS: THE ROLE OF THE PKC FAMILY OF ENZYMES

As discussed in the preceding, reduction of myoinositol levels per se likely does not underlie lithium's therapeutic effects. However, some of lithium's initial actions may occur through IMP inhibition, which initiates a cascade of secondary changes in the PKC signaling pathway and gene expression in the CNS, effects that are potentially responsible for lithium's therapeutic efficacy (reviewed in references 3–5 and 37). PKC exists as a family of closely related subspecies, has a heterogeneous distribution in the brain, and plays a major role in the regulation of neuronal excitability, neurotransmitter release, and long-term alterations in gene expression and plasticity (37–39). Lithium exerts significant effects on PKC in a number of cell systems, including the brain (3–5). Thus, lithium treatment has complex, biphasic effects on PKC, and chronic lithium administration at therapeutically relevant concentrations produces isozyme-specific decreases in PKC α and ε in the frontal cortex and hippocampus (40, 41). Furthermore, Lenox and associates (42) demonstrated that the levels of a critical

PKC substrate, myristoylated alanine-rich C kinase substrate (MARCKS), a key protein implicated in synaptic transmission and neuroplastic events, is also significantly reduced in the hippocampus after chronic lithium exposure. Valproate produces strikingly similar effects on the PKC signaling pathway, including MARCKS (41, 43, 44). These intriguing biochemical observations indicate that the PKC signaling pathway represents a common long-term target for both lithium and valproate, two agents with clinically proven antimanic and likely mood-stabilizing efficacy. It is interesting that preliminary studies suggest that chronic lithium and valproate regimens appear to regulate the PKC signaling pathway by distinct initiating mechanisms (43, 45). This finding is consistent with clinical observations that some patients show preferential response to one or other of the agents and that additive therapeutic effects are sometimes observed in patients.

LITHIUM'S EFFECTS ON IMMEDIATE EARLY GENES

The transcriptional activation of immediate early genes, including the *fos* and *jun* families, is a characteristic cellular response to extracellular stimuli such as hormones, growth factors, and neurotransmitters (46). The transcriptional activation is followed by cytoplasmic translation of Fos, Jun, and other proteins, which translocate into the nucleus and form a variety of protein complexes. AP-1 is a collection of homodimeric and heterodimeric complexes composed of products of *fos* and *jun* family members. These products bind to a common DNA site—12-O-tetradecanoylphorbol 13-acetate (TPA) response element (TRE)—in the regulatory domain of the gene and activate gene transcription. The genes regulated by AP-1 in the CNS include genes for various neuropeptides, neurotrophins, receptors, transcription factors, enzymes involved in neurotransmitter synthesis, and proteins that bind to cytoskeletal elements (46). The final result of this molecular cascade is alteration in the transcription of selected target genes bearing the specific DNA binding site on their regulatory regions.

It is noteworthy that both lithium and valproate, at therapeutically relevant concentrations, produce increases in AP-1 DNA binding activity in rat brain ex vivo and in cultured human neuroblastoma cells in vitro (5, 41, 47, 48). Furthermore, both lithium and valproate increase the expression of a luciferase reporter gene, effects that are markedly attenuated by mutations at the promoter AP-1 sites (41). While the reporter gene effects in vitro suggest that lithium-induced AP-1 activation does have functional effects, it is clearly necessary to demonstrate that they also occur in critical regions of the CNS in vivo. It is well established that the expression of tyrosine hydroxylase is mediated in large part by the AP-1 family of transcription factors (49). Thus, a study was undertaken to determine whether chronic lithium administration does, in fact, increase the CNS levels of a protein known to be regulated in large part by AP-1 (50). Consistent with AP-1 activation, chronic lithium administration significantly increased the levels of tyrosine hydroxylase in the frontal cortex, hippocampus, and striatum (50), three brain areas implicated in the pathophysiology of bipolar disorder (51–53). In view of the key roles of immediate early genes in long-term neuronal plasticity and cellular responsiveness, and the potential to regulate patterns of gene expression in critical neuronal circuits, these effects may play a major role in lithium's long-term therapeutic effects and are worthy of further study.

IDENTIFICATION OF NOVEL TARGETS

The preceding data suggest that lithium has the potential to regulate CNS gene expression, and indeed many genes have been suggested as targets for the actions of chronic lithium (3–6). However, the large number of genes expressed in a given cell at any time (10,000–15,000) opens up the opportunity for the identification of novel genes whose expression is affected by chronic drug treatment. In recent years, new methods have evolved to identify the differential expression of multiple genes (e.g., in pathological versus normal tissue or in control versus treated tissue); one such method that is being increasingly used is the reverse transcription polymerase chain reaction mRNA differential display (RT-PCR DD) (54, 55). By using this method, lithium was shown to increase 2′,3′-cyclic nucleotide 3′-phosphodiesterase mRNA levels in C6 glioma cells (56). In order to identify potentially therapeutically relevant changes in gene expression, we have used RT-PCR DD to concurrently investigate the effects of chronic lithium and valproate administration in intact animals (57). One of the transcripts whose levels were markedly increased by both lithium and valproate encodes a transcription factor—the β subunit of the polyomavirus enhancer-binding protein 2 (PEBP2β). In concert, the DNA binding activity of PEBP2αβ also increased in the rat frontal cortex. We therefore next investigated lithium's effects on the levels of a critical protein known to be regulated by PEBP2β—the major neuroprotective protein Bcl-2. We found that chronic lithium treatment of rats resulted in doubling of Bcl-2 levels in the frontal cortex, an effect accompanied by a marked increase in the number of Bcl-2 immunoreactive cells in frontal cortex layers II and III (22). The robust increase in Bcl-2 levels likely plays a major role in lithium's neuroprotective effects against a variety of insults both in vitro (including glutamate, calcium, and 1-methyl-4-phenylpiridinium [MPP^+]) and ex vivo (including irradiation, kainic acid, and ischemia) (discussed in references 20–22).

Are such putative neuroprotective effects relevant for mood disorders? There is now considerable evidence demonstrating significant reductions in regional CNS volume and cell numbers associated with mood disorders from both in vivo brain imaging studies and postmortem studies (51–53). It is intriguing that neuronal loss is especially pronounced in layer II of the rostral orbitofrontal region (53), an area with the largest lithium-induced increase in Bcl-2 immunoreactivity. Thus, overall, these data suggest that lithium's effects on CNS Bcl-2 levels (and accompanying neuroprotective effects) may be of considerable importance in the long-term treatment of mood disorders. It is noteworthy that several antidepressants increase the expression of brain-derived neurotrophic factor, findings that have led to the development of a heuristic molecular and cellular model of depression (58).

LIMITATIONS IN EXPERIMENTAL STUDY OF EFFECTS OF CHRONIC LITHIUM TREATMENT

Although the application of advanced cellular and molecular biologic methods to the study of lithium's actions has provided intriguing and unexpected new leads, several factors make it difficult to clearly attribute therapeutic relevance to these biochemical findings. To begin with, a suitable experimental model of manic-depression is currently not available. In this context, it is likely that the robust animal models of drug abuse have been instrumental in accelerating the pace of research on the underlying molecular events (8). Another inherent problem in the identification of lithium-target genes is the relative paucity of easily detectable phenotypic changes induced by chronic lithium treatment. This makes the task of ascribing functional significance to the multiple lithium-induced changes at the genomic level quite daunting. Moreover, the genetic basis of mood and affect as quantitative traits is still at its inception (59), and we therefore cannot focus on a group of genes known to be involved in affect regulation. In this regard, the observations that several genes encoding neuromodulatory peptides (prodynorphin, preprotachykinin, neuropeptide Y, and glucocorticoid receptor type II) are markedly affected by lithium treatment in the rat (3, 4) are still awaiting experimental validation of their functional significance in the treatment of mood disorders. In addition, as already discussed, chronic lithium treatment is also associated with side effects that could affect gene expression, including polyuria, polydipsia, and impairment of thyroid function. These observations illustrate the difficulties that the investigator faces in the search for therapeutically relevant lithium-target genes. Thus, overall, a growing body of evidence suggests that chronic lithium action is associated with a number of changes in gene expression. A difficulty arises, however, in testing the hypothesis that the altered expression of any given gene per se is involved in phenotypic changes associated with chronic lithium treatment.

Another factor worthy of consideration is the experimental systems used to study the mechanisms of chronic lithium action—these range from single cells to whole animals. The single cell models are attractive because of easy control over drug concentration and the possibility of intricately addressing cellular and molecular interactions. However, the cells generally do not exhibit readily detectable phenotypic alterations, even at concentrations much above the lithium levels that are toxic for the whole animal. Exceptions to this are the ultradian rhythms in yeast (30) and the protection against NMDA-induced apoptosis in dissociated neurons (20). Although cell culture systems lack normal cell-cell interactions, they offer the potential to identify genes that are direct cellular lithium targets.

Conversely, an example of a protein whose expression is significantly affected by chronic lithium administration in the whole rat but not in a cellular model is Gephyrin. Gephyrin clusters inhibitory postsynaptic membrane receptors (glycine and γ-amino-butyric-acid) in CNS neurons (60). Chronic lithium treatment (5 weeks but not 9 days) significantly increased Gephyrin levels in the frontal cortex but not the hippocampus; moreover, the increase in Gephyrin correlated well with the individual lithium plasma levels (61). By contrast, lithium treatment of human neuroblastoma cells (from 1 to 7 days) did not result in appreciable changes in Gephyrin levels. These data support the view that whole animal models are essential for the detection of certain long-term lithium-target genes whose expression depends on interacting neuronal networks.

However, the use of laboratory rodents also presents us with problems in interpreting the potential changes in gene expression because of chronic lithium-induced alterations in circadian rhythmicity. The latter problem is discussed in the following section.

CHRONIC LITHIUM TREATMENT AND CIRCADIAN RHYTHMS

Rhythmicity is a fundamental characteristic of living matter. When a variable is longitudinally monitored and the data series assessed by inferential statistics, the results are approximated with a sum of several rhythmic components with different periods and amplitudes. The most prominent rhythmic component under normal conditions has a period of 24 hours. Such a rhythm usually reflects a complex interaction between endogenous rhythmic and other (homeostatic, adaptive, pathological, etc.) mechanisms. The 24-hour rhythms with a proven endogenous component are called circadian, a term reflecting the observation that under constant external conditions the rhythms free-run with an endogenous period that is close to but significantly different from 24 hours (62). The circadian period of mammalian locomotor activity is controlled by a circadian clock located in the hypothalamic suprachiasmatic nucleus (63). Under synchronized conditions, all circadian rhythms appear with identical periods but have very different amplitudes and/or peak times (acrophases). Chronic (but not acute) lithium treatment prolongs the free-running period in almost all studied biological systems, including humans (16, 64). Lithium's effects under synchronized conditions

FIGURE 2. Molecular Model of Negative Feedback in the Circadian Clock of a Single *Drosophila* Cell[a]

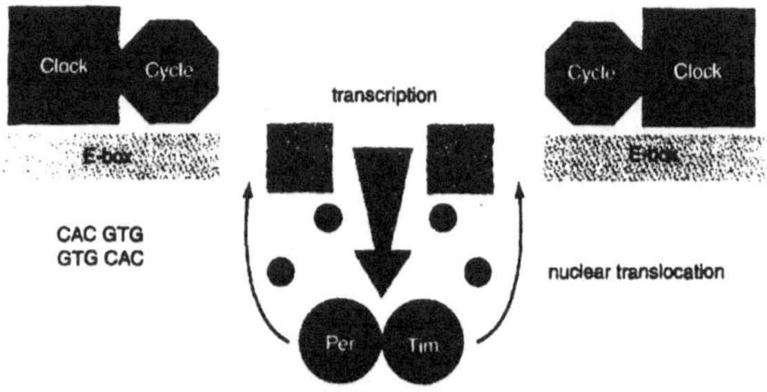

[a] Two proteins—Per and Tim—accumulate rhythmically (owing to rhythmicity at the level of their transcription), form heterodimers, and repress their own transcription when they reach a threshold level in the cell nucleus. This suppression is mediated by yet unknown interactions with the heterodimer of two other proteins—Clock and Cycle—shown to induce the transcription of the *per* (*period*) and *tim* (*timeless*) genes through interactions with E-boxes in their promoters. The model thus provides an explanation of the self-sustained circadian oscillations of Per and Tim, which are currently considered as a molecular basis of the evolutionary conserved cellular circadian clock.

are variable specific, with some variables showing significant acrophase delays and others exhibiting advances (65). The effects also depend on the timing of application, with evening application of lithium hydroxybutyrate for 10 days destabilizing circadian rhythms in the rat, in contrast to morning administration (66). The mechanism of lithium's action on the diverse circadian rhythms probably involves combined effects at the level of the circadian clock and at the level of integration of circadian rhythmicity with other regulatory systems. Experiments in a simple circadian model (*Neurospora crassa*) do not support the potential role of inositol depletion in lithium's effects on the circadian clock and its light synchronization (67).

Two recent breakthroughs are relevant to future approaches to the study of molecular and cellular mechanisms of lithium action. First, single dissociated suprachiasmatic nucleus neurons contain a circadian clock and express circadian rhythm in impulse activity (68). Second, a powerful combination of mutagenesis, isolation of behaviorally arrhythmic mutants, and molecular genetics was used to identify a set of four genes representing the molecular cogwheels of the cellular circadian clock in *Drosophila* (69) (figure 2). Two of the genes—*period* (*per*) and *timeless* (*tim*)—oscillate in a circadian fashion at both the mRNA and protein levels. It is important that the Per and Tim proteins form a cytosolic dimer, which translocates into the cell nucleus and suppresses their own transcription. The other two proteins—Clock and Cycle—also form a dimer in the nucleus. This dimer induces the transcription of *per* and *tim* mRNA by binding to E-boxes (5′-CACGTG-3′ sequence) located in the regulatory region of each gene. The activation of *per* and *tim* transcription may be suppressed by their own protein dimers, thus creating a molecular circadian clock based on a negative feedback loop (69). It is noteworthy that a mouse arrhythmic mutant has a single base mutation in the mammalian *clock* gene, which is highly homologous to the *clock* gene in *Drosophila*. The same holds true for the hamster BMAL1 gene—a partner of mammalian *clock* and homologous to the *Drosophila cycle* gene (69). Finally, mammals have three *Drosophila per* homologues with conservative E-boxes in their promoters (70). Overall, these observations imply that intracellular circadian clocks are based on evolutionary conserved molecular mechanisms. Together with the evolutionary conserved effects of chronic lithium treatment, this evidence suggests that the genes implicated in circadian clock function may also be targets for chronic lithium action. The potential consequences of chronic lithium treatment for circadian rhythms are illustrated by the following example. If we assume that lithium treatment results solely in a selective 6-hour acrophase delay, then a single-time-point study will be insufficient for properly characterizing the effect and possibly misleading; i.e., is the expression of the gene truly up or down, or simply phase-shifted? This cautionary note suggests that chronobiological studies are needed for many of lithium's putative molecular targets in order to determine whether the observed effects reflect changes in the spatiotemporal patterns of gene expression in critical neuronal circuits, effects that are likely to underlie the complex behavioral effects of lithium. Indeed, the importance of circadian factors and the sleep-wake cycle in bipolar disorder has been recognized for many years (discussed in reference 1).

CONCLUSIONS AND PERSPECTIVES

Lithium's profound effects on mood stabilization take several weeks to develop, a lag period that is most compatible with changes in the expression of critical neuronal genes. Although the indirect evidence is compelling, we cannot yet fully ascribe the therapeutic changes to alterations in the expression of any sets of genes per se. One of the major limitations is the absence of a good experimental model of bipolar disorder. Thus, the biological effects of lithium have, of necessity, been studied in "normal" experimental systems with the belief that the evolutionary conserved mechanisms of lithium's action are also relevant in the treatment of bipolar disorder. Indeed, abundant evidence indicates that many of lithium's effects are mediated through alterations in signal transduction pathways in critical neuronal circuits (3–5). Many of these signal transduction cascades are known to induce long-term cellular responses by means of regulated gene expression, and indeed, chronic lithium treatment is associated with changes in the expression of multiple genes. However, this reductive analysis is not yet complemented by evidence that these lithium-regulated genes are relevant to a particular lithium-induced phenotype. The few exceptions to this rule were studies that applied acute lithium treatment in early development (26) or in yeast (30). In conclusion, we have recently uncovered exciting new cellular and molecular leads concerning lithium's long-term therapeutic efficacy, but we await direct experimental evidence that a lithium-induced phenotypic change is based on selective alterations in gene expression. The additional use of systems with marked chronic lithium-induced phenotypic changes will greatly enhance the identification of experimentally tractable candidate lithium-target genes. The future approaches should also involve the evolutionary conserved effect of lithium on circadian rhythms. It is our firm belief that the use of a marked phenotype and chronobiologic approach, combined with the recent technological advances in the systems for identifying discordantly regulated genes and manipulating gene expression (including microarrays of DNA and oligonucleotides), holds much promise in the validation of chronic lithium-target genes in clinically relevant experimental systems and, ultimately, for the development of improved therapeutics.

REFERENCES

1. Goodwin FK, Jamison KR: Manic-Depressive Illness. New York, Oxford University Press, 1990
2. Baldessarini RJ, Tondo L, Hennen J: Effects of lithium treatment and its discontinuation in bipolar manic-depressive disorders. J Clin Psychiatry 1999; 60(suppl 2):77–84
3. Lenox RH, Manji HK: Lithium, in American Psychiatric Press Textbook of Psychopharmacology, 2nd ed. Edited by Schatzberg AF, Nemeroff CB. Washington, DC, American Psychiatric Press, 1998, pp 379–429
4. Manji HK, Potter WZ, Lenox RH: Signal transduction pathways: molecular targets for lithium's actions. Arch Gen Psychiatry 1995; 52:531–543
5. Jope RS: Anti-bipolar therapy: mechanism of action of lithium. Mol Psychiatry 1999; 4:117–128
6. Wang JF, Young LT, Li PP, Warsh JJ: Signal transduction abnormalities in bipolar disorder, in Bipolar Disorder: Biological Models and Their Clinical Applications. Edited by Young LT, Joffe RT. New York, Marcel Dekker, 1997, pp 41–80
7. Lenox RH: Role of receptor coupling to phosphoinositide metabolism in the therapeutic action of lithium. Adv Exp Biol Med 1987; 221:515–530
8. Hyman SE, Nestler EJ: Initiation and adaptation: a paradigm for understanding psychotropic drug action. Am J Psychiatry 1996; 153:151–162
9. Lifton RP: Genetic determinants of human hypertension. Proc Natl Acad Sci USA 1995; 92:8545–8551
10. Takahashi JS, Kornhauser JM, Koumenis C, Eskin A: Molecular approaches to understanding circadian oscillators. Annu Rev Physiol 1993; 55:729–754
11. Reisine T, Zatz M: Interactions among lithium, calcium, diacylglycerides, and phorbol esters in the regulation of adrenocorticotropin hormone release from AtT-20 cells. J Neurochem 1987; 49:884–889
12. Hokin LE, Dixon JF, Los GV: A novel action of lithium: stimulation of glutamate release and inositol 1,4,5 trisphosphate accumulation via activation of the *N*-methyl D-aspartate receptor in monkey and mouse cerebral cortex slices. Adv Enzyme Regul 1996; 36:229–244
13. Balla T, Enyedi P, Hunyady L, Spat A: Effects of lithium and angiotensin-stimulated phosphatidylinositol turnover and aldosterone production in adrenal glomerulosa cells: a possible causal relationship. FEBS Lett 1984; 171:179–182
14. Menkes HA, Baraban JM, Freed AN, Snyder SH: Lithium dampens neurotransmitter response in smooth muscle: relevance to action in affective illness. Proc Natl Acad Sci USA 1986; 83:5727–5730
15. Klein PS, Melton DA: A molecular mechanism for the effect of lithium on development. Proc Natl Acad Sci USA 1996; 93:8455–8459
16. Klemfuss H: Rhythms and the pharmacology of lithium. Pharmacol Ther 1992; 56:53–78
17. Richter-Levin G, Markram H, Segal M: Spontaneous recovery of deficits in spatial memory and cholinergic potentiation of NMDA in CA1 neurons during chronic lithium treatment. Hippocampus 1992; 2:279–286
18. Schmidt J: Lithium suppresses seizure susceptibility in pentylenetetrazol-kindled rats. Biomed Biochim Acta 1986; 45:1167–1172
19. Honchar MP, Olney JW, Sherman WR: Systemic cholinergic agents induce seizures and brain damage in lithium-treated rats. Science 1983; 220:323–325
20. Nonaka S, Hough CJ, Chuang DM: Chronic lithium treatment robustly protects neurons in the central nervous system against excitotoxicity by inhibiting *N*-methyl-D-aspartate receptor-mediated calcium influx. Proc Natl Acad Sci USA 1998; 95:2642–2647
21. Chen RW, Chuang DM: Long term lithium treatment suppresses p53 and Bax expression but increases Bcl-2 expression: a prominent role in neuroprotection against excitotoxicity. J Biol Chem 1999; 274:6039–6042
22. Manji HK, Moore GJ, Chen G: Lithium at 50: have the neuroprotective effects of this unique cation been overlooked? Biol Psychiatry (in press)
23. Dichtl B, Stevens A, Tollerey D: Lithium toxicity in yeast is due to the inhibition of RNA processing enzymes. EMBO J 1997; 16:7184–7195
24. Anai H, Ueta Y, Serino R, Bomura M, Kabashima N, Shibuya I, Takasugi M, Nakashima Y, Yamashita H: Upregulation of the expression of vasopressin gene in the paraventricular and supraoptic nuclei of the lithium-induced diabetes insipidus rat. Brain Res 1997; 772:161–166
25. Berridge MJ, Downes CP, Hanley MR: Neuronal and developmental actions of lithium: a unifying hypothesis. Cell 1989; 59:411–419
26. Hedgepeth CM, Conrad LJ, Zhang J, Huang HC, Lee VM, Klein PS: Activation of the Wnt signaling pathway: a molecular mechanism for lithium action. Dev Biol 1997; 185:82–91

27. Fisher SK, Heacock AM, Agranoff BW: Inositol lipids and signal transduction in the nervous system: an update. J Neurochem 1992; 58:18–38
28. Nahorski SR, Ragan CI, Challiss RAJ: Lithium and the phosphoinositide cycle: an example of uncompetitive inhibition and its pharmacological consequences. Trends Pharmacol Sci 1991; 12:297–303
29. Kofman O, Belmaker RH: Biochemical, behavioral and clinical studies of the role of inositol in lithium treatment and depression. Biol Psychiatry 1993; 34:839–852
30. Kippert F: Lithium affects the ultradian clock of *Schizosaccaromyces pombe* by inhibition of inositol monophosphatase. Biochem Soc Trans 1997; 25:S602
31. Jope RS, Williams MB: Lithium and brain signal transduction systems. Biochem Pharmacol 1994; 47:429–441
32. Moore GJ, Bebchuk JM, Parrish JK, Faulk MW, Arfken CL, Strahl-Bevacqua J, Manji HK: Temporal dissociation between lithium-induced frontal myo-inositol changes and clinical response in manic-depressive illness. Am J Psychiatry (in press)
33. Stambolic V, Ruel LR, Woodgett JR: Lithium inhibits glycogen synthase kinase-3 activity and mimics wingless signaling in intact cells. Curr Biol 1996; 6:1664–1668; correction, 1997; 7:196
34. Lucas FR, Goold RG, Gordon-Weeks PR, Salinas PC: Inhibition of GSK-3beta leading to the loss of phosphorylated MAP-1B is an early event in axonal remodelling induced by WNT-7a or lithium. J Cell Sci 1998; 111:1351–1361
35. Chen G, Huang LD, Jiang YM, Manji HK: The mood stabilizing agent valproate inhibits the activity of glycogen synthase kinase-3. J Neurochem 1999; 72:1327–1330
36. Lin A, Smeal T, Binetruy B, Deng T, Chambard JC, Karin M: Control of AP-1 activity by signal transduction cascades. Adv Second Messenger Phosphoprotein Res 1993; 28:255–260
37. Manji HK, Lenox RH: Long-term action of lithium: a role for transcriptional and posttranscriptional factors regulated by protein kinase C. Synapse 1994; 16:11–28
38. Nishizuka Y: Intracellular signaling by hydrolysis of phospholipids and activation of protein kinase C. Science 1992; 258:607–613
39. Stabel S, Parker PJ: Protein kinase C. Pharmacol Ther 1991; 51:71–95
40. Manji HK, Etcheberrigaray R, Chen G, Olds JL: Lithium decreases membrane-associated protein kinase C in hippocampus: selectivity for the alpha isozyme. J Neurochem 1993; 61: 2303–2310
41. Manji HK, Bebchuk JM, Moore GJ, Glitz D, Hasanat K, Chen G: Modulation of CNS signal transduction pathways and gene expression by mood stabilizing agents: therapeutic implications. J Clin Psychiatry 1999; 60(suppl 2):27–39
42. Lenox RH, Watson DG, Patel J, Ellis J: Chronic lithium administration alters a prominent PKC substrate in rat hippocampus. Brain Res 1992; 570:333–340
43. Lenox RH, McNamara RK, Watterson JM, Watson DG: Myristoylated alanine-rich C kinase substrate (MARCKS): a molecular target for the therapeutic action of mood stabilizers in the brain? J Clin Psychiatry 1996; 57(suppl 13):23–31
44. Chen G, Manji HK, Hawver DB, Wright CB, Potter WZ: Chronic sodium valproate selectively decreases protein kinase C α and ε in vitro. J Neurochem 1994; 63:2361–2364
45. Manji HK, Bersudsky Y, Chen G, Belmaker RH, Potter WZ: Modulation of PKC isozymes and substrates by lithium: the role of myo-inositol. Neuropsychopharmacology 1996; 15:370–382
46. Morgan JI, Curran TE: Proto-oncogenes: beyond second messengers, in Psychopharmacology: The Fourth Generation of Progress. Edited by Bloom FE, Kupfer DJ. New York, Raven Press, 1995, pp 631–642
47. Asghari V, Wang JF, Reiach JS, Young LT: Differential effects of mood stabilizers on Fos/Jun proteins and AP-1 DNA binding activity in human neuroblastoma SH-SY5Y cells. Brain Res Mol Brain Res 1998; 58:95–102
48. Ozaki N, Chuang DM: Lithium increases transcription factor binding to AP-1 and cyclic AMP-responsive element in cultured neurons and rat brain. J Neurochem 1997; 69:2336–2344
49. Kumer SC, Vrana KE: Intricate regulation of tyrosine hydroxylase activity and gene expression. J Neurochem 1996; 67:443–461
50. Chen G, Yuan PX, Jiang Y, Huang LD, Manji HK: Lithium increases tyrosine hydroxylase levels both *in vivo* and *in vitro*. J Neurochem 1998; 70:1768–1771
51. Drevets WC, Price JL, Simpson JR Jr, Todd RD, Reich T, Vannier M, Raichle ME: Subgenual prefrontal cortex abnormalities in mood disorders. Nature 1997; 38:824–827
52. Ketter TA, George MS, Kimbrell TA, Willis MW, Benson BE, Post RM: Neuroanatomical models and brain-imaging studies, in Bipolar Disorder: Biological Models and Their Clinical Application. Edited by Young LT, Joffe RT. New York, Marcel Dekker, 1997, pp 179–217
53. Rajkowska G, Miguel-Hidalgo JJ, Wei J, Dilley G, Pittman SD, Meltzer HY, Overholser JC, Roth BL, Stockmeier CA: Morphometric evidence for neuronal and glial prefrontal cell pathology in major depression. Biol Psychiatry 1999; 45:1085–1098
54. Liang P, Pardee AB: Differential display of eukaryotic messenger RNA by means of the polymerase chain reaction. Science 1992; 257:967–971
55. Ikonomov OC, Jacob MH: Preferential identification of differentially expressed mRNAs of moderate to low abundance in a microscopic system using selected primers, in Gene Cloning and Analysis by RT-PCR. Edited by Siebert P, Larrick JW. Natick, Mass, BioTechniques Books (Eaton Publishing), 1998, pp 171–181
56. Wang JF, Young LT: Differential display PCR reveals increased expression of 2′,3′-cyclic nucleotide 3′-phosphodiesterase by lithium. FEBS Lett 1996; 386:225–229
57. Manji HK, Zeng WZ, Huang LD, Ikonomov OC, Chen G: A new common transcriptional target for the mood-stabilizing agents lithium and valproic acid. Abstracts of the Society for Neuroscience 1997; 23:796.12
58. Duman RS, Heninger GR, Nestler EJ: A molecular and cellular theory of depression. Arch Gen Psychiatry 1997; 54:597–606
59. Flint J, Corley R: Do animal models have a place in the genetic analysis of quantitative human behavioral traits? J Mol Med 1996; 74:515–521
60. Kirsch J, Meyer G, Betz H: Synaptic targeting of ionotropic neurotransmitter receptors. Mol Cell Neurosci 1996; 8:93–98
61. Ikonomov OC, Zeng WZ, Jiang Y, Chen G, Manji HK: Gephyrin and ETO mRNA levels are differentially affected by chronic lithium treatment. Abstracts of the Society for Neuroscience 1997; 23:796.12
62. Ikonomov OC, Stoynev AG, Shisheva AC: Integrative coordination of circadian mammalian diversity: neuronal networks and peripheral clocks. Prog Neurobiol 1998; 54:87–97
63. Ralph MR, Foster RG, Davis FC, Menaker M: Transplanted suprachiasmatic nucleus determines circadian period. Science 1990; 247:975–978
64. Healy D, Waterhouse JM: The circadian system and the therapeutics of the affective disorders. Pharmacol Ther 1995; 65: 241–263
65. Subramanian P, Menon VP, Arokiam FV, Rajakrishnan V, Balamurugan E: Lithium modulates biochemical circadian rhythms in Wistar rats. Chronobiol Int 1998; 15:29–38
66. Zamoshchina TA, Matveenko AV, Saratikov AS: Effects of lithium hydroxybutyrate on circadian rhythms of rest-activity and sleep structure in experimental animals. Biull Eksp Biol Med 1992; 113:152–154
67. Lakin-Thomas PL: Evidence against a direct role for inositol phosphate metabolism in the circadian oscillator and the blue-light signal transduction pathway in *Neurospora crassa*. Biochem J 1993; 292:813–818
68. Welsh DK, Logothetis DE, Meister M, Reppert SM: Individual neurons dissociated from rat suprachiasmatic nucleus express independently phased circadian firing rhythms. Neuron 1995; 14:697–706
69. Schibler U: Circadian rhythms: new cogwheels in the clockworks. Nature 1998; 393:620–621
70. Zylka MJ, Shearman LP, Weaver DR, Reppert SM: Three period homologs in mammals: differential light responses in the suprachiasmatic circadian clock and oscillating transcripts outside of brain. Neuron 1998; 20:1103–1110

Signaling: Cellular Insights into the Pathophysiology of Bipolar Disorder

Husseini K. Manji and Robert H. Lenox

Clinical studies over the years have provided evidence that monoamine signaling and hypothalamic–pituitary–adrenal axis disruption are integral to the pathophysiology of bipolar disorder. A full understanding of the pathophysiology from a molecular to a systems level must await the identification of the susceptibility and protective genes driving the underlying neurobiology of bipolar disorder. Furthermore, the complexity of the unique biology of this affective disorder, which includes the predisposition to episodic and often progressive mood disturbance, and the dynamic nature of compensatory processes in the brain, coupled with limitations in experimental design, have hindered our progress to date. Imaging studies in patient populations have provided evidence of a role for anterior cingulate, amygdala, and prefrontal cortex in the pathophysiology of bipolar disorder. More recent research strategies designed to uncover the molecular mechanisms underlying our pharmacologic treatments and their interaction in the regulation of signal transduction as well as more advanced brain imaging studies remain promising approaches. This experimental strategy provides data derived from the physiologic response of the system in affected individuals and addresses the critical dynamic interaction with pharmacologic agents that effectively modify the clinical expression of the pathophysiology. Biol Psychiatry 2000;48:518–530 *© 2000 Society of Biological Psychiatry*

Key Words: Bipolar disorder, lithium, signal transduction, protein kinase C, G proteins, protein kinase A

Introduction

Clinical studies over the past 40 years have attempted to uncover the biological factors mediating the pathophysiology of bipolar disorder (BD) utilizing a variety of biochemical and neuroendocrine strategies. These studies have for the most part rested upon the conceptual foundation that monoamine signaling and hypothalamic–pituitary–adrenal axis disruption are integral to the pathophysiology of both depression and mania (Bowden 1997; Goodwin and Jamison 1990). Although such investigations have been heuristic over the years, they have been of limited value in elucidating the unique biology of this affective disorder, which must include an understanding of the underlying basis for the predilection to episodic and often profound mood disturbance that can become progressive over time. Kindling and progressive sensitization to seizures, taken from the epilepsy literature, has been very useful as a model for focusing attention to the long-term course of the illness, but thus far has been less useful in explicating the biological processes leading to instability in the regulation of mood; however, recent research characterizing the contributory roles of signaling pathways in various facets of kindling and sensitization holds promise in this regard. More recent research strategies designed to uncover the molecular mechanisms underlying our pharmacologic treatments coupled with more advanced brain imaging studies remain promising approaches as we enter the next millennium.

We should also keep in mind that a true understanding of the pathophysiology of BD must address its neurobiology at different physiologic levels (i.e., molecular, cellular, systems, and behavioral; Figure 1). Abnormalities in gene expression undoubtedly underlie the neurobiology of the disorder at the molecular level, and this will become evident as we identify the susceptibility and protective genes for BD in the coming years. Once this has been accomplished, however, the even more difficult work of examining the impact of the faulty expression of these gene products (proteins) on integrated cell function must begin. It is at these levels that we have identified some protein candidates using the psychopharmacologic strategies noted above and that will be more fully elucidated below. The precise manner in which these candidate molecular and cellular targets may or may not relate to the faulty expression of susceptibility gene products is yet to be determined. The task becomes even more daunting when one considers the possibility that a major component of the pathophysiology of BD may stem from discordant

From the Laboratory of Molecular Pathophysiology, Departments of Psychiatry and Behavioral Neurosciences, and Cellular and Clinical Neurobiology Program, Wayne State University School of Medicine, Detroit, Michigan (HKM) and the Molecular Neuropsychopharmacology Program, Departments of Psychiatry, Pharmacology, and Neuroscience, University of Pennsylvania School of Medicine, Philadelphia (RHL).

Address reprint requests to Husseini K. Manji, M.D., Wayne State University School of Medicine, 4201 St. Antoine, UHC 9B-29, Detroit MI 48201.

Received February 4, 2000; revised May 11, 2000; accepted May 17, 2000.

0006-3223/00/$20.00
PII S0006-3223(00)00929-X

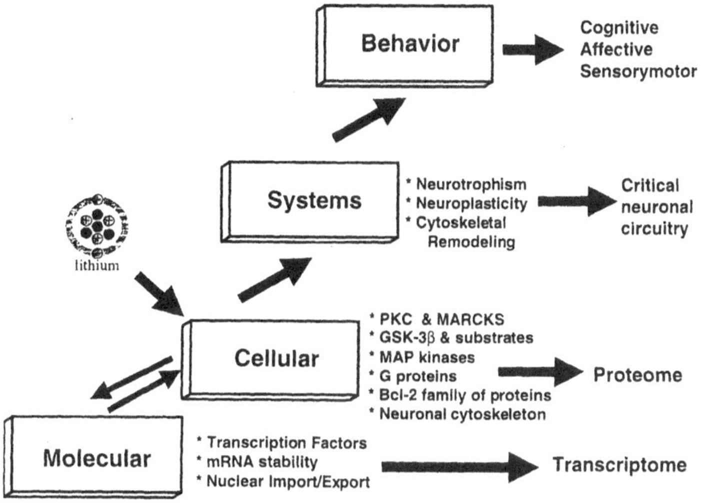

Figure 1. The pathophysiology of bipolar disorder (BD). This figure highlights the fact that a complete understanding of the pathophysiology of BD must address its neurobiology at different physiologic levels (i.e., molecular, cellular, systems, and behavioral). PKC, protein kinase C; MARCKS, myristoylated alanine-rich C kinase substrate; GSK-3, glycogen synthase kinase-3; MAP kinase, mitogen-activated protein kinase; Bcl-2, B-cell leukemia/lymphoma; proteome, the population of cellular protein species and their expression level; transcriptome, the population of cellular messenger RNA species and their expression level.

biological rhythms ranging from ultradian to infradian that ultimately drive the periodic recurrent nature of the disorder (Bunney and Bunney 2000; Ehlers et al 1988; Ikonomov and Manji 1999; Lenox and Manji 1998; Mandell et al 1984; Wehr and Goodwin 1983). The subsequent challenge for the basic and clinical neuroscientist will be the integration of these molecular/cellular changes to the systems and ultimately to the behavioral level, wherein the clinical expression of BD becomes fully elaborated.

Before critically reviewing the data relevant to the pathophysiology of BD, it is necessary to consider the complexity of our task (Table 1). To begin with, we would suggest that altered expression of critical proteins resulting from a series of susceptibility genes predisposes to a dysregulation of signaling in regions of the brain predisposing to periodic loss of homeostasis and clinical manifestation of affective symptomatology (i.e., mania and/or depression; Depue et al 1987; Goodwin and Jamison 1990). Thus the biological processes underlying the risk for mood cycling may be very distinct from the biology driving the clinical symptoms of mania or depression per se (Goodwin and Jamison 1990). In this regard it should be noted that there is increasing evidence for a shared genetic risk for both bipolar and unipolar disorders (Berrettini 2000), suggesting that the underlying pathophysiologic processes predisposing to recurrent mood disturbance may share common features. Furthermore, the clinical picture and system response are the result of a complex dynamic interaction between the dysregulated signaling systems and activation of existing physiologic feedback mechanisms designed to compensate for extreme changes (Post and Weiss 1999). In this way, the constellation of symptoms including not only mood but also autonomic, endo-

Table 1. The Pathophysiology of Bipolar Disorder: Constraints for Experimental Design

- Complex disease with diagnostic heterogeneity
- Episodic nature of symptoms and distinct symptom clusters
- The biology underlying recurrence/cyclicity may be distinct from that responsible for specific symptom clusters
- Disease progression dictates changes over the course of the illness
- Dynamic interaction between compensatory/adaptive changes in the brain and primary neurobiology of the disorder
- Effect of treatment and treatment withdrawal on measures
- Potential circadian rhythm abnormalities suggest that single time-point studies may be inadequate
- Relative inaccessibility of target organ and dependence on peripheral models
- Lack of suitable animal models
- The characterization of "mood" as a quantitative trait (quantitative trait locus analysis) has not yet been accomplished

crine, sleep/wake, and circadian activity determinants will reflect not only the stage and progression of illness, but also the unique individual characteristics conferring heterogeneity in clinical presentation and diagnosis. In light of this complexity and the dynamic properties of the system, research strategies examining biochemical and endocrine variables would be expected to be subject to a high degree of inherent variability not only when using cross-sectional analyses between patients, but also when utilizing longitudinal designs over time within individual patients. Furthermore, the use of peripheral sources of tissue and postmortem brains to address biochemical/neuroendocrine activity within patients' brains introduces another set of variables inherent in the experimental design and most often conferring significant constraints on data interpretation.

Table 2. Bipolar Disorder: A Putative Role for Signaling Pathways

- Regulate the functional balance and multiple neurotransmitter systems
- Dynamic regulation of complex signaling networks forms the basis for higher order brain function mediating mood and cognition
- Critical role in fine-tuning of signals (amplifiers, attenuators, and integrators of multiple signals)
- Critical role in maintaining cellular "memory" and long-term neuroplastic events
- Major targets for the actions of hormones, including gonadal steroids, thyroid hormones, and glucocorticoids
- Abnormalities are compatible with life (e.g., a variety of human diseases are from defects in G protein–coupled signal transduction pathways)
- Brain regional dysregulation and circumscribed symptomatology are indeed possible despite the ubiquitous expression of signaling proteins
- Signaling proteins have been identified as targets for medications that are most effective in the treatment of mood disorders

Classical Monoaminergic Neurotransmitter and Neuroendocrine Systems

The stimulus for the study of the biogenic amines in patients with BD was provided by the discovery of effective pharmacologic treatments for depression and mania (Goodwin and Jamison 1990). Although these pharmacologic agents have prominent effects on single episodes of depression and mania, even more pertinent to our discussion are the major effects that these agents exert on the long-term course of the illness (Goodwin and Jamison 1990; Manji and Potter 1997). Antidepressants in general, and tricyclics in particular, may increase the frequency of cycles and worsen long-term outcome (Wehr and Goodwin 1987). In addition to this compelling pharmacologic data, the biogenic amine neurotransmitter systems are distributed extensively in the limbic system, which is implicated in the regulation of sleep, appetite, arousal, sexual function, endocrine function, and emotional states such as fear and rage. The clinical picture of BD involves disruption of behavior, circadian rhythms, neurophysiology of sleep, and neuroendocrine and biochemical regulation within the brain (for reviews, see Goodwin and Jamison 1990; Holsboer 1995). Thus it is not surprising that clinical research strategies over the years have identified dysregulation of noradrenergic, dopaminergic, serotonergic, and cholinergic systems as well as the hypothalamic–pituitary axis in patients with BD. The behavioral and physiologic manifestations of the illness are complex and undoubtedly mediated by a network of interconnected neurotransmitter pathways (Lenox 1987; Manji 1992); the monoamine neurotransmitter systems are ideally placed to mediate such complex behavioral effects, and thus have represented attractive candidate systems underlying the pathophysiology of BD. The multiple functions of central neurotransmitter/neuroendocrine systems, however, make it difficult to conceptualize, let alone demonstrate, true specificity of detected abnormalities. Since these earlier studies have been amply reviewed elsewhere, in this perspectives article we focus upon more recent data linking signaling abnormalities with the underlying neurobiology of BD.

Signaling Networks: The Cellular Machinery Underlying Information Processing and Long-Term Neuroplastic Events

It is hardly surprising that abnormalities in multiple neurotransmitter systems and physiologic processes have been found in a disorder as complex as BD. Signal transduction pathways are in a pivotal position in the central nervous system (CNS), able to affect the functional balance between multiple neurotransmitter systems, and may therefore play a role in mediating the more "downstream" abnormalities in multiple neurotransmitter systems and physiologic processes. Moreover, recent research has clearly identified signaling pathways as therapeutically relevant targets for our most effective pharmacologic treatments (Table 2). Indeed, the molecular and cellular targets underlying lithium's ability to stabilize an underlying dysregulation of limbic and limbic-associated function strongly suggest that abnormalities in signaling pathways may also play a critical role in the pathophysiology of BD.

Multicomponent, cellular signaling pathways interact at various levels, thereby forming complex signaling networks that allow the cell to receive, process, and respond to information (Bhalla and Iyengar 1999; Bourne and Nicoll 1993). These networks facilitate the integration of signals across multiple time scales and the generation of distinct outputs depending on input strength and duration, and regulate intricate feed-forward and feedback loops (Weng et al 1999). These properties of signaling networks suggest that they play critical roles in cellular memory; thus, cells with different histories, and therefore expressing different repertoires of signaling molecules and transcription factors, interacting at different levels, may respond quite differently to the same signal over time. Given their widespread and crucial role in the integration, regulation, amplification, and fine-tuning of physiologic processes, it is not surprising that abnormalities in signaling pathways have now been identified in a variety of human diseases (Milligan and Wakelam 1992; Spiegel 1998; Weintraub 1995). Pertinent to the present discussion is the observation that a variety of diseases manifest relatively circumscribed symptomatology, despite the widespread, often ubiquitous expression of the affected signaling proteins.

Although complex signaling networks are likely present in all eukaryotic cells and control various metabolic, humoral, and developmental functions, they may be especially important in the CNS, where they serve the critical roles of first amplifying and "weighting" numerous extracellularly generated neuronal signals and then transmitting these integrated signals to effectors, thereby forming the basis for a complex information processing network (Bhalla and Iyengar 1999; Bourne and Nicoll 1993; Manji 1992). The high degree of complexity generated by these signaling networks may be one mechanism by which neurons acquire the flexibility for generating the wide range of responses observed in the nervous system (Table 2). These pathways are thus undoubtedly involved in regulating such diverse vegetative functions as mood, appetite, and wakefulness and are therefore likely to be involved in the pathophysiology of BD. We now turn to a discussion of the direct and indirect evidence supporting a role for abnormalities in signaling pathways in the pathophysiology of BD.

Alterations of Transmembrane Cellular Signaling Pathways in Animal Models of BD

The need to use caution in the appropriate application of animal models to an understanding of complex neuropsychiatric disorders has been well articulated (Einat et al, in press; Post and Weiss 1999), and in fact it is unlikely we will ever develop animal models that display the full range of symptomatology as clinically expressed in man. Two current models that have had reasonable heuristic value in the study of mood disorders are kindling and behavioral sensitization (Einat et al, in press; Post and Weiss 1999). In both of these paradigms, there is increased responsivity (either behavioral or electrophysiologic) to repeated "low dose" stimulation (pharmacologic or electric) over time. Indeed, the sensitized behavioral response has been reported to persist for months and years after discontinuation of drug administration. Considerable evidence implicates long-term alterations in midbrain dopaminergic transmission in the development of behavioral sensitization, but the cellular mechanism(s) underlying the long-term changes in excitability observed in kindled or stimulant-sensitized animals have not been fully elucidated. In recent years, an appreciation of the major role of signal transduction pathways in the regulation of neuronal excitability has led to extensive research into their involvement in kindling and behavioral sensitization, and a growing body of evidence implicates alterations in both protein kinase C (PKC; Table 3) and certain G proteins (especially G_i and G_o). Studies have demonstrated that pertussis toxin (which inactivates G_i and G_o) produces a significant augmentation of psychostimulant-induced motor activity, and dopamine release in the nucleus accumbens (Chen et al 1999; Steketee and Kalivas 1991). In keeping with these studies, specific decreases in $G\alpha_i$ and $G\alpha_i$ levels have been observed in response to chronic cocaine in the ventral tegmental area and nucleus accumbens (Nestler et al 1990), once again consistent with the hypothesis that regulation of G proteins represents part of the biochemical changes that underlie the effects of chronic psychostimulants. Similarly, injection of pertussis toxin into the amygdala of kindled rats markedly modifies kindled seizures, effects that appear to be mediated via an alteration in the after-discharge threshold.

Table 3. Protein Kinase C: Pathophysiology and Treatment of Bipolar Disorder

- Kindling produces dramatic increases in membrane-associated PKC in the hippocampus and amygdala
- Amphetamine produces increases in PKC activity, and GAP-43 phosphorylation (implicated in neurotransmitter release)
- PKC inhibitors block the biochemical and behavioral responses to amphetamine and cocaine and also block cocaine-induced sensitization
- Dexamethasone administration increases PKC activity, and increases the levels of PKC α and PKC ϵ in the rat frontal cortex and hippocampus
- Increased membrane/cytosol PKC partitioning in platelets from manic subjects; normalized with lithium treatment
- Increased PKC activity and translocation in bipolar disorder brains, as compared with control subjects
- Lithium and valproate regulate PKC activity, PKC α, PKC ϵ, and MARCKS
- Preliminary data suggest that PKC inhibitors may have efficacy in the treatment of acute mania
- Typical and atypical antipsychotics regulate the levels of PKC α and PKC ϵ in areas of the rat brain

PKC, protein kinase C; GAP, growth cone–associated protein; MARCKS, myristoylated alanine-rich C kinase substrate.

With respect to the PKC signaling system, dramatic increases in membrane-associated PKC have been observed in the bilateral hippocampus up to 4 weeks after the last kindled seizure and in the amygdala/pyriform cortex at 4 weeks after (Daigen et al 1991). Studies have also implicated alterations in PKC activity as mediators of long-term alterations in neuronal excitability in the brain following chronic stimulant use. Thus, both acute and chronic amphetamine produce an alteration in PKC activity, its cytosol relative to membrane distribution, and the phosphorylation of a major PKC substrate, growth cone–associated protein 43 (GAP-43), which has been implicated in long-term alterations of neurotransmitter release (Kantor and Gnegy 1998). Furthermore, PKC inhibitors have been shown to block the acute responses to both amphetamine and cocaine (as assessed by both behavioral and in vivo microdialysis studies) as well as cocaine-induced sensitization (Kantor and Gnegy 1998).

It is indeed striking that behavioral sensitization and kindling produce robust alterations in the PKC signaling pathway in critical limbic structures, since lithium and valproate (VPA) also target the very same biochemical targets (see below). Thus, although considerable caution clearly needs to be employed when extrapolating from the findings observed in these two models, the fact that they are associated with effects on PKC signaling that are the opposite of those observed with chronic lithium or VPA is compelling indeed.

Are G Protein–Coupled Signal Transduction Pathways Targets for Mood-Stabilizing Agents?

The cAMP/Protein Kinase A Signaling Pathway as a Target for the Actions of Mood Stabilizers and Antidepressants

As discussed above, dysregulation of cellular signaling networks in the brain likely underlies the oscillations in behavioral states observed in mood disorders. Thus, it is not surprising that increasingly recent research on the cellular mechanisms underlying lithium's therapeutic effects has focused on the transmembrane signaling pathways in the brain (for reviews, see Lenox and Manji 1998; Mork et al 1992; Post et al 2000).

Lithium and the AC System

It has been demonstrated that lithium exerts complex effects on the activity of adenylyl cyclase (AC), with the preponderance of the data demonstrating an elevation of basal AC activity but an attenuation of variety of receptor-mediated responses (Jope 1999a, 1999b; Manji et al 2000; Wang et al 1997). Lithium in vitro inhibits the stimulation of AC both by Gpp(NH)p (a poorly hydrolyzable analog of guanosine triphosphate [GTP]) and by Ca^{++}/calmodulin, suggesting that lithium in vitro is directly able to inhibit the catalytic unit of AC (Mork et al 1992; Newman and Belmaker 1987). Since these inhibitory effects of lithium in vitro can be overcome by Mg^{++}, it has been postulated that they are mediated (at least in part) by a direct competition with magnesium (whose hydrated ionic radius is similar to that of lithium) for a binding site on the catalytic unit of AC (Mork and Geisler 1989; Mork et al 1992; Newman and Belmaker 1987); however, the inhibitory effects of *chronic* lithium treatment on rat brain AC are not reversed by Mg^{++} and still persist after washing of the membranes, but are reversed by increasing concentrations of GTP (Mork and Geisler 1989; Mork et al 1992; Newman and Belmaker 1987). These results suggest that the effects of chronic lithium (those that are more likely to be therapeutically relevant) may be exerted at the level of signal-transducing G proteins at a GTP-responsive step (discussed below). These two distinct actions of lithium on the AC system may explain the differences in results that have been obtained by investigators using rat membrane preparations and those obtained with the use of rat slice preparations (Lenox and Manji 1998). This has led to an investigation of lithium's effects on the AC system in vivo, using microdialysis. These studies found that chronic lithium treatment produced a significant increase in basal and post–receptor stimulated (cholera toxin or forskolin) AC activity, while attenuating the β-adrenergic–mediated effect (Manji et al 2000; Masana et al 1992). Interestingly, chronic lithium treatment resulted in an almost absent cyclic adenosine monophosphate (cAMP) response to pertussis toxin, suggesting a lithium-induced attenuation of G_i function. It should be noted, however, that chronic lithium has been found to increase not only cAMP levels (Wiborg et al 1999), but also the levels of AC type I and type II messenger RNA (mRNA) and protein levels in the frontal cortex (Colin et al 1991; Jensen et al 2000), suggesting that lithium's complex effects on the system may represent the net effects of direct inhibition of AC, upregulation of AC subtypes, and effects on the stimulatory and inhibitory G proteins. Most recently, lithium's effects on the phosphorylation and activity of cyclic AMP response element–binding protein (CREB) have been examined in the rodent brain and in cultured human neuroblastoma cells, with somewhat conflicting results (Ozaki and Chuang 1997; Wang et al 1999).

A series of studies have also examined lithium's effects on AC in humans. In a longitudinal study of healthy volunteers (utilized to overcome the potentially confounding, significant effects of alterations in mood state–dependent biochemical and neuroendocrine parameters), 2 weeks of lithium administration was found to significantly increase platelet basal and post–receptor stimulated AC activity (Risby et al 1991), effects that are strikingly similar to those observed in the rodent brain. Consistent with a lithium-induced increase in basal cAMP and AC levels, a more recent study found that platelets obtained from lithium-treated euthymic bipolar patients exhibited enhanced basal and cAMP-stimulated phosphorylation of Rap1 (a protein kinase A [PKA] substrate), as well as another unidentified 38-kd phosphoprotein (Perez et al 2000a). Somewhat surprisingly, these investigators did not find similar effects of lithium in healthy subjects.

Carbamazepine and the AC System

The effects of carbamazepine (CBZ) on the AC system have been less extensively studied. It is noteworthy, however, that CBZ has been reported to decrease not only basal and stimulated cAMP production in rodents, but also cerebrospinal fluid levels of cAMP in manic patients (Post et al 2000). Recent studies have found that CBZ, at therapeutically relevant concentrations, inhibits both basal AC and FSK-stimulated cAMP accumulation in C6 glioma cells (Chen et al 1996). Furthermore, CBZ also inhibits both basal and FSK-stimulated activity of AC purified from the rat cortex, suggesting that CBZ inhibits cAMP production by acting directly on AC and/or through factor(s) that are tightly associated with and copurify with AC (Chen et al 1996). Carbamazepine's effects on cAMP-mediated transcriptional events have also been investigated, and CBZ has been found to inhibit forskolin-stimulated phosphorylation of CREB (Chen et al 1996) and c-fos expression (Divish et al 1991). Together, the results suggest that CBZ brings about a dampening of the AC system; these effects may play a role in both its antiepileptic and its antimanic effects, but such a contention requires extensive further validation.

Antidepressants and the AC System

The chronic administration of antidepressants (ADs) is known to bring about a variety of biochemical effects, including an enhanced coupling between $G\alpha_s$ and the catalytic unit of AC (Rasenick et al 2000). Several studies have also demonstrated that the postreceptor components of the cAMP system are regulated by long-term AD treatments, including cAMP-dependent protein kinase enzyme activity (Nestler et al 1989; Popoli et al 2000). Taken together, these results suggest that ADs, via their complex effects on G proteins and the AC signaling system, may attenuate β-adrenergic–mediated activation of G_s, while enhancing the effects of agents operating by pathways independent of the β-adrenergic receptor (βAR). Consistent with these results, ADs have been demonstrated to activate cAMP-dependent and calcium/calmodulin-dependent protein kinases, effects that are accompanied by increases in the endogenous phosphorylation of selected substrates (microtubule-associated protein 2 and synaptotagmin; Popoli et al 2000). Furthermore, recent data from Duman and associates (1997) have demonstrated that the chronic treatment of rats with a variety of ADs increases the levels of CREB mRNA, CREB, and CRE DNA binding activity in the hippocampus. The same laboratory has demonstrated that chronic AD treatment also increases the expression of two important genes known to be regulated by CREB—namely, brain-derived neuotrophic factor and its receptor trkB (Duman et al 1997). Preliminary postmortem human brain studies have also revealed increased CREB levels in patients treated with ADs, providing indirect support for the rodent and cell culture studies (Dowlatshahi et al 1998).

Lithium and G Proteins

Abundant experimental evidence has shown that lithium attenuates receptor-mediated second messenger generation in the absence of consistent changes in the density of the receptors themselves (Lenox and Manji 1998; Mork et al 1992). There is now considerable evidence that *chronic* lithium administration affects G protein *function* (Jope 1999a, 1999b; Lenox and Manji 1998; Wang and Friedman 1999); however, the preponderance of data suggests that lithium, at therapeutically relevant concentrations, does not have any *direct* effects on G proteins and does not consistently alter G protein subunit *levels* (Ellis and Lenox 1991; Lenox and Manji 1998). Although some studies have reported modest changes in the *levels* of G protein α subunits, the preponderance of the data suggests that the effects of chronic lithium on signaling pathways occur in the absence of changes in the levels of G protein subunits per se (Lenox and Manji 1998); however, chronic in vivo lithium treatment has been shown to produce a significant increase in pertussis toxin–catalyzed [^{32}P]adenosine diphosphate ([^{32}P]ADP) ribosylation in the rat frontal cortex. Since pertussis toxin selectively ADP-ribosylates the undissociated, inactive αβγ heterotrimeric form of G_i, these results suggest that lithium attenuates G_i function via a stabilization of the inactive conformation. These observations suggest that the removal of the "inhibitory tone" by lithium may be responsible for the elevations in basal AC and the responses to agents activating the stimulatory pathway *distal to the receptor* (Jope 1999b). Consistent with this hypothesis, lithium has been shown to potentiate the behavioral hyperactivity induced by intra-accumbens cholera toxin administration (which activates the stimulatory G proteins, G_s and G_{olf}; Kofman et al 1998).

Recent studies have also examined the effects of chronic lithium on G protein function in humans and have generally observed reduced receptor/G protein coupling (Lenox and Manji 1998; Risby et al 1991). The effects of 2 weeks of lithium administration on G protein measures has also been examined in healthy volunteers. Similar to the findings in the rat brain, lithium did not affect the levels of platelet G protein α subunits, but produced a significant increase in pertussis toxin–catalyzed [^{32}P]ADP ribosylation, once again suggesting a stabilization of the inactive undissociated $\alpha\beta\gamma$ heterotrimeric form of G_i. These long-term effects of chronic lithium on G protein are likely attributable to an indirect posttranslational modification of the G protein(s) and a relative change in the dynamic equilibrium of the active/inactive states of protein conformation. In this context, it is noteworthy that investigators have demonstrated that lithium alters the levels of endogenous ADP-ribosylation in C6 glioma cells (Young and Woods 1996) and in the rat brain (Nestler et al 1995), suggesting another novel mechanism by which chronic lithium may indirectly regulate the activity of these critical signaling proteins.

The Protein Kinase C Signaling Cascade

Over the last decade there have been major advances in our understanding of the critical role of the PKC signaling pathway as a therapeutically relevant target for the long-term actions of mood stabilizers. The "inositol depletion hypothesis" posited that lithium, as an uncompetitive inhibitor of inositol-1-phosphatase, produced its therapeutic effects via a depletion of neuronal *myo*-inositol (mI) levels. Although this hypothesis has been of great heuristic value, numerous studies have examined the effects of lithium on receptor-mediated phosphoinositide (PI) responses, and although some report a reduction in agonist-stimulated phosphatidylinositol 4,5-bisphosphate (PIP_2) hydrolysis in rat brain slices following acute or chronic lithium, these findings have often been small and inconsistent, and subject to numerous methodological differences (Jope and Williams 1994; Lenox and Manji 1998). Most recently, a magnetic resonance spectroscopy study has demonstrated that lithium-induced mI reductions are observed in the frontal cortex of BD patients after only 5 days of lithium administration, *at a time when the patients' clinical state is completely unchanged* (Moore et al 1999). Consequently, these and other studies suggest that whereas inhibition of inositol monophosphatase may represent an initiating lithium effect, reducing mI levels per se is not associated with therapeutic response. This led to our working hypothesis that some of the *initial* actions of lithium may occur with a relative reduction of mI—this reduction of mI initiates a cascade of secondary changes in the PKC signaling pathway and gene expression in the CNS, effects that are *ultimately* responsible for lithium's therapeutic efficacy.

Indeed, evidence accumulating from various laboratories has clearly demonstrated that lithium, at therapeutically relevant concentrations, exerts major effects on the PKC signaling cascade (Table 3). Currently available data suggest that acute lithium exposure facilitates a number of PKC-mediated responses, whereas longer exposure results in an attenuation of phorbol ester–mediated responses, which is accompanied by a downregulation of specific PKC isozymes (discussed in Manji and Lenox 1999). Studies in rodents have demonstrated that chronic (but not acute) lithium produces an isozyme-selective reduction in PKC α and ϵ in the frontal cortex and hippocampus, in the absence of significant alterations in the β, γ, δ, or ζ isozymes. Concomitant studies carried out in immortalized hippocampal cells in culture exposed to chronic lithium show a similar reduction in the expression of both the PKC α and ϵ isozymes in the cell as determined by immunoblot (Chen et al, in press; Manji and Lenox 1999).

A major strategy that has been utilized to investigate the downstream consequences of lithium-induced alteration in PKC isozymes is the examination of the effects of chronic lithium on endogenous PKC substrates in the brain. The most prominent substrate for PKC in the brain is an acidic protein, myristoylated alanine-rich C kinase substrate (MARCKS), which has been implicated in regulating long-term neuroplastic events. Lenox and associates (1992) provided the first evidence for the effects of chronic administration of lithium on the regulation of MARCKS in the rat brain. They demonstrated that chronic lithium administration dramatically reduced MARCKS expression in the hippocampus, effects that were not immediately reversed following lithium discontinuation. Subsequent studies carried out in immortalized hippocampal cells have demonstrated that this action of chronic lithium on MARCKS regulation is dependent upon both the inositol concentration and the level of receptor-mediated activation of PI hydrolysis (Watson and Lenox 1996). Although these effects of lithium on PKC isozymes and MARCKS are striking, a major problem inherent in neuropharmacologic research is the difficulty in attributing *therapeutic relevance* to *any* observed biochemical finding. It is thus noteworthy that the structurally dissimilar antimanic agent VPA produces effects strikingly similar to those of lithium on PKC isozymes and on the expression of the MARCKS protein (Manji and Lenox 1999; Watson et al 1998).

Are There Abnormalities in Signaling Pathways in BD?

The cAMP-Generating System

The data reviewed above strongly suggest that regulation of cellular signaling transduction pathways play a major role in the therapeutic effects of lithium and VPA. Do these clinically effective agents, in fact, *correct an underlying abnormality* in signaling pathways in BD? The future development of selective receptor and second messenger ligands for positron emission tomography studies may permit the direct assessment of CNS receptor and postreceptor sensitivity in humans. To date, however, studies of receptor and postreceptor function in mood disorders have been limited to indirect research strategies. The most commonly utilized strategy has been to characterize receptor function in readily accessible blood elements, and much clinical research has focused on the activity of the cAMP-generating system in mood disorders. Overall, the preponderance of the evidence suggests altered receptor and/or postreceptor sensitivity of the cAMP-generating system *in the absence of consistent alterations in the number of receptors themselves* (for a review, see Wang et al 1997). A consistently observed decrease in leukocyte βAR function in depression could reflect an inherited abnormality of the βAR/G_s/AC complex, as suggested by the findings utilizing immortalized (Epstein–Barr virus–transformed) lymphocytes (Wright et al 1984). These findings need to be replicated, however, and a number of additional confounding factors need to be considered. In this context, twin studies suggest that variations in isoproterenol-stimulated cAMP production are most likely due to "environmental" effects on the number or sensitivity of βARs (Ebstein et al 1986). A recent study found higher levels of cAMP-stimulated phosphorylation of a ~22-kd protein in platelets obtained from 10 treated euthymic BD patients, as compared with healthy subjects; by contrast, there was no significant difference in the basal phosphorylation between the groups (Perez et al 2000a, 2000b). Follow-up studies identified the ~22-kd protein as Rap1, and once again found higher cAMP-stimulated phosphorylation in the BD patients (Perez et al 2000a, 2000b).

Warsh and associates have undertaken the most thorough series of studies investigating the cAMP/PKA system in postmortem brains of BD patients. Due to the instability of cAMP in postmortem brain tissue, this research group has investigated downstream targets of cAMP. They found that the levels of PKA regulatory subunits (as assessed by [^{3}H]cAMP binding) were significantly lower in cytosolic fractions of BD frontal, temporal, occipital, and parietal cortices; cerebellum; and thalamus, as compared with matched control subjects (Rahman et al 1997). Furthermore, preliminary findings show that the reduction of regulatory subunits of PKA in the cytosolic fractions of the BD temporal cortex is accompanied by a higher basal kinase activity and significantly lower apparent activation constant for cAMP in the cytosolic fractions of the BD temporal cortex (Fields et al 1999). Whether such changes result in altered endogenous cAMP-stimulated phosphorylation in the brain, similar to what has been reported in platelets from euthymic BD patients (Perez et al 2000a, 2000b), remains to be demonstrated. Nevertheless, these observed changes in PKA provide additional important evidence for a potential dysregulation of the $G\alpha_s$-mediated cAMP signaling pathway in BD.

G Proteins in Mood Disorders

In view of the indirect evidence for abnormalities at postreceptor sites described above, it is not surprising that several independent laboratories have examined G proteins in patients with mood disorders (Chen et al 1999; Mathews et al 1997; Wang et al 1997; Warsh et al 2000). Young and associates (1993) were the first to report increased *levels* of $G\alpha_s$ in BD. Compared with control subjects matched with respect to age, postmortem interval, and brain pH, they found increased levels of $G\alpha_s$ in the frontal, temporal, and occipital cortices (but not in the hippocampus, thalamus, or cerebellum) in postmortem brain tissue from patients with BD. This group also found increases in forskolin-stimulated AC activity in postmortem brains of BD patients, compatible with enhanced G_s/AC signaling in BD (Warsh et al 2000). The findings of elevated $G\alpha_s$ levels and/or function are also supported by the recent observations of Friedman and Wang (1996), who found increased agonist-activated [^{35}S]GTPγS binding to G protein α subunits in frontal cortical membrane preparations from BD patients. Several studies have also examined G proteins in peripheral circulating cells and have found elevated levels of $G\alpha_s$ protein (Chen et al 1999; Wang et al 1997; Warsh et al 2000) and mRNA levels (Spleiss et al 1998), although the dependency on clinical state remains unclear. Similar to what has been observed in the CNS, one recent study has evaluated the role of platelet G proteins as "signal coincidence detectors," and has found this function to be impaired in depressed patients (Mooney et al 1998). Overall, the most consistent finding to emerge is that in both peripheral cells and postmortem brain tissue from BD patients elevations are observed in the *predominant* subspecies of $G\alpha_s$ present in the tissues examined. It should be emphasized, however, that there is at present *no evidence* to suggest that the alterations in the levels of $G\alpha_s$ are due to a mutation in the $G\alpha_s$ gene itself. Indeed, there are numerous transcriptional and posttranscriptional mechanisms that regulate the levels of G protein α subunits (Warsh et al 2000), and the elevated levels of $G\alpha_s$ could potentially represent the *indirect sequelae* of alterations in any one of these other biochemical pathways. Thus, at this point considerable caution is required in the interpretation of the data, since they derive primarily from peripheral cell models and postmortem studies involving a small number of patients.

Abnormalities of Calcium Signaling in BD

Acting via intracellular proteins such as MARCKS and calmodulin, and enzymes such as PKC, AC, and Ca^{++}/calmodulin-dependent kinase, calcium ions have been shown to regulate the synthesis and release of neurotransmitters, neuronal excitability, cytoskeletal remodeling, and long-term neuroplastic events. Thus, it is not surprising that a large number of studies have investigated intracellular Ca^{2+} in peripheral cells in BD (discussed in Dubovsky et al 1992; Emamghoreishi et al 1997; Wang et al 1997). In view of the caveats associated with studies of peripheral circulating cells, the remarkable consistency of the findings is surprising indeed. Studies have consistently revealed elevations in both resting and stimulated intracellular Ca^{2+} levels in platelets, lymphocytes, and neutrophils of patients with BD. The calcium abnormalities have been postulated to represent state-dependent findings (Dubovsky et al 1992), but recent studies using transformed lymphoblasts from BD patients have revealed similar abnormalities, suggesting that they may be trait dependent (Emamghoreishi et al 1997). The regulation of free intracellular Ca^{2+} is a complex, multifaceted process involving extracellular entry, release from intracellular stores following receptor-stimulated PI hydrolysis, uptake into specific organelles, and binding to specific proteins. Thus, the abnormalities observed in BD could arise from abnormalities at a variety of levels, and recent studies suggest that the abnormality lies beyond the receptor (Hough et al 1999). Interestingly, recent studies have demonstrated that Rap1 phosphorylation state is related to platelet intracellular calcium signaling (Magnier et al 1995), suggesting a possible relationship between these two documented abnormalities. Since PKC is also known to regulate calcium signaling at multiple levels (Ozaki et al 1997; Shibata et al 1996; Si-Tahar et al 1996), more recent studies have investigated the putative role of PKC in mediating the calcium abnormalities in BD; preliminary analysis suggests that alterations in tonic PKC activity may play an important role in mediating the abnormal intracellular calcium responses observed in BD (H.K. Manji and R.M. Post, unpublished observations, June 1998).

Are There Abnormalities of PKC Signaling in BD?

To date, there have only been a limited number of studies directly examining PKC in BD. Friedman and associates (1993) investigated PKC activity and PKC translocation in response to serotonin in platelets obtained from BD subjects before and during lithium treatment. They reported that the ratios of platelets membrane-bound to cytosolic PKC activities were elevated in the manic subjects. In addition, serotonin-elicited platelet PKC translocation was found to be enhanced in those subjects. With respect to brain tissue, Wang and Friedman (1996) measured PKC isozyme levels, activity, and translocation in postmortem brain tissue from BD patients; they reported increased PKC activity and translocation in BD brains, as compared with control subjects, effects that were accompanied by elevated levels of selected PKC isozymes in cortices of BD subjects.

In view of the pivotal role of the PKC signaling pathway in the regulation of neuronal excitability, neurotransmitter release, and long-term synaptic events, it was postulated that the attenuation of PKC activity may play a role in the antimanic effects of lithium and VPA. In a pilot study it was found that tamoxifen (a nonsteroidal antiestrogen known to be a PKC inhibitor at higher concentrations) may, indeed, possess antimanic efficacy (Bebchuk et al 2000). These data further support the potential role of the PKC pathway in mediating the pathophysiology of BD. The data implicating the PKC signaling system in the pathophysiology of BD are particularly compelling in view of the growing body of data suggesting that this signaling pathway represents a therapeutically relevant target for both lithium and VPA (see above). The complex effects of lithium on the PKC signaling pathway represent an attractive and heuristic mechanism by which the expression of various proteins involved in long-term neuronal plasticity and cellular response is modulated, thereby compensating for as yet genetically undefined physiologic abnormalities in critical regions of the brain. It is our strong conviction that it is at the cellular and molecular level that some of the most exciting advances in our understanding of the pathophysiology of BD will take place in the coming years. Current studies of the long-term lithium-induced changes of the PKC signaling pathway (including PKC isozyme regulation, post-translational modification of key phosphoproteins, and PKC-mediated alterations in gene and protein expression) are a most promising avenue for future investigation.

Concluding Remarks

As we have demonstrated, there is a considerable body of evidence both conceptually and experimentally in support of abnormalities in the regulation of signaling as integral to the underlying neurobiology of BD. The pathophysiology of this illness must account for not only the profound changes in mood but also a constellation of neurovegetative features derived from dysfunction in limbic-related regions such as the hippocampus, hypothalamus, and brain stem. The highly integrated monoamine and prominent neuropeptide pathways are known to originate and project heavily within these regions of the brain, and it is thus not surprising that abnormalities have been noted in their function across clinical studies. In fact, the contribution of these pathways to the pathophysiology of BD must be reasonably robust, given the variability that might be expected in assessing such dynamic systems under the constraints in experimental design imposed upon such research. Whereas in the past much of the research effort has been focused upon identifying which of these systems might be etiologic in nature, we suggest that we might be better served by addressing their relative contributions in the system response to the underlying neurobiology of the disease process. This will become particularly important as we begin to identify the susceptibility genes for BD in the coming years. More recently, investigators have begun to identify components of signal transduction pathways in the brain such as PKC that may not only play a role in the pathophysiology of the disease but also represent targets for the action of our most efficacious treatments (i.e., lithium and VPA). This experimental strategy may prove to be most promising, since it provides data derived from the physiologic response of the system in affected individuals and addresses the critical dynamic intereraction with pharmacologic agents that effectively modify the clinical expression of the pathophysiology. It is also noteworthy that a growing body of data is demonstrating significant reductions in regional CNS volume and cell numbers (both neurons and glia) in BD (Drevets et al 1997; Manji et al, in press; Rajkowska et al 1999). Furthermore, it has been increasingly recognized that for many patients there is a progressive decline in overall functioning; the potential role of cell death/atrophy in determining long-term outcome remains to be elucidated. Nevertheless, it is noteworthy that psychopharmacologic research strategies have most recently identified long-term actions of these mood stabilizers in the regulation of expression of genes implicated in processes involved in neuroplasticity, neuroprotection, and even neurogenesis (Chen et al, in press; Lenox and Watson 1994; Manji et al 1999, in press; Moore et al, in press). To what extent these long-term processes in the brain are critical to the ability of these drugs to compensate for the pathophysiology of BD as well as stabilize the clinical course and progression of BD has yet to be defined (Manji et al 1999).

The authors' research is supported by the National Institute of Mental Health (Grants Nos. RO1-MH57743 and RO1-MH59107 [HKM] and RO1-MH6247 [RHL]), Theodore and Vada Stanley Foundation (HKM, RHL), National Alliance for Research on Schizophrenia and Depression (HKM, RHL), and Joseph Young Sr. Research grants (HKM). Outstanding editorial assistance was provided by Celia Knobelsdorf. Space limitations necessitate our citing of review articles in many cases. A full reference list upon which this article was based is available upon request.

Aspects of this work were presented at the conference "Bipolar Disorder: From Pre-Clinical to Clinical, Facing the New Millennium," January 19–21, 2000, Scottsdale, Arizona. The conference was sponsored by the Society of Biological Psychiatry through an unrestricted educational grant provided by Eli Lilly and Company.

References

Bebchuk JM, Arfken CL, Dolan-Manji S, Murphy J, Manji HK (2000): A preliminary investigation of a protein kinase C inhibitor (tamoxifen) in the treatment of acute mania. *Arch Gen Psychiatry* 57:95–97.

Berrettini WH (2000): Are schizophrenic and bipolar disorders *related*? A review of family and molecular studies. *Biol Psychiatry* 48:531–538.

Bhalla US, Iyengar R (1999): Emergent properties of networks of biological signaling pathways. *Science* 283(5400):381–387.

Bourne HR, Nicoll R (1993): Molecular machines integrate coincident synaptic signals. *Cell* 72(suppl):65–75.

Bowden CL (1997): Toward an integrated biological model of bipolar disorder. In: Young LT, Joffe RT, editors. *Bipolar Disorder: Biological Models and Their Clinical Application.* New York: Marcel Dekker, 235–254.

Bunney WE, Bunney BG (2000): Molecular clock genes in man and lower animals. Possible implications for circadian abnormalities in depression. *Neuropsychopharmacology* 22:335–345.

Chen G, Hasanat KA, Bebchuk JM, Moore GJ, Glitz D, Manji HK (1999): Regulation of signal transduction pathways and gene expression by mood stabilizers and antidepressants. *Psychosom Med* 61:599–617.

Chen G, Hawver D, Wright C, Potter WZ, Manji HK (1996): Attenuation of adenylyl cyclases by carbamazepine in vitro. *J Neurochem* 67:2079–2086.

Chen G, Masana M, Manji HK (in press): Lithium regulates PKC-mediated intracellular cross-talk and gene expression in the CNS in vivo. *Bipolar Disord.*

Chen G, Rajkowska G, Du F, Seraji-Bozorgzad N, Manji HK (in press): Enhancement of hippocampal neurogenesis by lithium. *J Neurochem.*

Colin SF, Chang HC, Mollner S, Pfeuffer T, Reed RR, Duman RS, Nestler EJ (1991): Chronic lithium regulates the expression of adenylate cyclase and Gi-protein alpha subunit in rat cerebral cortex. *Proc Natl Acad Sci U S A* 88:10634–10637.

Daigen A, Akiyama K, Otsuki S (1991): Long-lasting change in the membrane-associated protein kinase C activity in the hippocampal kindled rat. *Brain Res* 545:131–136.

Depue RA, Karuss SP, Spoont MR (1987): A two-dimensional threshold model of seasonal bipolar affective disorder. In: Magnusson D, Ohman A, editors. *Psychopathology: An International Perspective.* Orlando, FL: Academic Press, 95–123.

Divish MM, Sheftel G, Boyle A, Kalasapudi VD, Papolos DF, Lachman HM (1991): Differential effect of lithium on fos protooncogene expression mediated by receptor and postreceptor activators of protein kinase C and cyclic adenosine monophosphate: model for its antimanic action. *J Neurosci Res* 28:40–48.

Dowlatshahi D, MacQueen GM, Wang JF, Young LT (1998): Increased temporal cortex CREB concentrations and antidepressant treatment in major depression. *Lancet* 2352(9142): 1754–1755.

Drevets WC, Price JL, Simpson JR Jr, Todd RD, Reich T, Vannier M, Raichle ME (1997): Subgenual prefrontal cortex abnormalities in mood disorders. *Nature* 386:824–827.

Dubovsky S, Murphy J, Christiano J, Lee C (1992): The calcium second messenger system in bipolar disorders: Data supporting new research directions. *J Neuropsychiatry Clin Neurosci* 4:3–14.

Duman RS, Heninger GR, Nestler EJ (1997): A molecular and cellular theory of depression. *Arch Gen Psychiatry* 54:597–606.

Ebstein RP, Oppenheim G, Ebstein BS, Amiri Z, Stessman J (1986): The cyclic AMP second messenger system in man: The effects of heredity, hormones, drugs, aluminum, age and disease on signal amplification. *Prog Neuropsychopharmacol Biol Psychiatry* 10:323–353.

Ehlers CL, Frank E, Kupfer DJ (1988): Social zeitgebers and biological rhythms. A unified approach to understanding the etiology of depression. *Arch Gen Psychiatry* 45:948–952.

Einat H, Kofman O, Belmaker RH (in press): Animal models of bipolar disorder: From a single episode to progressive cycling models. In: Myslobodsky MS, Weiner I, editors. *Contemporary Issues in Modeling Psychopathology.* Boston: Kluwer Academic.

Ellis J, Lenox RH (1991): Receptor coupling to G proteins: Interactions not affected by lithium. *Lithium* 2:141–147.

Emamghoreishi M, Schlichter L, Li PP, Parikh S, Sen J, Kamble A, Warsh JJ (1997): High intracellular calcium concentrations in transformed lymphoblasts from subjects with bipolar I disorder. *Am J Psychiatry* 154:976–982.

Fields A, Li PP, Kish SJ, Warsh JJ (1999): Increased cyclic AMP-dependent protein kinase activity in postmortem brain from patients with bipolar affective disorder. *J Neurochem* 73:1704–1710.

Friedman E, Hoau YW, Levinson D, Connell TA, Singh H (1993): Altered platelet protein kinase C activity in bipolar affective disorder, manic episode. *Biol Psychiatry* 33:520–525.

Friedman E, Wang HY (1996): Receptor-mediated activation of G proteins is increased in postmortem brains of bipolar affective disorder subjects. *J Neurochem* 67:1145–1152.

Goodwin FK, Jamison KR (1990): *Manic-Depressive Illness.* New York: Oxford University Press.

Holsboer F (1995): Neuroendocrinology of mood disorders. In: Bloom FE, Kupfer DJ, editors. *Psychopharmacology: The Fourth Generation of Progress.* New York: Raven, 957–969.

Hough C, Lu SJ, Davis CL, Chuang DM, Post RM (1999): Elevated basal and thapsigargin stimulated intracellular calcium of platelets and lymphocytes from bipolar affective disorder patients measured by a fluorometric microassay. *Biol Psychiatry* 46:247–255.

Ikonomov O, Manji HK (1999): Molecular mechanisms underlying mood-stabilization in manic-depressive illness: The phenotype challenge. *Am J Psychiatry* 156:1506–1514.

Jensen JB, Mikkelsen JD, Mork A (2000): Increased adenylyl cyclase type 1 mRNA, but not adenylyl cyclase type 2 in the rat hippocampus following antidepressant treatment. *Eur Neuropsychopharmacol* 10:105–111.

Jope RS (1999a): Anti-bipolar therapy: Mechanism of action of lithium. *Mol Psychiatry* 4:117–128.

Jope RS (1999b): A bimodal model of the mechanism of action of lithium. *Mol Psychiatry* 4:21–25.

Jope RS, Williams MB (1994): Lithium and brain signal transduction systems. *Biochem Pharmacol* 77:429–441.

Kantor L, Gnegy ME (1998): Protein kinase C inhibitors block amphetamine-mediated dopamine release in rat striatal slices. *J Pharmacol Exp Ther* 284:592–598.

Kofman O, Li PP, Warsh JJ (1998): Lithium, but not carbamazepine, potentiates hyperactivity induced by intra-accumbens cholera toxin. *Pharmacol Biochem Behav* 59:191–200.

Lenox RH (1987): Role of receptor coupling to phosphoinositide metabolism in the therapeutic action of lithium. *Adv Exp Med Biol* 221:515–530.

Lenox RH, Manji HK (1998): Lithium. In: Nemeroff CB, Schatzberg AF, editors. *American Psychiatric Press Textbook of Psychopharmacology,* 2nd ed. Washington, DC: American Psychiatric Press, 379–430.

Lenox RH, Watson DG (1994): Lithium and the brain: A psychopharmacological strategy to a molecular basis for manic depressive illness. *Clin Chem* 40:309–314.

Lenox RH, Watson DG, Patel J, Ellis J (1992): Chronic lithium administration alters a prominent PKC substrate in rat hippocampus. *Brain Res* 570:333–340.

Magnier C, Corvazier E, Aumont MC, Le Jemtel TH, Enouf J (1995): Relationship between Rap1 protein phosphorylation and regulation of Ca2+ transport in platelets: A new approach. *Biochem J* 310:469–475.

Mandell AJ, Knapp S, Ehlers C, Russo PV (1984): The stability of constrained randomness: Lithium prophylaxis at several neurobiological levels. In: Post RM, Ballenger JC, editors. *Neurobiology of Mood Disorders.* Baltimore: Williams & Wilkins, 744–776.

Manji HK (1992): G proteins: Implications for psychiatry. *Am J Psychiatry* 149:746–760.

Manji HK, Chen G, Hsiao JK, Masana MI, Moore GJ, Potter WZ (2000): Regulation of signal transduction pathways by mood stabilizing agents: Implications for the pathophysiology and treatment of bipolar affective disorder. In: Manji HK, Bowden CL, Belmaker RH, editors. *Bipolar Medications: Mechanisms of Action.* Washington, DC: American Psychiatric Press, 129–177.

Manji HK, Lenox RH (1999): Protein kinase C signaling in the brain: Molecular transduction of mood stabilization in the treatment of bipolar disorder. *Biol Psychiatry* 46:1328–1351.

Manji HK, Moore GJ, Chen G (1999): Lithium at 50: Have the neuroprotective effects of this unique cation been overlooked? *Biol Psychiatry* 46:929–940.

Manji HK, Moore GJ, Chen G (in press): Clinical and preclinical evidence for the neurotrophic effects of mood-stabilizing agents: Implications for the pathophysiology and treatment of manic-depressive illness. *Biol Psychiatry.*

Manji HK, Potter WZ (1997): Monoaminergic mechanisms. In: Joffe RT, Young LT, editors. *Bipolar Disorder: Biological Models and Their Clinical Application.* New York: Marcel Dekker, 1–40.

Masana MI, Bitran JA, Hsiao JK, Potter WZ (1992): In vivo evidence that lithium inactivates Gi modulation of adenylate cyclase in brain. *J Neurochem* 59:200–205.

Mathews R, Li PP, Young LT, Kish SJ, Warsh JJ (1997): Increased G alpha q/11 immunoreactivity in postmortem occipital cortex from patients with bipolar affective disorder. *Biol Psychiatry* 41:649–656.

Milligan G, Wakelam M (1992): *G Proteins: Signal Transduction & Disease.* San Diego: Academic Press.

Mooney JJ, Samson JA, McHale NL, Colodzin R, Alpert J, Koutsos M, Schildkraut JJ (1998): Signal transduction by platelet adenylate cyclase: Alterations in depressed patients may reflect impairment in the coordinated integration of cellular signals (coincidence detection). *Biol Psychiatry* 43: 574–583.

Moore GJ, Bebchuk JM, Parrish JK, Faulk MW, Arfken CL, Strahl-Bevacqua J, Manji HK (1999): Temporal dissociation between lithium-induced CNS myo-inositol changes and clinical response in manic-depressive illness. *Am J Psychiatry* 156:1902–1908.

Moore GJ, Bebchuk JM, Wilds IB, Chen G, Manji HK (in press): Pharmacologic increase in human gray matter. *Lancet.*

Mork A, Geisler A (1989): The effects of lithium in vitro and ex vivo on adenylate cyclase in brain are exerted by distinct mechanisms. *Neuropharmacology* 28:307–311.

Mork A, Geisler A, Hollund P (1992): Effects of lithium on second messenger systems in the brain. *Pharmacol Toxicol* 71(suppl 1):4–17.

Nestler EJ, Terwilliger RZ, Duman RS (1989): Chronic antidepressant administration alters the subcellular distribution of cyclic AMP-dependent protein kinase in rat frontal cortex. *J Neurochem* 53:1644–1647.

Nestler EJ, Terwilliger RZ, Duman RS (1995): Regulation of endogenous ADP-ribosylation by acute and chronic lithium in rat brain. *J Neurochem* 64:2319–2324.

Nestler EJ, Terwilliger RZ, Walker JR, Sevarino KA, Duman RS (1990): Chronic cocaine treatment decreases levels of the G protein subunits Gi alpha and Go alpha in discrete regions of rat brain. *J Neurochem* 55:1079–1082.

Newman ME, Belmaker RH (1987): Effects of lithium in vitro and ex vivo on components of the adenylate cyclase system in membranes from the cerebral cortex of the rat. *Neuropharmacology* 26:211–217.

Ozaki N, Chuang D-M (1997): Effect of lithium on transcription factor binding in cultured cerebellar granule cells and the brain of rats. *J Neurochem* 69:2336–2344.

Ozaki N, Manji HK, Luiberman V, Lu S, Rosenthal N, Goldman D (1997): A naturally occurring amino acid substitution of the human serotonin (5-HT) 2A receptor influences amplitude and timing of intracellular calcium mobilization. *J Neurochem* 68:2186–2193.

Perez J, Tardito D, Mori S, Racagni G, Smeraldi E, Zanardi R (2000a): Abnormalities of cAMP signaling in affective disorders: Implications for pathophysiology and treatment. *Bipolar Disord* 2:27–36.

Perez J, Tardito D, Mori S, Racagni G, Smeraldi E, Zanardi R (2000b): Altered Rap1 endogenous phosphorylation and levels in platelets from patients with bipolar disorder. *J Psychiatr Res* 34:99–104.

Popoli M, Brunello N, Perez J, Racagni G (2000): Second messenger-regulated protein kinases in the brain: Their functional role and the action of antidepressant drugs. *J Neurochem* 74:21–33.

Post RM, Chuang D-M (1991): Mechanism of action of lithium: Comparison and contrast with carbamazepine. In: Birch NJ, editor. *Lithium and the Cell: Pharmacology and Biochemistry.* London: Academic Press, 199–241.

Post RM, Weiss SRB (1999): Neurobiological models of recurrence in mood disorder. In: Charney DS, Nester EJ, Bunney BS, editors. *Neurobiology of Mental Illness.* New York: Oxford University Press, 365–384.

Post RM, Weiss SRB, Clark M, Chuang DM, Hough C, He L (2000): Lithium, carbamazepine and valproate in affective illness: Biochemical and neurobiological mechanisms. In: Manji HK, Bowden CL, Belmaker RH, editors. *Bipolar Medications: Mechanisms of Action.* Washington, DC: American Psychiatric Press, 219–248.

Rahman S, Li PP, Young LT, Kofman O, Kish SJ, Warsh JJ (1997): Reduced [3H] cyclic AMP binding in postmortem brain from subjects with bipolar affective disorder. *J Neurochem* 68:297–304.

Rajkowska G, Miguel-Hidalgo JJ, Wei J, Dilley G, Pittman SD, Meltzer HY, et al (1999): Morphometric evidence for neuronal and glial prefrontal cell pathology in major depression. *Biol Psychiatry* 45:1085–1098.

Rasenick MM, Chen J, Ozawa H (2000): Effects of antidepressant treatments on the G protein-adenylyl cyclase axis as the possible basis of therapeutic action. In: Manji HK, Bowden CL, Belmaker RH, editors. *Bipolar Medications: Mechanisms of Action.* Washington, DC: American Psychiatric Press, 87–108.

Risby ED, Hsiao JK, Manji HK, Bitran J, Moses F, Zhou DF, Potter WZ (1991): The mechanisms of action of lithium. *Arch Gen Psychiatry* 48:513–524.

Shibata K, Morita K, Kitayama S, Okamoto H, Dohi T (1996): Ca2+ entry induced by calcium influx factor and its regulation by protein kinase C in rabbit neutrophils. *Biochem Pharmacol* 52:167–171.

Si-Tahar M, Renesto P, Falet H, Rendu F, Chignard M (1996): The phospholipase C/protein kinase C pathway is involved in cathepsin G-induced human platelet activation: comparison with thrombin. *Biochem J* 313:401–408.

Spiegel AM (1998): *G Proteins, Receptors, and Disease.* Totowa, NJ: Humana Press.

Spleiss O, van Calker D, Scharer L, Adamovic K, Berger M, Gebicke-Haerter PJ (1998): Abnormal G protein alpha(s)- and alpha(i2)-subunit mRNA expression in bipolar affective disorder. *Mol Psychiatry* 3:512–520.

Steketee JD, Kalivas PW (1991): Sensitization to psychostimulants and stress after injection of pertussis toxin into the A10 dopamine region. *J Pharmacol Exp Ther* 259:916–924.

Wang HY, Friedman E (1996): Enhanced protein kinase C activity and translocation in bipolar affective disorder brains. *Biol Psychiatry* 40:568–575.

Wang HY, Friedman E (1999): Effects of lithium on receptor-mediated activation of G proteins in rat brain cortical membranes. *Neuropharmacology* 38:403–414.

Wang JF, Asghari V, Rockel C, Young LT (1999): Cyclic AMP responsive element binding protein phosphorylation and DNA binding is decreased by chronic lithium but not valproate treatment of SH-SY5Y neuroblastoma cells. *Neuroscience* 91:771–776.

Wang JF, Young LT, Li PP, Warsh JJ (1997): Signal transduction abnormalities in bipolar disorder. In: Joffe RT, Young LT, editors. *Bipolar Disorder: Biological Models and Their Clinical Application.* New York: Marcel Dekker, 41–79.

Warsh JJ, Young LT, Li PP (2000): Guanine nucleotide binding (G) protein disturbances in bipolar affective disorder. In: Manji HK, Bowden CL, Belmaker RH, editors. *Bipolar Medications: Mechanisms of Action.* Washington, DC: American Psychiatric Press, 299–329.

Watson DG, Lenox RH (1996): Chronic lithium-induced down-regulation of MARCKS in immortalized hippocampal cells: Potentiation by muscarinic receptor activation. *J Neurochem* 67:767–777.

Watson DG, Watterson JM, Lenox RH (1998): Sodium valproate down-regulates the myristoylated alanine-rich C kinase substrate (MARCKS) in immortalized hippocampal cells. A property of protein kinase C-mediated mood stabilizers. *J Pharmacol Exp Ther* 285:307–316.

Wehr TA, Goodwin FK (1983): Biological rhythms in manic-depressive illness. In: Wehr TA, Goodwin FK editors. *Circadian Rhythms in Psychiatry.* Pacific Grove, CA: Boxwood Press, 129–184.

Wehr TA, Goodwin FK (1987): Can antidepressants cause mania and worsen the course of affective illness? *Am J Psychiatry* 144:1403–1411.

Weintraub BD (1995): *Molecular Endocrinology: Basic Concepts and Clinical Correlations.* New York: Raven.

Weng G, Bhalla US, Iyengar R (1999): Complexity in biological signaling systems. *Science* 284(5411):92–96.

Wiborg O, Kruger T, Jakobsen SN (1999): Region-selective effects of long-term lithium and carbamazepine administration on cyclic AMP levels in rat brain. *Pharmacol Toxicol* 84:88–93.

Wright AF, Crichton DN, Loudon JB, Morten JE, Steel CM (1984): Beta-adrenoceptor binding defects in cell lines from families with manic-depressive disorder. *Ann Hum Genet* 48:201–214.

Young LT, Li PP, Kish SJ, Siu KP, Kamble A, Hornykiewicz O, Warsh JJ (1993): Cerebral cortex G_s α protein levels and forskolin-stimulated cyclic AMP formation are increased in bipolar affective disorder. *J Neurochem* 61:890–898.

Young LT, Woods CM (1996): Mood stabilizers have differential effects on endogenous ADP ribosylation in C6 glioma cells. *Eur J Pharmacol* 309:215–218.

NEWS AND VIEWS

Forty Years of Lithium Treatment

Mogens Schou, MD, DrMed, DrHCMult

This review is based on a lecture in which I was requested to present my personal experiences and views. Since its introduction into psychiatry more than 40 years ago, lithium treatment has in most countries gained wide acceptance in the prophylaxis of unipolar and bipolar affective disorders. At one time it was feared that lithium treatment might lead to a decrease in the glomerular filtration rate, but systematically collected data indicate that even long-term treatment does not induce renal insufficiency. During treatment, regular laboratory monitoring of serum lithium and creatinine concentrations is recommended. Recent studies suggest that long-term lithium treatment does not raise the mortality of manic-depressive patients and indeed may have a mortality-lowering and antisuicidal effect. Despite the availability of alternative therapies, lithium remains the treatment of choice for the prophylaxis of recurrent manic-depressive illness.
Arch Gen Psychiatry. 1997;54:9-13

THE SITUATION IN 1950 AND TODAY

In the late 1930s, the advent of electroconvulsive treatment of manic-depressive illness was received enthusiastically; now depressions and manias could be relieved and deaths due to acute delirium prevented. Thus, the treatment of manic-depressive patients had become markedly improved, but there was still a long way to go. Of the drug treatments, only opium drops and barbiturates, both entirely unsatisfactory, were available for treating depression and mania, respectively, and electroconvulsive treatment did not, at least as then given, prevent the recurrence of manic and depressive episodes.

During the 1950s, major developments occurred. Lithium salts and neuroleptic drugs were introduced for the treatment of mania, and tricyclic antidepressants, for depression. Between 1960 and 1970 the prophylactic effect of lithium in unipolar and bipolar affective illness was observed, tested, and substantiated. Antiepileptics and antidepressants were later found to be valid prophylactic alternatives. A new era had indeed dawned for manic-depressive patients; without these developments many more would have been hospitalized or might have died.

A number of studies from recent years have shown lithium treatment carried out under "naturalistic" or "clinical practice" conditions to be markedly less effective than found in studies from research establishments. Reasons for and remedies against this phenomenon have been discussed in detail elsewhere.[1]

See also pages 14, 16 and 21

Let us now consider current problems and controversies surrounding lithium treatment.

LITHIUM PROPHYLAXIS IN UNIPOLAR AFFECTIVE ILLNESS

Today, lithium prophylaxis is universally considered the treatment of choice for recurrent bipolar illness. Trials by Baastrup et al and myself[2,3] have demonstrated that lithium is also prophylactically effective in recurrent unipolar manic-depressive ill-

From the Psychiatric Hospital, Risskov, Denmark.

ness (recurrent major affective disorder), and, in most parts of the world, lithium has been used successfully for this indication.[4] In a recent comprehensive analysis of the literature Souza and Goodwin[5] concluded: "There is no reason to doubt the efficacy of lithium in the prophylaxis of unipolar depressive illness."

However, this view does not appear to be shared by American psychiatrists. Although in the early 1970s lithium was recognized by the US Food and Drug Administration as a prophylactic agent in recurrent bipolar illness, there has not been a similar recognition in recurrent unipolar illness. Moreover, three recent reviews[6-8] by American authors dealt with long-term management of recurrent depressions, two of which described maintenance treatment with antidepressants and electroconvulsive treatment but did not mention lithium.[6,7] The third review concluded that in unipolar depressive disorder "the routine use of lithium salts instead of, or in combination with, antidepressants does not appear well-justified as a first-line maintenance treatment."[8] In the third reviewer's opinion, lithium had been shown prophylactically ineffective in two studies: British psychiatrists found no advantage of treatment with amitriptyline plus lithium over treatment with amitriptyline alone,[9] and an American study found lithium no better than placebo in patients with a severe index episode.[10]

However, the British study reveals nothing about the value of lithium alone, and it is difficult to see how a single American study (based on pooling of patients from many clinics with consequent risk for "loose" diagnoses) can outweigh the evidence of more than 15 studies carried out over the last 25 years that show the prophylactic, recurrence-preventive action of lithium to be as effective in unipolar as in bipolar affective disorder.[5,11,12]

A German randomized multicenter study of 80 patients with unipolar illness has shown prophylactic superiority of lithium over amitriptyline (W. Greil, MD, unpublished data, 1994). However, the amitriptyline doses were rather low, and there is clearly room for further trials comparing lithium and antidepressants in the treatment of unipolar illness.

In recent years American research has proved that long-term treatment with antidepressants is prophylactically effective in recurrent depressions.[13,14] Although these are fine studies, lithium prophylaxis was not mentioned. I believe that patients who suffer from recurrent depressions without obvious psychosocial precipitating factors, have symptom-free intervals, and are without deviating character features, might benefit from first-line or second-line lithium maintenance treatment. The final choice of prophylactic agent must depend on how individual patients respond to and tolerate treatment with antidepressants and with lithium.

Possible reasons why antidepressants may be preferred to lithium as prophylactic agents may be that patients treated for acute depression are likely to be prescribed the same medication for maintenance treatment and that patients usually prefer to use medication that does not require monitoring by blood tests. Moreover, the new specific serotonin reuptake inhibiting antidepressants have few side effects, and they are being marketed aggressively (even to the extent of being called "happiness pills," which they are not).

Since an extensive controlled prophylactic trial has shown lithium to be significantly more effective than carbamazepine,[15] my view is that for patients with bipolar illness, lithium should be the first-choice prophylactic agent and carbamazepine a valid alternative. For patients with unipolar illness, the new antidepressants may, for the reasons given above, be preferable as first-choice agents, but lithium should not be forgotten as an effective alternative of proven efficacy.

LITHIUM TREATMENT AND KIDNEY FUNCTION

Long-term lithium treatment was at one time feared to damage kidney function and endanger patients' lives. These fears have been allayed. Lithium treatment does affect renal concentrating ability and patients must be warned against dehydration; however, according to extensive reviews in 1988 and 1989, lithium treatment, even when administered for many years, does not lead to changes in the glomerular filtration rate or to renal failure.[16,17]

During the last 5 years there have been a few cases in which lithium-treated patients experienced renal insufficiency with no perceivable cause other than, possibly, the treatment. von Knorring and associates[18] reported that a 71-year-old woman was given hemodialysis after a gradual rise in her serum creatinine level to higher than 500 µmol/L (5.7 mg/dL) during the second decade of lithium treatment. In a study by Gitlin,[19] three of 82 patients given lithium for an average period of 4.3 years experienced renal insufficiency (defined as serum creatinine concentrations consistently higher than 176 µmol/L [2.0 mg/dL]). One of the patients, a 48-year-old man who had been taking lithium for 16 years, needed hemodialysis. I know of a further case, a 72-year-old man who showed a gradual rise of serum creatinine levels to higher than 600 µmol/L (6.8 mg/dL) after 27 years of lithium treatment and who subsequently received hemodialysis (M. Schou, MD, unpublished observations, 1994).

It is difficult to know how to interpret such rare events. They may be late and exceptional adverse effects of lithium treatment, or they may be mere coincidences. Renal insufficiency without a known cause and that requires treatment has been known to occur in the general population. The incidence of renal failure among manic-depressive patients not treated with lithium is unknown.

In terms of practical consequences I agree with Gitlin,[19] who concluded that

> these findings do not imply that lithium treatment should be withheld from appropriate patients, nor do they imply that rises in creatinine levels up to 140 mmol/L or above warrant automatic lithium discontinuation. However, regular monitoring of the creatinine levels of lithium-treated patients, eg, every 6 months to 1 year, and medical consultation if the creatinine level rises much above this threshold would seem to be warranted.

Lithium-induced polyuria and, not always fully reversible, renal concentrating deficit, are well-known side effects of lithium treatment, but investigation of patients given lithium for up to 30 years has not revealed them as harbingers of reduction of glomerular filtration rate and renal insufficiency.[20]

MONITORING OF LITHIUM TREATMENT

Clinical and laboratory monitoring of lithium treatment is important to maintain effective and safe therapy and to keep side effects to a minimum. During the past years there has been debate about the need for, and the frequency of, routine serum lithium determinations.[21-26]

My own recommendations have varied over the years. For a long time I advocated regular serum lithium determinations as a safeguard against over-dosage, under-dosage, and reduction of the renal lithium clearance. The situation changed when extensive studies indicated that lithium treatment does not lower the glomerular filtration rate or the lithium clearance. Based on these observations, I found it important to counteract exaggerated fear of lithium-induced kidney damage and suggested that serum lithium levels need not be determined routinely.[27] However, at the same time I emphasized the importance of frequent contacts between patient and physician for discussion of treatment progress and possible personal and social problems associated with the illness or the treatment. On these occasions serum lithium, serum creatinine, and thyroid-stimulating hormone values might also be determined.

In recent years I have again recommended regular determinations of serum lithium levels. The serum lithium concentration is one of the issues that patient and physician may profitably discuss; this serves a didactic purpose and improves compliance as patients are made aware of their coresponsibility for the treatment. In addition, lithium concentrations should be determined in "at-risk" situations; on suspected impending intoxication; to check for noncompliance; and at shorter intervals during initial dosage adjustment.[28] In cases of litigation, the physician's position is stronger if he or she can show that the patient has been monitored regularly.

The frequency of routine checkups is debatable. In a recent set of recommendations, Birch et al[29] suggested serum lithium and creatinine deter- [illegible] natural that hospitals and clinics follow a certain routine, but the procedure should not be too rigid. I have, for example, a few patients whose serum lithium levels are determined only once or twice a year. But these patients are experienced; they know exactly which signs and symptoms to look for and under what circumstances to seek medical help.

As standard serum lithium concentrations for prophylaxis, I recommend levels of 0.5 to 0.8 mmol/L (identical in patients with bipolar and unipolar illness). This is in accordance with the study of Gelenberg et al,[30] in which serum lithium values of 0.4 to 0.6 mmol/L were found to have few side effects but also low efficacy, and values of 0.8 to 1.0 mmol/L were found to have marked efficacy but also many side effects. Concentrations lower than 0.5 mmol/L may be indicated in some elderly patients and concentrations higher than 0.8 mmol/L may be indicated in some young patients. Even within the recommended range, individual fine-tuning of dosage may be beneficial. Changes in serum lithium levels as small as 0.1 to 0.2 mmol/L, upward or downward, may substantially improve patients' quality of life during maintenance treatment.

Although I now recommend regular serum lithium and creatinine determinations (and determinations of serum thyroid-stimulating hormone once a year), I realize that certain risks are involved. Unless physicians are expressly warned when concentrations become too high or too low, or change too much (and this is not difficult with computer-controlled laboratory printouts), they may ignore routine laboratory results. Moreover, when physicians know that their patients are "under laboratory control," they may be tempted to neglect that careful observation of and attentive listening to patients is the best guarantee of safe and effective lithium treatment. Laboratory monitoring of lithium treatment is important, clinical monitoring essential.

MORTALITY OF PATIENTS GIVEN LONG-TERM LITHIUM TREATMENT

It has been demonstrated that the mortality of manic-depressive patients is markedly higher than that of the general population, and the increase is mainly, but not exclusively, caused by suicide. How does long-term lithium treatment affect this?

A number of mortality studies have been carried out on lithium-treated patients. Some are based on patients from single clinics[31-33] and others on pooled patient data from clinics in different countries, eg, those published by the International Group for the Study of Lithium-Treated Patients (IGSLI).[34-36]

With a single exception,[31] the studies have shown that the mortality of manic-depressive patients given long-term lithium treatment is markedly lower than that of patients not receiving such treatment.[32-36] In several of the studies, the mortality of the lithium-treated patients did not differ from that of the general population.

In the IGSLI studies, in which data were pooled from clinics in Risskov (Denmark), Berlin (Germany), Hamilton (Ontario), and Vienna (Austria), observations were based on a total of 5600 patient years. Standardized mortality ratios were calculated by dividing the number of observed deaths among the patients by the number of deaths expected in the general population after individual matching for sex, age, and observation period. In bipolar and unipolar manic-depressive patients, as well as in patients with schizoaffective disorder, the standardized mortality ratios did not differ from unity; in other words, the mortality ratios were not significantly higher than in the general population.

Studies of drug effects on mortality are more difficult to perform than those on morbidity. Death is such a rare event that very large numbers of patients must be treated and followed up over very long periods. Prospective mortality studies with random allocation to active drug and placebo treatment are obviously out of the question. Furthermore, while response can be studied before, during, and after treatment in the same group of patients in drug trials of morbidity, that is not possible in mortality studies, for a person can die only once. In studies without a randomized control group, subtle selection effects must be considered. For example, if patients with alcoholism or somatic illness have been excluded from prophylactic treatment, this could cause decreased mortality that need not be a result of the treatment.

The finding that the mortality of lithium-treated patients is not higher, or only moderately higher, than that of the general population does not prove, cannot prove, that lithium lowers mortality. The observation is, however, consistent with such an assumption.

Studies have also been carried out on patients who stopped taking lithium.[37-40] The mortality and suicide rates of these patients were significantly higher than those of the general population. As discontinuation of lithium treatment does not occur at random, we are again faced with the possibility that factors other than lithium treatment could have influenced mortality. I do not see how we can ever obtain conclusive evidence on this point, since seriously ill patients cannot be maintained on treatment with placebo.

However, one may compare lithium with prophylactic alternatives. In a German multicenter study, unfortunately only partly published, which lasted 2½ years, several hundred patients were randomly allocated to treatment with lithium or carbamazepine for bipolar illness and treatment with lithium or amitriptyline for unipolar illness.[41] Among the patients given the antidepressant drug, there were five suicides and no suicide attempts; among the carbamazepine-treated patients, there were four suicides and five suicide attempts; in the lithium-treated group, there were no suicides and no suicide attempts. The frequency of suicidal acts among the lithium-treated patients was significantly lower than the corresponding frequencies among those who were given antidepressants or carbamazepine (χ^2, $P<.001$ for both groups). These observations are consistent with the assumption that lithium treatment protects against suicidal behavior.

As scientists we must conclude that a mortality-lowering, antisuicidal effect of long-term lithium treatment has not been proved but remains a possibility.[42] As clinicians we must ask whether our patients and their relatives can afford that we disregard this possibility. As far as mortality is concerned, lithium seems currently the best remedy we can offer.

Let us, however, not forget what in my opinion is the most important outcome of the mortality investigations, and one on which there is agreement. All the studies have shown that long-term lithium treatment is *not* associated with *increased* mortality.

DISAPPOINTMENTS

In what ways do I feel disappointed with lithium after more than 40 years' experience?

I hoped for a long time that lithium could be rejected because something distinctly better emerged. That has not happened. I do not regard the current alternatives as generally better than lithium. They may be better for some patients and in special situations, but we are still waiting for something that is radically superior to lithium and its alternatives in terms of side effects and efficacy.

Another disappointment is that we still do not know the mechanism of action of lithium in affective illness. Many hypotheses exist, some of them ingenious and attractive, but none as yet proved correct. Moreover, in spite of what many believe, the same situation applies to antidepressants, anticonvulsants, and electroconvulsive treatment. As we do not know the pathophysiological basis of manic-depressive illness, we do not understand how treatments work; and as we do not know how treatments work, we cannot understand the pathophysiology of manic-depressive illness. The locked box with its key inside appears to present an insoluble problem. Nevertheless, in such situations a combination of perseverance and inspired guessing has before now borne fruit, and I trust that this may happen again.

PERSPECTIVES

Let us now consider various perspectives of lithium treatment. In 1969 Baastrup et al and I[3] carried out a randomized double-blind discontinuation trial to test lithium's prophylactic effect. Within 6 months, half of the patients receiving placebo relapsed, compared with none of the patients who continued taking lithium. The trial thus confirmed the prophylactic efficacy of lithium. The point I want to make, however, is that the patients all had a valid psychological explanation of why a recurrence had occurred at that particular time, eg, marital problems, transfer to a new apartment, or financial difficulties. The recurrences led to admission of the patients, and the ward staff, who apart from a single initiate did not know about the discontinuation trial, accepted unquestioningly the patients' psychological explanations.

This experience can be viewed in two ways. One can assume that recurrence in the placebo group was determined exclusively by the endogenous rhythm of the manic-depressive disease, and that lithium had corrected the anomaly. The patients' subjectively convincing psychological explanations thus represented a rationalization. On the other hand, it is conceivable that the recurrences in the placebo group were in fact provoked by environmental stress in persons with a particularly high vulnerability. In the patients given lithium, the treatment elevated the threshold for environmentally induced provocation of recurrences.

There is probably some truth in both scenarios. I find it difficult to conceive of a psychological phenomenon that is not accompanied by some biological change, neurophysiological or neurochemical. And there are presumably few biological processes that do not influence the mind, or psychological thresholds, to some extent. The day will presumably come when we succeed in finding out how our therapies work, and this may lead to new treatments with improved efficacy and even higher specificity.

What about the more distant future? If research should one day clarify the cerebral mechanisms that govern the endogenous mood level, this would raise the possibilities not only of *normalizing* mood but also of *manipulating* mood. It may, for example, become possible to adjust one's own mood, or that of others, to a particular level. This would enable people to choose spending their lives in a condition of light chronic mania, subjectively more alluring than even the most enjoyable alcohol- or crack cocaine–induced euphoria. Is this a happy vision? Or is it a frightening one? It is a possibility that forces us to ponder the central question: Should scientists under all circumstances reveal the secrets of nature, or are there doors that, because of the possible consequences, they should abstain from opening?

Another vexing question about the future is the following. If it becomes possible through gene manipulation to eradicate the disposition to manic-depressive illness, is that a desirable goal? It may be, and some Chinese legislators seem inclined to think so. Or it may not. Had eugenic measures of this kind been feasible and practiced in the past, then I myself might not have been in existence and able to express the views presented here.

Accepted for publication June 30, 1995.

This review was based on the first keynote address presented by the author at the First International Conference on Bipolar Disorder, Pittsburgh, Pa, June 23, 1994.

Reprint requests to The Psychiatric Hospital, 2 Skovagervej, DK-8240 Risskov, Denmark (Dr Schou).

REFERENCES

1. Schou M. Lithium prophylaxis: about 'naturalistic' or 'clinical practice' studies. *Lithium.* 1993;4:77-81.
2. Baastrup PC, Schou M. Lithium as a prophylactic agent: its effect against recurrent depressions and manic-depressive psychosis. *Arch Gen Psychiatry.* 1967;16:162-172.
3. Baastrup PC, Poulsen JC, Schou M, Thomsen K, Amdisen A. Prophylactic lithium: double-blind discontinuation in manic-depressive and recurrent-depressive disorders. *Lancet.* 1970;2:326-330.
4. Souza FGM, Mander AJ, Goodwin GM. The efficacy of lithium prophylaxis of unipolar depression: evidence from its discontinuation. *Br J Psychiatry.* 1990;157:718-722.
5. Souza FGM, Goodwin GM. Lithium treatment and prophylaxis in unipolar depression: a meta-analysis. *Br J Psychiatry.* 1991;158:666-675.
6. Nobler MS, Sackeim HA. Pharmacotherapy and electroconvulsive therapy for mood disorders. *Curr Opin Psychiatry.* 1993;6:10-15.
7. Kupfer DJ. Management of recurrent depression. *J Clin Psychiatry.* 1993;54(suppl 2):29-33.
8. Thase ME. Maintenance treatments of recurrent affective disorders. *Curr Opin Psychiatry.* 1993;6:16-21.
9. Johnstone EC, Owens DGC, Lambert MT, Crow TJ, Frith CD, Done DJ. Combination tricyclic antidepressant and lithium maintenance medication in unipolar and bipolar depressed patients. *J Affect Dis.* 1990;20:225-233.
10. Prien RF, Kupfer DJ, Mansky PA, Small JG, Tuason VB, Voss CB, Johnson WE. Drug therapy in the prevention of recurrences in unipolar and bipolar affective disorders. *Arch Gen Psychiatry.* 1984;41:1096-1104.
11. Goodwin FK, Jamison KR. *Manic-Depressive Illness.* Oxford, England: Oxford University Press; 1990.
12. Davis JM, Wang Z, Janicak PG. A quantitative analysis of clinical drug trials for the treatment of affective disorders. *Psychopharmacol Bull.* 1993;29:175-181.
13. Frank E, Kupfer DJ, Perel JM, Cornes C, Jarrett DB, Mallinger AG, Thase ME, McEachran AB, Grochocinski VJ. Three-year outcomes for maintenance therapies in recurrent depression. *Arch Gen Psychiatry.* 1990;47:1093-1099.
14. Kupfer DJ, Frank E, Perel JM, Cornes C, Mallinger AG, Thase ME, McEachran AB, Grochocinski VJ. Five-year outcome for maintenance therapies in recurrent depression. *Arch Gen Psychiatry.* 1992;49:769-773.
15. Greil W, Ludwig-Mayerhofer W, Steller B, Czernik A, Giedke H, Müller-Oerlinghausen B, Osterheider M, Rudolf GAE, Sauer H, Tegeler J, Wetterling T. Lithium-oder Carbamazepinprophylaxe bei affektiven Psychosen? Ergebnisse einer kontrollierten, multizentrischen Studie. In: Müller-Oerlinghausen B, Berghöfer A, eds. *Ziele und Ergebnisse der medikamentösen Prophylaxe affektiver Psychosen.* Stuttgart, Germany: Thieme; 1994:113-119.
16. Schou M. Effects of long-term lithium treatment on kidney function: an overview. *J Psychiatr Res.* 1988;22:287-296.
17. Waller DG, Edwards JG. Lithium and the kidney: an update. *Psychol Med.* 1989;19:825-831.
18. von Knorring L, Wahlin A, Nyström K, Bohman SO. Uraemia induced by long-term lithium treatment. *Lithium.* 1990;1:251-253.
19. Gitlin MJ. Lithium-induced renal insufficiency. *J Clin Psychopharmacol.* 1993;13:276-279.
20. Kallner G, Petterson U. Renal, thyroid and parathyroid function during lithium treatment: laboratory test in 207 people treated for 1-30 years. *Acta Psychiatr Scand.* 1995;91:48-51.
21. Aronson JK, Reynolds DJM. ABC of monitoring drug therapy: lithium. *BMJ.* 1992;305:1273-1276.
22. Hullin RP, Srinivasan DP, Birch NJ. Monitoring lithium treatment. *BMJ.* 1993;306:269.
23. Kehoe RF. Monitoring lithium treatment. *BMJ.* 1993;36:269-270.
24. Aronson JK, Reynolds DJM. Monitoring lithium treatment. *BMJ.* 1993;306:270.
25. Guscott R, Taylor L. Monitoring of lithium treatment. *Can J Psychiatry.* 1993;38:74.
26. Schou M. Monitoring of lithium treatment: reply to Guscott and Taylor. *Can J Psychiatry.* 1993;38:74.
27. Schou M. Relapse prevention in manic-depressive illness: important and unimportant factors. *Can J Psychiatry.* 1991;36:502-506.
28. Schou M. *Lithium Treatment of Manic-Depressive Illness: A Practical Guide.* 5th ed, revised. Basel, Switzerland: Karger; 1993.
29. Birch NJ, Grof P, Hullin RP, Kehoe RF, Schou M, Srinivasan DP. Lithium prophylaxis: proposed guidelines for good clinical practice. *Lithium.* 1993;4:225-230.
30. Gelenberg AJ, Kane JM, Keller MB, Lavori P, Rosenbaum JF, Cole K, Lavalle J. Comparison of standard and low serum levels of lithium for maintenance treatment of bipolar disorder. *N Engl J Med.* 1989;321:1489-1493.
31. Norton B, Whalley LJ. Mortality of a lithium-treated population. *Br J Psychiatry.* 1984;146:277-282.
32. Coppen A, Standish-Barry H, Bailey J, Houston G, Silcocks P, Hermon C. Long-term lithium and mortality. *Lancet.* 1990;335:1347.
33. Coppen A, Standish-Barry H, Bailey J, Houston G, Silcocks P, Hermon C. Does lithium reduce the mortality of recurrent mood disorders? *J Affect Dis.* 1991;23:1-7.
34. Müller-Oerlinghausen B, Ahrens B, Volk J, Grof P, Grof E, Schou M, Vestergaard P, Lenz G, Simhandl C, Thau K, Wolf R. Reduced mortality of manic-depressive patients in long-term lithium treatment: an international collaborative study by IGSLI. *Psychiatry Res.* 1991;36:329-331.
35. Müller-Oerlinghausen B, Ahrens B, Grof E, Grof P, Lenz G, Schou M, Simhandl C, Thau K, Volk J, Wolf R, Wolf T. The effect of long-term lithium treatment on the mortality of patients with manic-depressive or schizo-affective illness. *Acta Psychiatr Scand.* 1992;86:218-222.
36. Ahrens B, Müller-Oerlinghausen B, Schou M, Wolf T, Alda M, Grof E, Grof P, Lenz G, Simhandl C, Thau K, Vestergaard P, Wolf R, Möller H. Cardiovascular and suicide mortality of affective disorders may be reduced by lithium prophylaxis. *J Affect Dis.* 1995;33:67-75.
37. Nilsson A. Mortality in recurrent mood disorders during periods on and off lithium: a complete population study in 362 patients. *Pharmacopsychiatry.* 1995;28:8-13.
38. Müller-Oerlinghausen B, Müser-Causemann B, Volk J. Suicides and parasuicides in a high-risk patient group on and off lithium long-term medication. *J Affect Dis.* 1992;25:261-270.
39. Lenz G, Ahrens B, Denk E, Müller-Oerlinghausen B, Schratzberger-Topitz A, Simhandl C, Wancata J. Mortalität nach Ausscheiden aus der Lithiumambulanz. In: Müller-Oerlinghausen B, Berghöfer A, eds. *Ziele und Ergebnisse der medikamentösen Prophylaxe affektiver Psychosen.* Stuttgart, Germany: Thieme; 1994:49-52.
40. Felber W, Kyber A. Suizide und Parasuizide während und außerhalb einer Lithiumprophylaxe. In: Müller-Oerlinghausen B, Berghöfer A, eds. *Ziele und Ergebnisse der medikamentösen Prophylaxe affektiver Psychosen.* Stuttgart, Germany: Thieme; 1994:53-59.
41. Thies-Flechtner K, Seibert W, Walther A, Greil W, Müller-Oerlinghausen B. Suizide bei rezidivprophylaktisch behandelten Patienten mit affektiven Psychosen. In: Müller-Oerlinghausen B, Berghöfer A, eds. *Ziele und Ergebnisse der medikamentösen Prophylaxe affektiver Psychosen.* Stuttgart, Germany: Thieme; 1994:61-64.
42. Schou M. Mortality-lowering effect of prophylactic lithium treatment: a look at the evidence. *Pharmacopsychiatry.* 1995;28:1.

Conversions From Système International (SI) Units to Traditional Units (Modified From *The SI Manual in Health Care*)

System	Component	SI Reference Interval*	SI Unit	Conversion Factor (Divide by)	Traditional Reference Interval*	Traditional Unit
Serum	Lithium ion, therapeutic	0.50-1.50	mmol/L	0.001441	350-1050	μg/dL
		0.50-1.50	mmol/L	1.441	0.35-1.05	mg/dL

**These reference values are not intended to be definitive since each laboratory determines its own values. They are provided for illustration only.*

Forty Years of Lithium Treatment

THE article "Forty Years of Lithium Treatment"[1] represents a remarkable journey of 40 years by Schou, one of the pioneers in the treatment of manic-depressive illness and one of the most fervent advocates for lithium prophylaxis. Schou's article is based on a lecture given at the introductory plenary session of the First International Conference on Bipolar Disorder held in Pittsburgh, Pa, June 23-24, 1994.

The major purpose of this conference was to identify both current advances in the treatment of bipolar disorder and unresolved problems in both the short- and long-term treatment of this severe psychiatric disorder. Many of the speakers demonstrated their concern that as many as 40% of patients with bipolar disorder are not effectively treated with lithium. Since the development of alternative forms of therapy has become of increasing importance, it seems appropriate to review the current assets and liabilities of lithium treatment.

In this context, Schou's article represents a strong, articulate, and well-referenced review that is primarily focused on the positive aspects of lithium prophylaxis for bipolar and unipolar affective disorders. While he is concerned about recent studies that have suggested that there are a considerable number of people who do not respond to lithium treatment,[2,3] he is convinced that many of these studies represent naturalistic investigations, indicating lower levels of efficacy, probably as a result of compliance problems and patient selection criteria. Indeed, he is less concerned about the controversy of lithium indications in bipolar disorder than the indication for lithium in the long-term treatment of unipolar recurrent disorders. His own strong impression from the literature and his considerable clinical experience is that lithium represents a first line of treatment for unipolar prophylaxis. In contrast, some investigators have argued that lithium is not appropriate as a first-line treatment for recurrent unipolar disorders.[4] In one study, in which imipramine appeared superior to lithium in long-term prophylaxis, the initial treatment protocol necessitated successful response to the combination of imipramine and lithium and, thus, did not provide an adequate test of the question of whether patients who respond initially to lithium therapy can be maintained prophylactically on lithium regimen.[3] Perhaps, the field could use a controlled short-term and long-term trial comparing lithium vs tricyclic antidepressants vs SSRIs (selective serotonin reuptake inhibitors) in unipolar recurrent disorder. Schou does admit, however, that the ease of treatment and the increased level of compliance with routine antidepressants may lead to a greater use of alternatives to lithium in the treatment of recurrent unipolar illness.

See also pages 9, 16, and 21

Our own position is that while we would certainly agree that there are data supporting the use of lithium prophylaxis in unipolar recurrent illness, we believe that the studies on efficacy and the ease of use and adherence to either traditional tricyclic antidepressants or the newer SSRIs suggest that these agents represent a more useful alternative for the treatment of recurrent unipolar illness for both short- and long-term treatment.[5] Furthermore, in the United States, with the increasing treatment of recurrent unipolar illness by primary care practitioners, the antidepressants seem to be a more acceptable form of treatment than the use of lithium.

Turning to lithium administration, with respect to the notion of monitoring serum lithium, Schou feels that there is a need for regular determination of serum lithium only every 2 to 6 months. This recommendation represents a reduction in routine monitoring frequency compared with earlier suggestions. With respect to the appropriate dosage of lithium, Schou points to very small fine-tuning of dosage as beneficial in the long-term treatment. Therefore, the clinician has to be quite observant in examining the concentration and its effect on each patient, particularly those who are elderly.

Schou goes on to demonstrate that the use of lithium may lead to decreased mortality compared with other antidepressants. He also argues that the long-term side effects of lithium, such as kidney abnormalities, should not be of major continued concern. Schou refers to several German and Scandinavian studies[6-8] to support his argument that lithium treatment seems to be unrelated to suicide attempts and successful suicide. There are a number of areas that one would wish that Schou would have covered as important areas needing special attention in 1995. One of these areas is the treatment of bipolar depression. Clearly, neither the short- nor long-term treatment of bipolar depression is yielding the same level of efficacy as is obtained in the treatment of mania. Zornberg and Pope[9] have shown that, in contrast to the extensive data on the treatment of manic states, the paucity of data on the treatment of bipolar depression is appalling. Furthermore, the extant studies are limited or inconclusive. The major problem may be that the treatment strategies and efficacy rates do not seem to be as good as similar strategies for the treatment of unipolar depression. This has been confirmed by a number of studies by Keller and colleagues,[10] as well as in unpublished analyses of the current Pittsburgh protocol.

One key area of disappointment that we share with Schou has been that a better drug has not yet emerged. Some of this disappointment, we think, is related to the early belief that the introduction of lithium carbonate would "cure" this disorder. The reluctance of individuals to seek treatment and the stigma attached to the treatment of mood disorders have compounded the difficulty of inducing pharmaceutical companies to begin tackling the problem of finding antidepressants that would be especially useful in bipolar disorder. For that matter, even testing the antidepressants that the pharmaceutical companies are currently introducing (eg, SSRIs) to determine whether there is a specific indication for bipolar disorder has not happened. This appears to be in the face of evidence that the prevalence of bipolar depression is substantial, especially in female individuals.

Another disappointment that we share with Schou is that we still do not understand the mechanism of action of lithium in mood disorders. A very recent article on signal transduction pathways by Manji et al,[11] published in the ARCHIVES, represents an excellent review of the search for and identification of intracellular targets for lithium's action. These areas of interest, involving signal transduction pathways and, in particular, G proteins, suggest important potential breakthroughs in not only understanding the action of lithium but being in a better position to understand the action of all psychotropic agents in bipolar disorders.

The final disappointment or concern that Schou describes relates to one of ours: the future of genetics and molecular neurobiology in bipolar disorder. We believe that it is unlikely that a single gene will be found to account for all bipolar disorder, and that it is extremely likely that manic-depressive illness represents a complex polygenic genetic disorder. As such, a number of genes will ultimately be identified that contribute to the onset and development of this disorder. Both the molecular biologists and those clinicians and counselors who may eventually be involved in genetic counseling need to prepare for the period in time in which they will be put in a position of "prescribing" and counseling individuals and families with respect to bipolar illness. This represents both a set of problems and an important set of future opportunities for our field.

In closing, we believe that many of the disappointments that Schou enumerates will turn out to be the very fruits that need to be further investigated. We hope that there will be a follow-up to these very tough and important questions at the Second International Conference on Bipolar Disorder scheduled for June of 1997 in Pittsburgh.

David J. Kupfer, MD
Ellen Frank, PhD
Department of Psychiatry
University of Pittsburgh School of Medicine
Western Psychiatric Institute and Clinic
3811 O'Hara St
Pittsburgh, PA 15213

This study was supported in part by grants MH-29618 and MH-30915 from the National Institute of Mental Health and a grant from the Stanley Center for the Innovative Treatment of Bipolar Disorder.

REFERENCES

1. Schou M. Forty years of lithium treatment. *Arch Gen Psychiatry.* 1997;54:9-13.
2. Johnstone EC, Owens DGC, Lambert MT, Crow TJ, Frith CD, Done DJ. Combination tricyclic antidepressant and lithium maintenance medication in unipolar and bipolar depressed patients. *J Affect Disord.* 1990;20:225-233.
3. Prien RF, Kupfer DJ, Mansky PA, Small JG, Tuason VB, Voss CB, Johnson WE. Drug therapy in the prevention of recurrences in unipolar and bipolar affective disorders: report of the NIMH Collaborative Study Group comparing lithium carbonate, imipramine, and a lithium carbonate–imipramine combination. *Arch Gen Psychiatry.* 1984;41:1096-1104.
4. Thase ME. Maintenance treatments of recurrent affective disorders. *Curr Opin Psychiatry.* 1993; 6:16-21.
5. Frank E, Kupfer DJ, Perel JM, Cornes C, Jarrett DB, Mallinger AG, Thase ME, McEachran AB, Grochocinski VJ. Three-year outcomes for maintenance therapies in recurrent depression. *Arch Gen Psychiatry.* 1990;47:1093-1099.
6. Ahrens B, Müller-Oerlinghausen B, Schou M, Wolf T, Alda M, Grof E, Grof P, Lenz G, Simhandl C, Thau K, Vestergaard P, Wolf R, Möller H. Cardiovascular and suicide mortality of affective disorders may be reduced by lithium prophylaxis. *J Affect Disord.* 1995;33:67-75.
7. Nilsson A. Mortality in recurrent mood disorders during periods on and off lithium: a complete population study in 362 patients. *Pharmacopsychiatry.* 1995;28:8-13.
8. Schou M. Mortality-lowering effect of prophylactic lithium treatment: a look at the evidence. *Pharmacopsychiatry.* 1995;28:1.
9. Zornberg GL, Pope Jr, HG. Treatment of depression in bipolar disorder: new directions for research. *J Clin Psychopharmacol.* 1993; 13:397-408.
10. Keller MB, Lavori PW, Coryell W, Andreasen NC, Endicott J, Clayton PJ, Klerman GL, Hirschfeld RMA. Differential outcome of pure manic, mixed/cycling, and pure depressive episodes in patients with bipolar illness. *JAMA.* 1986; 255:3138-3142.
11. Manji HK, Potter WZ, Lenox RH. Signal transduction pathways: molecular targets for lithium's actions. *Arch Gen Psychiatry.* 1995;52: 531-543.

Cell, Vol. 59, 411–419, November 3, 1989, Copyright © 1989 by Cell Press

Neural and Developmental Actions of Lithium: A Unifying Hypothesis

Review

Michael J. Berridge,* C. Peter Downes,† and Michael R. Hanley‡
* AFRC Unit of Insect Neurophysiology and Pharmacology
Department of Zoology
Cambridge CB2 3EJ
England
† Smith Kline & French Research Ltd.
The Frythe, Welwyn
Hertfordshire AL6 9AR
England
‡ MRC Molecular Neurobiology Unit
University of Cambridge Medical School
Cambridge CB2 2QH
England

Lithium, with an atomic weight of 6.9, is the smallest of the alkali metals, yet this simple ion can exert a profound effect on both human behavior and early embryonic development. Manic-depressive psychosis, characterized by dramatic swings in mood, can be effectively controlled by maintaining a serum level of Li^+ of ~1 mM. Despite its therapeutic success, little is known about the way Li^+ can modify neurotransmission within the central nervous system (CNS). Many of the proposed mechanisms have suggested an inhibitory effect on components of various neurotransmitter signaling pathways, such as cyclic AMP formation, cyclic GMP formation, G proteins, or inositol phosphate metabolism (Hallcher and Sherman, 1980; Berridge et al., 1982). Only the latter provides a plausible explanation of the Li^+ conundrum, i.e., the reason this ion can selectively modulate neural activity within the CNS while having little effect on comparable signaling events within the periphery. We argued previously (Berridge et al., 1982) that Li^+ might act by reducing the supply of inositol required to maintain the membrane inositol lipids used to generate the second messengers inositol 1,4,5-trisphosphate ($Ins(1,4,5)P_3$) and diacylglycerol (DAG) (Berridge, 1987; Nishizuka, 1986, 1988). The unique sensitivity of the brain to Li^+ was explained by the low permeability of the blood–brain barrier to inositol, which thus places a heavy burden upon the mechanisms of synthesis and/or conservation to meet its requirements for inositol (Berridge et al., 1982).

Inositol can protect Xenopus embryos against the teratogenic effects of Li^+ (Busa and Gimlich, 1989), which indicates that the inositol depletion hypothesis may provide an equally plausible explanation for the way this ion disrupts early embryonic development. A better understanding of the way Li^+ acts may thus provide insights into the basic mechanisms underlying two major unsolved problems in biology—pattern formation in early development and the neural basis of human behavior.

Lithium, an Uncompetitive Inhibitor of Inositol Phosphate Metabolism

Cell surface stimulants control phosphoinositide metabolism by promoting the hydrolysis of inositol lipids to DAG and various inositol phosphates (Figure 1). The lipid that appears to be the principal target of activated phospholipase C is $PtdIns4,5P_2$ (Downes and Michell, 1985; but compare with Ackermann et al., 1987), and its breakdown

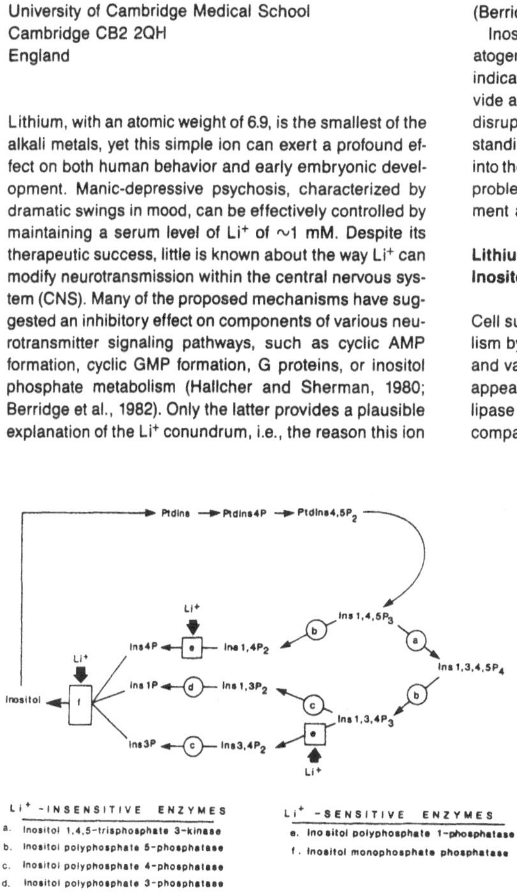

Figure 1. Lithium Inhibition of Phosphoinositide Metabolism

The agonist-dependent hydrolysis of $Ptd\text{-}Ins(4,5)P_2$ generates $Ins(1,4,5)P_3$, which is then metabolized through two separate pathways comprising both Li^+ insensitive and Li^+ sensitive enzymes. $Ins(1,4,5)P_3$ can be phosphorylated to $Ins(1,3,4,5)P_4$ by a kinase (a) or it can be hydrolyzed to $Ins(1,4)P_2$ by an inositol 5-phosphomonoesterase (b), which is also responsible for removing the 5-phosphate from $Ins(1,3,4,5)P_4$ to produce $Ins(1,3,4)P_3$. Another dual-acting enzyme is the Li^+ sensitive inositol polyphosphate 1-phosphatase (e), which hydrolyzes $Ins(1,3,4)P_3$ to $Ins(3,4)P_2$ and $Ins(1,4)P_2$ to Ins4P. The inositol polyphosphate 4 phosphatase (c), which hydrolyzes $Ins(1,3,4)P_3$ to $Ins(1,3)P_3$ and $Ins(3,4)P_2$ to Ins3P, is insensitive to Li^+. The $Ins(1,3)P_2$ is dephosphorylated to Ins1P by an inositol polyphosphate 3-phosphatase (d) that is also insensitive to Li^+. As a result of the three separate bisphosphatase activities the cell generates three inositol monophosphates (Ins1P, Ins3P, and Ins4P), all of which are hydrolyzed by a single inositol monophosphatase (f) whose activity is very sensitive to Li^+ inhibition.

generates the calcium-mobilizing second messenger $Ins(1,4,5)P_3$ (Berridge, 1987; Berridge and Irvine, 1984). However, at least three other phospholipids are potential substrates for hydrolysis during the initial response, producing DAG in all cases and $Ins(1,4)P_2$ from PtdIns4P, Ins1P from PtdIns, or $Ins(1,3)P_2$ from the newly identified lipid PtdIns3P (Whitman et al., 1988; Stephens et al., 1989). It has proved difficult to determine whether or not these lipids are being hydrolyzed, because the inositol phosphates they generate feed into the elaborate pathways responsible for metabolizing $Ins(1,4,5)P_3$ (Figure 1; Irvine et al., 1988; Majerus et al., 1988). The metabolism of inositol phosphates seems vastly more complex now than it did a few years ago, but viewed in a functional context, this complexity is more apparent than real. These metabolic pathways serve to terminate rapidly the activity of $Ins(1,4,5)P_3$, to conserve cellular supplies of *myo*-inositol, and potentially to diversify the informational messengers by providing cosignals such as $Ins(1,3,4,5)P_4$ (Irvine and Moor, 1986) and perhaps $Ins(1,3,4,5,6)P_5$ and $InsP_6$ (Vallejo et al., 1987; Hanley et al., 1988).

Much of the complication arises from the existence of more than one pathway for metabolizing $Ins(1,4,5)P_3$, each of which contains both Li^+ insensitive and Li^+ sensitive enzymes. The two Li^+ sensitive phosphatases have different K_i values depending on the substrate being hydrolyzed, but in practice the monophosphate phosphatase is more sensitive to Li^+ than the polyphosphate 1-phosphatase because of the high content of inositol monophosphates during stimulation (see below). The monophosphatase is the most widely studied enzyme of inositol phosphate metabolism and has been purified to homogeneity from bovine brain (Gee et al., 1988). The monophosphatase occupies a pivotal position in inositol homeostatic mechanisms because it resides at the confluence of two distinct pathways for the maintenance of intracellular inositol levels: the recovery of inositol following the activated breakdown of phosphoinositides, and a separate route for the de novo synthesis of inositol from glucose (see below).

Perhaps the most unusual aspect of Li^+ action on the sensitive enzymes is that it is *uncompetitive*, which means that it binds solely to the enzyme–substrate complex (Gee et al., 1988). Cornish-Bowden (1986) has discussed some of the remarkable consequences of such an inhibitory mechanism. For example, an increase in substrate concentration fails to compete out the inhibitor and actually enhances inhibition by providing more enzyme–substrate complex. Thus, a positive feedback loop is introduced into the inhibitory action of Li^+. An analogy to the inertia-reel mechanism of an automobile seatbelt may be made: as the forward momentum of inositol phosphate formation increases, so is the inhibitory braking power of Li^+ enhanced, which bears directly on the stimulus-dependence of this drug. Li^+ will selectively affect, in a graded fashion, those cells whose receptors are being actively stimulated.

In summary, the net effect of inhibiting inositol phosphate metabolism is that Li^+ suppresses the recycling of inositol by inhibiting the hydrolysis of intermediate inositol phosphates. Consistent with its identified sites of inhibition (Figure 1), the inositol phosphates that accumulate during chronic Li^+ treatment are the three inositol monophosphates (Ins1P, Ins3P, and Ins4P), $Ins(1,4)P_2$, and $Ins(1,3,4)P_3$. It is unlikely that Li^+ exerts its effects through these inositol phosphates, since none of these have any established biological messenger function with the possible exception of $Ins(1,4)P_2$, which has been suggested to activate a DNA polymerase (Sylvia et al., 1988). Li^+ can inhibit the accumulation of $Ins(1,3,4,5)P_4$ in stimulated brain slices after a short time lag, but the molecular basis and functional significance for this potentially important effect are not known (Whitworth and Kendall, 1988). A much more likely possibility concerning the action of Li^+ is that it interferes with inositol recovery to lower the level of free inositol; this forms the basis of the inositol depletion hypothesis outlined below.

Inositol Depletion Hypothesis

The agonist-dependent generation of phosphoinositide-derived second messengers DAG and $Ins(1,4,5)P_3$ depends on a continuous supply of the precursor lipid $PtdIns(4,5)P_2$. The latter is a minor inositol lipid whose level must be maintained by continuous lipid resynthesis, whereby free inositol is attached to CMP-PA (Figure 2). For this lipid resynthesis to occur, it is necessary for the cell to maintain a constant high level of inositol. Cells have access to three sources of inositol (Figure 2):

First, they can recycle the inositol from $Ins(1,4,5)P_3$, but it has first to be dephosphorylated through the pathways described earlier (Figure 1).

Second, inositol can be synthesised de novo by the cyclization of glucose-6-phosphate to L-inositol 1-phosphate, an alternative name for D-Ins3P, which is also formed during the metabolism of D-$Ins(1,3,4,5)P_4$ (Figure 1).

And finally, cells can take up inositol from the environment. Unlike the previous two mechanisms (recycling and synthesis), uptake of inositol is insensitive to the inhibitory action of Li^+ (Figure 2). As outlined later, cells may be restricted in their access to external inositol by either the presence of a blood–tissue barrier, the absence of a circulatory system (e.g., in the developing embryo), or the absence of a plasma membrane uptake system.

Lithium thus blocks at a convergence point the two mechanisms whereby the cell generates free cytoplasmic inositol, but it does not interfere with its ability to accumulate exogenous inositol. We argue, therefore, that cells or tissues sensitive to lithium are those that, for one reason or another, are unable to buffer internal inositol stores by uptake of external inositol.

Direct evidence that Li^+ led to a decrease in the level of *myo*-inositol was first obtained in brain (Allison and Stewart, 1971) but has been observed in stimulated parotid gland (Downes and Stone, 1986) and adrenal glomerulosa cells (Balla et al., 1984). We argue that the biological and therapeutic actions of Li^+ can be explained by a marked perturbation of the phosphoinositide signaling system that results from this reduction in the level of inositol. The immediate effect of lowering the level

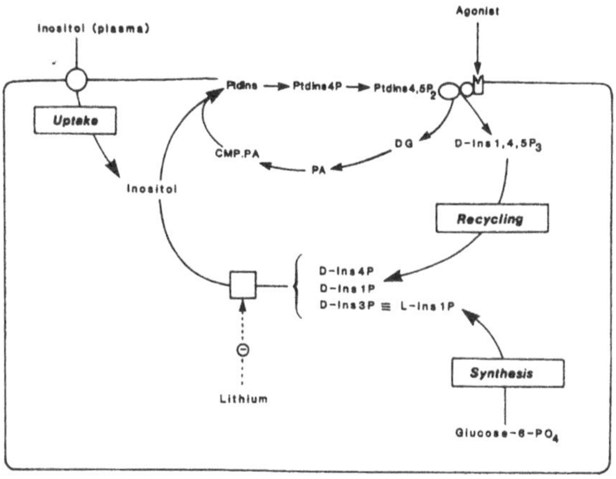

Figure 2. Summary of the Three Sources of Inositol

Inositol can be recycled via the pathways described in Figure 1, synthesized de novo from glucose-6-PO_4, or taken up from the plasma.

of inositol is that lipid synthesis will slow down, resulting in an accumulation of the precursors and a depletion of the product PtdIns. The CDP-diacylglycerol: *myo*-inositol transferase has a high K_m for inositol (2.5 mM in the case of liver; Takenawa and Egawa, 1977). Since the level of inositol in nerve is near the K_m, it seems that any reduction in the concentration of inositol will immediately slow down the rate of PtdIns synthesis. Any decline in the level of inositol will result in an immediate fall in the rate of synthesis and hence a decline in the level of PtdIns. During Li^+ treatment, large accumulations of the precursor CMP-PA have been detected in the parotid gland (Downes and Stone, 1986) and rat cerebral cortical slices (Godfrey, 1989). In GH_3 cells, Li^+ caused a significant accumulation of DAG (Drummond and Raeburn, 1984), perhaps because the accumulation of CMP-PA feeds back to cause increases in the levels of its immediate precursors, PA and DAG. Since the latter is an activator of protein kinase C (Nishizuka, 1986), one possible consequence of Li^+ is to enhance the DAG/protein kinase C limb of the bifurcating signal pathway.

Perhaps the most important consequence of lowering the level of *myo*-inositol is to slow down the synthesis of PtdIns. During the action of Li^+ there was a pronounced fall in the labeling of this lipid in GH_3 cells (Drummond and Raeburn, 1984), rat parotid gland (Downes and Stone, 1986), and glomerulosa cells (Balla et al., 1984). In none of these examples, however, was there clear evidence for any effects of Li^+ on the labeling of PtdIns4,5P_2. Indeed, in recent experiments the labeling of PtdIns4,5P_2 was significantly enhanced in rat cerebral cortex by chronic Li^+ treatment (Godfrey et al., 1989), which seems to argue against the idea that Li^+ may limit the supply of this precursor lipid. However, it is not clear to what extent the lipid labeled in these studies represents the presumptive hormone-sensitive pool in the plasma membrane that is used for signal generation. Of the total cellular pool of PtdIns, only a small proportion (~10%–20%) appears to be available for signaling, leading to the concept of a hormone-sensitive pool of precursor lipid (Fain and Berridge, 1979; Monaco and Woods, 1983). About half of the much smaller PtdIns(4,5)P_2 pool may also be unavailable for signaling (Koreh and Monaco, 1986). We would argue, therefore, that the dramatic fall in the level of PtdIns may result in the depletion of a distinct but small pool of PtdIns4,5P_2 required to generate the DAG and Ins(1,4,5)P_3 messengers.

A better way of assessing this prediction of the inositol depletion hypothesis is to study the effect of Li^+ on the agonist-dependent formation of Ins(1,4,5)P_3. Brain slices from Li^+ treated rats showed a marked reduction in inositol phosphate formation in response to norepinephrine and serotonin (Casebolt and Jope, 1989). Similar experiments in which individual inositol phosphates were measured revealed that Li^+ treatment suppressed the generation of both Ins(1,4,5)P_3 and Ins(1,3,4,5)P_4 (Batty and Nahorski, 1985; Whitworth and Kendall, 1988; Godfrey et al., 1989).

The Time-Dependence and Stimulus-Dependence of Li^+ Inhibition

Perhaps the most significant aspect of the inhibitory action of Li^+ is that it is both time- and stimulus-dependent. In the experiments on brain slices, Li^+ had no effect on Ins(1,4,5)P_3 and Ins(1,3,4,5)P_4 formation in the short term, but suppression becomes increasingly apparent during prolonged stimulation (Batty and Nahorski, 1985; Whitworth and Kendall, 1988). This time-dependence of Li^+ action is also apparent in numerous physiological studies, which indicate that short-term Li^+ treatment has no effect on a variety of phosphoinositide-mediated cellular responses. A typical example is the adrenal glomerulosa, where the formation of Ins(1,4,5)P_3 in response to Angiotensin II was normal for 5 min, but thereafter Li^+ markedly suppressed its formation (Balla et al., 1984).

This adrenal glomerulosa study is of particular interest because Li^+ had no effect on secretion up to about 30 min, but thereafter it caused a progressive decline in aldosterone secretion (Balla et al., 1984; Spat et al., 1988). This decline as a result of Li^+ was rapidly reversed upon addition of ACTH, which uses cyclic AMP as a second messenger. The inhibitory effect of Li^+ took time to develop and was specific for angiotensin II, whose receptors are coupled to the phosphoinositide system. Another example is the retardation of the relaxation rate following cholinergic-induced smooth muscle contraction (Menkes et al., 1986). The effect of Li^+ on relaxation was not apparent up to 30 min of stimulation but began to develop thereafter and was maximal after 2 hr. This time-dependence of Li^+ action is compatible with the inositol depletion hypothesis, because the cell has a considerable reserve of lipid that can be used to maintain signaling for a finite period before the Li^+ block on resynthesis begins to exert its inhibitory effect.

Another unique feature of Li^+ is that its action is stimulus-dependent. When the receptor is functioning within its normal operation range, the amount of $PtdIns4,5P_2$ that needs to be hydrolyzed to generate the second messengers DAG and $Ins1,4,5P_3$ is relatively small, which means a low rate of inositol recycling. Under these conditions, Li^+ has a small effect because of its uncompetitive action but becomes increasingly effective as the rate of $PtdIns4,5P_2$ hydrolysis is increased. In the case of cerebral cortical slices, Li^+ had no effect on the formation of $Ins1,4,5P_3$ at low concentrations of carbachol but began to suppress its formation as the concentration of carbachol was increased (Whitworth and Kendall, 1988). This phenomenon was also apparent in the studies on smooth muscle mentioned earlier, where Li^+ suppressed the rate of relaxation following prolonged stimulation with carbachol (Menkes et al., 1986). This effect of Li^+ on relaxation was very dependent on the extent of prior stimulation. Li^+ induced a larger reduction in the rate of relaxation following prestimulation with higher doses of carbachol, carbachol being more effective. In summary, Li^+ has little effect when receptors are operating normally but becomes increasingly effective the more the receptors become hyperactive. In this respect, Li^+ comes close to being a perfect drug in that its potency is tailored to the severity of receptor dysfunction. Put another way, it is a true homeostaticdrug that acts on hyperactive receptors to drive them back into their normal operating range.

Manic-Depressive Illness

Lithium is the major drug therapy currently in use to treat manic-depressive illness (Rosenthal and Goodwin, 1982) and is also finding a role in controlling some other neurological disorders, such as aggressive and self-mutilating behavior (Wickham and Reed, 1987) or cluster headache (Ekbom, 1981). Despite its widespread clinical application, very little is known about its mode of action. The inositol depletion hypothesis offers a plausible explanation of the way Li^+ may act that is consistent with both its therapeutic and pharmacological characteristics. The first point to emphasize is that the administration of Li^+ to rats leads to a decline in the level of inositol in the brain (Allison and Stewart, 1971). This fall may be accentuated for brain because, relative to its own synthetic capacity, there is little transport of inositol across the blood–brain barrier (Margolis et al., 1971; Lewin et al., 1976; Barkai, 1981). Barkai (1981) has estimated that only 2% of the inositol entering the cerebrospinal fluid of rats originates from the plasma, most of it coming from tissues within the brain. Neurones closeted behind the blood–brain barrier are sequestered from plasma inositol and are thus uniquely susceptible to lithium, which inhibits production of inositol via the two endogenous mechanisms of recycling and resynthesis (Figure 2). Moreover, resynthesis through glucose may be strictly confined to the blood side of the blood–brain barrier as the enzyme responsible for the conversion of glucose-6-phosphate to *myo*-inositol-1-phosphate is restricted to the cerebral vasculature (Wong et al., 1987). Cells in the periphery are protected against the effects of Li^+ by ready access to plasma inositol. It is the absence of this source of inositol that makes the CNS a unique target for Li^+. By blocking the supply of inositol, Li^+ will reduce lipid synthesis, leading to a reduction in the supply of $PtdIns4,5P_2$ for signaling.

The prediction of this hypothesis, therefore, is that Li^+ acts to attenuate phosphoinositide-dependent receptors whose hyperactivity is ultimately responsible for the exaggerated changes in mood. The identity and location of such aberrant activity remains to be identified, but recent attention has focused on serotonin receptors in limbic regions (Wood and Goodwin, 1987). One class of serotonin receptor (5-HT_2) is known to regulate phosphoinositide breakdown and signaling events (Pritchett et al., 1988). The fact that Li^+ is an uncompetitive inhibitor, which has little effect when receptors are operating normally, may explain why it has no central actions when administered to normal people. A corollary of this hypothesis is that Li^+ does not act on the gene product that is dysfunctional in manic-depression but rather modifies a downstream pathway to reestablish normal responses. It is not surprising, therefore, that human pedigrees have indicated that bipolar affective disorders are polygenic in origin (Robertson, 1987), since they may include alterations in genes for signal biosynthesis, signal inactivation, or receptors as candidate sites for lesions.

Li^+ and the Kindling Model of Epilepsy

Kindling is an animal model of neural plasticity and epilepsy. Repeated application of an appropriate electrical or chemical stimulus produces a progressive and long-lasting change in synaptic transmission that can culminate in a spontaneous epileptiform attack. The causes of the increased excitability responsible for epileptiform activity are still unknown, but studies using the electrical kindling model have suggested a possible role for an increase in the sensitivity of glutamate receptors that stimulate inositol lipid hydrolysis. The formation of inositol phosphate by the amygdala in response to a glutamate analog was significantly potentiated following electrical kindling, suggesting that the phosphoinositide-derived messengers $Ins1,4,5P_3$ and DAG may be part of the plastic change accompanying the enhanced excitability responsible for seizures (Iadorola et al., 1986). It is of some interest, therefore, to find that the onset of seizure susceptibility in kindled rats was completely suppressed if animals were kept on lithium (Schmidt, 1986).

In contrast to this suppression of seizures in kindled rats, Li^+ was found to enhance the onset of seizures in rats receiving systemic administration of cholinergic agonists such as physostigmine (Honchar et al., 1983). Indeed, the recognized human side effects of Li^+ treatment include a lowering of seizure threshold or the prolongation of evoked seizure activity. Recently, $Ins(1,3,4,5,6)P_5$ and $InsP_6$ were found to have potent neuroexcitant activity (Vallejo et al., 1987), and it was suggested that such an extracellular action might be involved in lithium-promoted seizure enhancement, perhaps by protecting the inositol polyphosphates from degradation upon release and thereby greatly intensifying their effect (Hanley et al., 1988). However, the extracellular inositol phosphatase most likely to break down any extracellularly acting inositol polyphosphates (Carpenter et al., 1989) is insensitive to Li^+.

Because we know so little concerning the neural basis of epilepsy, it is impossible to speculate why some seizures are suppressed while others are enhanced, but these effects of Li^+ are another reflection of its remarkable ability to modulate neural activity.

Lithium and Circadian Rhythms

Manic-depressive syndrome and cluster headache are periodic neural disorders; there is evidence linking lithium to the resetting of other, normal rhythmic phenomena. The behavior of single- and multi-cellular organisms is timed by intrinsic biological clocks. Indeed, the actions of lithium in altering the frequencies of physiological oscillators suggest that the phosphoinositide system may be part of the timing mechanism of biological clocks. In most organisms the diurnal or circadian clock is entrained to environmental cues (*zeitgeber*), normally the light–dark cycle. In the absence of such environmental signals, the rhythm free-runs, driven by an endogenous diurnal oscillator. When tested on such free-running rhythms, Li^+ invariably causes a lengthening of the period (Englemann, 1987) in a wide variety of organisms, including flowers, insects, and man. There are suggestions that the circadian system is altered in many individuals suffering from manic-depressive illness, which makes the effects of Li^+ on the circadian oscillator all the more interesting. Alterations in normal endocrine rhythms are also frequent side effects of chronic Li^+ treatment. In man there appear to be two oscillators that are somehow coupled together: the Y oscillator located in the suprachiasmatic nucleus of the hypothalamus drives the sleep–wake cycle, and the X oscillator located somewhere else in the CNS drives other physiological rhythms such as body temperature (Engelman, 1987). During free-running conditions these two oscillators become desynchronized, with the Y oscillator having a longer period than the X oscillator. Such abnormal phase relationships appear to characterize some of the diurnal alterations seen in endogenous depression. Li^+ seems to act by slowing down the X oscillator, thus bringing it back into phase with the Y oscillator.

Since the cellular basis of such oscillators is unknown, it is difficult to know whether or not the inositol depletion hypothesis can explain the effects of Li^+ on circadian rhythms. The hypothesis would predict that diurnal rhythms are somehow set by the rate of phosphoinositide turnover and Li^+ would slow down but not abolish such rhythms by depressing turnover. In keeping with its stimulus-dependent action, Li^+ slows down the X oscillator, which has the faster rhythm. Also it has been noted that Li^+ is particularly effective in those manic-depressive patients who have the fastest circadian rhythms (Engelmann, 1987). The characteristic time-dependence aspect of Li^+ action has also been described in that its period-lengthening effect often requires several days to appear (Kripke and Wyborney, 1980; Delius et al., 1984).

Lithium-Induced Teratogenesis

Lithium distorts pattern formation during early development, resulting in deformed embryos (Nieuwkoop, 1970). This teratogenic effect of Li^+ has been studied extensively in amphibia where the deformation can be traced back to a respecification of the dorso-ventral axis early in the blastula stage, but it has also been described in simpler organisms such as the sea urchin (Livingston and Wilt, 1989) and slime molds (Peters et al., 1989). In amphibia, the most sensitive period is the 32–64 cell stage during which a brief treatment with Li^+ results in a dorsalization of the embryo (Figure 3). The ventral regions have been respecified to form characteristic dorsal structures such as notochord and eye. In some cases, the embryo is radially symmetrical with a broad band of eye pigment and cement gland encircling the anterior part of the embryo (Kao and Elinson, 1989). UV irradiation of the zygote before the first cleavage has the opposite effect: it suppresses all dorsal structures and the embryo ends up as a radial ventral mass. Development of a normal embryo seems to depend on some positional variable set up in the form of a gradient along the dorso–ventral axis, which will direct the pattern of subsequent morphogenesis (Kao and Elinson, 1988). On the basis of various Li^+ injection experiments described later, it has been proposed that the phosphoinositide cycle and its accompanying second messengers may be important in specifying the dorso–ventral axis during normal frog embryogenesis (Busa, 1988; Busa and Gimlich, 1989). We would extend this proposal by suggesting that the ventral side has a high level of phosphoinositide turnover (represented by the degree of stippling in Figure 3), which then grades down toward a lower level at the dorsal side. Just how this gradient of phosphoinositide turnover is set up is unclear, but we note that the animal pole of the oocyte has a high density of muscarinic receptors (coupled to PtdIns turnover) (Kusano et al., 1982) and is also much more sensitive to injections of $Ins(1,4,5)P_3$ than is the vegetal pole

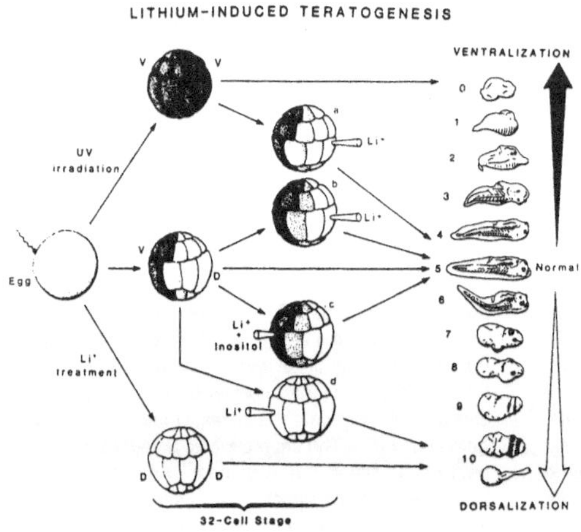

Figure 3. Teratogenic Effect of Li$^+$ Illustrated by Studies on the Development of Xenopus

Soon after fertilization the dorso–ventral axis is established, culminating in the development of a normal tadpole. The dorso–ventral axis can be distorted either by UV irradiation, leading to ventralization, or by Li$^+$, which has the opposite dorsalizing action. The gradation of axis deficiencies produced by these two treatments was taken from Figure 1 of Kao and Elinson (1988). The inositol depletion hypothesis would predict high phosphoinositide turnover in the ventral (V) region and a low level on the dorsal (D) side (stippling of the 32 cell blastula represents this proposed gradient of phosphoinositide turnover). UV irradiation may lead to a uniformly high level of turnover resulting in vegetalization (top), whereas Li$^+$ has the opposite effect—it reduces the gradient to a uniformly low level, resulting in dorsalization (bottom). See text for a description of the Li$^+$ injection experiments.

(Berridge, 1988). The hypothesis that best fits the available data is that a high level of phosphoinositide turnover specifies ventral structures, whereas low levels code for dorsal components. The two treatments of UV irradiation or Li$^+$ respecify the gradient toward the two extremes, producing ventralization and dorsalization, respectively (Figure 3).

The existence of a phosphoinositide gradient organized along the dorso–ventral axis is consistent with recent evidence concerning both the control of gap junctional permeability and the pattern of junctional communication within the developing Xenopus embryo. There is growing evidence that the permeability of gap junctions can be regulated by components of the phosphoinositide signaling pathway, such as calcium and protein kinase C (Randriamampita et al., 1988). The proposed phosphoinositide gradient predicts that junctions are closed in the ventral region, where turnover is high, but open in the presumptive dorsal region. This prediction was borne out by the observations of Guthrie et al. (1988). Using the transfer of Lucifer yellow as a probe for cell-to-cell communication, they found that dye passed readily between cells in the dorsal region, but there was little transfer in the ventral side. This pattern of junctional communication is not fixed but changed when the embryonic axis was respecified by either UV irradiation or treatment with Li$^+$ (Nagajski et al., 1989). The prediction based on the hypothesis outlined in Figure 3 is that UV irradiation results in a high phosphoinositide turnover throughout the embryo, which exactly fits the observation that junctional communication becomes uniformly low (Nagajski et al., 1989). Conversely, the uniformly high level of cell-to-cell coupling observed after treatment with Li$^+$ is entirely consistent with the notion that this ion depresses the normal gradient to the low value characteristic of the dorsal region. The pattern of junctional permeability and the changes that occur during treatment with UV or Li$^+$ are thus consistent with the early embryo's gradient of phosphoinositide turnover.

Postulating a gradient of phosphoinositide turnover can readily account for the teratogenic effects of Li$^+$ in Xenopus embryos (Figure 3). Since the early embryo lacks a vascular system, it must obtain all of its inositol from the Li$^+$ sensitive synthetic and recycling steps (Figure 2), which could explain why they are so sensitive to this ion. The intracellular Li$^+$ concentrations necessary to produce a maximal teratogenic effect lie in the 0.5–2.5 mM range (Breckenridge et al., 1987), which corresponds closely with the level required to inhibit the inositol phosphatases. On the basis of the inositol depletion hypothesis we propose that Li$^+$ may exert its teratogenic effect by inactivating the high rate of turnover in the ventral region, resulting in a flattened positional gradient and a uniform dorsal specification (Figure 3). It was argued earlier that UV-irradiated embryos may have a uniformly high turnover of phosphoinositides (Figure 3). Immersion of such embryos in 0.3 M Li$^+$ for 5 min during the 32–64 cell stage changes them from fully ventralized embryos to embryos showing extreme forms of dorsalization (Kao et al., 1986). In effect, the positional variable in such embryos had been switched from a uniformly high (ventral specification) to a uniformly low (dorsal specification) level. In a more subtle experiment, Li$^+$ was injected into one part of the UV-irradiated embryo (Figure 3, embryo a), leading to more normal embryos, presumably by reestablishing the gradient. While injecting Li$^+$ into the dorsal region of a normal embryo (Figure 3, embryo b) had no effect, as might be expected since this region already has a low level of phosphoinositide turnover, injection into the ventral region of a normal embryo (Figure 3, embryo d) led to dorsalization (Kao et al., 1986; Busa and Gimlich, 1989), presumably by reducing the gradient as discussed earlier. However, this teratogenic effect of injecting Li$^+$ into a ventral cell can be blocked by the coinjection of *myo*-inositol (Busa and Gimlich, 1989). This ability of *myo*-inositol to rescue embryos against the action of Li^+ provides the strongest evidence yet that the phosphoinositides are playing a role in early pattern formation.

The presence of such a positional gradient, perhaps based on a gradient of phosphoinositide turnover, may then set the stage for the action of the various morphogens originating from the vegetal region (Cooke and Smith, 1988). These morphogens resemble growth factors, such as basic fibroblast growth factor (bFGF) and transforming growth factor β (TGF-β) (Kimelman and Kirschner, 1987; Slack et al., 1987; Weeks and Melton, 1987). The observation that TGF-β can potentiate EGF-induced phosphoinositide metabolism and intracellular calcium levels in cultured cells (Muldoon et al., 1988) suggests that inducers such as TGF-β and bFGF may exert variable effects on cells, depending on the preexisting morphogenic gradient of varying phosphoinositide activity. As in the nervous system, Li^+ has a subtle action; it is not an inducer but it does act to modulate the responsiveness of cells to inductive signals (Nieuwkoop, 1970; Cooke et al., 1989; Kao and Elinson, 1989).

Li^+ has long been recognized as a mammalian teratogen as well. The exposure of animals to Li^+ has been linked to cleft palate and spina bifida, which are common abnormalities arising from embryonic teratogens. Although little is known about the possible inductive influences in palate or neural tube development, it is increasingly held that these processes in mammalian embryogenesis conform to a generalized pattern of inductive specification, possibly relying on diffusible or tissue-associated growth factors. Thus, the birth defects induced by Li^+ may, in a fashion analogous to actions in Xenopus embryonic development, imply that the modulation or induction of gradients based on the phosphoinositide system may be key steps in mammalian embryonic development. Although it is listed as a teratogenic agent in human beings (Shephard, 1986), there is relatively little evidence that Li^+ is a teratogen when administered at normal therapeutic doses (Schou et al., 1973).

Finally, lithium can interfere with the developmental program of the slime mold Dictyostelium. The multicellular slug that forms when the amoebae are starved differentiates into anterior prestalk cells and posterior prespore cells. Lithium modifies this simple anterior–posterior pattern by respecifying the prespore cells to become prestalk cells (Peters et al., 1989). More specifically, lithium seems to inhibit cyclic AMP-dependent gene expression through a mechanism independent of either cyclic AMP or cyclic GMP. A more likely possibility is that lithium interferes with the cyclic AMP-dependent stimulation of $Ins(1,4,5)P_3$ formation (Europe-Finner and Newell, 1987; Van Haastert et al., 1989). Indeed, both the resting and stimulated levels of this second messenger were reduced by lithium (Peters et al., 1989). These observations are consistent with the inositol depletion hypothesis and suggest that lithium might respecify the developmental program in Dictyostelium by interfering with the phosphoinositide signaling pathway.

Conclusion

A major challenge in modern biology is to understand the basic mechanisms controlling both neural activity and pattern formation during early development. The fact that both processes can be modulated by Li^+ is intriguing, especially as it seems it may be working through a common mechanism. Although a number of mechanisms of Li^+ action has been proposed, we feel that inhibition of inositol phosphate metabolism offers a very plausible explanation for both the neural and developmental effects of Li^+. The unusual uncompetitive nature of its inhibitory action implies that Li^+ will have little effect when the phosphoinositides are turning over slowly but will become increasingly effective as the level of signal generation increases. Li^+ acts like a pharmacological buffer by confining the activity of the messenger pathway within its normal operational range. This is exactly the property that fits with its therapeutic action of being able to dampen down manic-depressive episodes, while allowing most other neural mechanisms to occur normally. It is this subtle selective action of Li^+ that is also apparent in its teratogenic action: it allows embryogenesis to proceed but disrupts normal pattern formation by resetting the positional variable used to specify the dorso–ventral axis. Li^+ appears to modify the gradient by confining it to a narrower range such that all the cells receive a uniform dorsal specification.

The inositol depletion hypothesis suggests a mechanism for this subtle modulation of cellular activity. The specific proposal is that cells within the CNS or the developing embryo are denied access to plasma inositol and are thus uniquely sensitive to Li^+ inhibition of inositol formation by either recycling or de novo synthesis. Depletion of intracellular inositol will result in a reduction in the supply of inositol lipids required for signaling. This proposal is supported by the observation that inositol replacement can protect Xenopus embryos against the teratogenic action of Li^+ (Busa and Gimlich, 1989). A natural corollary of this hypothesis is that the phosphoinositide signaling system has a central role in controlling both neural signaling and early development. A role in the nervous system is not too surprising, because a large number of neurotransmitters are now known to act by stimulating the formation of $Ins(1,4,5)P_3$ and DAG. What is novel, however, is the possible role of these messengers in embryogenesis where they may act to set up a morphogenic field by regulating the responsiveness of cells to inducers resembling TGFβ or FGF.

Acknowledgments

M. R. H. is the recipient of a Research Award from the International Life Sciences Institute.

References

Ackermann, K. E., Gish, B. G., Honchar, M. P., and Sherman, W. R. (1987). Evidence that inositol 1-phosphate in brain of lithium-treated rats results mainly from phosphatidylinositol metabolism. Biochem. J. *242*, 517–524.

Allison, J. H., and Stewart, M. A. (1971). Reduced brain inositol in lithium treated rats. Nature New Biol. *233*, 267–268.

Balla, T., Enyedi, P., Hunyady, L., and Spät, A. (1984). Effects of lithium on angiotensin-stimulated phosphatidylinositol turnover and aldosterone production in adrenal glomerulosa cells: a possible causal relationship. FEBS Lett. *171*, 179–182.

Barkai, A. I. (1981). *Myo*-inositol turnover in the intact rat brain: increased production after d-amphetamine. J. Neurochem. *36*, 1485–1491.

Batty, I., and Nahorski, S. R. (1985). Differential effects of lithium on muscarinic receptor stimulation of inositol phosphates in rat cerebral cortex slices. J. Neurochem. *45*, 1514–1521.

Berridge, M. J. (1987). Inositol trisphosphate and diacylglycerol: two interacting second messengers. Annu. Rev. Biochem. *56*, 159–193.

Berridge, M. J. (1988). Inositol trisphosphate-induced membrane potential oscillations in *Xenopus* oocytes. J. Physiol. *403*, 589–599.

Berridge, M. J., and Irvine, R. F. (1984). Inositol trisphosphate, a novel second messenger in cellular signal transduction. Nature *312*, 315–321.

Berridge, M. J., Downes, C. P., and Hanley, M. R. (1982). Lithium amplifies agonist-dependent phosphatidylinositol responses in brain and salivary glands. Biochem. J. *206*, 587–595.

Breckenridge, L. J., Warren, R. L., and Warner, A. E. (1987). Lithium inhibits morphogenesis of the nervous system but not neuronal differentiation in *Xenopus laevis*. Development *99*, 353–370.

Busa, W. B. (1988). Roles for the phosphatidylinositol cycle in early development. Phil. Trans. Roy. Soc. (Lond.) B *320*, 415–426.

Busa, W. B., and Gimlich, R. L. (1989). Lithium-induced teratogenesis in frog embryos prevented by a polyphosphoinositide cycle intermediate or a diacylglycerol analog. Dev. Biol. *132*, 315–324.

Carpenter, D., Hanley, M., Hawkins, P., Jackson, T. R., Stephens, L., and Vallejo, M. (1989). The metabolism and functions of inositol pentakisphosphate and inositol hexakisphosphate in the nervous system. Biochem. Soc. Trans. *17*, 3–5.

Casebolt, T. L., and Jope, R. S. (1989). Long-term lithium treatment selectively reduces receptor-coupled inositol phospholipid hydrolysis in rat brain. Biol. Psychiatry *25*, 329–340.

Cooke, J., and Smith, E. J. (1988). The restrictive effect of early exposure to lithium upon body pattern in *Xenopus* development, studied by quantitative anatomy and immunofluorescence. Development *102*, 85–99.

Cooke, J., Symes, K., and Smith, E. J. (1989). Potentiation by the lithium ion of morphogenetic responses to a *Xenopus* inducing factor. Development *105*, 549–558.

Cornish-Bowden, A. (1986). Why is uncompetitive inhibition so rare? A possible explanation, with implications for the design of drugs and pesticides. FEBS Lett. *203*, 3–6.

Delius, K., Gunderoth-Palmowski, M., Krause, I., and Engelmann, W. (1984). Effects of lithium salts on the behaviour and the circadian system of *Mesocricetus auratus* W. J. Interdiscipl. Cycle Res. *15*, 289–299.

Downes, C. P., and Michell, R. H. (1985). In Molecular Mechanisms of Transmembrane Signalling, P. Cohen and M. Houslay, eds. (Amsterdam: Elsevier Science Publishers), pp 3–56.

Downes, C. P., and Stone, M. A. (1986). Lithium-induced reduction in intracellular inositol supply in cholinergically stimulated parotid gland. Biochem. J. *234*, 199–204.

Drummond, A. H., and Raeburn, C. A. (1984). The interaction of lithium with thryotropin-releasing hormone-stimulated lipid metabolism in GH_3 pituitary tumour cells. Biochem. J. *224*, 129–136.

Ekbom, K. (1981). Lithium for cluster headache. Headache *21*, 132–139.

Engelmann, W. (1987). Effects of lithium salts on circadian rhythms. In Neuropsychiatric Disorders and Disturbances in the Circadian System of Man, A. Halaris, ed. (Amsterdam: Elsevier Science Publishers), pp. 263–289.

Europe-Finner, G. H., and Newell, P. C. (1987). Cyclic AMP stimulates accumulation of inositol trisphosphate in *Dictyostelium*. J. Cell Sci. *87*, 221–229.

Fain, J. N., and Berridge, M. J. (1979). Relationship between phosphatidylinositol synthesis and recovery of 5-hydroxytryptamine-responsive Ca^{2+} flux in blowfly salivary gland. Biochem. J. *180*, 655–661.

Gee, N. S., Ragan, C. I., Watling, K. J., Aspley, S., Jackson, R. G., Reid, G. G., Gani, D., and Shute, J. K. (1988). The purification and properties of *myo*-inositol monophosphatase from bovine brain. Biochem. J. *249*, 883–889.

Godfrey, P. P. (1989). Potentiation by lithium of CMP phosphatidate formation in carbachol-stimulated rat cerebral cortical slices and its reversal by *myo*-inositol. Biochem. J. *258*, 621–624.

Godfrey, P. P., McClue, S. J., White, A. M., Wood, A. J., and Grahame-Smith, D. C. (1989). Subacute and chronic in vivo lithium treatment inhibits agonist- and sodium fluoride-stimulated inositol phosphate production in rat cortex. J. Neurochem. *52*, 498–506.

Guthrie, S., Turin, L., and Warner, A. E. (1988). Patterns of junctional communication during development of the early amphibian embryo. Development *103*, 769–783.

Hallcher, L. M., and Sherman, W. R. (1980). The effects of lithium ion and other agents on the activity of *myo*-inositol-1-phosphatase from bovine brain. J. Biol. Chem. *255*, 10896–10901.

Hanley, M. R., Jackson, T. R., Vallejo, M., Patterson, S. I., Thastrup, O., Lightman, S., Rogers, J., Henderson, G., and Pini, A. (1988). Neural function: metabolism and actions of inositol metabolites in mammalian brain. Phil. Trans. Roy. Soc. (Lond.) B *320*, 381–398.

Honchar, M. P., Olney, J. W., and Sherman, W. R. (1983). Systemic cholinergic agents induce seizures and brain damage in lithium-treated rats. Science *220*, 323–325.

Iadorola, M. J., Nicoletti, F., Naranjo, J. R., Putnam, F., and Costa, E. (1986). Kindling enhances the stimulation of inositol phospholipid hydrolysis elicited by ibotenic acid in rat hippocampal slices. Brain Res. *374*, 174–178.

Irvine, R. F., and Moor, R. M. (1986). Micro-injection of inositol (1,3,4,5) tetrakisphosphate activates sea urchin eggs by a mechanism dependent on external Ca^{2+}. Biochem. J. *240*, 917–920.

Irvine, R. F., Moor, R. M., Pollock, W. K., Smith, P. M., and Wreggett, K. A. (1988). Inositol phosphates: proliferation, metabolism and function. Phil. Trans. Roy. Soc. (Lond.) B *320*, 281–298.

Kao, K. R., and Elinson, R. P. (1988). The entire mesodermal mantle behaves as Spemann's organizer in dorsoanterior enhanced *Xenopus laevis* embryos. Dev. Biol. *127*, 64–77.

Kao, K. R., and Elinson, R. P. (1989). Dorsalization of mesoderm induction by lithium. Dev. Biol. *132*, 81–90.

Kao, K. R., Masui, Y., and Elinson, R. P. (1986). Lithium-induced respecification of pattern in *Xenopus laevis* embryos. Nature *322*, 371–373.

Kendall, D. A., and Nahorski, S. R. (1987). Acute and chronic lithium treatments influence agonist and depolarization-stimulated inositol phospholipid hydrolysis in rat cerebral cortex. J. Pharm. Exp. Ther. *241*, 1023–1027.

Kimelman, D., and Kirschner, M. (1987). Synergistic induction of mesoderm by FGF and TGF-β and the identification of an mRNA coding for FGF in the early Xenopus embryo. Cell *51*, 869–877.

Koreh, K., and Monaco, M. E. (1986). The relationship of hormone-sensitive and hormone-insensitive phosphatidylinositol to phosphatidylinositol 4,5-bisphosphate in the WRK-1 cell. J. Biol. Chem. *261*, 88–91.

Kripke, D. F., and Wyborney, V. G. (1980). Lithium slows rat circadian activity rhythms. Life Sci. *26*, 1319–1321.

Kusano, K., Miledi, R., and Stinnakre, J. (1982). Cholinergic and catecholaminergic receptors in the *Xenopus* oocyte membrane. J. Physiol. *328*, 143–170.

Lewin, L. M., Yanna, Y., Sulimovici, S., and Kraicer, P. F. (1976). Studies on the metabolic role of *myo*-inositol: distribution of radioactive *myo*-inositol in the male rat. Biochem. J. *156*, 375–380.

Livingston, B. T., and Wilt, F. H. (1989). Lithium evokes expression of vegetal-specific molecules in the animal blastomeres of sea urchin embryos. Proc. Natl. Acad. Sci. USA *86*, 3669–3673.

Majerus, P. W., Connolly, T. M., Bansal, V. S., Inhorn, R. C., Ross, T. S., and Lips, D. L. (1988). Inositol phosphates: synthesis and degradation. J. Biol. Chem. *263*, 3051–3054.

Margolis, R. V., Press, R., Altszuler, N., and Stewart, M. A. (1971). Inositol production by the brain in normal and alloxan-diabetic dogs. Brain Res. *28*, 535–539.

Menkes, H. A., Baraban, J. M., Freed, A. N., and Snyder, S. H. (1986). Lithium dampens neurotransmitter response in smooth muscle: relevance to action in affective illness. Proc. Natl. Acad. Sci. USA *83*, 5727–5730.

Monaco, M. E., and Woods, D. (1983). Characterization of the hormone-sensitive phosphatidylinositol pool in WRK-I cells. J. Biol. Chem. *258*, 15125–15129.

Montague, W., Morgan, N. G., Rumford, G. M., and Prince, C. A. (1985). Effect of glucose on polyphosphoinositide metabolism in isolated rat islets of Langerhans. Biochem. J. *227*, 483–489.

Muldoon, L. L., Rodland, K. D., and Magun, B. E. (1988). Transforming growth factor β modulates epidermal growth factor-induced phosphoinositide metabolism and intracellular calcium levels. J. Biol. Chem. *263*, 5030–5033.

Mustelin, T., Poso, H., Iivanainen, A., and Andersson, L. C. (1986). Myo-inositol reverses Li^+-induced inhibition of phosphoinositide turnover and ornithine decarboxylase induction during early lymphocyte activation. Eur. J. Immunol. *16*, 859–861.

Nagajski, D. J., Guthrie, S. C., Ford, C. C., and Warner, A. E. (1989). The correlation between patterns of dye transfer through gap junctions and future developmental fate in *Xenopus*: the consequences of u.v. irradiation and lithium treatment. Development *105*, 747–752.

Nieuwkoop, P. D. (1970). The formation of the mesoderm in urodelean amphibians III. The vegetalizing action of the Li ion. Roux's Arch. Dev. Biol. *166*, 105–123.

Nishizuka, Y. (1986). Studies and perspectives of protein kinase C. Science *233*, 305–312.

Nishizuka, Y. (1988). The molecular heterogeneity of protein kinase C and its implications for cellular regulation. Nature *334*, 661–665.

Otte, A. P., Koster, C. H., Snoek, G. T., and Durston, A. T. (1988). Protein kinase C mediates neural induction in *Xenopus laevis*. Nature *334*, 618–620.

Peters, D. J. M., Van Lookeren Campagne, M. M., Van Haastert, P. J. M., Spek, W., and Schaap, P. (1989). Lithium ions induce prestalk-associated gene expression and inhibit prespore gene expression in *Dictyostelium discoideum*. J. Cell Sci. *93*, 205–210.

Pritchett, D. B., Bach, A. W. J., Wozny, M., Taleb, O., Dal Toso, R., Shih, J. C., and Seeburg, P. H. (1988). Structure and functional expression of cloned rat serotonin 5HT-2 receptor. EMBO J. *7*, 4135–4140.

Randriamampita, C., Giaume, C., Neyton, J., and Trautmann, A. (1988). Acetylcholine-induced closure of gap junction channels in rat lacrimal glands is probably mediated by protein kinase C. Pflugers Arch. *412*, 462–468.

Robertson, M. (1987). Molecular genetics of the mind. Nature *325*, 755.

Rosenthal, N. E., and Goodwin, F. K. (1982). The role of the lithium ion in medicine. Annu. Rev. Med. *33*, 555–568.

Rubin, R. P. (1984). Stimulation of inositol trisphosphate accumulation and amylase secretion by caerulein in pancreatic acini. J. Pharm. Exp. Ther. *231*, 623–627.

Schmidt, J. (1986). Lithium suppresses seizure susceptibility in pentylenetetrazol-kindled rats. Biomed. Biochim. Acta *45*, 1167–1172.

Schou, M., Goldfield, M. D., Weinstein, M. R., and Villeneuve, A. (1973). Lithium and pregnancy-I, report from the Registrar of Lithium Babies. Br. Med. J. (April 21, 1973), 135–136.

Shephard, T. H. (1986). Catalog of Teratogenic Agents (Baltimore: Johns Hopkins University Press).

Slack, J. M. W., Darlington, B. G., Heath, J. K., and Godsave, S. F. (1987). Mesoderm induction in early *Xenopus* embryos by heparin-binding growth factors. Nature *326*, 197–200.

Spat, A., Balla, T., Enyedi, P., and Hunyady, L. (1988). Aldosterone production. In Lithium and the Endocrine System, F. N. Johnson, ed. (Basel: Karger), pp. 168–181.

Stephens, L., Hawkins, P. T., and Downes, C. P. (1989). Metabolic and structural evidence for the existence of a third species of polyphosphoinositide in cells: D-phosphatidyl-*myo*-inositol-3-phosphate. Biochem. J. *259*, 267–276.

Sylvia, V., Curtin, G., Norman, J., Stec, J., and Busbee, D. (1988). Activation of a low specific activity form of DNA polymerase α by inositol-1,4-bisphosphate. Cell *54*, 651–658.

Takenawa, T., and Egawa, K. (1977). CDP-diglyceride: inositol transferase from rat liver. J. Biol. Chem. *252*, 5419–5423.

Vallejo, M., Jackson, T., Lightman, S., and Hanley, M. R. (1987). Occurrence and extracellular actions of inositol pentakis- and hexakisphosphate in mammalian brain. Nature *330*, 656–658.

Van Haastert, P. J. M., De Vries, M. J., Penning, L. C., Roovers, E., Van Der Kaay, J., Erneux, C., and Van Lookeren Campagne, M. M. (1989). Chemoattractant and guanosine 5'[γ-thio]trisphosphate in *Dictyostelium* cells that are labelled with [^{3}H]inositol by electroporation. Biochem. J. *258*, 577–586.

Weeks, D. L., and Melton, D. A. (1987). A maternal mRNA localized to the vegetal hemisphere in Xenopus eggs codes for a growth factor related to TGF-β. Cell *51*, 861–867.

Whitman, M., Downes, C. P., Keeler, M., Keller, T., and Cantley, L. (1988). Type I phosphatidylinositol kinase makes a novel inositol phospholipid, phosphatidylinositol-3-phosphate. Nature 332, 644–646.

Whitworth, P., and Kendall, D. A. (1988). Lithium selectively inhibits muscarinic receptor-stimulated inositol tetrakisphosphate accumulation in mouse cerebral cortex slices. J. Neurochem. *51*, 258–265.

Wickham, E. A., and Reed, J. V. (1987). Lithium for the control of aggressive and self-mutilating behaviour. Int. Clin. Psychopharmacol. *2*, 181–190.

Wong, Y.-H. H., Kalmbach, S. J., Hartman, B. K., and Sherman, W. R. (1987). Immunohistochemical staining and enzyme activity measurements show *myo*-inositol-l-phosphate synthase to be localized in the vasculature of brain. J. Neurochem. *48*, 1434–1442.

Wood, A. J., and Goodwin, G. M. (1987). A review of the biochemical and neuropharmacological actions of lithium. Psychol. Med. *17*, 579–600.

Worley, P. F., Heller, W. A., Snyder, S. H., and Baraban, J. M. (1988). Lithium blocks a phosphoinositide-mediated cholinergic response in hippocampal slices. Science *239*, 1428–1429.

Proc. Natl. Acad. Sci. USA
Vol. 93, pp. 8455–8459, August 1996
Developmental Biology

This contribution is a part of the special series of Inaugural Articles by members of the National Academy of Sciences elected on April 25, 1995.

A molecular mechanism for the effect of lithium on development

PETER S. KLEIN* AND DOUGLAS A. MELTON†

*Howard Hughes Medical Institute and Department of Medicine (Hematology-Oncology) and Institute on Aging, University of Pennsylvania, Philadelphia, PA 19104; and †Howard Hughes Medical Institute and Department of Molecular and Cellular Biology, Harvard University, Cambridge, MA 02138

Contributed by Douglas A. Melton, May 6, 1996

ABSTRACT **Lithium, one of the most effective drugs for the treatment of bipolar (manic-depressive) disorder, also has dramatic effects on morphogenesis in the early development of numerous organisms. How lithium exerts these diverse effects is unclear, but the favored hypothesis is that lithium acts through inhibition of inositol monophosphatase (IMPase). We show here that complete inhibition of IMPase has no effect on the morphogenesis of *Xenopus* embryos and present a different hypothesis to explain the broad action of lithium. Our results suggest that lithium acts through inhibition of glycogen synthase kinase-3β (GSK-3β), which regulates cell fate determination in diverse organisms including *Dictyostelium*, *Drosophila*, and *Xenopus*. Lithium potently inhibits GSK-3β activity (K_i = 2 mM), but is not a general inhibitor of other protein kinases. In support of this hypothesis, lithium treatment phenocopies loss of GSK-3β function in *Xenopus* and *Dictyostelium*. These observations help explain the effect of lithium on cell-fate determination and could provide insights into the pathogenesis and treatment of bipolar disorder.**

Lithium has a profound effect on the development of diverse organisms, including *Dictyostelium*, sea urchins, zebrafish, and *Xenopus* (1–5). In *Dictyostelium*, lithium alters cell fate by blocking spore cell and promoting stalk cell development (1, 2). In *Xenopus*, lithium causes an expansion of dorsal mesoderm, leading to duplication of the dorsal axis or, in extreme cases, entirely dorsalized embryos lacking identifiably ventral tissues (3). Lithium also mimics insulin by stimulating glycogen synthesis (6) and is the most effective treatment for bipolar disorder (7, 8).

Several hypotheses have been advanced to explain the mechanism of lithium action, yet its molecular target in cell-fate determination and glycogen metabolism, as well as in the treatment of bipolar disorder, remains unclear (7–10). The most widely accepted model, the inositol depletion hypothesis, is based on the observation that lithium inhibits inositol monophosphatase (IMPase) and could thereby deplete the cell of an endogenous source of inositol (9, 11). Cells would become unable to generate inositol 1,4,5 trisphosphate ($InsP_3$) in response to extracellular signals and thus $InsP_3$-dependent responses would be blocked. In support of this hypothesis, microinjection of myo-inositol can prevent the effect of lithium in *Xenopus* (12), although this requires the coinjection of a high concentration of myo-inositol (0.3 M) with lithium (also at 0.3 M). However, the inositol depletion hypothesis does not explain why lithium alters cell fate in *Dictyostelium discoideum*, since mutants lacking the gene for phospholipase C, and thus unable to generate $InsP_3$ in response to extracellular signals, develop normally (13). It also does not explain simply the effect of lithium on glycogen synthesis or on cells that have an exogenous source of inositol.

A class of bisphosphonate compounds that are ≈1000-fold more potent than lithium in inhibiting IMPase has recently become available (14, 15). Using these inhibitors, we have reexamined the role of IMPase in the early development of *Xenopus*. We show here that complete inhibition of IMPase has no discernible effect on the morphogenesis of *Xenopus* embryos, ruling out this enzyme as the target of lithium-induced teratogenesis.

An alternative target of lithium is suggested by the close similarity between lithium action and the effect of ectopic expression of *wnt* genes in *Xenopus* embryos (3, 16). We have focused on a protein that appears to antagonize *wnt* signaling, the enzyme glycogen synthase kinase-3β (GSK-3β; ref.17), which plays a central role in the development of diverse organisms including *Drosophila* (18, 19), *Dictyostelium* (20), and *Xenopus* (21–23). In this paper, we show that lithium directly inhibits GSK-3β *in vitro* and propose that GSK-3β is the endogenous target of lithium in these diverse systems.

MATERIALS AND METHODS

Materials. Purified, bacterially expressed GSK-3β, casein kinase II (CKII), and phosphatase inhibitor 2 (I-2) were purchased from New England Biolabs. Glutathione *S*-transferase–extracellular signal-related kinase 1 (ERK-1) was a gift of Sandro Allesandrini and Ray Erickson (Harvard University). Protein kinase A (PKA) was from Sigma. L-690,330 was from Tocris Cookson (St. Louis). Tritium-labeled inositol-1-phosphate (1.0 Ci/mmol, 25 μCi/ml; 1 Ci = 37 GBq) was from American Radiolabeled Chemicals (St. Louis). [γ-^{32}P]ATP (3000 Ci/mmol) was from Amersham.

Embryos and Microinjection. Eggs were fertilized *in vitro* according to well-established protocols (24). Microinjections were done at 4–32 cell stages with 5–10 nl volumes. For lithium treatment, embryos were transferred to 0.3 M lithium chloride (LiCl) in 0.1× modified Ringer's solution (MMR; ref. 24) for 6 min, then washed in 0.1× MMR as described (3) or were microinjected into ventral vegetal blastomeres (C tier) at the 32-cell stage with 5 nl of 0.3 M LiCl (12). L-690,330 was dissolved in water at 0.1–10 mM, and 5–10 nl was injected into the ventral vegetal region of 4, 8, 16, and 32 cell embryos. All four cells of 4-cell stage embryos were also injected in separate experiments.

IMPase Activity. Thirty embryos at the 32-cell stage were washed in 1 ml of 50 mM Tris (pH 7.8), 250 mM KCl, and 3 mM $MgCl_2$ (IMPB) and then lysed in 300 μl of the same buffer. Lysates were centrifuged for 5 min at 20,000 × *g* at 4°C and supernatant was recovered. Water (2.5 μl), LiCl, or L-690,330 was added to 25 μl of lysate, which was then incubated at room temperature for 5 min. ^{3}H-inositol-1-phosphate (1 μl) was

Abbreviations: GSK-3β, glycogen synthase kinase-3β; IMPase, inositol monophosphatase; LiCl, lithium chloride; PKA, protein kinase A; CKII, casein kinase II; MAP, mitogen-activating protein; ERK-1, extracellular signal-related kinase 1.

added and the incubation was continued for 25 min. Samples were then diluted with 1.0 ml of 0.1× MMR, boiled for 5 min, and applied to Dowex columns as described (25). Inositol was present in the flow-through and inositol-1-phosphate was eluted by application of 3 ml of 0.1 M formic acid/1.5 M ammonium formate (25). Assays were repeated 2–4 times with similar results. LiCl (20 mM) also completely inhibited *in vitro* *Xenopus* IMPase activity (not shown). For *in vivo* measurement of IMPase activity, ^{3}H-inositol-1-phosphate was concentrated to 250 μCi/ml and mixed 1:1 with water, 10 mM L-690,330, or 0.6 M LiCl. Then 10 nl was injected into ventral-vegetal blastomeres at the 8- to 16-cell stage. After 10 min, 20 embryos were harvested by lysis in 1.0 ml of boiling 0.1× MMR with 20 mM LiCl. Lysates were prepared and applied to Dowex columns as above.

GSK-3β Activity. GSK-3β was obtained from New England Biolabs and assayed according to the supplier's protocol using 0.5–1.0 unit of GSK-3β per assay. The peptide substrate (GS-2) was present at 25 μM and incorporation of ^{32}P was measured by binding to P81 paper according to previously described methods (26). The peptide was synthesized with phosphate incorporated into the serine closest to the C terminus and had the sequence RPASYPPSPSLSRHSSPHQS(P)EDEEE (27). I-2 was present at 50 μg/ml and τ was 25 μg/ml. PKA, ERK-1 [mitogen-activating protein (MAP) kinase], and CKII were assayed under similar conditions as for GSK-3β except that

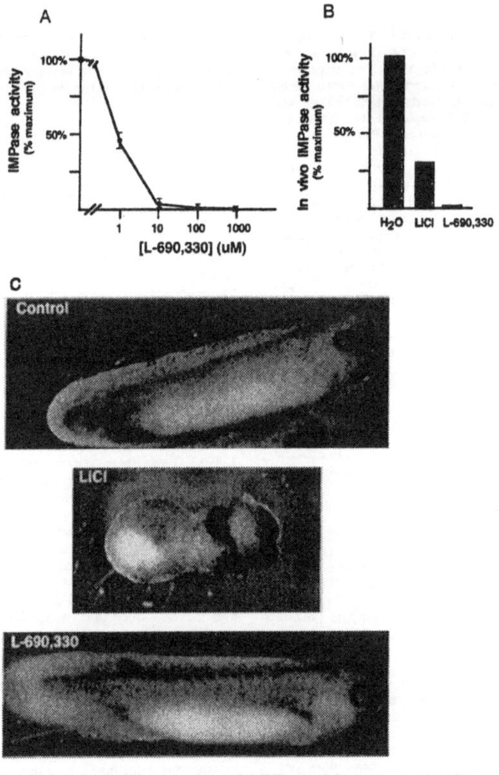

FIG. 1. Inhibition of IMPase does not dorsalize *Xenopus* embryos. (*A*) IMPase activity was measured as the amount of ^{3}H-inositol produced by hydrolysis of ^{3}H-inositol-1-phosphate in the presence of increasing concentrations of the bisphosphonate L-690, 330 in lysates of *Xenopus* embryos harvested at the 32-cell stage. (*B*) *In vivo* IMPase activity was measured by injecting a single ventral–vegetal blastomere at the 8- to 16-cell stage with 10 nl of ^{3}H-inositol-1-phosphate plus water, 5 mM L-690,330, or 0.3 M LiCl. Embryos were incubated for 10 min and then conversion to ^{3}H-inositol was measured. (*C*) Control, stage-30 embryo injected at 32-cell stage with water. LiCl, stage-30 embryo treated with 0.3 M lithium at the 32-cell stage, showing profound dorsalization with concentric cement gland, expanded anterior neural structures, and absent ventral and posterior structures. L-690,330, stage-30 embryo injected with 1 mM L-690,330 into a ventral–vegetal blastomere at the 16-cell stage (n = 55). Similar results were seen when ventral–vegetal blastomeres were injected at the 4-, 8-, or 32-cell stage or when each cell at the 4-cell stage was injected. L-690,330 was also injected at 10 mM. In no case was any evidence of dorsalization observed after injection of the IMPase inhibitor L-690,330.

2-mercaptoethanol was included in the PKA assays. For PKA assays, kemptide was 50 μM. For ERK-1 assays, myelin basic protein was present at 0.5 μg/μl. For CKII assays, casein was present at 50 μg/ml. (GSK-3β phosphorylation of I-2, but not GS-2 peptide or τ protein was partially inhibited by 20 mM KCl or NaCl, data not shown.)

RESULTS AND DISCUSSION

To test further the role of IMPase in *Xenopus* development, we have used a recently described competitive inhibitor of IMPase, the bisphosphonate L-690,330, which is ≈1000-fold more potent than lithium in inhibiting IMPase (14). As shown in Fig. 1, L-690,330 effectively inhibits IMPase activity from *Xenopus* embryos *in vitro* (50% inhibition at ≈1 μM). L-690,330 microinjected into blastomeres at the 4-cell, 8- to 16-cell, and 32-cell stages also completely inhibits IMPase activity *in vivo* (Fig. 1*B*). However, microinjection of L-690,330, in contrast to lithium, does not dorsalize embryos (Fig. 1*C*; $n = 55$) and has no discernible effect on development (at the highest injected doses mild nonspecific toxicity was observed, data not shown). These data show that inhibition of IMPase does not explain the effect of lithium on *Xenopus* development.

Because dorsalization by lithium is remarkably similar to ectopic expression of wingless/int-1 related genes (*wnt*) in *Xenopus* embryos (16), we have tested whether lithium might act on a component of the *wnt* signaling pathway. This pathway, which appears to be well conserved between vertebrates and invertebrates (21–23, 28), is inhibited in *Drosophila* by zeste white 3/shaggy (*zw3/sgg*), the homologue of the mammalian enzyme GSK-3β. Although GSK-3β was first described as an inhibitor of glycogen synthase (17, 29), it is likely that it regulates distinct substrates in other signal transduction pathways (17), including the *wnt* pathway. A central role has also been demonstrated for this gene in the development of diverse organisms including *Dictyostelium* and *Xenopus* (20–23). Therefore, we wished to test whether lithium acts by inhibiting GSK-3β directly, as this would be predicted to mimic *wnt* signaling.

To test our hypothesis, purified GSK-3β was assayed by using a peptide substrate (27, 30) and was found to be inhibited by lithium chloride with 50% inhibition (IC_{50}) at 2 mM (Fig. 2*A*). Little inhibition of phosphorylation was seen with NaCl, KCl, NH_4Cl, or CsCl at 20 mM (Fig. 2*B*), while lithium acetate showed inhibition nearly identical to LiCl (Fig. 2*B* and data not shown), indicating that the inhibition is mediated specifically by lithium ion and not by other monovalent cations or by chloride. LiCl inhibited GSK-3β-mediated phosphorylation of protein substrates, including protein phosphatase inhibitor-2 (31) and τ protein (32, 33) with an IC_{50} also near 2 mM (Fig. 3*A*, data not shown). Inhibition of GSK-3β is observed at concentrations well within the therapeutic range for lithium (0.5–1.5 mM) in the treatment of mania. In *Xenopus*, the effective internal concentration after lithium treatment is not known precisely but reaches a maximum of ≈8–9 mM (12).

The specificity of lithium inhibition was tested by assaying other protein kinases, including PKA, ERK-1/MAP kinase, and CKII, under similar conditions. Thus, at 20 mM lithium, PKA shows full activity toward kemptide (Fig. 3*B*) and casein (not shown). Similarly, lithium shows minimal inhibition of ERK-1/MAP kinase-mediated phosphorylation of myelin basic protein and CKII phosphorylation of casein (Fig. 3). These data indicate that lithium is not a general inhibitor of protein kinases in this dose range.

The kinetic nature of the inhibition of GSK-3β by lithium was investigated by measuring initial velocity as a function of substrate concentration at several concentrations of LiCl. The data, presented as double reciprocal plots (Fig. 4), show that the greatest effect is on the apparent V_{max}, and the plot of $1/V_{max}$ (*y*-intercept) versus lithium concentration is linear (not shown), suggesting that lithium acts as an uncompetitive inhibitor of GSK-3β. (K_i for LiCl = 2.1 ± 0.6 mM). Thus, inhibition of GSK-3β by lithium should not be overcome by increasing substrate concentration. The inhibition of IMPase by lithium is also uncompetitive (K_i = 0.8 mM), and it has been argued that this is an important feature for its therapeutic utility (9, 11) since the degree of inhibition is proportional to the concentration of substrate.

The hypothesis that GSK-3β is the endogenous target of lithium action is supported by genetic data as well as *in vivo* biochemical data. Thus inhibition of GSK-3β activity through expression of a dominant negative mutant of GSK-3β leads to dorsalization of *Xenopus* embryos, similar to lithium treatment (3, 21–23) and consistent with lithium inhibiting GSK-3β. In addition, disruption of GSK-3β in *Dictyostelium* (*gskA*) diverts cells normally fated to form spores to adopt the stalk-cell lineage (20), and this phenotype is also duplicated by lithium treatment (1). GSK-3β was first identified in mammals as the protein kinase responsible for the inhibitory phosphorylation of glycogen synthase (17, 29). Insulin is known to inhibit GSK-3β (30, 34), which in turn (together with activation of protein phosphatase) leads to increased glycogen synthesis. Lithium mimics insulin action by stimulating glycogen synthesis (6), and while the mechanism remains unknown, we suggest that lithium mimics insulin by inhibiting GSK-3β.

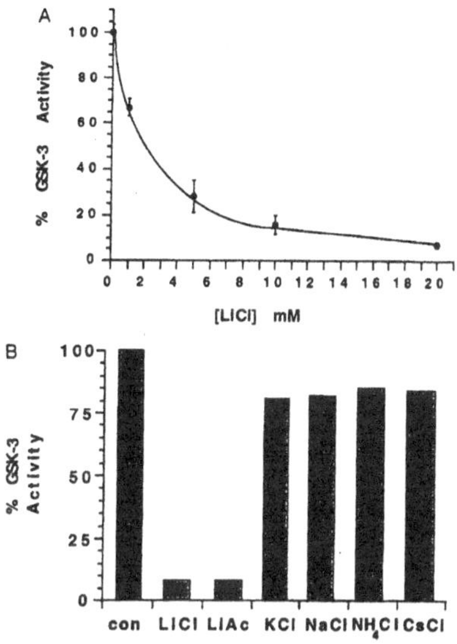

FIG. 2. GSK-3β activity is inhibited by lithium. (*A*) Purified GSK-3β was assayed by its ability to phosphorylate a peptide with a sequence derived from glycogen synthase (GS-2) in the presence of increasing concentrations of lithium chloride. Each data point represents the average of duplicate samples taken from three independent experiments and normalized to maximum GSK-3β activity. (*B*) GSK-3β was assayed as above without addition of monovalent cation (control) or in the presence of 20 mM monovalent cations as indicated in the figure. GSK-3β activity was normalized to the activity seen without added monovalent cations.

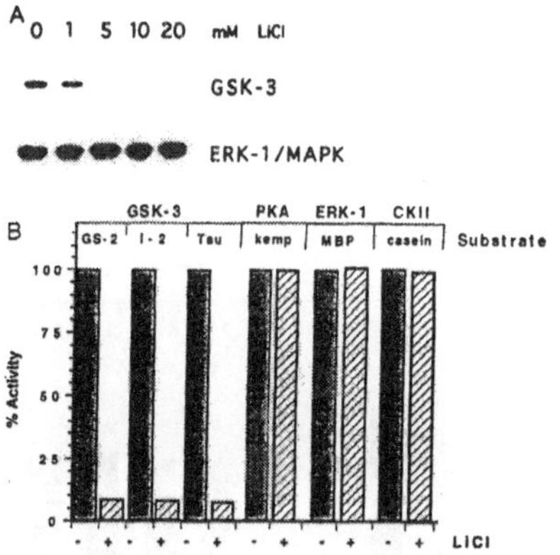

FIG. 3. Lithium does not inhibit cAMP-dependent protein kinase (PKA), ERK-1/MAP kinase, or CKII. (*A*) GSK-3β was assayed as above using protein phosphatase inhibitor-2 (I-2) as a substrate. ERK-1/MAP kinase was assayed under similar conditions using myelin basic protein (MBP) as substrate. Concentration of LiCl is indicated in the figure. Phosphorylated protein substrates were resolved by SDS/PAGE and visualized by autoradiography. (*B*) The activities of GSK-3β, PKA, ERK-1/MAP kinase, and CKII were measured in the absence or presence of 20 mM LiCl. Incorporation of ^{32}P was measured as in Fig. 1 (for GS-2 and kemptide) or by exposure of polyacrylamide gels to a Fuji BioImager and was normalized to incorporation in the absence of lithium. The substrates for GSK-3β were GS-2, I-2, and τ protein. For ERK-1, PKA, and CKII, the substrates were MBP, kemptide, and casein, respectively.

Our hypothesis offers a simple explanation for the effect of lithium on diverse systems and allows specific predictions, as well. For example, *wnt* signaling has been proposed to act through inhibition of GSK-3β (*zw3/sgg*) in *Drosophila* (28) and in *Xenopus*. If this pathway is conserved in other organisms, then lithium treatment should mimic *wnt* signaling in those systems as it does in *Xenopus* and zebrafish. In support of this, *wnt-4* has been shown to be required for the induction of mesenchymal condensation in the formation of renal epithelium in the mouse and ectopically expressed *wnt-1* can also induce mesenchymal condensation (35, 36). These effects of *wnts* are recapitulated by treating explanted renal mesenchyme with lithium (37), which also induces mesenchymal condensation. Furthermore, *wnts* were first identified in mammals by their ability to stimulate cell division and induce tumors in mammary cells (38); lithium can also stimulate cell division in primary mammary cell lines (39). It is not known how lithium exerts these effects in renal mesenchyme or mammary cell lines, but the correlation with *wnt* is compelling, given the other similarities of lithium to *wnt* actions.

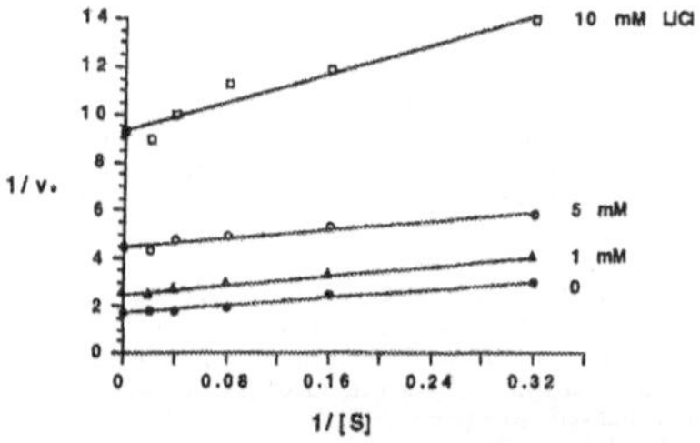

FIG. 4. Lithium is an uncompetitive inhibitor of GSK-3β. Initial velocity of GSK-3β phosphorylation at 3.125, 6.25, 12.5, 25, and 50 μM GS-2 peptide was measured in the presence of LiCl at 0, 1, 5, and 10 mM. The data are shown as a double-reciprocal plot. *Y*-intercepts ($1/V_{max}$) were extrapolated by linear regression. Reaction velocity was linear for up to 8 min and time points were taken at 5 min. The experiment was repeated four times with similar results. In addition, a plot of $1/V_{max}$ as a function of LiCl concentration was linear and allowed a calculation of the $K_i = 2.1 \pm 0.6$ mM (average from four separate experiments). However, it should be noted that kinetic analysis may be complicated by the fact that the peptide actually contains multiple GSK-3β phosphorylation sites that have different rates of phosphorylation (41).

Lithium has effects on numerous other organisms and it may have multiple physiological targets. However, the mechanism of lithium action in bipolar disorder remains uncertain. We propose that GSK-3β, which is abundantly expressed in brain (40), may serve a role in signal transduction in the brain, and that lithium inhibition of this pathway could explain its actions in manic-depressive illness in addition to its effects on development and its insulin-like activity.

We wish to thank Leslee Conrad for superlative technical assistance, Sandro Allesandrini for advice and reagents including glutathione *S*-transferase–ERK-1, Brian Anton for his advice on assaying GSK-3, and Betty Belmonte and Skip Brass for their advice on assaying IMPase. We thank Joseph Avruch and Albert Mildvan for very helpful discussions, and Min Ku and Dan Kessler for critically reading the manuscript. P.S.K. wishes to express special thanks to Betsy Wilder and to Min Ku for their ideas and experimental help.

1. Maeda, Y. (1970) *Dev. Growth Differ.* **12,** 217–227.
2. Van Lookeren Campagne, M. M., Wang, M., Spek, W., Peters, D. & Schaap, P. (1988) *Dev. Genet.* **9,** 589–596.
3. Kao, K. R., Masui, Y. & Elinson, R. P. (1986) *Nature (London)* **322,** 371–373.
4. Stachel, S. E., Grunwald, D. J. & Myers, P. Z. (1993) *Development (Cambridge, U.K.)* **117,** 1261–1274.
5. Livingston, B. T. & Wilt, F. H. (1989) *Proc. Natl. Acad. Sci. USA* **86,** 3669–3673.
6. Bosch, F., Gomez-Foix, A. M., Arino, J. & Guinovart, J. J. (1986) *J. Biol. Chem.* **261,** 16927–16931.
7. Price, L. H. & Heninger, G. R. (1994) *N. Engl. J. Med.* **331,** 591–598.
8. Goodwin, F. K. & Jamison, K. R. (1990) *Manic-Depressive Illness* (Oxford Univ. Press, New York).
9. Berridge, M. J., Downes, C. P. & Hanley, M. R. (1989) *Cell* **59,** 411–419.
10. Avissar, S., Schreiber, G., Danon, A. & Belmaker, R. H. (1988) *Nature (London)* **331,** 440–442.
11. Hallcher, L. M. & Sherman, W. R. (1980) *J. Biol. Chem.* **255,** 10896–10901.
12. Busa, W. B. & Gimlich, R. L. (1989) *Dev. Biol.* **132,** 315–324.
13. Drayer, A. L., Van der Kaay, J., Mayr, G. W. & Van Haastert, P. J. (1994) *EMBO J.* **13,** 1601–1609.
14. Atack, J. R., Cook, S. M., Watt, A. P., Fletcher, S. R. & Ragan, C. I. (1993) *J. Neurochem.* **60,** 652–658.
15. Atack, J. R., Prior, A. M., Fletcher, S. R., Quirk, K., McKernan, R. & Ragan, C. I. (1994) *J. Pharmacol. Exp. Ther.* **270,** 70–76.
16. McMahon, A. P. & Moon, R. T. (1989) *Cell* **58,** 1075–1084.
17. Woodgett, J. R. (1991) *Trends Biochem. Sci.* **16,** 177–181.
18. Siegfried, E., Perkins, L. A., Capaci, T. M. & Perrimon, N. (1990) *Nature (London)* **345,** 825–829.
19. Bourouis, M., Moore, P., Ruel, L., Grau, Y., Heitzler, P. & Simpson, P. (1990) *EMBO J.* **9,** 2877–2884.
20. Harwood, A. J., Plyte, S. E., Woodgett, J., Strutt, H. & Kay, R. R. (1995) *Cell* **80,** 139–148.
21. Pierce, S. B. & Kimelman, D. (1995) *Development (Cambridge, U.K.)* **121,** 755–765.

22. He, X., Saint-Jeannet, J.-P., Woodgett, J. R., Varmus, H. E. & Dawid, I. B. (1995) *Nature (London)* **374**, 617–622.
23. Dominguez, I., Itoh, K. & Sokol, S. Y. (1995) *Proc. Natl. Acad. Sci. USA* **92**, 8498–8502.
24. Peng, H. B. (1991) in *Methods in Cell Biology*, eds. Kay, B. K. & Peng, H. B. (Academic, San Diego), pp. 657–662.
25. Berridge, M. J., Dawson, R. M. C., Downes, C. P., Heslop, J. P. & Irvine, R. F. (1983) *Biochem. J.* **212**, 473–482.
26. Stokoe, D., Campbell, D. G., Nakielny, S., Hidaka, H., Leevers, S. J., Marshall, C. & Cohen, P. (1992) *EMBO J.* **11**, 3985–3994.
27. Fiol, C. J., Mahrenholz, A. M., Wang, Y., Roeske, R. W. & Roach, P. J. (1987) *J. Biol. Chem.* **262**, 14042–14048.
28. Siegfried, E., Wilder, E. L. & Perrimon, N. (1994) *Nature (London)* **367**, 76–80.
29. Cohen, P., Yellowlees, D., Aitken, A., Donella-Deana, A., Hemmings, B. A. & Parker, P. J. (1982) *Eur. J. Biochem.* **124**, 21–35.
30. Sutherland, C., Leighton, I. A. & Cohem, P. (1993) *Biochem. J.* **296**, 15–19.
31. Hemmings, B. A., Resnick, T. J. & Cohen, P. (1982) *FEBS Lett.* **150**, 319–324.
32. Hanger, D. P., Hughes, K., Woodgett, J. R., Brion, J.-P. & Anderton, B. H. (1992) *Neurosci. Lett.* **147**, 58–62.
33. Mandelkow, E. M., Drewes, G., Biernat, J., Gustke, N., Van, L. J., Vandenheede, J. R. & Mandelkow, E. (1992) *FEBS Lett.* **314**, 315–321.
34. Welsh, G. I. & Proud, C. G. (1993) *Biochem. J.* **294**, 625–629.
35. Stark, K., Vainio, S., Vassileva, G. & McMahon, A. P. (1994) *Nature (London)* **372**, 679–683.
36. Herzlinger, D., Qiao, J., Cohen, D., Ramakrishna, N. & Brown, A. M. (1994) *Dev. Biol.* **166**, 815–818.
37. Davies, J. A. & Garrod, D. R. (1995) *Dev. Biol.* **167**, 50–60.
38. Nusse, R., van Ooyen, A., Cox, D., Fung, Y. K. & Varmus, H. E. (1984) *Nature (London)* **307**, 131–136.
39. Ptashne, K., Stockdale, F. E. & Conlon, S. (1980) *J. Cell. Physiol.* **103**, 41–46.
40. Woodgett, J. R. (1990) *EMBO J.* **9**, 2431–2438.
41. Fiol, C. J., Wang, A., Roeske, R. W. & Roach, P. J. (1990) *J. Biol. Chem.* **265**, 6061–6065.

A Randomized, Placebo-Controlled 12-Month Trial of Divalproex and Lithium in Treatment of Outpatients With Bipolar I Disorder

Charles L. Bowden, MD; Joseph R. Calabrese, MD; Susan L. McElroy, MD; Laszlo Gyulai, MD; Adel Wassef, MD; Frederick Petty, MD, PhD; Harrison G. Pope, Jr, MD; James C.-Y. Chou, MD; Paul E. Keck, Jr, MD; Linda J. Rhodes, MD; Alan C. Swann, MD; Robert M. A. Hirschfeld, MD; Patricia J. Wozniak, PhD; for the Divalproex Maintenance Study Group

Background: Long-term outcomes are often poor in patients with bipolar disorder despite treatment; more effective treatments are needed to reduce recurrences and morbidity. This study compared the efficacy of divalproex, lithium, and placebo as prophylactic therapy.

Methods: A randomized, double-blind, parallel-group multicenter study of treatment outcomes was conducted over a 52-week maintenance period. Patients who met the recovery criteria within 3 months of the onset of an index manic episode (n = 372) were randomized to maintenance treatment with divalproex, lithium, or placebo in a 2:1:1 ratio. Psychotropic medications were discontinued before randomization, except for open-label divalproex or lithium, which were gradually tapered over the first 2 weeks of maintenance treatment. The primary outcome measure was time to recurrence of any mood episode. Secondary measures were time to a manic episode, time to a depressive episode, average change from baseline in Schedule for Affective Disorders and Schizophrenia–Change Version subscale scores for depression and mania, and Global Assessment of Function scores.

Results: The divalproex group did not differ significantly from the placebo group in time to any mood episode. Divalproex was superior to placebo in terms of lower rates of discontinuation for either a recurrent mood episode or depressive episode. Divalproex was superior to lithium in longer duration of successful prophylaxis in the study and less deterioration in depressive symptoms and Global Assessment Scale scores.

Conclusions: The treatments did not differ significantly on time to recurrence of any mood episode during maintenance therapy. Patients treated with divalproex had better outcomes than those treated with placebo or lithium on several secondary outcome measures.

Arch Gen Psychiatry. 2000;57:481-489

ALTHOUGH MOST treatment studies of bipolar disorder have focused on acute episodes, the maintenance phase of treatment dominates clinical treatment. Maintenance studies conducted a quarter of a century ago concluded that lithium was effective in preventing both manic and depressive episodes of bipolar disorder,[1-5] but more recent open-label studies of lithium have reported less favorable treatment outcomes.[6-10]

See also page 490

No placebo-controlled studies of maintenance therapy for bipolar disorder have been conducted in more than 25 years. Even these early studies had limitations: most failed to employ established diagnostic criteria or outcome measures and included not only patients with bipolar disorder, but also those with recurrent unipolar depression.[1] Often, data were analyzed only for patients completing the trials, and the reasons for premature termination were inadequately described, preventing critical evaluation of possible sources of bias. In addition, artifactual differences between lithium and placebo treatment may have been created in some studies because of abrupt discontinuation of lithium at the point of randomization to placebo.[1,3-5]

Double-blind, randomized controlled trials have demonstrated that divalproex is superior to placebo and comparable with lithium in reducing or eliminating manic symptoms.[11,12] Although open-label studies[13-15] also suggest that valproate reduces the frequency and intensity of recurrent manic and depressive episodes, to our knowledge, no double-blind, controlled maintenance studies of valproate in bipolar disorder have been reported until now. Our randomized double-blind, parallel-group trial compared the efficacy of divalproex with that of placebo and lithium in preventing new bipolar epi-

The affiliations of the authors appear in the acknowledgment section at the end of the article. A list of members of the Divalproex Maintenance Study Group appears on page 488.

PATIENTS AND METHODS

PATIENTS

To enter the initial open-label phase of the study, patients had to be between ages 18 and 75 years, meet the *DSM-III-R*[16,17] criteria for bipolar disorder, have an index manic episode as diagnosed by the Structured Clinical Interview for *DSM-III-R*,[16] and have had at least 1 other manic episode in the previous 3 years. Patients could be enrolled in the open-label phase while manic, partially recovered from the manic episode, or euthymic after the episode, but not while depressed. Patients had to be randomized to double-blind maintenance treatment within 3 months of the onset of the index episode. Randomization criteria included scores of 11 or less on the Mania Rating Scale (MRS), 13 or less on the Depressive Syndrome Scale (DSS), and more than 60 on the Global Assessment Scale (GAS) on 2 consecutive occasions at least 6 days apart; the second evaluation took place on the day of randomization.[18,19]

Exclusion criteria included a history of intolerance of divalproex or lithium; alcohol abuse within the previous 6 months; current substance dependence or positive results on a urine toxicology test; concomitant drug treatment that could confound study results; the presence of any central nervous system, neuromuscular, or uncontrolled systemic disorders; serious suicidal risk; ongoing individual psychotherapy; or evidence of failure to adhere to the open-phase protocol. Female patients could not be pregnant.

After enrollment in the maintenance phase, patients were terminated from the study if they required hospitalization for depression or mania, had an MRS score of 16 or more, experienced intolerable side effects or other evidence of medical danger, became pregnant, or had a Schedule for Affective Disorders and Schizophrenia suicide item score of 4 or more. If any of the above occurred, they were referred for treatment.

Patients signed informed consent forms approved by the centers' institutional review boards.

STUDY DESIGN

This randomized, placebo-controlled, double-blind, parallel-group study was designed to compare the efficacy and safety of divalproex sodium therapy primarily with that of placebo and secondarily with that of lithium carbonate therapy. The initial open phase lasted 3 months or less, followed by a 52-week randomized maintenance phase. During the open phase, the index manic episode was treated at the discretion of the investigator, except that depot neuroleptics and electroconvulsive treatments were prohibited. The criteria for randomization could be met with or without drug treatment during the open phase. Any drugs other than divalproex or lithium given during the open phase were discontinued by the day before randomization.

Patients were randomized to divalproex, lithium, or placebo in a 2:1:1 ratio. Those taking divalproex or lithium on the day of randomization had the drug gradually reduced and withdrawn during the first 2 weeks of maintenance treatment. Patients who had received both drugs had to have one discontinued before randomization. The study drug was administered 3 times daily and the dose gradually increased based on body weight. Unless adverse events intervened, serum trough concentrations were maintained at 71 to 125 µg/mL for valproate and 0.8 to 1.2 mmol/L for lithium. Study visits were scheduled weekly or every other week for the first 12 weeks of the maintenance phase, then monthly.

Two courses of lorazepam were permitted: up to 6 mg/d for a 14-day maximum during the first month and no more than 7 days for the remainder of the study. Up to 10 mg of

sodes in patients whose disease was in remission. In addition, the relationship between acute treatment of a manic episode and subsequent maintenance therapy outcomes was studied, as this is the first prophylactic study with treatment of an acute bipolar episode.

RESULTS

COMPARABILITY OF TREATMENT GROUPS

Of 571 patients enrolled in the open phase, 372 were randomized to maintenance treatment. The reasons for exclusion of the other 199 patients from randomization are shown in **Table 1**. Because multiple reasons for failure could be reported, many patients were listed in the *other* category. Review of comments indicates that most patients in the other and noncompliant categories had uncontrolled manic symptoms as a major factor contributing to their discontinuation. During the open phase, 117 of the 372 subsequently randomized patients had been treated with divalproex only, 124 with lithium only, 50 with both drugs (usually sequentially), and 81 with neither drug; 187 of 372 were subsequently randomized to divalproex, 91 to lithium, and 94 to placebo. Two patients randomized to lithium never received the drug and one randomized to placebo was noncompliant, reducing the intent-to-treat sample to 369 patients. Twenty-five of the 37 participating centers randomized at least 1 patient to each of the 3 treatment groups; 80% of those in the intent-to-treat sample were treated at 16 centers. For purposes of comparisons across centers, the data from centers that enrolled fewer than 3 patients were pooled and treated as data from a single center. No significant treatment-investigator interactions were found in either baseline or mean change scores on the MRS or DSS.

Demographic characteristics were comparable among treatment groups in the intent-to-treat sample (**Table 2**), with 61% having at least one previous psychiatric hospitalization and 18% hospitalized for the index episode. Illness at the screening visit, conducted prior to open-phase treatment, was significantly less severe for randomized patients than for those not qualifying for randomization (MRS: 10.8 ± 9.5 vs 14.1 ± 10.5; $t_{559} = -3.69$; $P = .002$) (DSS: 12.1 ± 9.4 vs 14.5 ± 11.0; $t_{559} = -2.68$; $P = .008$). Baseline scores were also similar in the subsets of patients taking divalproex or lithium at the point of randomization.

haloperidol daily was permitted during the second consecutive week of lorazepam use in the first month only. These rescue medications were allowed to minimize the recurrence of manic symptoms caused by withdrawal of open-label medication. Neither lorazepam nor haloperidol was allowed within 8 hours before behavioral assessments.

OUTCOME MEASURES

The primary outcome measure was time to either a manic or depressive episode, subsequently referred to as *any mood episode*. The secondary measures were time to a manic episode, time to a depressive episode, and average change from baseline in scores on the MRS, DSS, and GAS during maintenance therapy. (Outcome measures were revised at the suggestion of reviewers.) A manic episode was defined as one accompanied by an MRS score of 16 or more or requiring hospitalization. A depressive episode was defined as one requiring antidepressant use or premature discontinuation from the study because of symptoms. Patients with DSS scores of 25 or higher were treated with sertraline or paroxetine, and their data were censored from the analyses of time to mania relapse on the day that antidepressant treatment began. Symptom severity was measured by the Schedule of Affective Disorders and Schizophrenia–Change Version, augmented to include all 11 items of the MRS.[11,19] Subgroups of patients with elated and depressive manic symptoms were established using the depressive mania criteria of Swann et al[20] based on open-phase ratings at the point of the highest open-phase MRS score. Additional details of the study design and rationale appear elsewhere.[21,22]

STATISTICAL ANALYSES

All tests were 2 tailed. Analyses were performed with the SAS system.[23] Values of $P \leq .05$ were considered significant, with the following exception: a Bonferroni adjustment was made for the 3 pairwise efficacy and adverse effect comparisons, yielding an adjusted *P* value of .02 (equivalent to an unadjusted value of .05); this adjustment was also made for comparisons of adverse effects related to laboratory findings (adjusted $P = .03$).

All randomized patients were evaluated for safety and reasons for premature discontinuation. Comparability of groups at baseline was assessed by one-way analysis of variance and Kruskal-Wallis tests. Differences between treatment groups in categorical measures were examined with Cochran-Mantel-Haenszel and Fisher exact tests. Survival analyses of time to occurrence of a manic or depressive episode were performed for the intent-to-treat sample (all patients receiving at least one dose of study drug). Life-table methods were employed to compare survival curves using the Wilcoxon test because of its sensitivity to early group differences.[24] Two-way analysis of variance models were used to evaluate differences in the change from baseline to the average of all scores on the Schedule for Affective Disorders–Change Version subscales and the GAS during the randomized phase. The first analysis of variance model included effects for treatment, center, and treatment-center interaction; the second included effects for treatment, mania type (depressive vs elated), and their interaction. The COSTART terms[25] were used to categorize treatment-emergent adverse events, defined as any event starting or worsening in severity after administration of the first dose of blinded study drug. Mean changes in laboratory values between treatment groups from baseline to final evaluation were compared using one-way analysis of variance. Sample-size estimation was based on a projected rate of manic relapse of 55% in the placebo group and 35% in the divalproex group, yielding an estimated power of 0.8 for a 2-tailed value of $\alpha = .05$ for an overall sample of 350 patients.

By day 30 of randomized treatment, the median and mean ± SD serum concentrations were 83.9 and 84.8 ± 29.9 µg/mL, respectively, for valproate and 0.9 and 1.0 ± 0.48 mEq/L for lithium; concentrations remained stable in succeeding months. The minimum and maximum concentrations for the entire study were 0.6 to 156 µg/mL for valproate and 0.1 to 2.7 mEq/L for lithium.

Premature termination rates for all reasons tended to be lower in the divalproex group than in the lithium and placebo groups ($P = .03$ and $P = .05$, respectively) (**Table 3**). The lithium group had significantly higher termination rates for study drug intolerance and noncompliance than the placebo group ($P = .001$), but more patients given placebo were prematurely dropped from the study for other reasons, including administrative reasons and loss to follow-up ($P = .01$). Patients in the divalproex group had a significantly lower termination rate for recurrent mania or depression than the placebo group ($P = .02$), and they were significantly less likely to be dropped from the study because of depressive episodes ($P = .02$).

Patients treated with divalproex continued treatment significantly longer than those treated with lithium (mean ± SD, 198 ± 152 days vs 152 ± 148 days) ($F_{1,366} = 5.96$; $P = .02$) and showed a trend toward longer treatment duration than the placebo group (mean ± SD, 165 ± 140 days) ($F_{1,366} = 3.11$; $P = .08$).

OUTCOME MEASURES

The time to development of any mood episode did not differ significantly among treatment groups, although a trend was observed favoring divalproex over lithium ($P = .06$; Wilcoxon $\chi^2_1 = 3.54$) (**Figure**). The median times to 50% survival without any mood episode, based on 4-week intervals, were 40 weeks for divalproex, 24 weeks for lithium, and 28 weeks for placebo.

The time in maintenance treatment before the occurrence of a protocol-defined manic episode did not differ significantly among groups. The time elapsed before development of depression tended to be longer in the divalproex group than in the lithium group ($P = .08$; Wilcoxon $\chi^2_1 = 3.11$).

The mean changes in the MRS during maintenance treatment were small and did not differ significantly for either the center effects or mania subtype model (**Table 4**). Treating the initial screening MRS score as a

Table 1. Reasons Open-Phase Patients Failed to Achieve Randomization Into the Maintenance Phase of the Study

Reason	No. (%)
Continuing or recurrent manic symptoms	28 (14.1)
Depressive symptoms	11 (5.5)
Noncompliant in open phase	31 (15.6)
Withdrew consent	15 (7.5)
Intolerant of divalproex or lithium	10 (5.0)
Other illness	8 (4.0)
Drug abuse	6 (3.0)
Other*	90 (45.2)
Total	199 (100)

**Most patients listed in the* other *category had uncontrolled manic symptoms as a factor in their termination.*

covariate resulted in no significant differences between treatment groups for mean change in scores.

The mean change from baseline in DSS scores using the center effects model indicated a trend for less deterioration in depressive symptoms in the divalproex group than in the placebo group ($F_{1,289}$ = 2.86; *P* = .09). With the mania subtype model, DSS scores worsened less for the divalproex group than for the lithium group ($F_{1,358}$ = 11.58; *P*<.001) and less for the placebo group than for the lithium group ($F_{1,358}$ = 5.20; *P* = .02). The interaction effect between treatment and mania subtype ($F_{1,358}$ = 11.38; *P*<.001) indicated that the treatment difference was a function of a poorer response to lithium prophylaxis among patients without depression in the index manic episode. Results were similar when either screening or baseline DSS was treated as a covariate.

The mean change in GAS scores showed somewhat less worsening in the divalproex group than in the lithium group with the center effects model ($F_{1,262}$ = 2.60; *P* = .12). With the mania subtype model, GAS scores worsened less for the divalproex group than for the lithium group ($F_{1,325}$ = 11.22; *P* = .001) and less for the placebo group than for the lithium group ($F_{1,325}$ = 4.92; *P* = .03), with the interaction between treatment and mania subtype ($F_{1,325}$ = 4.71; *P* = .03) indicating worse prophylactic response to lithium among patients without depression during the index manic episode.

RELATIONSHIP OF TREATMENT OUTCOME TO OPEN-PHASE TREATMENT

Among patients taking divalproex at the end of the open phase, those randomized to divalproex had a 46% longer duration of prophylaxis in the maintenance phase (*P* = .03) than those randomized to placebo; they were also 42% less likely to be prematurely dropped from the study for any major affective episode (*P* = .04) and 32% less likely to be prematurely terminated for any reason (*P* = .002) (**Table 5**). The divalproex group showed a trend for longer time to recurrence of any major affective episode than the lithium group. Among patients taking lithium as their last open-phase drug, no significant differences were observed in the 3 randomized treatment groups in premature discontinuation rates or time to recurrence of any affective episode (Figure). There was a trend (*P* = .07)

Table 2. Characteristics of Patients in the Intent-to-Treat Sample Before Treatment*

	Treatment Group†		
Characteristic	Divalproex (n = 187)	Lithium (n = 90)	Placebo (n = 92)
Age, y‡	38.9 ± 12.7	40.3 ± 9.8	38.7 ± 11.9
Sex, No. (%)			
Male	93 (50)	43 (48)	44 (48)
Female	94 (50)	47 (52)	48 (52)
Race, No. (%)			
White	168 (90)	82 (91)	87 (95)
Black	10 (5)	4 (4)	1 (1)
Other	9 (5)	4 (4)	4 (4)
Prior manic episodes, No. (%)§			
1-10	96 (51)	44 (51)	40 (44)
11-20	29 (16)	9 (10)	11 (12)
>20	62 (33)	34 (39)	39 (43)
Prior depressive episodes, No. (%)‖			
0	7 (4)	5 (6)	6 (7)
1-10	81 (44)	45 (51)	39 (43)
>10	96 (52)	38 (43)	46 (50)
Age at first manic episode, y‡¶	24.1 ± 10.4	25.4 ± 11.0	24.4 ± 10.9
Age at first depressive episode, y‡#	21.0 ± 9.9	23.1 ± 10.3	21.1 ± 9.8
Time since first manic episode, y‡**	14.9 ± 11.4	15.0 ± 10.1	14.7 ± 10.9
Use of divalproex in open phase, No. (%)††	70 (37)	41 (46)	38 (41)
Use of lithium in open phase, No. (%)††	79 (42)	31 (34)	32 (35)
Time of open phase, d§§	35.7 (24.6)	38.3 (24.7)	35.8 (23.6)
Time from start of index episode to randomization, d§§	74.2 (22.9)	75.1 (21.5)	72.8 (24.0)
MRS at baseline‡	3.4 ± 3.7	3.2 ± 3.7	3.4 ± 3.4
DSS at baseline‡	4.6 ± 4.6	4.5 ± 4.6	5.3 ± 4.2
GAS at baseline‡	69.8 ± 8.2	70.4 ± 7.7	70.5 ± 7.4

**MRS indicates Mania Rating Scale; DSS, Depressive Syndrome Scale; and GAS, Global Assessment Scale.*

†Percentages may not add to 100% due to rounding.

‡Values are mean ± SD.

§One hundred eighty-seven patients were randomized to divalproex; 87 to lithium; and 90 to placebo.

‖One hundred eighty-four patients were randomized to divalproex; 88 to lithium; and 91 to placebo.

¶One hundred eighty-seven patients were randomized to divalproex; 86 to lithium; and 90 to placebo.

#One hundred seventy-seven patients were randomized to divalproex; 83 to lithium; and 85 to placebo.

***One hundred eighty-seven were randomized to divalproex; 89 to lithium; and 92 to placebo.*

††Based on use closest to randomization.

§§Values are mean (SD).

for longer mean duration of prophylaxis with divalproex than with lithium (Table 5).

ADVERSE EFFECTS

The divalproex group had a significantly higher incidence of tremor and weight gain than the placebo group (**Table 6**). Tremor was significantly more common in the lithium group than in the placebo group. The divalproex group also had a significantly higher incidence of sedation, infection, and tinnitus than the lithium group.

Table 3. Reasons for Premature Termination for Randomized Patients*

	Treatment Group†			
	Divalproex (n = 187)	Lithium (n = 91)	Placebo (n = 94)	Significant Differences (*P*)‡
Reason				
Any mood episode	45 (24)	28 (31)	36 (38)	Divalproex < placebo (.02)
Mania	33 (18)	19 (21)	21 (22)	
Depression	12 (6)	9 (10)	15 (16)	Divalproex < placebo (.02)
Intolerance or noncompliance	41 (22)	32 (35)	11 (12)	Divalproex > placebo (.05) Lithium > placebo (<.001) Divalproex < lithium (.02)
Other§	30 (16)	9 (10)	24 (25)	Lithium < placebo (.01)
Total terminations	116 (62)	69 (76)	71 (75)	Divalproex < placebo (.05) Divalproex < lithium (.03)
Relapse time				
Time to 50% relapse with any mood episode, d (95% CL)	275 (167, NC)	189 (88, NC)	173 (101, NC)	
Time to 25% relapse with mania, d (95% CL)	>365 (NC)	293 (71, NC)	189 (84, NC)	
Time to 25% relapse with depression, d (95% CL)	126 (100, 204)	81 (33, 234)	101 (55, 190)	

**CL indicates confidence limits; NC, not calculable.*
†Values are presented as No. (%) unless otherwise indicated.
‡By Fisher exact test.
§Lost to follow-up, intercurrent illness, administrative reasons, or other reasons.

Patients treated with lithium had a significantly higher incidence of polyuria and thirst than those treated with divalproex. When compared with patients in the placebo group, patients in the divalproex group had significant reductions in platelet count ($-53 \pm 52.1 \times 10^9$/L vs $3.4 \pm 44.5 \times 10^9$/L) and white blood cell count ($-1.1 \pm 2.0 \times 10^9$/L vs $-0.3 \pm 2.2 \times 10^9$/L) ($F_{1,233} = 69.7$, $P<.001$, and $F_{1,234} = 6.91$, $P = .009$, respectively). Reductions below normal values were observed in 6.5% of patients for platelet count and 9.1% for white blood cell count. When compared with the placebo group, the lithium group had significant increases in white blood cell count ($1.2 \pm 1.7 \times 10^9$/L vs $-0.3 \pm 2.2 \times 10^9$/L) ($F_{1,145} = 20.82$; $P<.001$); uric acid level (0.03 ± 0.08 vs -0.001 ± 0.07 mmol/L [0.49 ± 1.3 vs -0.16 ± 1.1 mg/dL]) ($F_{1,145} = 10.85$; $P = .001$); creatinine level (3.5 ± 11.5 vs -1.8 ± 12.4 µmol/L [0.04 ± 0.13 vs -0.02 ± 0.14 mg/dL]) ($F_{1,145} = 8.99$; $P = .003$); and calcium level (0.04 ± 0.10 vs -0.12 ± 0.11 mmol/L [0.16 ± 0.40 vs -0.05 ± 0.43 mg/dL]) ($F_{1,145} = 9.14$; $P = .003$). Increases to above-normal values were observed in 10.8% of patients for white blood cell count, 11.9% for uric acid level, and 3.1% for calcium level; no above-normal increases were observed in creatinine level. No significant differences in hepatic enzyme changes were observed among groups.

RELATIONSHIP OF OUTCOME MEASURES TO SERUM VALPROATE AND LITHIUM LEVELS

Serum lithium levels were unrelated to average change in MRS (n = 74) ($r = 0.08$) or DSS ($r = 0.01$) scores; valproate serum levels correlated with average change in MRS score (n = 169; $r = 0.17$; $P = .03$). Serum lithium levels above 1.5 mEq/L correlated with the incidence of diarrhea and tremor. Weight gain was associated with serum valproate levels above 125 µg/mL; serum valproate levels correlated with reductions in white blood cell count (n = 154; $r = -0.27$; $P<.001$) and platelet count (n = 153; $r = -0.32$; $P \leq .001$).

COMMENT

Our study is the first randomized, blinded clinical trial to compare divalproex with placebo and lithium in the maintenance treatment of patients with bipolar disorder. Our data indicated no greater efficacy for divalproex than for placebo or lithium in preventing the recurrence of mania sufficiently severe to require hospitalization and/or associated with an MRS score of 16 or more, the development of a depressive episode, or the development of the first mood episode of either type. However, divalproex was significantly more effective than either placebo or lithium on several other outcome measures, including the rates of recurrence of affective episodes severe enough to warrant patients' discontinuation from the study. Divalproex was somewhat more effective than lithium in controlling subsyndromal depressive symptoms. Among patients treated with divalproex during the open phase of the study, continued administration of divalproex as the randomized treatment was more effective than placebo treatment in terms of patients' ability to continue in the maintenance phase.

The effectiveness of lithium was less than that reported in other placebo-controlled studies, but consistent with the outcomes of naturalistic studies of lithium as maintenance therapy in bipolar disorder over the past decade.[8-10,26,27] Several factors may have contributed to the unexpectedly poor response to lithium. First, the lithium group had a larger proportion of patients dropped from the study for intolerance to treatment or noncompliance than the divalproex or placebo group. In addition, fewer patients were randomized to the lithium group than to the divalproex group, reducing the power for lithium-placebo comparisons; lithium was included in

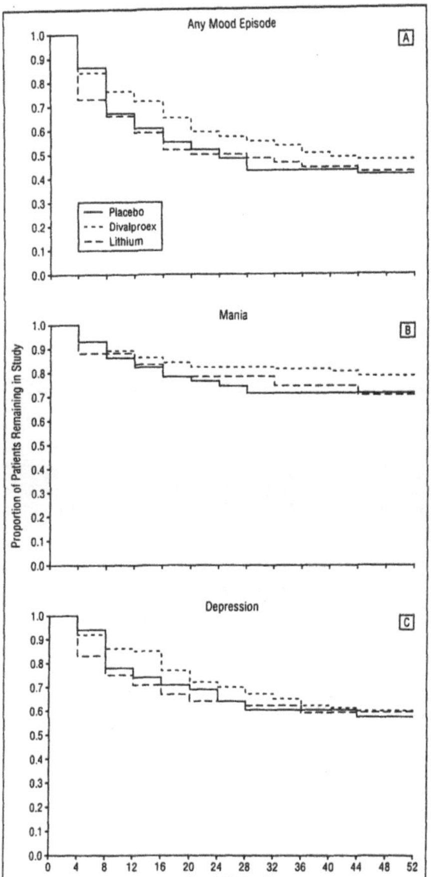

A, Time to any affective episode: Kaplan-Meier survival curves (placebo, n = 92; divalproex, n = 187; lithium, n = 90). Wilcoxon χ^2_1 = 0.95, P = .33 for divalproex vs placebo; Wilcoxon χ^2_1 = 1.03, P = .31 for lithium vs placebo; and Wilcoxon χ^2_1 = 3.54, P = .06 for divalproex vs lithium. B, Time to mania, censoring for antidepressant use: Wilcoxon χ^2_1 = 0.69, P = .41 for divalproex vs placebo; Wilcoxon χ^2_1 = 0.26, P = .61 for lithium vs placebo; and Wilcoxon χ^2_1 = 1.74, P = .19 for divalproex vs lithium. C, Time to depression: Wilcoxon χ^2_1 = 0.47, P = .49 for divalproex vs placebo; Wilcoxon χ^2_1 = 1.30, P = .25 for lithium vs placebo; and Wilcoxon χ^2_1 = 3.11, P = .08 for divalproex vs lithium.

the study primarily for comparison purposes, as it is considered the standard prophylactic treatment for bipolar disorder.

Mean serum levels of lithium were relatively high in patients treated with lithium but were unrelated to changes in depressive or manic symptoms. Possibly the high serum levels of lithium had an adverse effect on efficacy measures in a manner not revealed by statistical analyses. Among patients treated with divalproex, serum valproate levels correlated positively with manic symptoms. While this relationship may be causal, it probably also reflects increases in divalproex dosage prescribed by investigators to deal with continuing manic symptoms in some patients.

Table 4. Mean Changes From Baseline in Mania Rating Scale (MRS), Depressive Syndrome Scale (DSS), and Global Assessment Scale (GAS) Scores for Randomized Patients

		Treatment Group, Mean ± SD		
Measure	Model	Divalproex	Lithium	Placebo
MRS	Center effects	3.1 ± 10.6	3.0 ± 10.5	3.4 ± 9.5
	Mania subtype	1.7 ± 6.3	2.6 ± 7.1	2.7 ± 6.5
DSS	Center effects	3.9 ± 10.7	5.7 ± 10.7	6.1 ± 9.7
	Mania subtype	3.6 ± 6.9	7.0 ± 8.0	4.4 ± 7.2
GAS	Center effects	−4.7 ± 14.7	−7.8 ± 13.8	−5.7 ± 13.2
	Mania subtype	−4.7 ± 12.1	−10.8 ± 13.7	−6.2 ± 12.5

A placebo group was included in our study in part because no placebo-controlled maintenance study of pharmacotherapy for bipolar disorder had been conducted in more than 25 years, and the outcomes in these early studies may have been biased against placebo because of risk of early relapse associated with the abrupt withdrawal of lithium at the point of randomization to placebo.[28-30] In our study, the risk of relapse associated with the withdrawal of active drug in the placebo group was reduced by tapering the dose of open-phase lithium or divalproex over the first 2 weeks of randomized treatment. In addition, adjunctive medications were permitted in the first month of maintenance to minimize symptoms related to withdrawal of any open-phase drug. We found no evidence of rebound symptoms in patients withdrawn from one drug and randomized to another, as judged by lack of significant differences in treatment-emergent manic or depressive episodes between patients taking the same drugs during the open and maintenance phases and those switched to another drug or placebo.

Several factors may have contributed to the surprisingly good outcomes in the placebo group.[22] Patients with mild forms of bipolar disorder may have been selected for the study because of the enrollment requirement that 2 consecutive GAS scores had to be above 60. Bias may also have been introduced by the requirement that remission of mania had to be achieved within 3 months of the manic episode, as failure to meet this criterion was a major reason for exclusion from randomization. Also, some patients were randomized whose manic episodes resolved without specific treatment. In addition, a number of study candidates with histories of severe illness were reluctant to enroll in the study because of the chance of receiving placebo for up to 1 year, with minimal use of rescue medications. Moreover, the index episodes of mania seemed to be more severe in patients who failed to qualify for randomization than in those randomized. Drug-placebo differences are known to be greater when patients with more severe forms of illness are studied.[31-33] Another factor influencing the favorable outcomes in the pla-

Table 5. Outcome Measures Among Patients Receiving Divalproex or Lithium in the Open Phase

	Treatment Group*		
	Divalproex	Lithium	Placebo
Divalproex in open phase (n = 149)†			
Time in maintenance phase of study, d, mean ± SD	209 ± 155‡	162 ± 146	143 ± 123
Early termination for mania or depression	20 (29)§	15 (37)	19 (50)
Early termination for intolerance to study drug or noncompliance	12 (17)	14 (34)	7 (19)
Early termination for any reason	41 (59)‖	31 (76)	33 (87)
Lithium in open phase (n = 142)¶			
Time in maintenance phase of study, d, mean ± SD	188 ± 150	130 ± 146	183 ± 151
Early termination for mania or depression	12 (15)	10 (32)	12 (38)
Early termination for intolerance to study drug or noncompliance	15 (20)#	10 (32)**	1 (3)
Early termination for any reason	51 (65)	25 (81)	21 (66)

*Values are No. (%) unless otherwise indicated.
†Seventy patients were randomized to divalproex; 41 to lithium; and 38 to placebo.
‡$F_{1,145}$ = 5.01; P = .03 for divalproex vs placebo.
§P = .07 by Fisher exact test for divalproex vs placebo.
‖P = .002 by Fisher exact test for divalproex vs placebo.
¶Seventy-nine patients were randomized to divalproex; 31 to lithium; and 32 to placebo.
#P = .02 by Fisher exact test for divalproex vs placebo.
**P = .003 by Fisher exact test for lithium vs placebo.

cebo group may have been the structured therapeutic environment in which patients received treatment, the high level of support and encouragement given by study personnel, the ready access of patients and their families to educational information about bipolar disorder, and staff attention to patient compliance. In addition, bias favoring the placebo group may have been introduced by the relatively high rate of premature terminations associated with protocol violations and loss to follow-up; this may have resulted in lowering the proportion of those remaining at risk for developing mania or depression. Survival analysis of an intent-to-treat sample may inflate placebo response rates, since premature study terminations for withdrawn consent and protocol violations tend to occur disproportionately in patients receiving placebo. The aggregate result of these factors was a lower proportion of manic relapses in the placebo group than projected, yielding inadequate power to test the primary outcome variable (ie, 0.3 rather than the planned power of greater than 0.8).

Perhaps outcome measures resembling those used in previous bipolar maintenance studies would have provided greater sensitivity to group treatment differences than our primary outcome measure, time to any mood episode. In placebo-controlled studies of lithium published in the 1970s, the duration of symptom-free maintenance therapy was used as the strongest evidence of lithium efficacy.[1,2,4,5,34,35] For example, Fieve et al[35] reported that patients treated with lithium remained in treatment for 40.1 months compared with 18.2 months for those treated with placebo ($P<.01$). Greil et al[36] found no significant difference between lithium and carbamazepine in survival time to an affective episode, but when the outcome criteria were broadened to include the time to use of concomitant medication, lithium was superior to carbamazepine. Variations in severity of illness in different patient populations contribute to difficulties in interpreting outcome measures. For example, in the open

Table 6. Incidence of Adverse Effects With Significantly Greater Frequency by Treatment Group

	Treatment Group, No. (%)			
Adverse Effect	Divalproex (n = 187)	Lithium (n = 94)	Placebo (n = 94)	Significant Differences (*P*)*
Nausea	79 (42)	41 (45)	29 (31)	Lithium > placebo (.05)
Diarrhea	65 (35)	42 (46)	28 (30)	Lithium > placebo (.02)
Tremor	77 (41)	38 (42)	12 (13)	Lithium > placebo (<.001) Divalproex > placebo (<.001)
Sedation	78 (42)	24 (26)	33 (35)	Divalproex > lithium (.02)
Weight gain	39 (21)	12 (13)	7 (7)	Divalproex > placebo (.004)
Polyuria	15 (8)	17 (19)	9 (10)	Lithium > divalproex (.01)
Thirst	11 (6)	14 (15)	7 (7)	Lithium > divalproex (.01)
Alopecia	30 (16)	7 (8)	6 (6)	Divalproex > placebo (.03)
Infection	51 (27)	12 (13)	18 (19)	Divalproex > lithium (.009)
Tinnitus	11 (6)	0 (0)	1 (1)	Divalproex > lithium (.01)
Tachycardia	1 (<1)	4 (4)	1 (1)	Lithium > divalproex (.04)
Akathisia	1 (<1)	4 (4)	1 (1)	Lithium > divalproex (.04)
Dry eyes	0 (0)	3 (3)	0 (0)	Lithium > divalproex (.03)

*By Fisher exact test.

17-year maintenance study reported by Harrow et al,[6] all patients were initially hospitalized for mania, indicating severe disease; indeed, 78% were considered psychotic. Although placebo controls would not have been possible among such severely ill patients, the authors reported an outcome similar to that found in our study (ie, the occurrence of new affective episodes in more than half of patients, with recurrence rates unrelated to lithium treatment).[22]

In the aggregate, the time patients were able to continue receiving maintenance therapy was longer in the divalproex group than in either the placebo or lithium group. Although only some comparisons were significant, our findings were consistent with those of open-label studies in which valproate was found to be

The Divalproex Maintenance Study Group

The following members of the study group took part in this study: Paul E. Alexander, MD, Psychiatric Foundation for Research and Education, Warwick, RI; Jeffrey Clothier, MD, University of Arkansas Medical School, Little Rock; Robert Cooke, MD, Clarke Institute of Psychiatry, Toronto, Ontario; William Coryell, MD, University of Iowa Hospitals and Clinics, Iowa City; Scott Crow, MD, University of Minnesota Hospital, Minneapolis; Pedro Delgado, MD, University of Arizona College of Medicine, Tucson; Dwight Evans, MD, University of Florida College of Medicine, Gainesville; Arlene F. Frank, MD, Brookside Hospital, Nashua, NH; Robert Gerner, MD, University of California Center for Mood Disorders, Los Angeles; William J. Giakas, MD, Rockford Psychiatric Medical Services, Rockford, Ill; Ira David Glick, MD, Stanford University School of Medicine, Stanford, Calif; Steven Parker James, MD, Yorba Hills Medical Plaza, Yorba Linda, Calif; Philip G. Janicak, MD, Illinois State Psychiatric Institute, Chicago; James W. Jefferson, MD, Dean Foundation for Health, Research, and Education, Madison, Wis; Barbara L. Kennedy, MD, PhD, University of Louisville, Louisville, Ky; K. Ranga Rama Krishnan, MD, Duke University Medical Center, Durham, NC; B. Raj Nakra, MD, Washington University School of Medicine, St Louis, Mo; Henry A. Nasrallah, MD, Ohio State University College of Medicine, Columbus; Charles B. Nemeroff, MD, Emory University School of Medicine, Atlanta, Ga; William M. Patterson, MD, Birmingham Research Group Inc, Birmingham, Ala; Samuel Craig Risch, MD, Medical University of South Carolina, Charleston; Alan H. Rosenbaum, MD, Comprehensive Psychiatric Services, Farmington Hills, Mich; David Vincent Sheehan, MD, University of South Florida Psychiatry Center, Tampa; Richard L. Wang, MD, Milwaukee County Medical Complex, Milwaukee, Wis; Richard H. Weisler, MD, Raleigh, NC; Phillip Wilner, MD, Payne Whitney Psychiatric Clinic, New York, NY; John Downs, MD, University of Tennessee, Memphis.

effective in preventing new episodes of both mania and depression.[13-15] Our results also indicated complex relationships between illness characteristics and treatments during the index manic episode and subsequent maintenance treatments (to be addressed in forthcoming articles). We recommend that future studies of prophylactic therapy for bipolar disorder focus on more sensitive indicators of drug efficacy than time to relapse with a full bipolar episode. Such measures should include subsyndromal symptoms, time spent in remission, and time to premature discontinuation for any reason.

Accepted for publication September 17, 1999.

From the Departments of Psychiatry, University of Texas Health Science Center at San Antonio, San Antonio, Tex (Drs Bowden and Rhodes), Case Western Reserve University School of Medicine, Cleveland, Ohio (Drs Calabrese), University of Cincinnati College of Medicine, Cincinnati, Ohio (Drs McElroy and Keck), University of Pennsylvania Medical Center, Philadelphia (Dr Gyulai), and the University of Texas Health Science Center (Dr Wassef) and Medical School (Dr Swann), Houston; Psychiatry Service, Veterans Affairs Medical Center, Dallas, Tex (Dr Petty); Biological Psychiatry Laboratory, McLean Hospital, Belmont, Mass, and the Department of Psychiatry, Harvard Medical School, Boston, Mass (Dr Pope); Nathan S. Kline Institute, Orangeburg, NY (Dr Chou); Department of Psychiatry and Behavioral Sciences, University of Texas Medical Branch, Galveston (Dr Hirschfeld); and Clinical Statistics, Pharmaceutical Products Division, Abbott Laboratories, Abbott Park, Ill (Dr Wozniak). A list of members of the Divalproex Maintenance.

This multicenter collaborative trial was sponsored by Abbott Laboratories, North Chicago, Ill.

Corresponding author: Charles L. Bowden, MD, University of Texas Health Science Center at San Antonio, Department of Psychiatry, 7703 Floyd Curl Dr, San Antonio, TX 78284-7792 (e-mail: bowdenc@uthscsa.edu).

REFERENCES

1. Baastrup PC, Poulsen JC, Schou M, Thomsen K, Amdisen A. Prophylactic lithium: double-blind discontinuation in manic-depressive and recurrent-depressive disorders. *Lancet.* 1970;2:326-330.
2. Coppen A, Noguira R, Bailey J, Burns BH, Swani MS, Hare EH, Gardner R, Maggs R. Prophylactic lithium in affective disorders. *Lancet.* 1971;2:275-279.
3. Cundall RL, Brooks PW, Murray LG. A controlled evaluation of lithium prophylaxis in affective disorders. *Psychol Med.* 1972;2:308-311.
4. Melia PI. Prophylactic lithium: a double-blind trial in recurrent affective disorders. *Br J Psychiatry.* 1970;116:621-624.
5. Prien RF, Caffey EM Jr, Klett CJ. Prophylactic efficacy of lithium carbonate in manic-depressive illness: report of the Veterans Administration and National Institute of Mental Health collaborative study group. *Arch Gen Psychiatry.* 1973; 28:337-341.
6. Harrow M, Goldberg JF, Grossman LS, Meltzer HY. Outcome in manic disorders: a naturalistic follow-up study. *Arch Gen Psychiatry.* 1990;47:665-671.
7. O'Connell RA, Mayo JA, Flatow L, Cuthbertson B, O'Brien BE. Outcome of bipolar disorder on long-term treatment with lithium. *Br J Psychiatry.* 1991;159:123-129.
8. Tohen M, Waternaux CM, Tsuang MT. Outcome in mania: a 4-year prospective follow-up of 75 patients utilizing survival analysis. *Arch Gen Psychiatry.* 1990; 47:1106-1111.
9. Coryell W, Winokur G, Solomon D, Shea T, Leon A, Keller M. Lithium and recurrence in a long-term follow-up of bipolar affective disorder. *Psychol Med.* 1997; 27:281-289.
10. Vestergaard P, Licht RW, Brodersen A, Rasmussen NA, Christensen H, Arngrim T, Gronvall B, Kristensen E, Poulstrup I. Outcome of lithium prophylaxis: a prospective follow-up of affective disorder patients assigned to high and low serum lithium levels. *Acta Psychiatr Scand.* 1998;98:310-315.
11. Bowden CL, Brugger AM, Swann AC, Calabrese JR, Janicak PG, Petty F, Dilsaver SC, Davis JM, Rush AJ, Small JG, Garza-Trevino ES, Risch SC, Goodnick PJ, Morris DD, for the Depakoke Mania Study Group. Efficacy of divalproex vs lithium and placebo in the treatment of mania. *JAMA.* 1994;271:918-924.
12. Pope HG Jr, McElroy SL, Keck PE Jr, Hudson JI. Valproate in the treatment of acute mania: a placebo-controlled study. *Arch Gen Psychiatry.* 1991;48:62-68.
13. Lambert PA, Venaud G. Comparative study of valpromide versus lithium in the treatment of affective disorders. *Nervure.* 1992;5:57-65.
14. Calabrese JR, Delucchi GA. Spectrum of efficacy of valproate in 55 patients with rapid-cycling bipolar disorder. *Am J Psychiatry.* 1990;147:431-434.
15. McElroy SL, Keck PE Jr, Pope HG Jr. Sodium valproate: its use in primary psychiatric disorders. *J Clin Psychopharmacol.* 1987;7:16-24.
16. Spitzer RL, Williams JBW, Gibbons M, First MB. *Structured Clinical Interview for the DSM-III-R.* Washington, DC: American Psychiatric Press Inc; 1990.
17. American Psychiatric Association. *Diagnostic and Statistical Manual of Mental Disorders, Revised Third Edition.* Washington, DC: American Psychiatric Association; 1987.
18. Secunda S, Katz MM, Swann A, Koslow SH, Maas JW, Chuang S, Croughan J. Mania: diagnosis, state measurement and prediction of treatment response. *J Affect Disord.* 1985;8:113-121.
19. Endicott J, Spitzer RL. A diagnostic interview: the schedule of affective disorders and schizophrenia. *Arch Gen Psychiatry.* 1978;35:837-844.
20. Swann AC, Bowden CL, Morris D, Calabrese JR, Petty F, Small J, Dilsaver SC,

Davis JM. Depression during mania: treatment response to lithium or divalproex. *Arch Gen Psychiatry.* 1997;54:37-42.
21. Bowden CL, Calabrese JR, Wallin BA, Swann AC, McElroy SL, Risch SC, Hirschfeld MA. Who enters therapeutic trials: illness characteristics of patients in clinical drug studies of mania. *Psychopharmacol Bull.* 1995;31:103-109.
22. Bowden CL, Swann AC, Calabrese JR, McElroy SL, Morris D, Petty FL, Hirschfeld RM, Gyulai L. Maintenance clinical trials in bipolar disorder: design implications of the divalproex-lithium-placebo study. *Psychopharmacol Bull.* 1997; 33:693-699.
23. *SAS/STAT User's Guide, Version 6.* 4th ed. Cary, NC: SAS Institute Inc; 1989.
24. Lawless JF. *Statistical Models and Methods for Lifetime Data.* New York, NY: John Wiley & Sons; 1982:423.
25. *COSTART: Coding Symbols for Thesaurus of Adverse Reaction Terms.* 3rd ed. Rockville, Md: Division of Drug and Biological Product Experience, Center for Drugs and Biologics, Food and Drug Administration, Dept of Health and Human Services; 1989.
26. Maj M, Pirozzi R, Kemali D. Long-term outcome of lithium prophylaxis in patients initially classified as complete responders. *Psychopharmacology.* 1989; 98:535-538.
27. Goldberg JF, Harrow M, Grossman LS. Course and outcome in bipolar affective disorder. *Am J Psychiatry.* 1995;152:379-384.
28. Suppes T, Baldessarini RJ, Faedda GL, Tohen M. Risk of recurrence following discontinuation of lithium treatment in bipolar disorder. *Arch Gen Psychiatry.* 1991;48:1082-1088.
29. Faedda GL, Tondo L, Baldessarini RJ, Suppes T, Tohen M. Outcome after rapid vs gradual discontinuation of lithium treatment in bipolar disorders. *Arch Gen Psychiatry.* 1991;50:448-455.
30. Baldessarini RJ, Tondo L, Floris G, Rudas N. Reduced morbidity after gradually discontinuing lithium in bipolar I and II disorders: a replication study. *Am J Psychiatry.* 1997;154:551-553.
31. Uhlenhuth EH, Matuzas W, Warner TD, Thompson PM. Growing placebo response rate: the problem in recent therapeutic trials? *Psychopharmacol Bull.* 1997; 33:31-39.
32. Fisher S, Lipman RS, Uhlenhuth EH, Rickels K, Park LC. Drug effects and initial severity of symptomatology. *Psychopharmacologia.* 1965;7:57-60.
33. Benjamin LS. Statistical treatment of the Law of Initial Values (LIV) in autonomic research: a review and recommendation. *Psychosom Med.* 1963;25:556-566.
34. Hullin RP, McDonald R, Allsopp MN. Further report on prophylactic lithium in recurrent affective disorders. *Br J Psychiatry.* 1975;126:281-284.
35. Fieve RR, Kumbaraci T, Dunner DL. Lithium prophylaxis of depression in bipolar I, bipolar II, and unipolar patients. *Am J Psychiatry.* 1976;133:925-929.
36. Greil W, Ludwig-Mayerhofer W, Erazo N, Schöchlin C, Schmidt S, Engel RR, Czernik A, Giedke H, Müller-Oerlinghausen B, Osterheider M, Rudolf GA, Sauer H, Tegeler J, Wetterling T. Lithium versus carbamazepine in the maintenance treatment of bipolar disorders: a randomised study. *J Affect Disord.* 1997;43:151-161.

Clozapine for Treatment-Refractory Mania

Joseph R. Calabrese, M.D., Susan E. Kimmel, M.D., Mark J. Woyshville, M.D., Daniel J. Rapport, M.D., Carl J. Faust, M.A., Paul A. Thompson, Ph.D., and Herbert Y. Meltzer, M.D.

Objective: The efficacy of clozapine for treatment-resistant mania was examined in a prospective trial for patients with bipolar or schizoaffective disorder. Method: The subjects were 25 acutely manic patients with either bipolar disorder (N=10) or schizoaffective disorder—bipolar subtype (N=15) for whom lithium, anticonvulsants, and neuroleptics had been ineffective, had produced intolerable side effects, or both. After a 7-day washout, the patients were treated with clozapine monotherapy. They were evaluated over 13 weeks with the Young Mania Rating Scale and the Brief Psychiatric Rating Scale (BPRS). Results: Of the 25 patients, 18 (72%) exhibited marked improvement on the Young Mania Rating Scale, and eight (32%) exhibited marked improvement on the BPRS. The bipolar patients as compared to schizoaffective patients, and the nonrapid as compared to rapid cyclers, had significantly greater improvement in total BPRS score. Conclusions: These results suggest that clozapine is an effective therapy for treatment-resistant bipolar and schizoaffective mania.

(Am J Psychiatry 1996; 153:759–764)

Clinical experience accumulated over the last two decades indicates that 20%–40% of patients in the acute phase of bipolar disorder fail to respond to lithium and that 72%–82% of patients with the rapid-cycling type of bipolar disorder are resistant to lithium (1, 2). In addition, many patients with refractory bipolar or schizoaffective disorder are given maintenance neuroleptic treatment in order to control psychopathology and are, thus, at risk for tardive dyskinesia (3). Data suggest that more severe mania predicts poor response not only to lithium but also to carbamazepine (4) and valproate (5), the two other mood-stabilizing drugs most frequently used to treat bipolar mood disorder. Because of the large number of manic patients with refractory psychotic and mood disorder symptoms and poor social function, more-effective therapies for these patients are needed.

Data from retrospective studies suggest that clozapine, a novel atypical antipsychotic drug effective for up to 60% of patients with neuroleptic-resistant schizophrenia (6), is effective in treating schizoaffective and bipolar disorders (7–13). Earlier we reported two cases in which clozapine decreased rapid cycling in two bipolar patients whose disorders were refractory to all conventional treatments, including typical neuroleptic drugs (14). This report indicated that rapid cycling, a traditional predictor of lithium failure, did not preclude response to clozapine. Furthermore, some reports suggest the potential usefulness of clozapine in the treatment of nonpsychotic (8, 15, 16) and psychotic (17, 18) depression. These findings, together with our preliminary data, provided the rationale for this prospective study of the efficacy of clozapine for patients with refractory bipolar or schizoaffective mania.

METHOD

Subjects

Twenty-five patients meeting the DSM-III-R criteria for the manic phase of either bipolar disorder (N=10) or schizoaffective disorder (N=15) were given a prospective open trial of clozapine (table 1). The patients were healthy men (N=16) and women (N=9), and their mean age was 38.5 years (SD=9.2, range=25–67). These patients either had not responded adequately to a 6-week trial of lithium (plasma level, ≥0.8 meq/liter) or had not been able to tolerate lithium. Similarly, all

Received Dec. 23, 1992; revisions received April 30, 1993, June 23 and Oct. 4, 1994, and Dec. 1, 1995; accepted Feb. 13, 1996. From the Mood Disorders Program, Case Western Reserve University School of Medicine. Address reprint requests to Dr. Calabrese, Mood Disorders Program, Case Western Reserve University School of Medicine, Suite 200, 11400 Euclid Ave., Cleveland, OH 44106.
Supported by a grant from Sandoz Pharmaceuticals Corp.

TABLE 1. Clinical Features of Manic Patients in a Prospective Trial of Clozapine for Treatment-Resistant Bipolar Disorder or Schizoaffective Disorder

Patient	Age (years)	Sex	Lifetime Episodes		Experience With Lithium	Maximum Clozapine Dose (mg/day)	Change in Score During Study[a]	
			Manic	Depressive			Young Mania Rating Scale	BPRS
Bipolar disorder								
Rapid cycling								
1	37	M	—[b]	—[b]	Poor response	650	34	20
2	47	F	—[b]	—[b]	Poor response	400	17	11
3	42	F	—[b]	—[b]	Poor response	350	33	15
4	35	M	—[b]	—[b]	Poor response	400	23	8
5	36	M	5	6	Intolerance	800	27	22
6	48	M	15	—[b]	Poor response	525	7	18
7	36	M	—[b]	3	Poor response	800	5	12
Nonrapid cycling								
8	39	M	5	2	Intolerance; poor response	650	14	13
9	27	M	4	0	Intolerance; poor response	500	47	42
10	30	M	7	2	Intolerance; poor response	500	34	49
Schizoaffective disorder								
Rapid cycling								
11	40	F	—[b]	—[b]	Poor response	400	31	11
12	43	F	—[b]	—[b]	Poor response	350	12	–6
13	48	M	—[b]	2	Poor response	250	28	23
14	51	M	16	15	Poor response	550	32	15
Nonrapid cycling								
15	25	M	20	20	Poor response	350	25	13
16	29	F	—[b]	10	Poor response	400	20	17
17	42	F	8	7	Poor response	400	27	10
18	35	F	—[b]	—[b]	Intolerance	625	21	22
19	29	M	12	—[b]	Poor response	400	30	24
20	67	M	5	6	Intolerance; poor response	400	6	–3
21	36	F	6	1	Poor response	700	12	28
22	29	M	—[b]	2	Poor response	450	3	–5
23	31	M	—[b]	—[b]	Poor response	500	9	3
24	37	F	—[b]	—[b]	Poor response	400	37	33
25	43	M	—[b]	—[b]	Poor response	600	18	17

[a]Difference between baseline and endpoint raw total scores; a positive value represents a decrease in total score, i.e., improvement.
[b]Too numerous to count.

had had poor responses to individual trials of either carbamazepine (plasma level, ≥6 μg/ml) or valproate (plasma level, ≥50 μg/ml) or had been unable to tolerate either. In addition, all had less than satisfactory remission of manic symptoms after two courses of typical antipsychotic agents (6 weeks of 20 mg/day of haloperidol or its equivalent), as determined by inability to resume normal function or inability to tolerate the antipsychotic agents. Thus, all patients in the study either responded poorly to or were intolerant of lithium, at least two neuroleptics, and either valproate or carbamazepine. Seventeen patients had had unsuccessful prior trials of carbamazepine. Of the 17, 10 had responded poorly, three had not been able to tolerate it, and four had had both poor tolerance and poor responses. Fifteen patients had had unsuccessful prior trials of valproate; 12 had had poor responses, one had not been able to tolerate valproate, and two had had both poor tolerance and poor responses. Fourteen patients who had previously received a combination of lithium and one of the anticonvulsants had responded poorly. Poor compliance with at least one medication before the clozapine trial had been observed in 11 of the 25 patients.

Each of the 25 patients had had at least one episode of mania in the past 2 years. Eleven patients exhibited rapid cycling, as defined by four or more episodes in the 12 months before study entry; seven of the rapid cyclers had bipolar disorder, and four had schizoaffective disorder. Six patients had been continuously manic for the past 6 months, i.e., had experienced no period of full remission of manic symptoms lasting more than 2 weeks. Before study entry, the mean number of hospitalizations was 14.9 (SD=17.1). None of the patients exhibited evidence of substance abuse in the 6 months before study entry, but 12 patients had lifetime histories of substance abuse.

Procedure

All patients provided written informed consent. Before the drug washout period the patients were evaluated with the Schedule for Affective Disorders and Schizophrenia—Change Version (SADS-C) (19), based on the Research Diagnostic Criteria (RDC) (20), and the Young Mania Rating Scale (21). The patients were required to have taken no depot neuroleptics for at least 8 weeks, and the washout period lasted at least 7 days. After the washout, any patient who showed a 20% or greater reduction in score on the Young scale would have been excluded; none of the patients in this study met that criterion. Minimum scores of 25 on the Young scale and 4 on the Clinical Global Impression (CGI) were required for inclusion in the trial.

Clozapine treatment was initiated according to a semifixed titration schedule (Sandoz Pharmaceuticals Corp.). Maximum dose was achieved by a mean of 10.8 weeks (SD=11.7). Efficacy was assessed by administration of the SADS-C, Young Mania Rating Scale, Brief Psychiatric Rating Scale (BPRS), and Global Assessment Scale (GAS) (22), weekly for the first 6 weeks and at weeks 9, 11, and 13. Efficacy was further assessed with the two subscales of the SADS-C mania scale: the manic syndrome screening items and the behavior and ideation subscale. Adjunctive medications were given for insomnia: clonazepam (one patient, 2 mg/day), lorazepam (23 patients, 2–13 mg/day), and chloral hydrate (15 patients, 500–3500 mg/day). A decrease of 50% or greater in the score on either the Young mania scale or BPRS was considered to indicate a marked response.

Statistical Analysis

We used a split-plot analysis of variance, with a within-subject factor of time (11 levels), a between-subjects factor of diagnosis (schizoaffective or bipolar), and a between-subjects factor of cycling (rapid or nonrapid). The time factor involved an observation before washout (termed "previous medication"), one observation after washout (termed "baseline"), and nine observations during treatment with clozapine. The effects of time, diagnosis, and cycling on the various psychological evaluations were examined by using the unbalanced repeated measures method, as implemented in PROC MIXED. The method enables the statistician to examine all present data points, without listwise deletion of cases. In the present study, the data were analyzed by using an unconstrained structure for the within-subject covariance matrix (23, 24).

Although ratings on seven scales (Young Mania Rating Scale, GAS, BPRS total, BPRS positive symptom subscale, SADS-C mania subscale, SADS-C manic syndrome screening items, and SADS-C behavior and ideation subscale) were obtained, only the Young Mania Rating Scale and BPRS total scores will be presented (other results, which were entirely consistent, may be obtained from the authors). Since many hypotheses were tested, we took care to ensure that falsely significant effects were not found frequently, using the Bonferroni adjustment method and considering the two primary variables for the analysis (thus, $alpha_1$=alpha/2=0.025 for most analyses). Because of the large number of results examined and the large number of dependent variables, only significant results are presented. The term "cycling" will refer to the comparison of rapid cyclers and nonrapid cyclers, while the term "diagnosis" will refer to the comparison of patients with schizoaffective disorder and those with bipolar disorder.

RESULTS

Of the 25 patients, 22 (88%) completed the 13-week drug trial. Of the three (12%) who did not complete the trial, one prematurely left the study at week 9 because of poor compliance (defined as missing more than three consecutive doses of clozapine), one withdrew at week 9 because of poor outcome, and one withdrew at week 5 because of a change in residence. No patients were excluded from study participation because of a decrease in mania score of greater than 20% at the end of the washout phase. There was a 25% or greater increase in manic symptoms during the washout period in 18 (72%) of the 25 patients and a 50% or greater increase in manic symptoms in 12 patients (48%). Across groups, the mean peak dose of clozapine was 494 mg/day (SD=145, range=250–800); however, within diagnostic groups, a trend toward a higher mean peak clozapine dose was observed in the bipolar group (mean=558 mg/day, SD=162) than in the schizoaffective group (mean=452 mg/day, SD=120). Table 1 shows the maximum doses of the individual patients.

Response to Clozapine

Eighteen (72%) of the 25 patients exhibited marked improvement on the Young Mania Rating Scale, while eight (32%) exhibited marked improvement on the BPRS. To determine whether the four groups differed over time, the interactions of diagnosis and cycling with time were examined. For the BPRS, the diagnosis-by-time interaction was significant (F=5.23, df=9, 175, p=0.0001), but the interaction for the Young mania scale was not. That is, the patients with bipolar disorder improved more on the BPRS than did the patients with schizoaffective disorder. The baseline mean score for the total bipolar group was 35.50 (SD=10.92), and their score at the end of the study was 14.50 (SD=7.88); the baseline and endpoint mean scores for the schizoaffective group were 36.00 (SD=9.28) and 20.47 (SD=7.96), respectively. The cycling-by-time interaction was also significant for the BPRS (F=16.85, df=9, 175, p=0.0001) but not for the Young mania scale. That is, the patients with nonrapid cycling showed greater improvement on the BPRS than the rapid cyclers. The baseline mean score for the total group of nonrapid-cycling patients was 37.75 (SD=10.84), and their score at the end of the study was 16.50 (SD=7.89); the baseline and endpoint mean scores for the rapid cyclers were 33.64 (SD=8.48) and 20.09 (SD=8.78). When the cycling-by-diagnosis-by-time interaction was evaluated, a significant effect was again observed with the BPRS (F=5.56, df=9, 175, p=0.0001) but not the Young mania scale. The patients with nonrapid-cycling bipolar disorder improved more than the patients with nonrapid-cycling schizoaffective disorder. The latter, in turn, improved more than the bipolar rapid cyclers. Schizoaffective rapid cyclers responded less than did the bipolar rapid cyclers.

Figure 1 presents the mean scores on the BPRS and Young mania scale at each time point. The main analy-

FIGURE 1. Scores Over Time on the BPRS and Young Mania Rating Scale for 25 Manic Patients Receiving Clozapine for Treatment-Resistant Bipolar or Schizoaffective Disorder

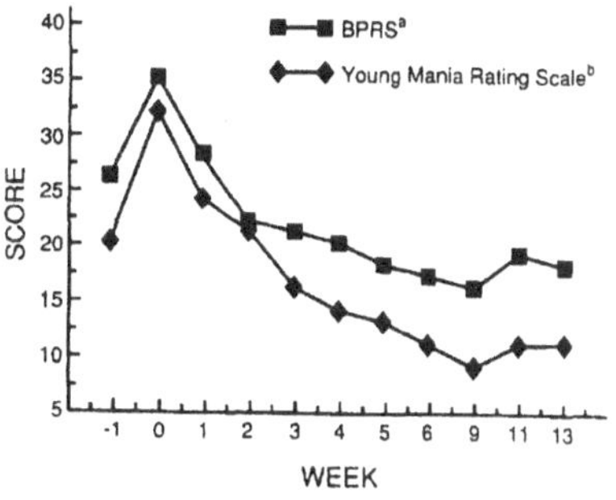

[a]Significant change over time (F=14.90, df=10, 175, p=0.0001) and significant difference between prewashout and clozapine treatment (F=8.18, df=9, 175, p=0.0001).

[b]Significant change over time (F=17.05, df=9, 188, p=0.0001) and significant difference between prewashout and clozapine treatment (F=4.91, df=9, 188, p=0.0001).

sis of time compared baseline ratings to later ratings and did not include the time point before washout. The overall effect of time was examined by using the unbalanced repeated measures method, and it revealed significant change over time for each measure. Moreover, the ratings on both instruments after clozapine treatment were also found to be significantly better than those obtained at the prewashout time point (figure 1).

In light of the overall interactions found, the time effect was examined separately for each group. In the comparison of baseline with the time points during clozapine treatment, significant time effects for the Young Mania Rating Scale were found within each of the four groups: bipolar rapid cyclers (F=8.48, df=9, 188, p=0.0001), bipolar nonrapid cyclers (F=6.76, df=9, 188, p=0.0001), schizoaffective rapid cyclers (F=3.96, df=9, 188, p=0.0001), and schizoaffective nonrapid cyclers (F=5.77, df=9, 188, p=0.0001). A similar pattern of significant results was also observed with the BPRS (data available on request). Between before and after washout there were no differences across the four groups in illness severity as reflected by scores on the Young scale and the BPRS.

When comparing the baseline rating to those obtained during the course of clozapine therapy, the point at which the rating changes significantly can be ascertained by using the Bonferroni-adjusted alpha ($alpha_T$= alpha/9=0.0056). Significant changes were found at week 1 for both the BPRS (F=10.58, df=1, 175, p=0.001) and the Young mania scale (F=10.43, df=1, 188, p=0.002). When clozapine was compared to the prior medication before the washout, a significant clozapine effect did not occur until week 9, and it continued for the duration of the study (Young Mania Rating Scale: F=18.57, df=1, 188, p=0.0001; BPRS: F=10.96, df=1, 175, p=0.001). When the Young mania scale was used as the measure of manic symptoms, there was no correlation between clozapine response (from postwashout baseline to study endpoint) and the degree of deterioration observed during the washout (r=0.36, N=25, n.s.). When the BPRS was used to measure psychotic symptoms, there was a significant correlation (r=0.64, N=25, p=0.001).

Side Effects

The side effects experienced included hypersialorrhea (88% of the patients, N=22), sedation (84%, N=21), constipation (56%, N=14), diarrhea (40%, N=10), aches and pains (40%, N=10), dizziness or lightheadedness (36%, N=9), decrease in WBC count to below normal (4,800–10,800 cells/mm^3) (28%, N=7), increased appetite or weight gain (28%, N=7), headaches (28%, N=7), urinary incontinence (24%, N=6), tachycardia (20%, N=5), orthostatic hypertension (20%, N=5), and sweating (16%, N=4). No episodes of agranulocytosis were observed. One patient experienced transient leukopenia. There was no difference between baseline and endpoint in score on the Abnormal Involuntary Movement Scale (AIMS) (25) (baseline: mean=1.85, SD=2.40; endpoint: mean=2.05, SD=3.36) or the Simpson Angus scale (26) (baseline: mean=3.46, SD=3.53; endpoint: mean=3.75, SD=3.01). Of the six patients (24%) who exhibited mild symptoms of tardive dyskinesia at study entry, all exhibited marked improvement, as determined by clinical assessment. For these six patients, the AIMS score decreased from a baseline mean of 2.8 (SD=2.6) to 0.8 (SD=2.0) at study endpoint (n.s.).

Follow-Up

Since the study endpoint, 22 patients (11 bipolar and 11 schizoaffective) have continued to take clozapine for maintenance therapy for an average of 15 months (range=4–46). Five patients with bipolar disorder (23%) and two with schizoaffective disorder (9%) required increases in their doses of clozapine for treatment of early signs of relapse into mania. Four bipolar patients and one schizoaffective patient required hospitalizations, which occurred, respectively, at week 58, at both weeks 13 and 64, at both weeks 19 and 63, at both weeks 22 and 50, and at week 29. Three of the four bipolar patients hospitalized for depression were diagnosed as rapid cyclers. During the 15-month follow-up period, the mean number of hospitalizations was 0.48 (SD=0.65). Five bipolar and five schizoaffective patients developed major depression that required treatment with antidepressants, which included fluoxetine, sertraline, nortriptyline, and imipramine. Of the 10 patients who became depressed, three exhibited moderate to marked response, as indicated by a 30% or greater improvement in the Beck Depression Inventory score. Three patients with schizoaffective disorder exhibited return of mild psychotic symptoms without major mood swings; the psychotic symptoms responded to an increase in the dose of clozapine. The absolute total number of episodes of mania during the 15-month follow-up period was seven.

DISCUSSION

The major finding of this study was that clozapine is effective in decreasing mania in patients poorly responsive to or intolerant of separate trials of lithium, carbamazepine or valproate, and at least two typical antipsychotic agents. The data of figure 1 show a rapid response to clozapine, in both antipsychotic effects and specific antimanic effects. Marked response was defined as a 50% improvement in score on either the Young Mania Rating Scale or the BPRS. Seventy-two percent of the patients exhibited marked improvement on the Young scale, and 32% showed marked response on the BPRS. The rate of improvement on the Young scale compares favorably with findings from a recently published 21-day double-blind comparison of valproate and lithium to placebo for 179 patients with bipolar mania (27). Marked response in that study was defined as a 50% improvement on the SADS-C mania rating scale, and about 50% of both the valproate and lithium cohorts exhibited this degree of improvement. These data also indicate a more profound and rapid response than we found for treatment-resistant schizophrenia or schizoaffective disorder—mainly schizophrenic subtype, which was usually 30% in a 6-week period, when only a 20% decrease in BPRS total score was used as the criterion for response (28). The rate of marked response with the BPRS was probably lower because many items on that scale have less relevance to mania, whereas the Young Mania Rating Scale is more specific to mania.

The worsening of symptoms during the washout probably indicates that the patients were experiencing a substantial but limited therapeutic effect from aggressive combination therapy before the treatment trial. However, the mean prewashout (during prior drug treatment) scores on the Young mania scale (mean=19.9, SD=11.9) and the BPRS (mean=26.5, SD=13.9) indicate that the average patient was experiencing a moderately severe episode of mania at the time of washout. Thus, these patients may be considered nonresponders to aggressive combination therapy. Most commonly, five different psychotropic medications were being prescribed concomitantly at the time of study entry.

Side effects during this 13-week trial were noteworthy and appeared to be related to the rate at which the medication was titrated at the beginning of the trial. The bipolar patients appeared to be less tolerant of rapid titration. The more clinically significant side effects included sedation, dizziness, weight gain, urinary incontinence, and tachycardia. Hypersialorrhea was the most common side effect, but it was not severe enough to result in drug discontinuation in any case. Sedation was also commonly reported. However, this resulted in drug discontinuation for only one patient. This rate is in contrast to the 11 of the 25 study patients who had exhibited poor compliance due to side effects from the combination of medications used immediately before this trial. Dizziness occurred in 36% of the patients and was directly related to the dose of clozapine and the rate of titration. For these patients the dose of clozapine was decreased, and after 4–5 days this side effect disappeared; it usually did not return with subsequent increases in dose. Weight gain occurred in 28% of the patients but did not result in drug discontinuation. One patient experienced a weight gain of 65 lb during the 15-month follow-up period, but this patient wanted to continue maintenance therapy. Urinary incontinence occurred in 24% of the patients, was not associated with age, and appeared most commonly in the more severely disorganized manic patients while secluded. Tachycardia was subclinical, did not exceed 120 beats/minute, and did not require dose alteration or symptomatic treatment with beta blockers. Of the six patients who entered the trial with overt evidence of tardive dyskinesia, all exhibited marked improvement within 30–45 days.

These results suggest that the efficacy of clozapine for treatment-resistant psychotic patients is not restricted to patients who meet the DSM-III-R criteria for schizophrenia alone. Clozapine was effective in decreasing both manic symptoms and psychotic symptoms, rated by the Young Mania Rating Scale and BPRS, respectively. In addition, the response of our bipolar patients on the BPRS, but not the Young mania scale, was superior to that of the schizoaffective patients. This finding is consistent with a prior report that showed that bipolar patients with psychotic features responded better to clozapine than did patients with either subtype of schizoaffective disorder (11). The fact that the BPRS, but not the Young mania scale, differentiated the responses of the bipolar and schizoaffective patients is probably due to the fact that the Young scale has fewer items devoted to the assessment of psychosis.

These data are also consistent with our prior report of the potential role of clozapine in the treatment of rapid-cycling bipolar disorder (14). Although patients with the rapid-cycling variant of bipolar disorder improved significantly over the course of the study, they did not do as well as those without a history of rapid cycling. It is noteworthy that the gender distribution of our rapid cyclers was not different from that of our nonrapid cyclers, a finding suggesting that this group of rapid cyclers differs from the usual one, in which women are more common than men (29). Since rapid cycling is widely recognized as predicting poor response to lithium (1, 2), clozapine's efficacy in the management of this refractory variant of illness, as well as other variants that do poorly with lithium, may prove to be particularly valuable. Since 21 of the 23 nonresponders to lithium who were enrolled in the study exhibited at least a moderate response to clozapine, these data further support the conclusion that the predictors of response to clozapine may complement those for lithium.

This report provides prospective data that confirm prior findings (7–13). Randomized controlled trials are needed to definitively establish the efficacy of clozapine in treatment-resistant mania vis-à-vis the full gamut of standard treatments. Without a parallel control group treated with standard therapy for mania, conclusions regarding the efficacy of clozapine should be viewed as preliminary. If findings from such studies are consistent with the results observed here, they would suggest the need to further consider shared biological mechanisms in treatment-resistant bipolar disorder and schizophrenia, especially since some treatments, such as lithium and carbamazepine, are much more effective in nonresistant bipolar disorder than in schizophrenia.

REFERENCES

1. Dunner DL, Fieve RR: Clinical factors in lithium carbonate prophylaxis failure. Arch Gen Psychiatry 1974; 30:229–233
2. Kukopolos A, Reginaldi D, Laddomada P, Floris G, Serra G, Tondo L: Course of the manic depressive cycle and changes caused by treatment. Pharmacopsychiatria 1980; 13:156–167
3. Davis KL, Berger PA, Hollister LE: Tardive dyskinesia and depressive illness. Psychopharmacology Communications 1976; 2: 125–130
4. Small JG, Klapper MH, Milstein V, Kellams JJ, Miller MJ, Mar-

henke JD, Small IF: Carbamazepine compared with lithium in the treatment of mania. Arch Gen Psychiatry 1991; 48:915–921
5. Calabrese JR, Woyshville MJ, Kimmel SE, Rapport DJ: Predictors of valproate response in bipolar rapid cycling. J Clin Psychopharmacol 1993; 13:280–283
6. Meltzer HY: Dimensions of outcome with clozapine. Br J Psychiatry 1992; 160:46–53
7. Nahunek K, Svestka J, Misurec J, Rodova D: [Experiences with clozapine.] Cesk Psychiatr 1975; 71:11–21 (Czech)
8. Klik J, Kraausova J, Krizova K, Maresova H, Vencovsky E: [Experience with clozapine in psychiatric home practice.] Cesk Psychiatr 1976; 72:197–200 (Czech)
9. Muller P, Heipertz R: [Treatment of manic psychosis with clozapine.] Fortschr Neurol Psychiatr 1977; 45:420–424 (German)
10. Naber D, Hippius H: The European experience with use of clozapine. Hosp Community Psychiatry 1990; 41:886–890
11. McElroy SL, Dessain EC, Pope HG, Cole JO, Keck PE, Frankenberg FR, Aizley HG, O'Brien S: Clozapine in the treatment of psychotic mood disorders, schizoaffective disorder, and schizophrenia. J Clin Psychiatry 1991; 52:411–414
12. Suppes T, McElroy SL, Gilbert J, Dessain EC, Cole JO: Clozapine in the treatment of dysphoric manic. Biol Psychiatry 1992; 32:270–280
13. Cole JO, Zarate CA, Banov MD, Green AI: Clozapine in affective disorders (abstract), in Proceedings of the 1993 Annual Meeting of the American College of Neuropsychopharmacology. Nashville, ACNP, 1993, p 69
14. Calabrese JR, Meltzer HY, Markovitz PJ: Clozapine prophylaxis in rapid-cycling bipolar disorder. J Clin Psychopharmacol 1991; 11:396–397
15. Kogan W, Nikolaenko N: [New drugs in the treatment of nervous and mental disease.] Reports of Leningrad Bechterev Psychoneurological Research Institute, 1974, p 40–41 (Russian)
16. Nahunek K, Svestka J, Misurec J, Rodova D: [Experiences with clozapine.] Cesk Psychiatr 1975; 71:11–20 (Czech)
17. Parsa M, Ramirez LF, Loula EC, Meltzer HY: Effect of clozapine on psychotic depression and parkinsonism. J Clin Psychopharmacol 1991; 11:330–331
18. Dassa D, Kaladjian A, Azorin JM, Giudicelli S: Clozapine in the treatment of psychotic refractory depression. Br J Psychiatry 1993; 163:822–824
19. Spitzer RL, Endicott J: Schedule for Affective Disorders and Schizophrenia—Change Version, 3rd ed. New York, New York State Psychiatric Institute, Biometrics Research, 1978
20. Spitzer RL, Endicott J, Robins E: Research Diagnostic Criteria (RDC) for a Selected Group of Functional Disorders, 3rd ed. New York, New York State Psychiatric Institute, Biometrics Research, 1978
21. Young RC, Biggs JT, Ziegler VE, Meyer DA: A rating scale for mania: reliability, validity and sensitivity. Br J Psychiatry 1978; 133:429–435
22. Endicott J, Spitzer RL, Fleiss JL, Cohen J: The Global Assessment Scale: a procedure for measuring overall severity of psychiatric disturbance. Arch Gen Psychiatry 1976; 33:766–771
23. Jennrich RI, Schluchter MD: Unbalanced repeated measures models with structured covariance matrices. Biometrics 1986; 42:805–820
24. SAS Technical Report P-229, SAS/STAT Software: Changes and Enhancements, release 6.07. Cary, NC, SAS Institute, 1992
25. Guy W (ed): ECDEU Assessment Manual for Psychopharmacology: Publication ADM 76-338. Washington, DC, US Department of Health, Education, and Welfare, 1976, pp 534–537
26. Simpson GM, Angus JWS: A rating scale for extrapyramidal side effects. Acta Psychiatr Scand (Suppl) 1970; 212:11–19
27. Bowden CL, Brugger AM, Swann AC, Calabrese JR, Janicak PG, Petty F, Dilsaver SC, Davis JM, Rush AJ, Small JG, Garza-Trevino ES, Risch SC, Goodnick PJ, Morris DD: Efficacy of divalproex vs lithium and placebo in the treatment of mania: the Depakote Mania Study Group. JAMA 1994; 271:918–924; correction, 271:1830
28. Meltzer HY, Burnett S, Bastani B, Ramirez LF: Effect of six months of clozapine treatment on the quality of life of chronic schizophrenic patients. Hosp Community Psychiatry 1990; 41:892–897
29. Bauer MS, Calabrese J, Dunner DL, Post R, Whybrow PC, Gyulai L, Tay LK, Younkin SR, Bynum D, Lavori P, Price RA: Multisite data reanalysis of the validity of rapid cycling as a course modifier for bipolar disorder in DSM-IV. Am J Psychiatry 1994; 151:506–515

Interpersonal and Social Rhythm Therapy: Managing the Chaos of Bipolar Disorder

Ellen Frank, Holly A. Swartz, and David J. Kupfer

Interpersonal and social rhythm therapy is an individual psychotherapy designed specifically for the treatment for bipolar disorder. Interpersonal and social rhythm therapy grew from a chronobiological model of bipolar disorder postulating that individuals with bipolar disorder have a genetic predisposition to circadian rhythm and sleep–wake cycle abnormalities that may be responsible, in part, for the symptomatic manifestations of the illness. In our model, life events (both negative and positive) may cause disruptions in patients' social rhythms that, in turn, perturb circadian rhythms and sleep–wake cycles and lead to the development of bipolar symptoms. Administered in concert with medications, interpersonal and social rhythm therapy combines the basic principles of interpersonal psychotherapy with behavioral techniques to help patients regularize their daily routines, diminish interpersonal problems, and adhere to medication regimens. It modulates both biological and psychosocial factors to mitigate patients' circadian and sleep–wake cycle vulnerabilities, improve overall functioning, and better manage the potential chaos of bipolar disorder symptomatology. Biol Psychiatry 2000;48:593–604 © *2000 Society of Biological Psychiatry*

Key Words: Psychotherapy, bipolar disorder, mood disorders, circadian rhythms, life events, interpersonal psychotherapy

Introduction

During the second half of the 20th century, new treatments for bipolar disorder focused primarily on somatic therapies. The discovery of lithium carbonate as a treatment for "psychotic excitement" by Cade in 1949 (Cade 1949) and advances in research supporting the heritability of bipolar disorder led investigators to conceptualize bipolar disorder as a purely biological process amenable to pharmacotherapy alone. Furthermore, clinical lore mistakenly led practitioners to believe that most patients with bipolar disorder recover fully from mania or depression, remain asymptomatic between episodes, and experience no decline in functional status over time. Psychotherapy for bipolar disorder was considered superfluous and was largely neglected as a treatment strategy for many years (Benson 1975). Beginning in the 1980s, however, reports appeared in the literature suggesting that outcomes with lithium alone were suboptimal. Cumulative data suggest that pharmacotherapy alone fails to prevent recurrence in 50 to 70% of patients over a 2- to 3-year period (Markar and Mander 1989; Prien et al 1984) and that overall functioning of bipolar patients remains low even after the resolution of fully syndromal episodes (Coryell et al 1993; Goldberg et al 1995). Researchers and clinicians became increasingly cognizant that the chronic course of bipolar disorder may, in the absence of appropriate interventions, lead to unremitting symptoms and a downward psychosocial spiral.

A Disorderly Disorder

As depicted in Figure 1, the course of recurrent unipolar disorder, although often debilitating, is unidirectional and relatively easy to describe: patients become depressed, recover, have a period of remission, and then may or may not become depressed again at some point in the future (Kupfer 1991). Although a small percentage of the population experiences refractory depression, most patients, in the absence of significant comorbidity, eventually respond to treatment and achieve a euthymic state. By contrast, the course of bipolar disorder is typically hectic and variable. A "roller coaster" for both patients and clinicians, extreme highs and lows intermingle with mixed states and subsyndromal symptom flurries to create hybrid symptom states that defy easy labels. As depicted in Figure 2, hypomania can surge into a fully syndromal mania and then plummet into a debilitating major depression. A fall from mania can lead to endless months of major depression, with brief excursions into minor depression providing only relative relief from unrelenting dysphoria, anergia, and hypersomnia. Treatments for those intolerable depressions may send a patient's mood back into the manic range, only to plunge back down into depression. Although we distinguish between the treatment of acute symptomatology (labeled

From the Department of Psychiatry, University of Pittsburgh, Western Psychiatric Institute and Clinic, Pittsburgh, Pennsylvania.
Address reprint request to Ellen Frank, Ph.D., University of Pittsburgh Medical Center, Western Psychiatric Institute and Clinic, 3811 O'Hara Street, Pittsburgh PA 15213-2593.
Received March 3, 2000; revised June 14, 2000; accepted June 22, 2000.

0006-3223/00/$20.00
PII S0006-3223(00)00969-0

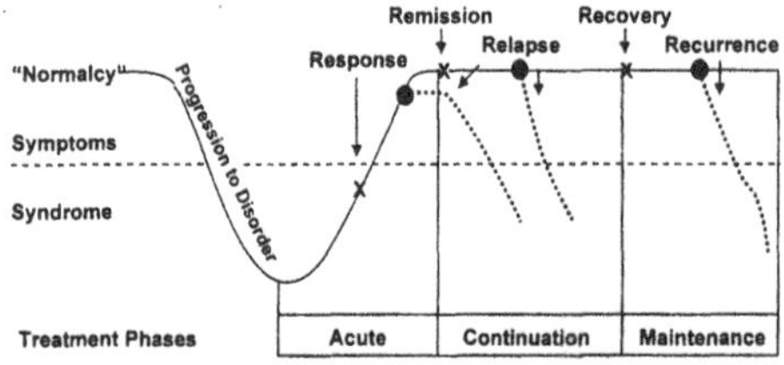

Figure 1. Response, remission recovery, relapse, and recurrence: phases of treatment in unipolar disorder. (Reproduced with permission from Kupfer 1991.)

Preliminary Phase in Figure 2) and prophylactic treatment following remission (labeled *Preventative Phase*), we recognize that these distinctions are often arbitrary and inaccurate. In fact, patients in a nonacute phase of treatment often experience on-going symptom fluctuations. Depressive symptoms, in particular, seem especially difficult to eradicate completely (Hlastala et al 1997). Thus, the holy grail of sustained euthymia in bipolar disorder may remain an elusive goal in the absence of sophisticated treatments that address both the biological and psychological aspects of this disorder.

Pathways to Recurrence

Goodwin and Jamison's definitive textbook on bipolar disorder (Goodwin and Jamison 1990) acknowledges the important interplay between biological and psychosocial factors in determining the course of bipolar disorder. Recognizing the primacy of biology, they hypothesized that "the genetic defect in manic depressive illness involves the circadian pacemaker or systems that modulate it" (Goodwin and Jamison 1990, 589) but then further postulated that psychosocial factors will interact with biology to create three probable pathways to recurrence of bipolar illness: 1) stressful life events; 2) disruptions in social rhythms; and 3) medication nonadherence. As envisioned by Goodwin and Jamison, these routes to illness are interconnected. Their model suggests that individuals with bipolar disorder are fundamentally vulnerable to disruptions in circadian rhythms. Psychosocial stressors then interact with this biological vulnerability to cause symptoms. For instance, stressful life events disrupt social rhythms, which causes disturbances in circadian integrity, which, in turn, may lead to recurrence. Alternately, problematic interpersonal relationships or disordered schedules contribute to a patient's difficulty adhering to a medication regimen which, again, may lead to recurrence. As a direct consequence of this model, one would assume that helping patients learn to take their medication regularly, lead more orderly lives, and resolve interpersonal problems more effectively would promote circadian integrity and minimize risk of recurrence.

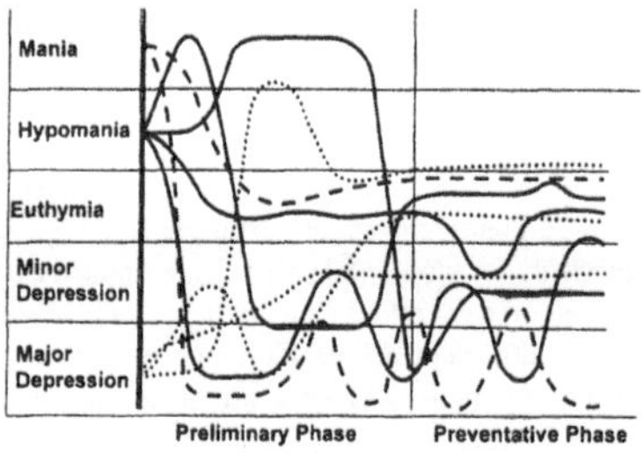

Figure 2. Response, remission, recovery, relapse, and recurrence: phases of treatment of bipolar disorder.

Treating Bipolar Disorder

As depicted in Figure 2, bipolar illness is a disorderly disorder. Characterized by erratic sleep–wake cycles and dramatic symptom fluctuations, the clinical course is unpredictable and rarely static. Needless to say, treating this "moving target" creates many interesting—and sometimes problematic—challenges. For instance, lithium monotherapy is still considered the "gold standard" of pharmacotherapy for bipolar disorder. As patients move through the various phases of the disorder, however, most psychiatrists find themselves treating patients with a range of mood stabilizers in combination with neuroleptics, sedative-hypnotics, and antidepressants (Sachs et al 2000). Efforts to simplify regimens are often thwarted by unsatisfactory treatment response, resulting in years of complex polypharmacy. Vacillating symptomatology, impaired psychosocial functioning, and problematic medication side effects converge to create unique clinical challenges for both patients and health care professionals. Considering the complexities of this illness, it is not surprising that pharmacotherapy alone does not address the multiple needs of patients with bipolar disorder. Although there are many excellent review papers discussing extant psychosocial approaches to bipolar disorder (Colom et al 1998; Johnson et al 2000; Miklowitz and Frank 1999), there are surprisingly few data supporting their efficacy (Craighead et al 1998; Swartz and Frank, in press). The absence of well-designed, empirically tested psychotherapies in the literature led us to develop and test a model of individual psychotherapy that would be used in conjunction with medication to enhance functioning and diminish recurrences in patients with bipolar I disorder.

Theoretical Context for Interpersonal and Social Rhythm Therapy

Interpersonal and social rhythm therapy (IPSRT) is a treatment that is specifically designed for patients with bipolar disorder. As elaborated below, the genesis of IPSRT rests in a psycho-chronobiological theory of affective illness that we articulated in a series of papers in the 1980s and early 1990s (Ehlers et al 1988, 1993; Monk et al 1991, 1990). Its design was also strongly influenced by the instability model of bipolar disorder proposed by Goodwin and Jamison (1990) and our evolving understanding of the relationship between stressful life events and bipolar episodes.

Circadian Rhythms, Sleep–Wake Cycles, and Mood Disorders

Researchers have identified reciprocal relationships among circadian rhythms, sleep–wake cycles and mood. Wehr and colleagues have demonstrated that sleep reduction can lead to mania in bipolar subjects (Leibenluft et al 1996; Wehr et al 1987). Sleep deprivation has significant (if transient) antidepressant effects in both unipolar and bipolar depressed subjects (Barbini et al 1998; Leibenluft et al 1993; Leibenluft and Wehr 1992), and PET studies have demonstrated localized effects of sleep deprivation in the medial prefrontal cortex (Wu et al 1999). The purpose of IPSRT is to regulate both circadian rhythms and sleep–wake cycles. It must be noted, however, that the relationship between bipolar disorder and circadian rhythms is less well characterized than its relationship to sleep–wake disturbances. By targeting social factors that modulate these rhythms, IPSRT is presumed to alter the underlying neuronal circuitry involved in the pathogenesis of bipolar symptomatology.

The theoretical underpinnings of IPSRT began with our efforts to better understand the psycho-chronobiological determinants of unipolar disorder. In 1988, we proposed an etiologic model of major depression that focused on the role of disrupted social rhythms in the emergence of a depressive episode in biologically vulnerable individuals (Ehlers et al 1988). Noting that the established biological correlates of affective disorder include disrupted sleep electroencephalogram recordings (Kupfer et al 1991) and phasic changes in the circadian secretions of pituitary hormones (Carroll et al 1980), we hypothesized that disruptions in the social cues that entrain these cycles may act as triggers for mood episodes. We argued that *social Zeitgebers,* that is, personal relationships, social demands, or tasks that entrain biological rhythms, may serve as the link between the biological and psychosocial processes that place an individual at risk for developing mood symptoms. We hypothesized that losing a social Zeitgeber could trigger an episode by causing the dysregulation of biological rhythms. For instance, the loss of a spouse through death or divorce results in the loss of a social Zeitgeber that may have previously determined sleep–wake times, rest periods, and meal times. In an individual with the genetic predisposition to depression, the physiologic and chronobiological disturbances produced by losing the social cues for sleep and meal times could be as important in the genesis of an episode as the psychologic distress generated by the event.

We subsequently extended this model of mood disorders to include the concept of Zeitstörers (time disturbers; Ehlers et al 1993). As defined above, social Zeitgebers are persons, social demands, or tasks that set the biological clock. By contrast, Zeitstörers are physical, chemical, or psychosocial events that disturb the biological clock. For instance, travel across time zones represents a prototypical Zeitstörer. The abrupt change in the timing of light exposure, meal times, and sleep times can produce a range of symptoms from mild "jet lag" to a full-blown affective episode in predisposed individuals. Other examples of potential Zeitstörers include newborn babies, marital separations, work deadlines (e.g., a college student who stays up all night to complete a term paper), and rotating shift work. Each of these disruptions has the potential to significantly alter an individual's circadian and sleep–wake rhythms that we argue, in turn, could result in an affective episode. In the context of our exploration of social Zeitgebers and Zeitstörers, our group developed an instrument to quantify an individual's social rhythms (Monk et al 1990). The Social Rhythm Metric (SRM) was designed as both a means of categorizing interindividual differences in social rhythm regularity and as a therapeutic tool to track decline into and recovery from an affective episode. We hypothesized that a psychotherapy that helps regulate social rhythms could help a vulnerable individual reduce the risk of developing mood symptoms.

Stressful Life Events and Mood

We formulated IPSRT at a time when there was a great deal of interest in the relationship between stressful life events and bipolar episode onset (Ellicott et al 1990). Given the probable role of circadian rhythm disruption in the genesis of bipolar episodes, our research group was particularly interested in the effects of those life events that caused a significant disruption in social rhythms. These theories, however, had not been subject to methodologically rigorous testing at the inception of IPSRT. Therefore, simultaneous with our early testing of IPSRT, we began an on-going study to assess the relationship between life events and bipolar episode onset with a reliable and valid life stress instrument, the Bedford College Life Event and Difficulty Schedule (LEDS).

In our research program, each life event of any severity identified by LEDS criteria was subject to an additional rating devised by our group to reflect the degree to which any given event is likely to have an acute effect on social routines, particularly those that might disrupt the sleep–wake cycle. The Social Rhythm Disruption (SRD) ratings, like the LEDS rating, were contextually determined by consensus panel and guided by clearly delineated criteria and a dictionary of examples. In an initial report based on 39 subjects with bipolar I disorder who were assessed with the LEDS/SRD protocol, we found evidence that life events (regardless of severity of threat) characterized by a high degree of social disruption were associated with the onset of manic but not depressive episodes (Malkoff-Schwartz et al 1998). Severely stressful life events (regardless of SRD rating) were related to the onset of both manic and depressive bipolar episodes. In a follow-up study, we interviewed bipolar subjects with purely manic ($n = 21$), purely depressed ($n = 21$), and mixed or cycling ($n = 24$) episodes and compared this bipolar sample with 44 patients with recurrent unipolar depression (Malkoff-Schwartz et al 2000). We again found that life events associated with a high degree of social disruption occurring in the 8 weeks before the onset of an episode were more frequently associated with the onset of manic episodes relative to bipolar cycling, bipolar depressed, or unipolar depressive episodes. Severely life-threatening events were more frequently associated with the onset of manic episodes relative to bipolar cycling episodes. We conclude that SRD and severe events are associated with manic episode onsets in a manner distinct from the association between SRD and severe events in bipolar depressed, bipolar cycling, and unipolar depressed onsets.

Origins of Interpersonal and Social Rhythm Therapy

Interpersonal Psychotherapy of Depression

Interpersonal psychotherapy (IPT) is a time-limited, focused psychotherapy developed in the 1970s by Klerman, Weissman, and colleagues for the treatment of unipolar depression (Klerman et al 1984). Unlike many other psychotherapies, IPT is designed to treat a specific disorder (depression) and has been systematically evaluated in several randomized, controlled research trials. IPT was envisioned as an acute (12–16 weeks) treatment for depression but has also been tested in an 8-month continuation study (Klerman et al 1974) and as a long-term maintenance strategy for patients with recurrent depression (Frank et al 1990). The basis of IPT is the premise that depression occurs in a psychosocial and interpersonal context. Akin to the social Zeitgeber hypothesis, the philosophy of IPT posits that in biologically vulnerable individuals, stressful interpersonal events may contribute to the onset of depression. It also argues that depressive symptoms can interfere with an individual's capacity to successfully negotiate interpersonal conflict or find constructive solutions to interpersonal dilemmas. Interpersonal psychotherapy is a "here and now" treatment that focuses on the relationship between the patient's current interpersonal milieu and his or her depressive symptoms. Treatment focuses on one of four IPT problem areas: grief, role disputes, role transitions, or interpersonal deficits.

Integrating the Behavioral, Interpersonal, and Psychoeducational Models

In the context of adapting IPT for the maintenance treatment of recurrent unipolar depression, we saw the potential utility of this treatment for another highly recurrent affective illness, bipolar disorder. We established that patients with recurrent unipolar disorder could recover from depression with an acute course of IPT and then decrease the risk of having another episode by receiving monthly sessions of maintenance IPT (Frank et al 1990). We began to conceptualize a similar kind of maintenance treatment for bipolar I disorder; however, given extant theories about the relationship between circadian rhythms and bipolar episodes and subsequent data linking SRD events to mania (Malkoff-Schwartz et al 1998, 2000), we decided to augment IPT with behavioral strategies designed to stabilize daily routines. We borrowed traditional cognitive-behavioral techniques such as self-monitoring, realistic goal-setting, and graded task assignment to help patients follow more consistent patterns of eating, sleeping, and social stimulation.

We expected IPT to contribute a specific antidepressant effect and hypothesized that helping patients stabilize their social rhythms would decrease the risk of new affective (especially manic) episodes. Nonetheless, we were aware that there is tremendous overlap between interpersonal stress and social rhythm disruption: a disturbance in the social milieu (such as a new job or conflict with a spouse) often acts as a Zeitstörer which, in turn, can lead to changes in daily routines. We therefore envisioned IPSRT as a truly integrated therapy that would allow these strategies to function synergistically. Thus, we expected that the IPT-induced resolution of interpersonal conflict would also contribute to more stable rhythms and more stable daily routines would promote more stable life circumstances (jobs, relationships, etc.).

The third component of IPSRT is psychoeducation. Recalling that the Goodwin and Jamison model (Goodwin and Jamison 1990) predicts three probable pathways to recurrence in bipolar disorder, including medication nonadherence, a cogent psychotherapy for bipolar disorder also necessarily addresses medical issues such as side effects, discontinuation risks, and relapse warning signs. Psychoeducation helps patients understand bipolar disorder and their medications, thereby decreasing denial and improving adherence to pharmacotherapeutic regimens. Indirect routes to medication adherence in IPSRT include regulating social routines (e.g., routinizing times of day when medications are administered) and addressing interpersonal problems (e.g., helping a patient find time for treatment in the setting of a demanding new job). Thus, IPSRT integrates behavioral, interpersonal, and psychoeducational approaches to prevent the onset of new episodes of bipolar disorder.

Interpersonal and Social Rhythm Therapy: Treatment Description

Interpersonal and social rhythm therapy is a manual-based psychotherapy (E. Frank et al, unpublished data, 1999) focusing on 1) the link between mood and life events, 2) the importance of maintaining regular daily rhythms as elucidated by the SRM, 3) the identification and management of potential precipitants of rhythm dysregulation with special attention to interpersonal triggers, 4) the facilitation of mourning the lost healthy self, and 5) the identification and management of affective symptoms. The therapy process is divided into four phases: initial phase, intermediate phase, preventative phase, and termination. We describe each phase of treatment below.

Initial Phase

In the initial phase, the clinician 1) obtains a history of the illness, 2) conducts an interpersonal inventory, 3) identifies an interpersonal problem area, 4) educates the patient about the disorder, and 5) initiates the SRM. Treatment may be initiated while the patient is fully symptomatic, subsyndromal, or euthymic. Because the medical management of a patient's acute symptoms may slow the initiation of the key features of IPRST, the duration of the initial phase may vary from several weeks to several months, depending on the severity of the patient's current symptoms. During this period, the patient and therapist meet weekly for 45-minute sessions.

The therapist begins by conducting a thorough psychiatric and medical history. In addition to the traditional psychiatric amanuensis, the therapist attempts to elicit in great detail the events leading up to current and previous episodes, searching for evidence of alterations or disruptions in the patient's daily routines and interpersonal interactions that preceded the development of symptoms. From Malkoff-Schwartz et al (1998), we know that manic episodes in particular are likely to be preceded by a social rhythm disrupting event. These historic details will help the therapist understand the patient's patterns of illness and aid in the identification of potential episode triggers. As the therapist elicits this information, he or she begins to clarify for the patient the relationship between the disrupting event and the onset of symptoms.

In accordance with the principles of IPT, the therapist also conducts an assay of the important individuals in the patient's life, known as the interpersonal inventory. A more interpersonally focused search for an episode precipitant, the interpersonal inventory consists of a review of all important past and present relationships as they relate to the current episode. The therapist asks about the patient's life circumstances and requests a description of the important people in his or her life. In addition to outlining the "cast of characters" in the patient's life, the therapist probes the quality of those relationships, asking the patient to describe satisfying and unsatisfying aspects of relationships, unmet expectations of others, and aspects of relationships that the patient would like to change. The therapist listens closely for omissions, such as the unemployed young adult who lives at home but does not mention his parents, or the "happily" married housewife who labels her marriage to an absent, high-powered executive as "fine," but does not volunteer details. The therapist listens for perturbations in relationships that may correspond temporally to the onset or maintenance of mood symptoms. Understanding the relationship between interpersonal difficulties and the onset of affective symptoms will help the therapist identify an appropriate treatment focus for the intermediate phase of treatment. In IPT, there are four possible treatment foci or interpersonal problem areas that are discussed in detail in the section entitled "Interpersonal Strategies."

After establishing a diagnosis, the therapist begins to educate the patient about his or her disorder. The educational component includes information about bipolar symptoms, prescribed medications, medication side effects, and so forth. The therapist also begins to help the patient understand the possible role of social and circadian rhythm disruption in precipitating his or her episode. Finally, the therapist initiates a revised version of the SRM (SRM-II) (Frank et al 1994). This 17-item self-report form (Figure 3) requires patients to record daily activities (e.g., time out of bed, first contact with another person, meal times, bedtime), whether each occurred alone or with others present, and how stimulating (i.e., quiet vs. interactive) these others were. The patient also rates his or her mood each day. After becoming familiar with the forms, patients spend 5 to 15 minutes per day completing the SRM. In our experience, most patients (about 85%) are willing and able to fill out the forms most (about 80%) of time. Therapists encourage patients to complete the forms by reminding them of their importance in the therapy and

THE SOCIAL RHYTHM METRIC (SRM)
MacArthur Foundation Mental Health Research Network I

Please Fill This Out At The End Of The Day

Respondent #: Day of Week: Date:

PEOPLE
0 = Alone
1 = Others just present
2 = Others actively involved
3 = Others very stimulating

ACTIVITY	TIME	AM or PM	S	M	T	W	T	F	S
TAKE AN AFTERNOON NAP	Earlier								
	Exact Earlier Time								
	2:00								
	2:15								
	2:30								
	2:45						0		
mid-point of your normal range →	3:00	PM						0	0
	3:15								
	3:30								
	3:45		0						
	4:00								
	Later								
	Exact Later Time								
	Check if did not do			✓	✓	✓			
HAVE DINNER	Earlier								
	Exact Earlier Time								
	5:30								
	5:45								
	6:00								
	6:15								
mid-point of your normal range →	6:30	PM			2		2	2	
	6:45			1		2			
	7:00								
	7:15								
	7:30		0						
	Later								3
	Exact Later Time								9:00
	Check if did not do								

Figure 3. Sample page from the Social Rhythm Metric.

reviewing the week's SRM at each session. Working with the SRM, the patient begins to see the dynamic interplay among instabilities in daily routines, patterns of social stimulation, sleep–wake times, and mood fluctuations. In the initial phase of IPSRT, however, no effort is made to regulate these daily rhythms.

Many individuals with bipolar disorder have suffered with their illness for many years before entering treatment

(Goodwin and Jamison 1990). The toll it takes on one's psyche cannot be underestimated. Importantly, the initial phase of treatment allows the therapist to establish the so-called "nonspecific" factors of therapy (Frank 1971). The therapist offers the patient hope and a human connection in the midst of an affective storm. Interpersonal and social rhythm therapy provides an affectively meaningful forum in which to begin an exploration of the effects of the illness on the patient's life trajectory, interpersonal relationships, and self-esteem.

Intermediate Phase

The intermediate phase of treatment is conducted weekly over several months. During this period, the therapist helps the patient develop strategies to manage affective symptoms, stabilize daily rhythms, and resolve the selected interpersonal problem area. The therapist also provides a forum for the patient to mourn lost "highs," struggle with denial, and find a balance between spontaneity and stability.

Social Rhythm Strategies

During the intermediate phase of treatment, IPSRT uses a behavioral approach to help the patient alter those activities that promote rhythm irregularities. The patient and therapist review the first 3 or 4 weeks of "free-running" SRMs to find those rhythms that seem to be particularly unstable. For example, is the patient going to bed at 10 PM one night, 2 AM the next night, and midnight the third night? Is there evidence of regularity during the week but extreme deviation on the weekend? Every effort is made to determine whether the patient's social rhythm instability results from untreated/prodromal bipolar symptoms or from a self-imposed lifestyle choice. In either case, the therapist will encourage the patient to work toward stabilization. If the rhythm instability is related to symptoms, the therapist helps the patient understand that stabilizing his or her rhythms can help diminish these symptoms. The therapist also encourages the patient to address the issue with his or her psychiatrist in the event that a medication change might help reduce the symptoms. If the therapist determines that the rhythm instability is a lifestyle choice, the therapist explains that disrupting circadian integrity may prevent a complete recovery. Therapist and patient discuss general strategies for regulating rhythms (e.g., minimizing overstimulation, monitoring the frequency and intensity of social interactions) and identify specific SRM goals. Goals are graded and include short term (i.e., adhering to a 7 AM wake-up time for 7 consecutive days), intermediate (i.e., sustaining a regular sleep–wake cycle for a month), and long-term (i.e., finding regular employment) objectives. The therapist of course allows for modifications of goals as the therapy proceeds.

Following from our Zeitstörer hypothesis, the therapist attends not only to the patient's daily rhythms but also to the larger environmental stressors that might result in a circadian rhythm derailment. The search for triggers of rhythm disruption leads the IPSRT therapist to comb the patient's history in search of external sources of rhythm disruption (Zeitstörers); IPSRT then encourages the patient to make relatively significant life changes in order to protect the integrity of his or her circadian rhythms and sleep–wake cycle. For instance, a factory worker who alternated between a night shift and a day shift became manic and needed to be hospitalized following the insomnia-inducing transition from day shift to night shift. The patient and therapist evaluated the risks of rotating shift work and determined that the frequent shifts in sleep schedule would be incompatible with reasonably stable social rhythms. Ultimately, the patient decided to change to a slightly less lucrative—but more regular—day job.

At some point in the recovery process, most patients with bipolar disorder question the need for protecting the integrity of their social rhythms. To someone with a long history of fluctuating mood states and erratic social rhythms, a very regular lifestyle can seem "boring" and unappealing. The therapist addresses this crucial issue on several levels. First, the therapist can help the patient find a healthy balance between stability and spontaneity. This process requires a spirit of careful experimentation on the parts of both therapist and patient to determine how much sleep, stimulation, and regularity are associated with an optimal mood state for each individual. Extreme inactivity, on one hand, can contribute to isolation and depressive symptoms; excess stimulation, on the other hand, may precipitate a mania. It is helpful to pursue this aspect of treatment over many months because seasonal variation in mood and energy often occurs in bipolar patients (Goodwin and Jamison 1990). Some patients, for instance, may find they benefit from a busier schedule during the winter months when they would typically tend toward depression but must learn to curtail these same activities during the summer months when they are at increased risk for a mania.

Changes in routine are an inexorable part of life. Some changes are predictable (e.g., a vacation or a professional conference); others are not (e.g., job loss or physical illness). Another goal in IPSRT is to help patients adapt to changes in routine. In the event of a predictable change, the therapist can help the patient modify his or her activity level to modulate potential disruptions in social rhythms. For example, a young, unemployed woman had finally demanded that her abusive, substance-abusing boyfriend move out of her apartment as of a specified date. Although both therapist and patient viewed this change as positive, they both recognized that his departure would create great upheaval in the patient's routines. She relied on her boyfriend to wake her up in the mornings and scheduled mealtimes around his evening routines. Because of his jealous nature, she had greatly limited her social contacts during their relationship. In preparation for his departure, the patient began using an alarm clock to determine her own waking time. She planned social outings during the day that would not involve her boyfriend (e.g., meeting an old friend at the mall) and "practiced" these interactions as part of planning for the move. Helping the patient to gradually entrain her rhythms to a new schedule mitigated against the disruptive effects of the lost social Zeitgeber. Unanticipated changes, however, may require considerable effort from the therapist to address both the unexpected alterations in social Zeitgebers and the psychological meaning of the event.

Interpersonal Strategies

The interpersonal techniques employed in IPSRT are similar to those described in Klerman and colleagues' definitive description of IPT for unipolar depression (Klerman et al 1984). As described previously, the therapist identifies an interpersonal problem area during the initial phase of treatment that will serve as the interpersonal treatment focus. Each problem area is associated with a set of IPT techniques that are fully described in the Klerman et al (1984) text. In the section that follows, we will briefly describe each problem area and focus on the ways in which IPRST employs traditional IPT strategies to meet the specific needs of patients with bipolar disorder.

1. *Grief.* Grief or complicated bereavement refers to symptoms that result from incomplete mourning or unresolved feelings about the death of an important person in the patient's life. Symptoms must exceed in duration and intensity those characteristic of the normal mourning process. In IPT, the problem area of grief is not typically invoked when the patient experiences symbolic losses such as the loss of a job or loss of function from physical illness. In most cases, these issues would be handled as role transitions. Patients with bipolar disorder, however, frequently grieve for the person they were before the illness or the person they could have become if they did not suffer from bipolar disorder. In IPSRT, we call this grieving for the lost healthy self and utilize the IPT techniques associated with grief to help the patient mourn this loss. The therapist encourages the patient to express painful feelings about lost hopes, ruined relationships, interrupted careers, and passed opportunities. As the patient mourns the passing of a "former self," the therapist encourages the patient to develop new relationships, establish new, more realistic goals, and focus on future opportunities.
2. *Interpersonal role disputes.* An interpersonal dispute refers to any close relationship in which there are nonreciprocal expectations. Examples include a college student who wants to live in the dorms but whose parents want her to live at home, and a construction worker who became symptomatic in the context of pressure from his girlfriend of 7 years to propose marriage. Individuals with bipolar disorder are frequently involved in interpersonal disputes. Bipolar symptoms may contribute to interpersonal disputes or interpersonal disputes may overstimulate patients, which may, in turn, precipitate episodes or exacerbate mood symptoms. The former scenario is illustrated by a treatment-nonadherent man with bipolar disorder who became hypomanic, spent excessive sums of money on unnecessary computer equipment, and engaged in promiscuous extramarital behaviors. Even though the behaviors subsided with reinitiation of medication, his angry spouse moved into her mother's house and threatened to leave the marriage. The therapist helped the patient understand the role of medication nonadherence in the evolution of these behaviors and encouraged the patient to accept more responsibility for his treatment. With the help of his therapist, the patient was able to express his contrition to his partner and admit to her his ambivalence about taking medication. The couple was able to reconcile with the understanding that the patient would accept and adhere to treatment as part of the terms of the marriage.
3. *Role transition.* A role transition is any major life role change. This category subsumes many potential stressors, including new employment, unemployment, matriculation, graduation, retirement, marriage, divorce, giving birth, and so forth. The profoundly disruptive nature of bipolar disorder may cause significant interpersonal upheaval in a patient's life. A destructive mania can result in a job loss or tremendous financial debt. Entrenched depressions can lead to ruptured social ties and loss of socioeconomic status. In IPSRT, these life changes are handled under the rubric of role transitions. The therapist should be especially sensitive to these issues and probe for the status of important relationships pre- and postepisode. Another transition confronting newly stable bipolar patients is the loss of previously pleasurable, baseline hypomania. The allure of the lost euphoric state may tempt patients to seek transient mood elevation by either discon-

tinuing medications or manipulating social rhythms to produce insomnia. The therapist must help the patient relinquish this aspect of the "former self" to maintain overall stability. It is important to remind the patient of the negative consequences of hypomania and to encourage the patient to identify rewarding life goals (i.e., an enduring and stable marriage) that may constitute a suitable alternative to the seductive and dangerous pleasures of hypomania.

4. *Interpersonal deficits.* Patients with interpersonal deficits suffer from a long-standing history of impoverished or contentious social relationships and are unable to identify a single acute interpersonal stressor associated with the onset of their episode. Most bipolar patients' problems will fall into one of the three categories previously discussed; however, a minority of individuals will benefit from an interpersonal deficits focus. These patients may include individuals whose illness-dependent grandiosity, social withdrawal, or extreme mood fluctuations contribute to multiple failed relationships, recurrent patterns of conflict with coworkers, or constricted social networks.

In addition to focusing on the interpersonal meaning of each problem area, the therapist attends to the role of these kinds of problems in promoting or disrupting social rhythm regularity. For instance, the death of a loved one may result in complicated bereavement but will also result in the loss of an important Zeitgeber. The on-going interpersonal disputes of a husband and wife may lead to prebedtime fighting and subsequent decrease in sleep. The requirements of a new job may involve changing wake times or interfere with previously regular exercise routines. In IPSRT, the therapist generally encourages social rhythm regularity first and then explores the interpersonal meaning of an event.

Preventative Phase

Because IPSRT is designed, above all, to prevent future mood episodes and enhance functioning during relatively euthymic periods, the preventative phase is a crucial component of this treatment. In our conceptualization of a preventative therapy, treatment frequency decreases to monthly and lasts 2 or more years. The patient is provided with an opportunity to consolidate treatment gains and increase confidence in his or her capacity to apply IPSRT techniques outside of sessions. For instance, before entering treatment, an academic scholar developed an episode of mania during a professional conference in another time zone. She became very stimulated, did not sleep well, and soon required hospitalization for a psychotic mania. The acute phase of treatment focused on recovery from the episode and making lifestyle changes to balance her personal and professional lives. During the preventative phase of treatment, the patient wanted to pursue career goals more intensively. She worked with her therapist to monitor her career choices to preserve her sleep and maintain regular social rhythms. For instance, the patient learned that she could tolerate demanding individual projects (e.g., writing papers) but became overly stimulated in group settings (e.g., committee meetings in her department). A year after the beginning of treatment, the patient wished to return to the conference that led to her first hospitalization. Both patient and therapist were concerned about the conference's potential for provoking a recurrence. The therapist helped the patient develop a strategy for diminishing stimulation at the conference (e.g., attending only selected meetings, avoiding the late-night social events) that permitted her to participate in the event, but in a controlled manner. Thus, in the preventative phase, the therapist continues to encourage the patient to maintain regular social rhythms and addresses problems as they arise. The patient works on his or her interpersonal problem area(s), although the specific interpersonal focus may differ from that of the acute phase. The preventative phase of treatment may require occasional additional crisis sessions to address either a symptom exacerbation or an interpersonal dilemma.

Termination

The final phase of treatment facilitates termination of the psychotherapy. The therapist reviews treatment successes, as well as the patient's potential vulnerabilities, helping the patient identify strategies for future management of interpersonal difficulties and symptom flares. Termination is handled gradually, occurring over four to six monthly sessions. Because bipolar disorder is a chronic condition, patients often approach termination with some trepidation. It is important to remind them about available resources for treatment should symptoms flare in the future while offering encouragement about their ability to exercise their new skills independently. At the end of treatment, patients can usually be congratulated on the tremendous strides they have made in both relationships and social rhythm stability during the course of IPSRT. In some cases, treatment may continue for an indefinite period at a reduced frequency, given the chronic nature of the disorder and the likelihood that a patient will be maintained on medications indefinitely.

Empirical Data Supporting the Efficacy of IPSRT

We are currently conducting an on-going randomized clinical trial at the University of Pittsburgh testing the efficacy of IPSRT as an adjunctive maintenance treatment for bipolar I disorder (Maintenance Therapies in Bipolar Disorder; MH29618, E. Frank, PI). After giving written, informed consent, acutely ill bipolar patients are treated with medication and randomly assigned to either IPSRT or intensive clinical management (CM). Once stabilized, patients are reassigned to either IPSRT or CM (in conjunction with a stable medication regimen) for 2 years of monthly preventative treatment. Although the study is not yet complete, we have published several reports of preliminary findings from this trial.

As further evidence of the complexities of treating bipolar disorder, we have discovered that departures from our protocol pharmacotherapy are the norm rather than the exception. In theory, we attempt to treat all patients with lithium plus specified neuroleptics or antidepressants administered transiently in the acute phase according to a specified protocol. Our study design specified a goal of lithium monotherapy in the preventative phase. But, among the first 91 subjects to enter the preventative phase, only 23% entered on lithium alone. Also of interest, only 63% of subjects presenting with mania, and 22% of subjects presenting with depression were able to follow the specified pharmacotherapy algorithm to achieve stabilization. The demands of the disorder routinely resulted in substantial deviation from our carefully planned model. By contrast, the psychotherapy condition has remained quite "pure," with raters who are unaware of treatment assignment distinguishing reliably between audio tapes of IPSRT and CM sessions.

Our first published report from the Maintenance Therapies in Bipolar Disorder (MTBD) protocol demonstrated that patients in IPSRT can be taught to maintain stability in their daily routines over the course of acute treatment (Frank et al 1997). Over time (up to 52 weeks), subjects receiving IPSRT (n = 18) and CM (n = 20) had comparable changes in symptomatology, but the IPSRT group showed significantly greater stability of daily routines with increasing time in treatment (p = .047). The mean number of weeks of data included in these analyses were 24.8 ± 13.8 and 26.7 ± 15.0 for IPSRT and CM subjects, respectively.

We next reported on 42 subjects treated acutely with either IPSRT or CM, demonstrating that manic subjects achieved clinical remission significantly more quickly than did depressed subjects (Hlastala et al 1997). Although we found no statistically significant effects of treatment assignment, among the 22 depressed subjects, median time to remission was 21 weeks with IPSRT versus 40 weeks with CM. This statistically nonsignificant but clinically interesting finding suggests that IPSRT may hasten recovery from a depression more effectively than a nonspecific "medication clinic" intervention.

We have most recently reported on the first 82 subjects to enter the preventative phase of treatment in this protocol (Frank et al 1999). We found that groups of subjects who received the same treatment for both acute and preventative phases (either CM followed by CM or IPSRT followed by IPSRT) had lower rates of recurrence (<20% vs. >40%) and levels of symptomatology over the subsequent 52 weeks than those reassigned to the alternate modality (either IPSRT followed by CM or CM followed by IPSRT). The polarity of the episode for which a subject was treated before entering the preventative phase did not affect the relative risk of recurrence in the groups receiving altered versus stable treatments. Subsequent analyses, however, have suggested that the loss (as opposed to gain) of IPSRT put subjects at particular risk for a depressive recurrence. We concluded that even relatively minor disruptions in the psychosocial treatment plan contribute to worse outcomes in bipolar disorder. These analyses provide additional data to support the hypothesis that instability contributes to morbidity in bipolar disorder.

As described previously, our research has demonstrated a correlation between life events associated with a high degree of social rhythm disruption and the onset of manic—but not depressive—episodes (Malkoff-Schwartz et al 1998). One might predict that a psychotherapy promoting regular social rhythms would have a selectively prophylactic effect on mania. Although we are still in the process of collecting data, our impression is that the opposite may be true: patients assigned to IPSRT in the preventative phase seem to suffer fewer depressive symptoms than those assigned to CM but have the same rate of manic recurrences (Frank 1999). These paradoxical findings may reflect the multiple sites of action of IPSRT and the as yet unclear effects of this multifaceted treatment on a complex disorder.

Conclusion

Among medical treatments, psychotherapies have the dubious distinction of being among the least well tested and most "cultish" prescriptions offered to patients. Although the field is beginning to redress this wrong, IPSRT is among only a handful of psychotherapies utilizing techniques derived from sound scientific theory, the efficacy of which will be evaluated in a randomized controlled trial This rational treatment rests firmly on the circadian rhythm theory of bipolar disorder and our explication of social Zeitgebers and Zeitstörers as the putative "bridges" between biological processes and the patients' interpersonal experiences. When the preventative phase of our MTBD study concludes, we will be in a position to answer the most urgent question: Does IPSRT prevent episode recurrence in patients with bipolar I disorder? Until that time, we work with the smaller pieces of the puzzle thus far unearthed.

To date, we have established that IPSRT helps patients achieve more stable social rhythms (Frank et al 1997). We also have demonstrated a clear link between life events associated with social rhythm disruption and the onset of manic episodes (Malkoff-Schwartz et al 1998). In an ironic twist, the cross-over design of our study has provided additional data to support Goodwin and Jamison's instability model of bipolar disorder (Frank et al 1999). Given these converging reports that continue to implicate circadian instability as an important precipitant of bipolar episodes and our preliminary data demonstrating that IPRST can help stabilize social rhythms, we have reason to believe that a psychosocial intervention that promotes rhythm integrity and aids in the resolution and prevention of interpersonal distress is likely to enhance course and outcome in bipolar disorder.

Before the identification of lithium as a treatment for bipolar disorder, pharmacologic options were limited and largely inadequate. By default, psychotherapy was the mainstay of treatment. In the absence of effective medications, psychotherapies of the day (mostly insight-oriented therapies) were also unsuccessful (Fromm-Reichmann 1949). A discouraging era of psychotherapy treatments was followed by a disappointing "biological era" in which scientists, abandoning psychotherapy, struggled with medications alone to optimize outcomes. The challenge facing contemporary investigators of bipolar disorder is to develop treatments that address both the biological and psychologic aspects of the illness. The strength of IPSRT lies in its ability to utilize psychosocial strategies to address the underlying biology of bipolar disorder. Deployed in combination with thoughtful pharmacotherapy, IPSRT appears to successfully integrate biological and psychosocial models of bipolar disorder and, we hope, ultimately to lessen the impact of this devastating illness on patients' lives.

Supported in part by National Institute of Mental Health Grants Nos. MH-30915 (DJK), MH-29618 (EF), and MH-60473 (HAS).

Aspects of this work were presented at the conference "Bipolar Disorder: From Preclinical to Clinical, Facing the New Millennium," January 19–21, 2000, Scottsdale, Arizona. The conference was sponsored by the Society of Biological Psychiatry through an unrestricted educational grant provided by Eli Lilly and Company.

References

Barbini B, Colombo C, Benedetti F, Campori E, Bellodi L, Smeraldi E (1998): The unipolar-bipolar dichotomy and the response to sleep deprivation. *Psychiatry Res* 79:43–50.

Benson R (1975): The forgotten treatment modality in bipolar illness: Psychotherapy. *Dis Nerv Syst* 36:634–638.

Cade J (1949): Lithium salt in the treatment of psychotic excitement. *Med J Aust* 2:349–352.

Carroll BJ, Greden JF, Feinberg M (1980): Neuroendocrine disturbances and the diagnosis and aetiology of endogenous depression. *Lancet* 1:321–322.

Colom F, Vieta E, Martinez A, Jorquera A, Gasto C (1998): What is the role of psychotherapy in the treatment of bipolar disorder? *Psychother Psychosom* 67:3–9.

Coryell W, Scheftner W, Keller M, Endicott J, Maser J, Klerman GL (1993): The enduring psychosocial consequences of mania and depression. *Am J Psychiatry* 150:720–727.

Craighead WE, Miklowitz DJ, Vajk FC, Frank E (1998): Psychosocial treatments for bipolar disorder. In: Nathan PE, Gorman JM, editors. *A Guide to Treatments That Work.* New York: Oxford University Press, 240–248.

Ehlers CL, Frank E, Kupfer DJ (1988): Social zeitgebers and biological rhythms. *Arch Gen Psychiatry* 45:948–952.

Ehlers CL, Kupfer DJ, Frank E, Monk TH (1993): Biological rhythms and depression: The role of zeitgebers and zeitstorers. *Depression* 1:285–293.

Ellicott A, Hammen C, Gitlin M, Brown G, Jamison K (1990): Life events and the course of bipolar disorder. *Am J Psychiatry* 147:1194–1198.

Frank E (1999): Interpersonal and social rhythm therapy prevents depressive symptomatology in bipolar I patients. *Bipolar Disord* 1:13.

Frank E, Hlastala S, Ritenour A, Houck P, Tu XM, Monk TH, et al (1997): Inducing lifestyle regularity in recovering bipolar disorder patients: Results from the maintenance therapies in bipolar disorder protocol. *Biol Psychiatry* 41:1165–1173.

Frank E, Kupfer DJ, Ehlers CL, Monk TH, Cornes C, Carter S, Frankel D (1994): Interpersonal and social rhythm therapy for bipolar disorder: Integrating interpersonal and behavioral approaches. *Behav Therapist* 17:143–149.

Frank E, Kupfer DJ, Perel JM, Cornes C, Jarrett DB, Mallinger AG, et al (1990): Three-year outcomes for maintenance therapies in recurrent depression. *Arch Gen Psychiatry* 47: 1093–1099.

Frank E, Swartz HA, Mallinger AG, Thase ME, Weaver EV, Kupfer DJ (1999): Adjunctive psychotherapy for bipolar disorder: effects of changing treatment modality. *J Abnorm Psychol* 108:579–587.

Frank J (1971): Therapeutic factors in psychotherapy. *Am J Psychother* 25:350–361.

Fromm-Reichmann F (1949): Intensive psychotherapy of manic-depressives. *Confinia Neurol* 9:158–165.

Goldberg JF, Harrow M, Grossman LS (1995): Course and outcome in bipolar affective disorder: A longitudinal follow-up study. *Am J Psychiatry* 152:379–384.

Goodwin F, Jamison K (1990): *Manic-Depressive Illness.* New York: Oxford University Press.

Hlastala SA, Frank E, Mallinger AG, Thase ME, Ritenour AM, Kupfer DJ (1997): Bipolar depression: An underestimated treatment challenge. *Depression Anxiety* 5:73–83.

Johnson SL, Greenhouse W, Bauer M (2000): Psychosocial approaches to the treatment of bipolar disorder. *Curr Opin Psychiatry* 13:69–72.

Klerman GL, Dimascio A, Weissman M, Prusoff B, Paykel ES

(1974): Treatment of depression by drugs and psychotherapy. *Am J Psychiatry* 131:186–191.

Klerman GL, Weissman MM, Rounsaville BJ, Chevron ES (1984): *Interpersonal Psychotherapy of Depression.* New York: Basic Books.

Kupfer DJ (1991): Long-term treatment of depression. *J Clin Psychiatry* 52:28–34.

Kupfer DJ, Ehlers CL, Frank E, Grochocinski VJ, McEachran AB (1991): EEG sleep profiles and recurrent depression. *Biol Pyschiatry* 30:641–655.

Leibenluft E, Albert PS, Rosenthal NE, Wehr TA (1996): Relationship between sleep and mood in patients with rapid-cycling bipolar disorder. *Psychiatry Res* 63:161–168.

Leibenluft E, Moul DE, Schwartz PJ, Madden PA, Wehr TA (1993): A clinical trial of sleep deprivation in combination with antidepressant medication. *Psychiatry Res* 46:213–227.

Leibenluft E, Wehr TA (1992): Is sleep deprivation useful in the treatment of depression? *Am J Psychiatry* 149:159–168.

Malkoff-Schwartz S, Frank E, Anderson B, Sherrill JT, Siegel L, Patterson D, Kupfer DJ (1998): Stressful life events and social rhythm disruption in the onset of manic and depressive bipolar episodes. *Arch Gen Psychiatry* 55:702–707.

Malkoff-Schwartz S, Frank E, Anderson BP, Hlastala SA, Luther JF, Sherrill JT, et al (2000): Social rhythm disruption and stressful life events in the onset of bipolar and unipolar episodes. *Psychol Med* 30:1005–1016.

Markar H, Mander A (1989): Efficacy of lithium prophylaxis in clinical practice. *Br J Psychiatry* 155:496–500.

Miklowitz DJ, Frank E (1999): New psychotherapies for bipolar disorder. In: Goldberg JF, Harrow M, editors. *Bipolar Disorders: Clinical Course and Outcome.* Washington, DC: American Psychiatric Press, 57–84.

Monk TH, Kupfer DJ, Frank E, Ritenour AM (1991): The Social Rhythm Metric (SRM): Measuring daily social rhythms over 12 weeks. *Psychiatry Res* 36:195–207.

Monk TK, Flaherty JF, Frank E, Hoskinson K, Kupfer DJ (1990): The Social Rhythm Metric: An instrument to quantify the daily rhythms of life. *J Nerv Ment Dis* 178:120–126.

Prien RF, Kupfer DJ, Mansky PA, Small JG, Tuason VB, Voss CB, Johnson WE (1984): Drug therapy in the prevention of recurrences in unipolar and bipolar affective disorders: Report of the NIMH Collaborative Study Group comparing lithium carbonate, imipramine, and a lithium carbonate-imipramine combination. *Arch Gen Psychiatry* 41:1096–1104.

Reynolds CF III, Frank E, Perel JM, Imber SD, Cornes C, Miller MD, et al (1999): Nortriptyline and interpersonal psychotherapy as maintenance therapies for recurrent major depression: A randomized controlled trial in patients older than 59 years. *JAMA* 281:39–45.

Sachs GS, Printz DJ, Kahn DA, Carpenter D, Docherty JP (2000): The expert concensus guidline series: Medication treatment of bipolar disorder 2000. *Postgrad Med* April:1–104.

Swartz HA, Frank E (in press): Psychotherapy for bipolar depression: A phase-specific strategy? *Bipolar Disord.*

Wehr TA, Sack DA, Rosenthal NE (1987): Sleep reduction as a final common pathway in the genesis of mania. *Am J Psychiatry* 144:201–204.

Wu J, Buchsbaum MS, Gillin JC, Tang C, Cadwell S, Wiegand M, et al (1999): Prediction of antidepressant effects of sleep deprivation by metabolic rates in the ventral anterior cingulate and medial prefrontal cortex. *Am J Psychiatry* 156:1149–1158.

Acknowledgments

Sachs, G.S. "A 25-Year-Old Woman with Bipolar Disorder." *JAMA* 285 (2001): 454–462. Copyright 2001. The American Medical Association.

Kessler, R.C., Rubinow, D.R., Holmes, C., Abelson, J.M., and Zhao, S. "The Epidemiology of DSM-III-R Bipolar Disorder in a General Population Survey." *Psychological Medicine* 27 (1997): 1079–1089. Reprinted with the permission of Cambridge University Press.

Osby, U., Brandt, L., Correia, N., Ekbon, A., and Sparen, P. "Excess Mortality in Bipolar and Unipolar Disorder in Sweden." *Arch Gen Psychiatry* 58 (2001): 844–850. Reprinted with the permission of American Medical Association.

Craddock, N., and Jones, I. "Genetics of Bipolar Disorder." *J Med Genet* 36 (1999): 585–594. Reprinted with the permission of BMJ Publishing House.

Berrettini, W.H. "Are Schizophrenic and Bipolar Disorders Related? A Review of Family and Molecular Studies." *Biol Psychiatry* 48, 6 (2000): 531–538. Reprinted with the permission of Elsevier Science. Copyright 2000 by the Society of Biological Psychiatry.

Potash, J.B., Willour, V.L., Chiu, Y.F., Simpson, S.G., MacKinnon, D.F., Pearlson, G.D., DePaulo, J.R., Jr., and McInnis, M.G. "The Familial Aggregation of Psychotic Symptoms in Bipolar Disorder Pedigrees." *Am J Psychiatry* 158, 8 (2001): 1258–1264. Copyright 2001, the American Psychiatric Association. Reprinted by permission.

Angst, J., and Sellaro, R. "Historical Perspectives and Natural History of Bipolar Disorder." *Biol Psychiatry* 48 (2000): 445–457. Reprinted with the permission of Elsevier Science. Copyright 2000 by the Society of Biological Psychiatry.

Coryell, W., Turvey, C., Endicott, J., et al. "Bipolar I Affective Disorder: Predictors of Outcome after 15 Years." *J Affect Disord* 50 (1998): 109–116. Reprinted with the permission of Elsevier Science. Copyright 1998.

Ellicott, A., Hammen, C., Gitlin, M., Brown, G., and Jamison, K. "Life Events and the Course of Bipolar Disorder." *Am J Psychiatry* 147 (1990): 1194–1198. Copyright 1990, the American Psychiatric Association. Reprinted by permission.

Kilzieh, N., and Akiskal, H.S. "Rapid-Cycling Bipolar Disorder: An Overview of Research and Clinical Experience." *Psychiatr Clin North Am* 22, 3 (1999): 585–607. Reprinted with the permission of the W.B. Saunders Company.

Altshuler, L.L., Post, R.M., Leverich, G.S., et al. "Antidepressant-Induced Mania and Cycle Acceleration: A Controversy Revisited." *Am J Psychiatry* 152 (1995): 1130–1138. Copyright 1995, the American Psychiatric Association. Reprinted by permission.

Jamison, K.R. "Suicide and Bipolar Disorder." *J Clin Psychiatry* 61, supp. 9 (2000): 47–51. Copyright 2000, Physicians Postgraduate Press. Reprinted by permission.

Geller, B., and Luby, J. "Child and Adolescent Bipolar Disorder: Review of the Past 10 Years." *J Am Acad Child Adolesc Psychiatry* 36 (1998): 1168–1176. Reprinted with the permission of Williams & Wilkins.

National Institute of Mental Health. "National Institute of Mental Health Research Roundtable on Prepubertal Bipolar Disorder." *J Am Acad Child Adolesc Psychiatry* 40, 8 (2001): 871–878. Reprinted with the permission of Williams & Wilkins.

Sanchez, L., Hagino, O., Weller, E., and Weller, R. "Bipolarity in Children." *Psychiatr Clin North Am* 22, 3 (1999): 629–648. Reprinted with the permission of the W.B. Saunders Company.

Wilson, D.R. (1998) "Evolutionary Epidemiology and Manic Depression." *Br J Med Psychol* 71, Pt 4 (1999): 375–395. Reprinted with permission from the British Journal of Medical Psychology and the British Psychological Society.

Blumberg, H.P., Stern, E., Martinez, D., Ricketts, S., de Asis, J., White, T., Epstein, J., McBride, P.A., Eidelberg, D., Kocsis, J.H., and Silbersweig, D.A. "Increased Anterior Cingulate and Caudate Activity in Bipolar Mania." *Biol Psychiatry* 48 (2000): 1045–1052. Reprinted with the permission of Elsevier Science. Copyright 2000 by the Society of Biological Psychiatry.

Leibenluft, E., Albert, P.S., Rosenthal, N.E., and Wehr, T.A. "Relationship between Sleep and Mood in Patients with Rapid-Cycling Bipolar Disorder." *Psychiatry Res* 31 (1996): 161–168. Reprinted with the permission of Elsevier Science Ireland Ltd.

Ikonomov, O.C., and Manji, H.K. "Molecular Mechanisms Underlying Mood Stabilization in Manic-Depressive Illness: The Phenotype Challenge." *Am J Psychiatry* 156 (1999): 1506–1514. Copyright 1999, the American Psychiatric Association. Reprinted by permission.

Manji, H.K., and Lenox, R.H. "Signaling: Cellular Insights into the Pathophysiology of Bipolar Disorder." *Biol Psychiatry* 48 (2000): 518–530. Reprinted with the permission of Elsevier Science. Copyright 2000 by the Society of Biological Psychiatry.

Schou, M. "Forty Years of Lithium Treatment." *Arch Gen Psychiatry* 54, 1 (1997): 9–13, discussion 14–15. Reprinted with the permission of American Medical Association.

Berridge, M.J., Downes, C.P., and Hanley, M.R. "Neural and Developmental Actions of Lithium: A Unifying Hypothesis." *Cell* 59 (1989): 411–419. Reprinted with permission from Elsevier Science.

Klein, P.S., and Melton, D.A. "A Molecular Mechanism for the Effect of Lithium on Development." *Proc Natl Acad Sci USA* 93 (1996): 8455–8459. Copyright 1996 National Academy of Sciences, U.S.A.

Bowden, C.L., Calabrese, J.R., McElroy, S.L., et al. "A Randomized, Placebo Controlled 12-Month Trial of Divlaproex and Lithium in Treatment of Outpatients with Bipolar I Disorder." *Arch Gen Psychiatry* 57 (2000): 481–489. Reprinted with the permission of American Medical Association.

Calabrese, J.R., Kimmel, W.E., Woyshville, M.J., et al. "Clozapine for Treatment Refractory Mania." *Am J Psychiatry* 154 (1996): 759–764. Copyright 1996, the American Psychiatric Association. Reprinted by permission.

Frank, E., Swartz, H.A., and Kupfer, D.J. "Interpersonal and Social Rhythm Therapy: Managing the Chaos of Bipolar Disorder." *Biol Psychiatry* 48 (2000): 593–604. Copyright 2000 by the Society of Biological Psychiatry.